HANDBOOK OF HYPNOSIS
FOR PROFESSIONALS

HANDBOOK
of
HYPNOSIS
for
PROFESSIONALS

Second Edition

Roy Udolf

JASON ARONSON INC.
Northvale, New Jersey
London

THE MASTER WORK SERIES

First softcover edition 1995

Copyright © 1992, 1987 by Roy Udolf

Library of Congress Cataloging-in-Publication Data

Udolf, Roy.
    Handbook of hypnosis for professionals.

    Originally published : New York: Van Nostrand
Reinhold Co., ©1987. (ISBN: 0-442-28531-0)
    Includes bibliographical references and indexes.
    1. Hypnotism I. Title. II. [DNLM: 1. Hypnosis.
WM 415 U21h 1987a].
BF1141.U36   1992   154.7   92-27304
ISBN 1-56821-727-7

Manufactured in the United States of America. Jason Aronson Inc. offers books and cassettes. For information and catalog write to Jason Aronson Inc., 230 Livingston Street, Northvale, New Jersey 07647.

To Beaty Kadis, a great aunt in every sense of the term, who deserves a book dedicated to her, and to Mary Joan Demarco, supersecretary, to nurture her well-deserved feelings of guilt for deserting the author when he needed her to work on this edition.

Contents

Foreword   ix
Preface   xiii
Acknowledgments   xvii

1. Introduction   1

History of Hypnosis, 2   Preliminary Formulations Concerning the
Nature of Hypnosis, 10   Common Misconceptions Concerning
Hypnosis, 13

2. Hypnotic Susceptibility   21

Tests of Hypnotic Susceptibility, 25   Factors Related to Hypnotic
Susceptibility, 33   Personality Tests as Predictors of Hypnotic
Susceptibility, 42   Lateral Eye Movements, 45   Situational Variables
in Hypnotizability, 45   Preinduction "Tests" of Hypnotizability, 47

3. Induction and Deepening Procedures   55

Arm Levitation Method, 58   Braidism, 63   Cognitive Inductions, 65
Progressive Relaxation Method, 66   Flower's Method, 67
Trance Induction by Poetry, 69   Mechanical Aids, 69   New Methods
and Combinations of Methods, 71   Hypnotic *Passes* and *Stroking*, 74
"Instant" Hypnosis, 75   Hypnotic Induction during Sleep, 78
Authoritative Versus Permissive Dimension, 78   Signs of Hypnosis, 79
Deepening Techniques, 83   Terminating a Trance, 86

4. Hypnotic Phenomena   89

Physiological Effects of Hypnosis, 91   Hypnotically Induced Emotional
States, 98   Hallucinations, 100   Trance Logic, 108   Hypnotic
Analgesia and Anesthesia, 109   Posthypnotic Amnesia, 121
Hypnotic Hypermnesia and Effects on Learning, 140   Hypnosis
and Creativity, 149   Hypnotic Age Regression and Revivification, 152
Hypnotic Distortion of Subjective Time, 159   Posthypnotic

Suggestions, 163   Hypnotic Dissociation, 172   Hypnotically
Induced Dreams, 175

5. Practical Applications of Hypnosis   ·   181

Hypnosis in Psychotherapy, 182   Hypnosis in Medicine and
Dentistry, 237   Nontherapeutic Applications of Hypnosis, 274

6. Self-Hypnosis   293

Advantages and Disadvantages of Self-Hypnosis, 298   Techniques
of Authohypnosis, 299   Problems with Self-Hypnosis, 304

7. Psychological, Legal, and Legislative Problems
and Alleged Dangers of Hypnosis   307

Psychological Problems in Hypnosis, 308   Self-Destructive, Antisocial,
Immoral, or Criminal Behavior as Possible Results of Hypnotic
Suggestion, 317   Legal and Legislative Problems in Hypnosis, 328

8. Hypnosis in Perspective   341

Glossary   351

References and Bibliography   365

Author Index   479

Subject Index   495

Foreword

Developed two centuries ago and based upon ideas even then millennia old, Franz Anton Mesmer's theory of animal magnetism was one of the most significant markers on the long path that has led to our modern day understanding of the total person. Although his basic assumptions were soon disproved by his contemporaries, it is noteworthy that Mesmer's major contribution was that he interested and stimulated later generations of researchers, clinicians, and others to study and use what has ultimately come to be known as hypnosis. While we do not as yet have a definitive understanding of what hypnosis is, and although the very name of the modality is a misnomer (based as it is upon the etymological root for sleep and termed as such in 1821 by d'Henin de Cuvilliers), the waves of scientific, clinical, and lay interest that have always accompanied hypnosis have not been deterred. There is something about the process that has continued to attract and intrigue many, possibly because hypnosis is a fundamental aspect of the human experience.

What we do know is that in working with patients of all ages and from all backgrounds, hypnosis has numerous applications in the various health specialties. The finding that negative side-effects are virtually nonexistent has served to enhance the importance of this therapeutic tool. In the management of pain, it is an increasingly used technique, and post-surgical problems such as nausea and vomiting can be reduced. Recent accounts in which burn victims have been aided are impressive, as are reports that hypnosis can be useful in working in different ways with cancer patients. In dermatology, it has long been known that hypnotherapy can be helpful in a variety of disorders, including those caused by viruses such as herpes and warts. The latter application suggests even broader uses. In childbirth, the method has been employed with success for more than a century by giving the patient greater and easier control over the process. In dentistry, there are important uses in diminishing bleeding, gagging, and salivation. Hypnosis can also aid the retention of dental tools and appliances. In ophthalmology, the relaxation necessary during laser treatment has been facilitated, and the overall easing of anxiety and fear in any patient can only serve to assist the professional. For the terminal patient, hypnosis can help make that person more comfortable in his or her last days. An important implication for future use is the possiblity that hypnosis can impact positively upon the body's immune system. In general, then, there is considerable empirical evidence that the applications of the modality in medicine can be extremely helpful when employed in appropriate cases by qualified practitioners.

For the psychotherapist, as well, the method may be used with effect in many disorders. For psychosomatic dysfunctions, phobias, psychosexual problems, and conversion symptomatology, hypnosis is a treatment that can be short term, successful, and cost-effective. In these days of changes in the health care provider system, the last is no small benefit. In overcoming repression and other forms of resistance, the technique can at times be dramatic in its effects. Direct positive suggestions for improvement and remission can be effective in certain cases. Maladaptive habits such as smoking and weight management, which are significant public health problems, can also be treated. Certain unusual disorders, such as multiple personality, have been treated with good results, and even some psychotic reactions can be affected.

There are other areas where hypnosis can be utilized. The retrieval or refreshment of memories with victims of and witnesses to crime is not without controversy in terms of admissibility in courts of law, but it is evident that the method can often be useful in the resolution of law enforcement cases in real-life situations, that is, non-laboratory settings. Other areas where hypnosis has been successfully utilized include the facilitation of learning and the enhancement of performance in sport activities.

There have been literally thousands of books, pamphlets, scientific articles, and other publications over the past 200 years that have discussed hypnosis and its applications. Indeed, this plethora of words poses an increasingly difficult task for the serious student, for in order to remain current and comprehend fully the significance of present reports, one must at the same time have an appreciation for that which preceded them. How many of those who are interested in hypnosis have ready access to the vast and comprehensive literature that exists? And how many have the time to pursue those books and papers in full? These questions underlie the real importance of Professor Roy Udolf's book.

In 1981, a most important service for the field was performed when Udolf published the first edition of his *Handbook of Hypnosis for Professionals*. His goal was

to acquaint the reader with the factual basis and techniques of hypnotism and to suggest to him some of the practical applications of this phenomenon in a variety of fields both clinical and otherwise. No book on any clinical technique can take the place of personal experience under supervision; but it is hoped that this book will provide the necessary practical and theoretical understanding to make such subsequent personal instruction more effective and to enable the reader to decide if hypnosis is likely to be helpful to him in his work. A major goal of this book is to bring together in one source a variety of material and ideas that the beginning hypno-therapist needs to be familiar with prior to gaining professional experience in hypnosis.

Udolf succeeded admirably in his chosen task, and it was no surprise that the book quickly became one of the leading sources of its kind, since within its pages were made available what in essence was one of the most compre-hensive overviews of the literature ever prepared. Furthermore, this accom-plishment was managed in a smoothly flowing, well researched, and easy to read style, so that the reader was greatly helped in getting the most out of the book. Of course, any author's work necessarily has to have a cutoff point, and this was no exception. Since the publication of the first edition, the field of hypnosis has continued a pattern of rapidly expanding growth, which has characterized it for the past several decades. Increasing numbers of psy-chologists, physicians, and others are finding that the modality is helpful in a wide array of clinical and other applications, and the output of research continues to be impressive as well. Consequently, the second edition of the handbook is welcome indeed, for it affords a more up-to-date review of the field for both beginning and experienced readers. Not only is it comprehen-sive in its coverage of the field, but it is done with objectivity and clarity.

As one who has worked with hypnosis and studied it since graduate school days, I have looked forward to this revision. Now that it is here, I am con-fident that my colleagues will also share my enthusiasm for what is inevitably bound to be a very useful aid to anyone who is interested in hypnosis and its applications.

MELVIN A. GRAVITZ, Ph.D. *
Clinical Professor of Psychiatry
and Behavioral Sciences
George Washington University

---

* Past president of the American Society of Clinical Hypnosis, past president of the American Board of Psychological Hypnosis, and past editor of the *American Journal of Clinical Hypnosis.*

Preface

Hypnosis has been known in one form or another since the beginning of recorded history. In the past, it has been associated with religious ceremonies, magic, the supernatural, and many erroneous theories. Today it is officially recognized as a legitimate tool in medicine, dentistry, and psychotherapy, but much concerning its mechanism of operation is still unknown, and there is even more disagreement among experts with respect to what phenomena can and cannot be elicited by hypnotic suggestion. The research, even when properly designed and controlled, often yields seemingly inconsistent results and is amenable to many theoretical interpretations.

Since the first edition of this book was published in 1981, hypnosis has continued to be a topic of considerable interest to both reseachers and clinicians, as well as to a number of other professional groups, including lawyers and law enforcement agencies. Psychotherapists and other professional people interested in investigating the possible value of hypnosis in their work find themselves beset by many difficulties. Training facilities are usually limited to weekend-type seminars or, more rarely, an opportunity for a postdoctoral fellowship in an institute specializing in hypnotherapy. Such fellowship experience is often impractical for an established practitioner. Although there are a few excellent books on some limited aspects of the subject (such as Weitzenhoffer's *General Techniques of Hypnotism,* Hull's classic report of his experimental work in *Hypnosis and Suggestibility,* and Hilgard's more recent review of the experimental literature in *The Experience of Hypnosis*), there is no one source available to acquaint interested professional readers with all of the varied aspects of hypnotic phenomena that they need to know to evaluate its potential for practical application in their own work.

As a result, practitioners inadequately trained in the uses and limitations of hypnotic suggestion often attempt the impossible. For example, even experienced therapists have made such posthypnotic suggestions as, "Your symptoms will disappear, and you will feel happier and more secure," as if, in spite of their knowledge to the contrary, hypnosis were a form of magic, and a desired end result could be obtained by simply enunciating it to a hypnotized subject. A subject who was capable of effectuating such a suggestion probably would not be in psychotherapy in the first place.

Effective hypnotherapists must learn the essential nature of hypnotic sug-gestibility and what types of suggestions a hypnotized person is capable of effectuating. Then they must learn to make these suggestions in such a man-ner to produce a desired end result that cannot·effectively be suggested di-rectly. Hypnosis, however, has far more to offer as an aid to psychotherapy than the mere implanting of therapeutic suggestions, or it would not be worth reading a book about. Every hypnotic phenomenon obtainable can be used to further the progress of psychotherapy if utilized in an imaginative manner by a creative therapist. Furthermore, these phenomena may find application in radically different methods of therapy ranging from classical psychoanalysis to behavior modification.

Therapists who limit their efforts to suggesting therapeutic end results soon accumulate an impressive collection of failures. They conclude that hypnosis is not worthwhile, and abandon its use. Had they been trained to ap-preciate its full potential as well as its limitations, they might have found it a useful adjunct to their standard therapeutic methods, although certainly not the panacea that some overenthusiastic writers proclaim. Indeed, one of the major obstacles to the acceptance and utilization of hypnosis in clinical prac-tice is the exaggerated and totally unjustifiable claims made for it in some of the popular, and occasionally even the scientific, literature.

Although the first edition of this book was originally intended as a primer for clinicians and other professionals desiring to explore the potential of hyp-nosis as a tool in their work rather than as a source book, it developed in the latter direction. The goal of this book is to acquaint readers with the factual basis and techniques of hypnotism and to suggest some of the practical ap-plications of this phenomenon in a variety of fields, clinical and otherwise. No book on any clinical technique can take the place of personal experience under supervision, but it is hoped that this book will provide the necessary practical and theoretical understanding to make such subsequent personal instruction more effective and to enable readers to decide if hypnosis is likely to be helpful to them in their work. A major objective of this book is to bring together in one source a variety of material and ideas that beginning hyp-notherapists need to be familiar with prior to gaining professional experience in hypnosis. It is intended as a book on hypnosis and hypnotic phenomena per se, not on hypnotherapy, the effective practice of which requires knowl-edge of hypnotism plus training in conventional methods of psychotherapy. However, readers trained in psychotherapy will find suggestions in this book for the utilization of hypnotic phenomena in the course of several different psychotherapeutic approaches.

In order to maintain the book's usefulness as a source of reference ma-terial, it was decided that it was time to revise it to take into account some 600-odd references that have appeared since the first edition. A large ma-jority of these articles have been cited as additional references in appropriate places in the text, and many of them have been discussed briefly. All that were relevant to any major issue in hypnosis, whether referred to or not, appear in the bibliography. The criterion for the incorporation of new reference material into the text was basically its importance and its applicability to the areas covered. The author was satisfied that the organization of the original edition achieved his objectives for this book and, except for the addition of a few new sections, did not believe that this organization needed to be altered. In no case was the decision to include or exclude a reference based on the extent to which such reference agreed with any position taken in this book. In fact, wherever possible, articles with opposing viewpoints were included in order to give readers a balanced view of the material.

The reviews of the first edition of this book that the author is aware of were all fair, constructive, and sometimes very perceptive. Many were also quite generous. All comments by reviewers were considered in preparing this revision, but in some cases the author did not agree with the opinions of the reviewer. For example, one reviewer referred to the tendency of the book to go into "long enthusiastic digressions into classical psychology." If anything, this edition has more of this type of material, for one of the major goals of this book is to put hypnosis in context as part of a larger body of psychological knowledge rather than treat it, as many other books do, as though it were some isolated esoteric phenomenon.

In short, the basic goals and structure of the book remain unchanged, but it has been updated to keep pace with the current explosion of literature. In addition, it has been reviewed carefully in an effort to weed out as many unclear or ambiguous statements as possible to improve readability. It is still intended as a book on hypnosis per se rather than clinical hypnosis, although clinicians will find a great deal of material of value to them in spite of the absence of a detailed how-to-do-it approach.

The focus of the book is empirical and practical as opposed to theoretical. Theoretical positions are discussed in relation to research findings when necessary for an understanding of the research issues or design rather than as a separate topic.

There are still, as one reviewer noted, major differences in goals and styles between chapters. Chapter 1 is a general introduction and orientation to hypnosis, while Chapter 2 is a detailed review of hypnotic susceptibility and the instruments for its measurement. Chapter 3 is a less formal discussion of the mechanics of hypnotic induction and trance management. Chapter 4 is essentially a collection of 13 minichapters that review the experimental literature, and Chapter 5 is a review of the clinical and applied literature. Chapter 6 covers self-hypnosis from both experimental and practical clinical viewpoints, and Chapter 7 takes the same approach for the psychological and legal problems encountered in working with hypnosis. Chapter 8 is a brief concluding chapter.

Like any other book this one reflects the author's own interests, attitudes, and limitations. It still falls short of the perfect attainment of its objectives, but it is hoped that this revision will make it more useful to the reader.

ROY UDOLF, J. D., Ph.D.

Publisher's Note: Masculine pronouns were used throughout the text to avoid awkward sentence structure. They should be understood to refer to both females and males.

Acknowledgments

Richard O'Brien, Ph.D., of the Psychology Department and Alfred Cohn, Ph.D., of the New College of Hofstra University reviewed the entire manuscript of this book and made many valuable suggestions for its improvement. They both expended an enormous amount of time and energy on this task, and, if there were any justice in the world, they would appear as coauthors.

John Baum, M.D., of the University of Rochester School of Medicine and Dentistry also took time out from a busy schedule to review all of the material on the medical applications of hypnosis.

The author is grateful to these consultants for the generous contribution of their time and expertise to this undertaking. However, their suggestions were not always followed, and they are in no way responsible for any remaining errors or any of the opinions expressed in this book.

Joan Dale and Veronica Estler typed the entire manuscript from illegible, misspelled notes with skill, dispatch, and unfailing good humor.

Finally, the author would like to give substantial negative credit to the members of the Ninety-fourth Congress who enacted the current copyright law whose inane provisions doubled the amount of effort required to obtain copies of most of the articles referred to in this edition and made it impossible to obtain many relevant materials formerly available through interlibrary loans.

CHAPTER 1

Introduction

The logical way to write a book about hypnotism would be to define hypnosis at the beginning, describe its theory and mechanism of operation, and then go on to discuss its practical uses and limitations. Unfortunately, it is not possible to do that because we do not know the essential nature or mechanism of hypnosis, although there is much mutually contradictory theorizing on the subject by many competent professionals in the field. The approach taken in this book is first to describe the phenomena associated with hypnosis and its induction and then to discuss some of the practical ways in which these phenomena may be utilized. Theoretical explanations and models will be referred to in connection with research findings and practical applications as appropriate.

In this chapter, the modern history of hypnosis will be outlined briefly. Readers will then be introduced to a few of the basic theoretical positions concerning hypnosis to alert them to the issues that must ultimately be resolved by the data. Last, some common misconceptions about hypnosis that exist among potential subjects and patients, and even in some cases among psychologists or psychiatrists, will be described. Although it is difficult to say exactly what hypnosis is, it may be easier to set the record straight by describing what it is not.

HISTORY OF HYPNOSIS

Genesis 2:21-22 contains what some claim is the earliest recorded description of the use of hypnoanesthesia: "And the Lord God caused a deep sleep to fall upon Adam, and he slept; and He took one of his ribs, and closed up the flesh instead thereof; And the rib, which the Lord God had taken from man, made He a woman."

It would be difficult, if not impossible, to assess accurately how large a role hypnotic phenomena played in the lives of ancient peoples, particularly those who failed to develop a written language to record their experiences. From what we know of the ancient Egyptian and Greek dream-incubation centers (where people with problems came to fast and pray, hoping that they might have a dream that could be interpreted to give them the guidance they sought), it is probable that many of the dreams generated were hypnotically induced (Stam and Spanos, 1982; Machovec, 1979a). A study of primitive cultures today suggests that hypnotic phenomena probably played a large role in religious experience and healing in ancient cultures. Even in highly civilized countries like our own, faith healing, similar or identical in nature to hypnotic suggestion, still flourishes. An adequate treatment of the ancient history of hypnosis would be a major undertaking in its own right and would probably result in a work many times the size of this one. Although such an account would prove fascinating, it is not necessary for our purposes, and we will begin our historical review with more modern times.

Paracelsus (1493-1541), as he is commonly known (he was born Philip Aureolus Theothrastus Bombastus Von Hohenheim), was a Swiss physician who is of interest to students of hypnosis primarily because he believed in the astrological idea that the stars influence human beings. He developed the theory that the influence of the stars came from their magnetic nature, and he believed that all magnets influenced the human body by means of invisible emanations. This idea is similar to notions of an invisible "ether" that filled all space and was regarded by an earlier generation of engineers as the medium by which radio waves were propagated (by analogy to sound waves, which need some medium such as air in which to travel). Although it is fashionable now to treat this theory of a magnetic fluid with condescension, even today many sophisticated students of physics regard the concept of a magnetic or an electric field as an explanation of the action of a magnet or a charged body through a distance, when in fact it is nothing more or less than a mathematical description of such action.

Van Helmont (1577-1644) expanded on Paracelsus' concept of a magnetic fluid to include the notion of an "animal magnetism" that emanated from the human body with the potential to influence the minds and bodies of others. The idea of the influence and potential healing power of magnets on people led to a great many magnetic healers practicing over the next hundred or so years, some of whom are reputed to have produced dramatic cures. Because of the belief in animal magnetism, the technique of "laying on of hands" developed. This technique is still in use today by faith healers, although they now ascribe its efficacy to God's power rather than to animal magnetism. Even Freud used this technique as a method of treatment prior to the development of psychoanalysis. Two of the more famous magnetic healers were an Irishman named Greatrakes (1629-1683), and Father Maximilian Hell (1720-1792), a Viennese Jesuit.

The most notorious of all magnetic healers and the man with whom most modern historical descriptions of hypnosis begin was an Austrian physician by the name of Friedrich (Franz) Anton Mesmer (1734-1815). Mesmer received his medical degree from the University of Vienna in 1776. The title of his doctoral dissertation was "The Influence of the Stars and Planets on Curative Powers." Mesmer became interested in the curative effects of magnets after experimenting with some given to him by Father Hell. Influenced by Paracelsus' theories, he believed that an invisible magnetic fluid emanated from the stars and influenced people and their health. In his view, illness was caused by an imbalance of this fluid, and by redistributing it under the influence of magnets, health could be restored. Later in his practice he discovered that magnets were unnecessary and that the same effects could be obtained by making passes over the afflicted parts of the patient's body with his hands alone. Rather than abandon the theory of magnetism altogether, he simply concluded that the curative effect was due to the animal magnetism contained in his own body and hands.

Mesmer was moderately successful in Vienna, and in 1778 he came to Paris at the invitation of the king. There he became so successful that he had to develop group therapy techniques to accommodate all of the patients clamoring to be treated by him. He was quite a showman; during his group sessions, he wore flowing lilac robes and flourished a wand. The treatment room was dimly lit and had reflecting mirrors and background music. Patients were seated around a large oaken vat or *baquet* filled with chemicals and iron magnets, and they would hold hands in a circle very much like at a seance. Mesmer would then move about from patient to patient making passes with his hands and touching them with magnets.

Often his technique was overtly sexual (the majority of his patients were women). He would touch or stroke the patient, sometimes in the hypochondria or ovarian area. The patient's knees were held between Mesmer's, and the lower parts of their bodies were in close contact. Barber (1978d) describes Mesmer's induction procedure as primarily nonverbal.

What Mesmer was doing without knowing it was inducing a state of hypnosis, but the type of hypnotic reaction he obtained was different from that produced by a modern hypnotist. The standard reaction obtained, called a *crisis*, amounted to a convulsive reaction often accompanied by laughing,

crying, or unconsciousness—similar to what would be called a hysterical reaction today.

At the beginning of his work Mesmer reported his findings to various scientific societies, most of which ignored him. It was said that when he became
famous the French government offered him a large sum of money in exchange for his secret, which he refused to disclose (because he did not know
it). He became so notorious that in 1784 a committee of the French Academy
of Science was appointed to investigate him and his methods. This committee, presided over by the American ambassador to France, Benjamin Franklin, included such prominent people as Lavoisier, the renowned chemist, and
Guillotin, the inventor of the guillotine (McConkey and Perry, 1985; Perry and
Laurence, 1983b). After careful investigation, this committee concluded that
$\longrightarrow$ magnets produced no cures unless the patients knew that they were being
magnetized, and hence the effects obtained were due to the patient's imagination and belief rather than to magnetism.

It may seem incredible to readers that a committee of distinguished scientists would depreciate as worthless a method of treatment that empirically
$\longrightarrow$ was shown to have produced dramatic cures in cases of chronic pain and
other hysterical symptoms simply because the theory behind it was correctly
perceived as erroneous. However, the prevailing *zeitgeist* in the scientific
community of the day has to be appreciated. It was a time when scientists
sought to explain all natural phenomena in terms of physical or chemical
principles based on scientifically controlled observations. Any explanation that
appeared to be based on imagination or other "mentalistic" or subjective factors was repugnant to the emergent spirit of scientific rigor. Indeed, the attitude was not very different from the present one of some behaviorists toward
many psychoanalytic concepts.

The committee went beyond merely pronouncing Mesmer's methods
worthless; they denounced them as potentially harmful because of the convulsions produced, as well as the close physical contact between patient and
therapist, which they believed stimulated sexual feelings in both parties and
was therefore immoral.

The effect of these findings was to discourage reputable scientists from
working with hypnosis, or mesmerism as it was then called, and to create
difficulties with the medical organizations of the time for the few physicians
who did pursue the subject. Even prior to the commission report, Mesmer
had problems with the medical establishment, who disapproved of his
magician-like methods. Following the report Mesmer fell into complete dis-
repute and had to leave Paris. He died penniless in Switzerland in 1815.

The Marquis Armand de Puységur (1751–1825), a retired military man,
was a pupil of Mesmer who discovered that the dramatic *crises* were neither
inevitable nor necessary. When the hypnotist talked to the patient and suggested relaxation and calmness, the patient developed a tranquil trance, which

he referred to as artificial somnambulism or a "sleeping" trance. In this tranquil state the patient could talk and be given instructions.

John Elliotson (1791–1868) was an English surgeon with a reputation as a radical in medicine. For example, he began using the stethoscope, which was invented on the Continent for use in listening to the hearts of patients (without the necessity of the doctor placing his ear on the chest of a frequently filthy patient). He had heard of Mesmer's work, and in 1837, when he was a professor of surgery at University College in London, he began to use mesmerism at his hospital to perform painless surgery. This practice led to difficulties with both the administration of his hospital and the prestigious British medical journal *Lancet*, which denounced him as a fraud. In 1838 he was forced to leave his hospital post over this issue, and in 1846 he gave a Harvey lecture bitterly denouncing what he considered obstacles being placed in the path of medical progress. In 1843 Elliotson founded *Zoist*, a journal dealing with hypnosis.

James Esdaile (1808–1859), a Scottish surgeon practicing in India, read Elliotson's work and began to use hypnosis to control surgical pain. Between 1845 and 1850 he performed over 300 major surgical procedures painlessly using only hypnosis as an anesthetic. The most common of these operations involved the excision of massive scrotal tumors, and nineteen were amputations. He found that hypnosis was not only an effective anesthetic but that it also reduced surgical shock. Patients were relaxed and quiet during the operations when formerly they would have had to be held down while writhing in pain. Mortality rates for scrotal tumor removal dropped from 50% to 5% (Pulos, 1980). In spite of these impressive results most medical journals refused to publish his results, and one went so far as to claim that the Indian peasants enjoyed having the surgery done on them and pretended not to feel pain to please Esdaile!

One of the reasons that hypnosis did not find widespread acceptance as an anesthetic at the time was the fortuitous development of chemical anesthetics—nitrous oxide in 1844 and ether in 1846. These agents, although more dangerous than hypnosis, were easier to administer, and susceptibility to them was universal. Finally, chloroform was introduced into India and contributed to the decline in the use of mesmerism even in that relatively receptive country. Esdaile ultimately returned to Scotland, where he died in 1859.

James Braid (1795–1860) was an English physician who had a profound effect on the history of hypnotism. It was he who coined the name *hypnotism*, which replaced the old term *mesmerism*, with all of its associations to Mesmer and the kind of showmanship that most medical men of the time found unprofessional and repugnant. He was as different a person from Elliotson as possible. Far from being a radical, he was an accepted and conservative member of the medical community.

His first exposure to mesmerism came in 1841 when he attended a demonstration by a Swiss magnetizer by the name of Lafontaine, in Manchester. After witnessing the first demonstration Braid was convinced that it was a fraud and denounced it as such, but at the second meeting, the demonstrations of analgesia and eye catalepsy convinced him of the reality of the phenomenon, and he began to investigate it.

He originally believed that a hypnotic trance was related to sleep and is generally credited with coining the term *neurohypnology*, which means "nervous sleep." This was modified and shortened by usage to *hypnosis*, although Gravitz and Gerton (1984a) trace the term *hypnosis* to prior sources. Braid believed that the induction of the trance state was brought about by fatigue of the eye muscles caused by prolonged fixation. Hence he developed a technique of hypnotic induction called *Braidism,* which involved fatiguing the eye musculature by having the subject fixate on a point somewhat above his or her normal line of vision. Today we know that this idea is erroneous; mere fixation and fatigue of the eye muscles do not produce a trance.

With time, Braid began to believe that the hypnotist influenced the subject by suggestion rather than by any direct physiological effects. He also realized that it was inaccurate to refer to hypnosis as a nervous sleep because it was really quite different from ordinary sleep. He then developed the view that the essence of the hypnotic experience is the narrowing of the subject's perceptual field by concentrating on a single idea. Hence, he tried, unsuccessfully, to change the name from *hypnosis* to the more descriptive *monoideism.* He also discovered that it was possible to induce a hypnotic state without any formal or ritualistic induction procedure.

The real importance of Braid's work was in his making hypnosis more acceptable to the medical community of his time. His publications were opposed by many in the medical establishment, but his conservative approach minimized their opposition. The term *neurohypnosis* implied a physiological basis for the phenomenon, which made it more palatable to physicians, and the mesmerists' opposition to Braid's approach, along with the deprecating remarks made about it in *Zoist,* also aided its acceptance by orthodox medicine. The term *hypnosis* permitted an emotional divorce between the phenomenon and its past flamboyant history.

A. A. Liébeault (1823-1904) was a country doctor who settled in Nancy, France, in 1864. He became interested in hypnosis in 1860 and used it in the treatment of his peasant patients for over twenty years. (Barber makes the point that most eighteenth- and nineteenth-century hypnotists were well-educated professional men or powerful aristocrats, and most patients were illiterate peasants. Hence, the hypnotists of the time tended to use authoritative induction procedures, no longer effective with today's better-educated subjects.)

In 1866, he published the results of his successful treatments in a book entitled *Du Sommeil,* which may hold the all-time record for being the least successful book ever published. It is reputed to have sold only one copy, although Gravitz, (1985d), noting the frequency with which this work was cited by contemporary scholars, doubts this. Liébeault was considered an eccentric by his medical colleagues. Possibly to avoid the label of charlatan, he would not charge patients for treatment by hypnosis, but if they wished to be treated with medicines, he charged his normal fee.

Hippolyte Bernheim (1837–1919), a prominent neurologist practicing in Nancy, originally thought that Liébeault was a fraud and wanted to expose him as such. But he became converted to Liébeault's point of view when the latter was successful in the hypnotic treatment of a case of sciatica that Bernheim had treated unsuccessfully for six years.

Liébeault and Bernheim collaborated and jointly treated over 12,000 patients. They believed that hypnosis was based on the patient's increased suggestibility. Like Charcot, they found that hysterical symptoms could be induced and removed by suggestion, but unlike Charcot, they recognized that this could be done with normal people and not just hysterics.

Bernheim founded the Nancy School of Hypnosis, which stood in opposition to the views of Charcot's Paris School until the latter's conversion to Bernheim's viewpoint. In 1884 Bernheim published *De La Suggestion* in which, like Braid before him, he recognized suggestion as the basis of hypnosis. In 1886 he added two chapters on hypnotherapy for hysteria and psychosomatic disorders (Weitzenhoffer, 1980a).

Jean Charcot (1825–1893) was one of the most distinguished neurologists of the nineteenth century. He was the director of the neurological clinic at the Salpêtrière in Paris (Chertok, 1984b). He found that all hysterical symptoms (physical symptoms without any organic etiology) such as paralysis, deafness, and even the anatomically impossible condition known as glove anesthesia (where sensation is lost over the region of the hand normally covered by a glove) could be both produced and relieved by hypnosis.

Based on these observations he erroneously concluded that hypnosis was a phenomenon related to hysteria and could be produced only in hysterical patients. This theory was opposed to Bernheim's and the more modern view that hypnosis is a normal phenomenon produced by suggestion. Charcot also believed that hypnosis was an organic condition and could be induced by purely physical manipulations. He talked of three well-defined stages of hypnosis—lethargy, catalepsy, and somnambulism—and their elicitation by neurological stimulation. Ultimately, to his credit, Charcot was convinced of the correctness of Bernheim's views by the weight of the evidence presented by the latter—an analysis of over 10,000 cases. Charcot's major contribution to hypnosis was not in his theories but in the fact that such a highly esteemed medical authority as he considered hypnosis a respectable phenomenon worthy of study. He thus completed the process, begun but not finished by Braid, of making hypnosis acceptable to the medical community.

Pierre Janet (1859-1947) received his medical degree in 1893. He was Charcot's student and successor as director of the psychological laboratory at the Paris hospital of the Salpêtrière. He believed that hypnosis concentrated the field of consciousness of the subject, a theory reminiscent of Braid's conception of hypnosis as monoideism. Morton Prince (1854-1929) espoused Janet's views in the United States.

Sigmund Freud's (1856-1939) influence on hypnosis was probably as negative as Charcot's was positive. The reason for this unfortunate state of affairs was simply the greatness of the man. When Freud ultimately abandoned the use of hypnosis in the treatment of neurotics and went on to develop his own method of treatment, psychoanalysis, hypnotherapy was set back several generations. Indeed Freud's work has been so influential that it has probably set psychology itself back to a similar degree. This is not to depreciate the value of Freud's contributions, but it is a fact that whenever a theory becomes so well entrenched that all new ideas are evaluated against it, it must of necessity have an impeding effect on innovations and progress.

Freud studied under Charcot in 1885 and later under Bernheim (Chertok, 1977, 1984a). Prior to developing the method of psychoanalysis, he utilized hypnosis in the psychotherapy of neurotic patients. He was never particularly comfortable with this method of treatment and has been described by some as a poor hypnotist, although Orne (1982) describes his knowledge of hypnosis as profound and his writings on the subject as brilliant. He ultimately abandoned the use of hypnosis for a number of reasons:

1. He found that not all patients were capable of being hypnotized to the necessary depth.
2. Often the patient would not be benefited when informed, after awakening, of material discovered. The patient had to participate actively in the discovery process, and the method of free association was much better suited to this than hypnosis.
3. Hypnosis stripped patients of their defenses while they still needed them.
4. Even when symptoms were relieved, the cure was often not permanent.
5. Hypnosis was too time-consuming.
6. Hypnosis had an objectionable seductive quality about it.

Orne (1982) characterized the first objection as bizarre. He finds it comparable to saying that penicillin is not a useful drug because it cannot be given to all patients.

The notion that hypnosis was too time-consuming suggests that at the time Freud raised this objection, he was unduly optimistic about the development of a method of treatment that could be accomplished in a short time span.

Classical psychoanalysis requires seeing a patient a minimum of three (preferably five) times a week for a period of several years. Even if it had a 100% cure rate, it would remain totally valueless to the vast majority of patients who need psychotherapy but could not afford such an expensive method of treatment. One of the major values of hypnosis as an adjunct to any type of psychotherapy is its capacity to shorten the required length of treatment.

With respect to the last objection, Kline cites a story about a patient who awoke from a trance and threw her arms around Freud just as a maid serving coffee entered his consulting room. This atypical reaction probably caused him a great deal of embarrassment. However, the generation of inappropriate and often intense positive or negative emotional feelings directed at the analyst (transferences) are a necessary part of psychoanalytic treatment, although they are not required for hypnosis per se.

Most of the early work in hypnosis was done by medically trained people and arose out of the practical problems of medical practice. This was a natural state of affairs because psychology, which developed out of a marriage between physiology and philosophy, is only about 100 years old. With the advent of the science of psychology in the twentieth century, more and more work in hypnosis is being done by psychologists specifically trained in research methodology, either exclusively or in addition to clinical training.

Thus in 1933, Clark L. Hull (1884-1952), the creator of one of the most influential behavioristic theories of learning, published his classic work, *Hypnosis and Suggestibility: An Experimental Approach,* which describes his own methodical attempts at controlled experimentation covering a wide range of hypnotic phenomena. The book is available today as a reprint and is still worth reading. Although Hull's theoretical views may be out of date, the empirical facts of human behavior and the requirements of good experimental design have not changed. The book is particularly worth reading by modern psychologists who have been spoiled by the ready availability of oscilloscopes and a whole host of other equipment, for it shows how human ingenuity was able to make precise measurements in the absence of sophisticated recording and measuring equipment (Triplet, 1982).

Hull was quite critical in this book of the quality of the research done in hypnosis by Alfred Binet (1857-1911), the developer of the first modern intelligence test in 1904, the derivatives of which are still in widespread use. Binet and Féré were both students of Charcot, and they published a book on hypnosis called *Animal Magnetism,* which Hull castigated as being based on a series of "wretched experiments."

Another psychologist prominent in the fields of learning and hypnosis is Ernest R. Hilgard, who has published influential reviews of the literature in both areas. His book *Hypnotic Susceptibility* was shortened and republished as *The Experience of Hypnosis* in 1965. He is still active in this area at Stanford University's Laboratory of Hypnotic Research. A great deal of research, theoretical formulations, and clinical applications are being developed by the present generation of American psychologists.

It was not until 1955 that the British Medical Society officially recognized hypnosis as a legitimate medical tool, followed by the American Medical Association in 1958 (Schneck, 1985; Mutter, 1985). The American Psychological Association recognized it as a respectable entity in 1958, and certifying boards were set up for both the experimental and clinical usage of hypnosis in 1960.

PRELIMINARY FORMULATIONS CONCERNING THE NATURE OF HYPNOSIS

Although it is not possible to define precisely the nature of hypnosis, it will prove helpful to give some general formulations about what some investigators have regarded as the essential characteristics of the hypnotic state. Most of these notions are not mutually exclusive; indeed all may be involved in hypnosis to some extent. Whether any one of them is the essence of the hypnotic experience, however, is another matter.

Some view the hypnotic state simply as one of a variety of possible *altered states of consciousness* (e.g., sleep, coma, drunkenness, meditation) (Fromm, 1977*a*, 1977*b*; McCabe, Collins and Burns, 1978, 1979; Barmark and Gaunitz, 1979). This view may be true; many hypnotic subjects report feeling different when hypnotized, but it is not a very illuminating theory. Others characterize hypnosis primarily as a profound state of relaxation, and indeed certain methods of induction such as the progressive relaxation method are designed to produce just this result (Benson, 1983). To Braid and Janet, it was primarily the narrowing of the subject's perceptual field and total concentration on a single idea or image—that is, monoideism.

A common explanation of hypnosis today is Bernheim's notion that it is a heightened state of suggestibility, although such a statement actually explains nothing, merely substituting the word *suggestibility* for the word *hypnosis*. Some modern workers use such terms as *task motivation* (Barber), *demand characteristics* (Orne), or *social roles* (Coe and Sarbin) to explain hypnotic phenomena (Sarbin, 1984; Cescato, 1981; Coe and Sarbin, 1977). Task motivation implies that the subject produces the phenomena that he does under hypnosis because of his motivation to comply with the hypnotist's instructions rather than because of the existence of a hypnotic state. It implies that the hypnotist is perceived as an authority figure; and as Milgram's (1963) studies have demonstrated, there is a powerful motive in most people to please authority figures.

The notion of hypnosis as a social role, wherein the subject acts the way he believes he is supposed to act or is influenced by the demand characteristics of the situation, can be seen quite readily in the case of stage hypnotists, who routinely elicit behavior from subjects that would be difficult or impossible to get in the laboratory because of the social influence of the other subjects and the presence of an audience. Barber's notion that hypnosis involves an interpersonal situation between subject and hypnotist is related to all of these viewpoints.

Some regard hypnosis as a learned phenomenon, (Smyth, 1981a) or a form of conditioning (Salter, 1973), and believe that how a subject reacts in a trance is determined by his previous experience with hypnosis and his expectations. In support of this view, the wide amount of variation obtainable in the trance states of different subjects should be noted, ranging from the hysterical type of reaction of Mesmer's *crisis* to a stuporous state. The issue is often confused by the question of whether different trance reactions reflect different degrees of the same phenomenon or are in fact different kinds of reactions: that is, is a light hypnoidal state different in nature or degree from a profound somnambulistic state? This view implies that the trance itself is merely a reaction to suggestions, like most other hypnotic phenomena, rather than a special state of consciousness that produces or facilitates the development of other phenomena; that is, a hypnotic trance is primarily an effect, not a cause, although to some extent it may be both. This is a view for which the present author has considerable sympathy.

Another view of hypnosis is that it is a dissociative state wherein different mental functions are isolated from each other. Some workers share Charcot's view that hypnosis may be a physiological phenomenon and that there may be brain centers involved in hypnosis as there are in the hypothalamus for primary drives (Reyher, 1977a). Graham (1978) believes that hypnosis is a function of the activity of the nondominant cerebral hemisphere, which is more concerned with emotions and imagery, rather than the dominant hemisphere, which is involved more with speech and logical thought. (Carter, Elkins, and Kraft, 1982; MacLeod-Morgan, 1982; Graham, 1977; Crawford, Crawford, and Koperski, 1983; Frumkin, Ripley, and Cox, 1978; Levine, Kurtz, and Lauter, 1984; Sackeim, 1982; Graham and Pernicano, 1979).

H. J. Crawford (1982) finds support for this position in preliminary evidence that there are changes in cognitive functioning during hypnosis in the realms of ego functioning, imagery, creativity, and the nature of cognitive strategies employed that are in consonance with the functions of the dominant and nondominant hemispheres. Gruzelier and his co-workers (1984) report evidence that emphasizes the inhibition of the activity of the dominant hemisphere as the major occurrence that follows a hypnotic induction procedure.

Some medical hypnotists, such as Robert London and Herbert Spiegel, also believe that there is a physiological basis for hypnosis and that it is possible to predict hypnotic susceptibility by what superficially appears to be purely physiological measurements, such as the amount of eye roll produced in response to a request to look up. Certainly, to the extent that the brain is the organ of thought, all psychological activities must ultimately have a physiological or physical explanation.

Some explanations of hypnosis refer to it as a state in which the unconscious may be communicated with directly or in which the unconscious mind comes to the surface. Such explanations are often found in books by lay hypnotists and are particularly unfortunate for several reasons. First, a hypnotized subject is not unconscious in any sense of the term and is fully aware of everything going on around him. This type of explanation has a tendency to obscure that fact.

Second, the statement is basically meaningless. What does it mean to communicate directly with the unconscious? The term *unconscious* is used to mean so many different things by different people (or even by the same person at different times) that it is often quite meaningless. Sometimes the term *unconscious* is used to mean ideas that are not freely available to conscious awareness but that cause an affective response that affects the person's behavior. Sometimes it is used to refer to motives for behavior that the person is unaware of. Sometimes it is used to refer to complete, logical sequences of thought carried on without conscious awareness, often involving the use of childlike prototypic thought processes. Frequently it is used to refer to various combinations of the foregoing and to other forms of mental activity.

Third, the concept of the unconscious is unnecessary to describe what occurs in the hypnotic state. If a subject is given a posthypnotic suggestion and is then told to forget having been given this suggestion, it seems simpler to say that he merely forgot as suggested rather than to talk about communicating with his unconscious mind.

Although it is difficult and probably impossible to propose an explanation of the essential nature of hypnosis with which all experts would agree, it is possible to find agreement concerning what hypnosis is not. Thus some attention will now be devoted to dealing with certain misconceptions concerning the nature of hypnosis. Although most readers are probably sophisticated enough not to believe most of these erroneous ideas, it is important for them to be aware that they exist. They will find some of them to be quite common among potential patients, experimental subjects, and even mental health professionals, and such beliefs may interfere with the development of the proper hypnotic state unless the therapist takes the time to recognize them in patients and adequately dispel them (Channon, 1984*a*; McIntosh and Hawney, 1983; Vingoe, 1982*a*; Kraft and Rodolfa, 1982). It is not possible to get good results either in hypnotic induction or in the subsequent utilization of a trance without the active cooperation of the patient, and this requires his fears and reservations to be recognized and allayed (Garver, Fuselier, and

Booth, 1981). To a large extent, a hypnotized subject does behave in a manner consistent with his expectations.

COMMON MISCONCEPTIONS
CONCERNING HYPNOSIS

Misconception 1:   Hypnosis is a condition induced in the subject by the hypnotist.

This erroneous idea is the natural result of our use of English. We colloquially refer to hypnotizing subjects, and books are written and courses are given to train therapists and others "to hypnotize" subjects. Actually all hypnosis is self-hypnosis in the sense that any effect produced, including the trance state itself, is produced by the concentration and imagination of the subject, not the operator. The real role of the hypnotist is to guide and teach the subject how to think and what to do to produce the desired result. The operator no more imposes this state on a subject than a teacher learns the content of a course for a student. Both teacher and hypnotist can only facilitate the efforts of the student or subject.

Once a trance state is induced, the hypnotist may seem to utilize it for whatever result is sought, but even in the area of trance utilization, whatever phenomena occur do so because of the imagination of the subject, not the operator. For this reason the term *trance capacity* is preferable to the more common term *hypnotic susceptibility* to refer to the likelihood of a given subject's achieving a given trance depth. The latter term implies that the subject is having the state imposed on him, while the former recognizes that the capacity to achieve a given trance level is an ability of the subject, not the operator.

This is not to imply that the hypnotist is not important or does not have to be highly skilled. Self-hypnosis is extremely difficult to achieve without help and training from an external hypnotist in the beginning. Even with experience in self-hypnosis, it is always easier to achieve and utilize the trance state with the help of an external operator.

Inexperienced subjects should always be advised that they, not the hypnotist, are responsible for producing whatever results are obtained. This will have the effect of taking the onus of any difficulty in induction away from the operator and preventing the subject from losing the confidence in the hypnotist's ability that is so essential to a successful induction. Also, it is the truth. Some feel it undermines the probability of success in the induction if the hypnotist uses such equivocal language as "We will try to hypnotize you," or "We will see how deep a state you can attain." They believe that the hypnotist should always speak as though the induction is certain to be successful. If the responsibility for the success of the induction is placed fully on the subject, such unprofessional assurances of success are unnecessary. It is possible to reflect confidence in the subject's success by both word and manner without adopting the unwarranted behavior of a charlatan.

Misconception 2:   A hypnotist must be a dynamic, forceful, or charismatic person.

Since the subject and not the hypnotist is ultimately responsible for the induction of the trance state, it follows that the abilities of the subject and his motivation for hypnosis are more important than the personality of the hypnotist—unless this personality is such that it is incompatible with the needs or expectations of the subject. Different subjects require different types of hypnotists or different techniques. Some subjects can respond successfully to a wide range of hypnotists; others may require a specific type of approach to be successful. Certainly if the hypnotist is personable and has a good rapport with the subject, it is a positive factor. On the other hand, some outstanding hypnotists are not very good speakers and often have poor diction or marked accents. These characteristics evidently do not interfere with their success.

Kroger (1977*b*) makes the point that hypnosis is a "prestige" type of phenomenon and that it is the belief in the imminence of hypnosis that produces it. Hence, it is an advantage to a hypnotist to be known to the subject as an authority in the field or to have a title like "Doctor," for this will enhance the subject's expectations of success. For this reason, psychotherapists who use hypnosis frequently in their practice would do well to have their diplomas and degrees on exhibition in their office or waiting room.

Misconception 3:   Hypnosis involves a battle of wills with the hypnotist, who needs a stronger will than the subject.

This is a common misconception of many subjects that probably came from watching old Bela Lugosi movies. Unless it is dispelled, it can make the induction of hypnosis difficult or impossible since the subject will see it is an admission of inferiority.

If a subject comes to the therapist's office with the attitude that he is challenging the latter to be able to hypnotize him, he must be informed that there is no contest and if he chooses to resist hypnosis he will, of course, be successful. He must be made to understand that the hypnotic state can be produced only with his active cooperation and help.

Incidentally, it is possible to achieve a hypnotic state without the subject's being aware that he is being hypnotized. This can be done simply by avoiding the use of the words *hypnosis* or *sleep* in the induction procedure, or by saying that what the hypnotist is trying to do is get him to relax deeply. On the surface, this may seem as if the operator is unethically hypnotizing a subject without his consent, but bear in mind that no effect will occur unless the subject is willing to produce it. Such a procedure may be justified in the case of a patient who could profit from hypnosis but who cannot get over his fear of being hypnotized because of some unfounded ideas he has about it. A good question to ask at this point is whether there is any real difference between a deep state of relaxation as produced by the Jacobson method (see p. 66) and hypnosis? In other words, what is being suggested is that hypnosis often occurs in therapy when even the therapist does not consciously intend to produce it. In any event, this issue deals more with names than with reality. Not only is the ability to be hypnotized not a sign of a weak will, gullibility, or stupidity, but it in fact requires a good degree of intelligence in order to be able to concentrate and to think in the unfamiliar manner that the operator requests. Generally the author has found that bright people make good subjects, and it is a good idea to so inform subjects prior to induction attempts.

Misconception 4: Hypnosis is an unusual, abnormal, or artificial condition.

With a little thought, readers will be able to think of dozens of examples of spontaneously induced mental states that are highly similar or identical to a hypnotic trance. The common experience of daydreaming while commuting to work or becoming completely absorbed in a book to the exclusion of everything else going on around you are common examples. There is a condition called highway hypnosis, which is produced by a driver staring straight ahead on a monotonously straight road, possibly with the added influence of windshield wipers in steady operation. This phenomenon is probably responsible for an unknown number of highway accidents each year. Good human engineering of highways requires taking this phenomenon into account by providing enough turns in a road to break up the monotony of travel. A straight line may be the shortest distance between two points, but it is not always the best roadway design. Other common examples of spontaneously induced trance states may be found in a person's staring at a television set or reading a book without noticing what he is watching or reading. Most members of a movie audience exhibit many of the characteristics of people in a hypnotic state.

Misconception 5: Hypnosis is a form of sleep.

There are several reasons for this common misconception. First, the word *hypnosis* itself is a misnomer (Goldstein, 1982). It derives from Hypnus, the name of the Greek god of sleep. Second, the lack of facial expression and spontaneous movement coupled with slumping of the head or body frequently seen in hypnotized people is suggestive of sleep. Last, many methods of induction make use of exhortations directing the subject to sleep. Indeed, it is possible to bore a subject to the point where he will actually fall into a real state of sleep instead of hypnosis.

In spite of the superficial similarity between a hypnotic trance and normal sleep, the two states are quite different (Evans, 1977, 1982). During stage 1 sleep (the phase in which vivid visual dreams are most common), the skeletal musculature is effectively paralyzed, and, thus, reflexes like the knee jerk are diminished. However, under hypnosis, there is no paralysis (unless suggested), and there is no diminution of the basic reflexes or muscle tone.

Electroencephalograph (EEG) patterns are often said to be different for the hypnotic state and for sleep, but during stage 1 sleep, the EEG pattern is similar to the normal waking state except for the presence of rapid eye movements (REMs). Hence, stage 1 sleep is called arousal or paradoxical sleep. In stage 2, sleep spindles appear on the EEG record. Delta waves begin to appear in stage 3, becoming over 50% of the record by the deeper stage 4. None of these events occurs under hypnosis, where the EEG record is consistently similar to the waking state.

Misconception 6:   The subject is under the control of the hypnotist and can be made to do things that he ordinarily would not do or to reveal secrets.

This misconception makes it difficult for some subjects to permit themselves to be hypnotized because they fear loss of control. It is also the subject of much controversy and will be dealt with in more detail later. The weight of the evidence seems to support the notion that if a subject is directly requested to do something that is objectionable to him, he will simply refuse to do it or in some cases "awaken" from the trance. On the other hand, it may be possible to get a subject to perform an act he would not normally do by deceiving him into believing a situation is different than it actually is. For example, he may be told that a person that he is being asked to attack is about to harm him.

All subjects should be informed prior to an induction that they will be in complete control; and if the hypnotist suggests anything that offends them, they will be free not to follow the suggestion. Such an instruction will allay the fears of the subject and will also serve to protect the hypnotist from charges of misconduct or of exercising undue influence over the subject. There is no legitimate reason in therapy why a subject would ever be asked to do something repugnant to him. Indeed, one of the great advantages of a passive therapist is that he or she permits a patient to limit the production of anxiety-producing material to what the patient feels he can currently tolerate. This is a built-in safety valve. If the therapist is to make the decision about how much anxiety a patient can handle, he or she had better be an extremely good prognosticator or there is a risk of driving the patient out of therapy.

Although a hypnotist does not have complete control over a subject (and, in fact, if he or she did, hypnosis would be a dangerous procedure at best), the hypnotic state creates an atmosphere where suggestions, if acceptable to the subject, are more influential than they would be if the subject were not hypnotized. However, it must be kept in mind that people do influence the behavior of other people with words, whether their listeners are hypnotized or not. Although hypnosis does not produce a zombie-like dependence on a hypnotist, words can be potent and have the power to cure or harm, whether the recipient is hypnotized or awake. The danger lies not in the hypnotic state but in the use made of it. If any method of psychotherapy has the potential to help a patient, it must necessarily also have the power to harm him if not competently handled.

As an example of the misuse of a valid psychological technique, the practice of a certain industrial plant that utilized a psychological screening test to select its employees may be cited. An applicant had to have a certain personality profile on this instrument before being hired. The net result of this selection process was the hiring of an undue number of neurotic employees and the failure to hire many potentially productive people. The reason for this regrettable state of affairs was not that this particular test or psychological tests in general are not useful. In fact, it was a very good test; for if it caused the selection of neurotic candidates, it could just as readily have been used to exclude them. The real difficulty in this case was caused by the incompetent use of a valid test by an untrained personnel manager. The same is true in the case of many examples cited to show the dangers of hypnosis, which are really examples of the danger of its incompetent use.

Misconception 7: Hypnosis may be harmful to the subject.

There are many specific dangers postulated under this general heading. Some of those more frequently expressed include the following:

The subject may become unduly dependent on or influenced by the hypnotist.
The subject may not awaken from the trance.
A susceptible subject may develop a serious mental or physical illness.
Repeated hypnosis may weaken the subject's "will."

The first of these misconceptions can be illustrated by the nineteenth-century novel *Trilby*, by Du Maurier, about the power-hungry Svengali who hypnotized an artist's model and made her his virtual slave (Schneck, 1978b). While normally she had no singing voice, under Svengali's influence she became a famous singer. When Svengali became ill, her voice disappeared; when he died, she became hopelessly demented, as if he had destroyed her soul by hypnosis and rendered her a mere automaton, completely dependent on him.

This story illustrates a common nineteenth-century belief about hypnosis that has not totally disappeared. There is no evidence to support the idea that continued hypnosis causes a person to become unduly dependent on a hypnotist, but the same kind of transference reactions that occur in any form of psychotherapy can occur with hypnotherapy. Far from being a disadvantage, a transference is a vital tool for the psychotherapist. The misuse of a transference reaction by a lay hypnotist is not a danger of hypnosis but of untrained people doing psychotherapy.

The second "danger"—that the subject will be difficult to awaken— is extremely rare. The author has never had a subject display the slightest difficulty in awakening. Probably the most common reason for difficulties in awakening a subject is the use of ambiguous suggestions by the hypnotist, coupled with the average subject's literal interpretation of instructions. For example, if the hypnotist wants to be sure that the subject does not awaken spontaneously during a surgical procedure, he or she may suggest to the subject that he will not awaken until he is instructed to do so. (This suggestion may or may not be effective, but it should never be relied on to the exclusion of other precautions.) If he intends to convey this suggestion but uses the words "You will not awaken," then in effect the subject is simply following the suggestion literally when he refuses to awaken. This situation is easily dealt with as discussed in Chapter 3.

Fear is often expressed about what would happen to the subject if the hypnotist suddenly died. Experiments in which the hypnotist simply walked out of the room have answered this question (Evans and Orne, 1971). As soon as the subject realizes the operator has left, he comes out of the trance and leaves himself. Indeed the fear that a subject may not maintain a trance for as long as necessary may be more justified. Maintaining a trance for a prolonged period of time, as in a surgical procedure, often requires a constant flow of suggestions to the subject. Ending a trance is usually extremely easy.

The fear that hypnosis will produce a mental or physical illness is often based on statements by physicians, usually untrained in hypnosis, who are nevertheless anxious to establish it as an exclusively medical technique. The author knows of no reliable report of a psychosis or other mental illness proved to have been caused by hypnosis per se. If a patient has a brittle enough personality to have a psychosis triggered by hypnosis, it would almost certainly be triggered by the ordinary stresses of everyday life in any event. On the other hand, a certain number of people will develop mental and physical illnesses in the normal course of events; if these closely follow or occur during a hypnotic session, the hypnotist may well be accused of precipitating them and must be prepared to justify the procedures used. Although hypnosis per se will not produce a physical or mental illness, if a stage hypnotist causes a subject to exert himself unduly or suggests emotionally upsetting experiences, these could conceivably induce a heart attack or other acute problems. Again, the danger is not the hypnosis but its mismanagement. The same effects could be produced in a waking subject, as was illustrated by fatal heart attacks alleged to have been precipitated in two young soldiers by having them perform unusually strenuous punishment exercises in basic training.

With respect to the notion that repeated hypnosis may weaken the subject's *will*, this fear probably dates back to the theories of the phrenologists concerning faculties of the mind and their location in the brain. One of these faculties was labeled the *will*. The concept of *will* is totally meaningless in modern psychology, but people expressing fears about its weakening are probably concerned about the possibility of the hypnotist's acquiring undue influence over the subject. This is no more likely with hypnosis than with other methods of psychotherapy and is possibly less likely because of the shorter treatment time involved.

Misconception 8:   Hypnosis is a form of treatment or is beneficial by itself.

Hypnosis is simply a natural psychological phenomenon that is neither helpful nor harmful in itself. It is a technique that may be useful, in a proper case, as a supplement to a variety of standard psychotherapeutic techniques. As Kline (1977) pointed out, one does not treat a patient with hypnosis; one treats him under hypnosis.

Misconception 9:   A subject develops enhanced physical, mental, or ESP powers under hypnosis.

A subject under hypnosis is not capable of any physical act that he could not perform when awake if motivated enough. If he cannot play the piano when awake, he cannot play it under hypnosis. There is no credible evidence that he (or anybody else) develops any ESP powers.

Certainly if a subject is put into a rigid state of catalepsy by a stage hypnotist and his body is supported between two chairs by his shoulders and ankles while the hypnotist stands on his stomach, he is likely to suffer grievous physical injuries. Merely being in a cataleptic state does not make him immune to injuries; it only gives that impression to the naive observer. (A waking subject can also be supported between two chairs in this manner if properly instructed.) Also, if a subject is made to lift a very heavy weight, he is just as likely to develop a severe muscle strain or even a hernia whether in the hypnotized state or awake.

There is some evidence, to be discussed later, that memory may be improved and some perceptual effects may be obtained under hypnosis, but the extent of this enhancement and the advantages of the hypnotic state, as opposed to a high degree of motivation while awake, in producing these effects are still matters of considerable controversy.

CHAPTER 2

Hypnotic Susceptibility

Hypnotic susceptibility or trance capacity refers to the ability of a subject to achieve a given level of trance. This in turn makes two assumptions:

1. There is such a phenomenon as a trance state.
2. This state can be meaningfully measured along a depth scale from shallow (hypnoidal) to deep (somnambulistic).

With respect to the first issue, Sutcliffe (1961) has oriented theoretical views about the nature of hypnosis on a scale ranging from "credulous" to "skeptical." At the credulous end of the scale are the "hypnotic state" theorists, who regard a trance state as a phenomenon that enhances the suggestibility of a hypnotized subject. At the skeptical end of the scale are theorists like Barber, who take the view that a hypnotic state is neither a necessary nor sufficient condition to produce the classic effects of hypnosis, or Gibbons, who refers to the notion of a trance state as a "shared delusion" (Gibbons, 1982a, 1982b; Moon, 1982; Vingoe, 1982a; Wagstaff, 1982a). Barber points out that well-motivated subjects who have not been hypnotized can produce all of these phenomena, while some subjects in a deep trance cannot (Barber, 1958b; Chaves, 1968; Dalal, 1966; Spanos, 1970).

It is important for readers to bear in mind that this controversy relates specifically to the use of the term *hypnosis* as an independent variable or an explanation for the increased suggestibility of a subject. In this regard, Barber believes that what we should study are the specific antecedent events capable of producing such hypnotic phenomena as age regression, positive and negative hallucinations, amnesia, and so on. He believes that many of these antecedents are part of the hypnotic induction procedure but would be effective without hypnosis.

On the other hand, if the term *hypnosis* is used not as an explanation for the behavior of hypnotized subjects but as a form of behavior or a phenomenon that requires an explanation in its own right (i.e., as a dependent variable), then these theoretical controversies have no application. There is little conflict among the most credulous or skeptical of theorists concerning the types of behavior obtainable under hypnosis or their range and characteristics. *Trance state* is a convenient term or metaphor to describe a series of responses produced by a subject following procedures designed to produce hypnosis. These responses are easy to produce and demonstrate, and there is little controversy among theorists concerning the reality of the responses that collectively make up this state. Whether this state is a causative factor in other hypnotic behavior or merely another example of suggested responses is an unresolved issue that pragmatically may not be as important as the theoretical literature may indicate. As Cescato (1981) suggested, the important clinical question is whether hypnosis is useful in therapy, not the basis for its empirical effectiveness.

With respect to the second question, trance depth is conventionally measured in terms of the kinds of phenomena that the subject is capable of producing. This implies that some phenomena are more difficult to elicit than others, and the more difficult the phenomena, the deeper the trance that presumably permitted them to occur.

One immediate problem with this approach is that the difficulty of eliciting a given hypnotic phenomenon is a statistical concept. Thus, the fewer hypnotized subjects who are able to produce a given effect, like a negative hallucination, the more difficult it is said to be and the deeper the trance it is said to require. While enabling us to make excellent predictions about groups, statistics have no legitimate application to individual subjects. Thus, it is not uncommon to find a hypnotized subject who is capable of producing some effects thought to require a very deep trance (e.g., negative hallucinations) who fails to produce much easier phenomena (e.g., arm catalepsy). This, of course, casts doubt upon statistically obtained hierarchies of response difficulty as true ordinal scales and suggests that, to some extent at least, they are artifacts of group data (very much like Hull's lawful-appearing group learning curves). The fact that any hypnotic phenomenon can be obtained from a certain percentage of nonhypnotized subjects casts further doubt on their validity as a measure of the depth of a hypnotic state.

However unsatisfactory it may be theoretically, elicitable hypnotic phenomena are used to estimate trance depth because it is of practical value and permits good estimates of what can be expected from large groups of hypnotic subjects, if not from a single individual.

Trance capacity or hypnotic susceptibility is usually regarded as an organismic variable or an individual characteristic of a subject in the same manner that artistic ability or intelligence is. It is measured by using a standardized induction procedure to produce a trance state and then measuring the depth of the trance produced by the hypnotic phenomena elicited. Since the induction procedure is identical for all subjects, differences in depth of hypnosis may logically be assigned to differences in susceptibility rather than to differences in induction procedures. Thus, in using any susceptibility scale, the hypnotist must strive to adhere strictly to the standardized procedure and not make changes in an attempt to produce a deeper trance, since any changes would invalidate the measure. It should be noted that any scale designed to measure hypnotic susceptibility in conjunction with a standardized induction procedure is also capable of measuring the depth of a trance produced with any procedure. Hence, it is a double-edged tool.

When examples of specific susceptibility scales are discussed, readers may wonder why they are needed since they all necessarily involve the induction of hypnosis and often take more time than it would simply to hypnotize a patient and try out a proposed procedure. To answer this question, the situation in clinical practice, where hypnotic phenomena are being utilized for some practical purpose, must be distinguished from the case involving research in hypnotic phenomena. In a clinical situation, it is often simpler to proceed directly on the theory that the best predictor of hypnosis is hypnosis unless the clinician believes that a failure will undermine his relationship with the patient. Frankel and his associates, who advocate the use of susceptibility tests in clinical practice, state that the great majority of over 300 patients subjected to testing with the Stanford Hypnotic Susceptibility Scales forms A and B found it to be a positive experience and that therapy was not generally adversely affected by failure on some items in spite of the initial apprehension on the part of the therapists (Frankel et al., 1979).

In hypnotic research, on the other hand, it is often necessary to have some a priori estimate of subject hypnotizability so that experimental and control groups may be balanced in this regard. In some experiments, a second control group made up of low-susceptibility subjects may be desirable to guard against inadvertent hypnosis produced by the instructions. Also, if the experimenter desires to study a particular phenomenon, such as age regression, he or she might not only want to select subjects high in susceptibility in general but also subjects who are capable of producing this specific phenomenon.

A hypnotic susceptibility scale is a psychological test and, like any other good psychological test, requires the following characteristics:

1. Reliability or consistency in measurement.
2. Validity or assurance that it is measuring what it purports to measure.
3. Ease in administration and scoring.

Although the third requirement is self-evident, a few remarks concerning the first two are in order for the reader trained in some discipline other than psychology.

Reliability is customarily expressed as either the correlation between the two sets of scores obtained by giving the same test twice over a period of time to the same subjects (stability method) or the correlation between the two sets of scores obtained by the concurrent administration of two equivalent forms of the same test to the same subjects (equivalence method). If only one form of the test is available, the equivalence method can be achieved by dividing the test into two halves and treating each half as an equivalent test (*split-half method*). In any of these methods, the correlation coefficient obtained is called a *reliability coefficient* (r). A good psychological test should have a reliability coefficient of 0.8 or above.

Reliability demonstrates that a test is measuring something and therefore may be valid. If an instrument is unreliable, it is measuring nothing and thus cannot measure what it purports to, or be valid. If reliability has been established, validity may be demonstrated in a variety of ways.

Scores on the instrument being tested may be correlated with scores obtained by the same subjects on a criterion measure of established validity. This method is called *concurrent validity* if the criterion measure is made at the same time as the test score is obtained and *predictive validity* if the criterion does not become available until some time in the future. The logic behind this method is that if the two sets of scores are highly correlated, then they are essentially measuring the same thing, and if the criterion is valid, then the test must also be. An example of concurrent validity would be to validate a new test of susceptibility against an older established one. An example of predictive validity would be to validate a scholastic aptitude test, to be used as a college admission screening device, against grade-point averages obtained four years later.

Another way of validating a test is called *construct validity*. Here an instrument is said to be valid because it is based on a hypothetical construct. For example, a scale of susceptibility may be said to be valid because it is based on the concept that greater hypnotic ability is reflected in the performance of more difficult or lower probability tasks.

The more common specific tests of hypnotic susceptibility will now be described. Some of these tests, like the Stanford Hypnotic Susceptibility Scale, are individual tests, and some, like the Harvard Group Scale of Hypnotic Susceptibility, are group tests suitable for the rapid screening for groups of potential subjects.Some of these measures are sensitive enough for research applications, while others, like the Hypnotic Induction Profile, yield a cruder estimate, which is usually adequate for clinical work.

TESTS OF HYPNOTIC SUSCEPTIBILITY

Stanford Hypnotic Susceptibility Scale (SHSS)

The Stanford Hypnotic Susceptibility Scale (SHSS) was developed by Weitzenhoffer and Hilgard primarily for use in hypnotic research, but the manual contains slight modifications in the initial procedures for the establishment of rapport with the subject, rendering the instrument suitable for clinical use as well. While intended for use on subjects with no prior hypnotic experience, the test has two equivalent forms, A and B, which make it possible to take before and after measurements in research designed to assess the effects of procedures intended to alter hypnotic susceptibility. The test-retest reliability coefficient between equivalent forms A and B averages 0.83. The test is an individual one that takes approximately 45 minutes to administer: 5 minutes for an introductory interview and the establishment of rapport, 30 minutes for a standard induction procedure and testing, and 10 minutes for a final inquiry phase. Standardized scoring forms are provided, with scoring criteria given for a plus or minus score on all 12 items. Thus, test scores can range from 0 to 12. In addition to a numerical score, the scale provides a profile of the kinds of phenomena that the subject is or is not capable of producing. The following items are tested on this instrument:

1. Postural sway (falling backward).
2. Eye closure (during induction).
3. Hand lowering (on suggestion of heaviness).
4. Arm immobilization (inability to lift arm when heaviness is suggested).
5. Finger lock (inability to separate hands with fingers intertwined).
6. Arm rigidity (inability to bend arm).
7. Hands moving together (or apart—form B).
8. Verbal inhibition (inability to speak one's name [or name of town—form B]).

9. Visual hallucination (fly [or mosquito—form b]).
10. Eye catalepsy (inability to open eyes when challenged).
11. Posthypnotic suggestion accepted (changes chairs [or stands up—form B]).
12. Amnesia (recalls three or fewer items of the test during the posthypnotic inquiry phase).

The test is administered in such a manner that the subject is given a minimum sense of failure when he does not produce an effect being tested (in an effort to avoid having a failure on one item influence the results of future items). Hence, when a subject fails an item, the tester points up partial success and tries to get the subject to suppose he is performing according to expectations. Forms A and B were standardized on a sample of 124 Stanford University students (64 men and 60 women).

As a result of experience with forms A and B, the authors developed form C of the test, which arranges the items tested in order of increasing difficulty (on a statistical basis) and includes new items of greater difficulty. Since form C still consists of 12 items, some items, such as postural sway, verbal inhibition, posthypnotic suggestion, and finger lock, were eliminated, and eye closure is noted but not scored. All of the items except amnesia are arranged in order of difficulty in an attempt to produce a Guttman-like scale (where the passing of any item implies that all earlier items would be passed and the failing of any item implies that all later items will be failed). Since item difficulty is assessed from group data, it follows that for an individual subject, such predictions are not possible, and the scale is not a true Guttman scale. But in situations where testing time is limited, an abbreviated test might be given, subject to greater errors in prediction. The final item tested, amnesia, must of necessity be at the end of the test and hence is out of sequence. The following items are scored on form C of the SHSS:

1. Hand lowering.
2. Moving hands apart.
3. Mosquito hallucination.
4. Taste hallucination (sweet and sour).
5. Arm rigidity.
6. Dream induction.
7. Age regression (to fifth grade in school).
8. Arm immobilization.
9. Anosmia to ammonia.
10. Hallucinated voice (which asks the subject questions over a "loudspeaker").
11. Negative visual hallucination (failure to see one of three colored boxes on a table).
12. Posthypnotic amnesia.

Unlike forms A and B, form C requires some apparatus beyond a stop-watch to administer it: a pad and pencil for the age-regression task, three colored boxes for the negative visual hallucination, and a bottle of household ammonia. This form of the SHSS was standardized on a sample of 101 male and 102 female Stanford undergraduates. Its split-half reliability coefficient is 0.85, and it correlates 0.85 with form A.

Weitzenhoffer (1980*b*), the senior author of the SHSS, has recently crit-icized these scales for their emphasis on objective behavior and hence their failure to tap what he calls the "classic suggestion effect," which he conceives as involving both a response to a suggestion and the subject's experiencing the response as nonvolitional. He also questioned the appropriateness of in-cluding several easy items and suggested that susceptibility should be mea-sured by the difference between pretrance and post-induction responsiveness to suggestions.

Weitzenhoffer's view is similar to Spanos's position that hypnosis is a so-cially supported strategic enactment having the central demand characteristic that the subject view his or her actions as involuntary "happenings" rather that self-initiated behaviors (Spanos, 1982; Spanos and Gorassini, 1984). Wagstaff (1977*a*) notes that the incorporation of goal-directed fantasies into hypnotic suggestions increases the probability that subjects will experience their responses as nonvolitional.

Several researchers have investigated Weitzenhoffer's criticisms and, while recognizing their validity in part, have concluded that in spite of imperfect items, on balance, scores on the SHSS correlate well with indexes of invol-untary or nonvolitional responding (P. Bowers, 1982; K. Bowers, 1981*a*, 1981*b*; Farthing, Brown, and Venturino, 1983; Hilgard, 1981*a*). (For further discussion of experienced involuntariness of responses to hypnotic sugges-tions, see Spanos, Rivers, and Ross, 1977.)

Hilgard, Crawford, Bowers, and Kihlstrom (1979) describe a modification of the SHSS form C to enable its use to determine a specific hypnotic ability, as well as a general susceptibility score. This modification produces what they call a "tailored SHSS:C," which is less time-consuming than using the SPSHS for this purpose.

Stanford Profile Scales of Hypnotic Susceptibility (SPSHS)

The Stanford Profile Scales of Hypnotic Susceptibility (SPSHS) have two forms, I and II, and were designed to supplement forms A, B, and C of the SHSS. These scales were designed more to provide a profile of different hypnotic abilities than a mere susceptibility score; thus, although the two forms are equivalent, the authors recommend giving both scales to provide a full diagnosis of specific hypnotic abilities. There are nine items on each form, and each may receive a score ranging from 0 to 3; hence total scores range from 0 to 27.

Form I uses a standard method of induction involving arm levitation and scores the following phenomena:

1. Hand analgesia.
2. Hallucination of music.
3. Anosmia to ammonia.
4. Recall of a meal of a week or two ago.
5. Hallucination of a light.
6. Dream about an unspecified subject.
7. Agnosia for *house*.
8. Impairment of arithmetic ability.
9. A posthypnotic verbal compulsion.

Form II uses a standardized hypnotic procedure based on suggested arm heaviness and lowering. It scores the following phenomena:

1. Heat hallucination.
2. Selective deafness.
3. Hallucination of ammonia.
4. Regression to tenth birthday.
5. Negative hallucination of missing watch hand.
6. A dream about hypnosis.
7. Agnosia for *scissors*.
8. Personality alteration.
9. Posthypnotic automatic writing.

Both of these tests require standardized apparatus and test stimuli to administer. The standardization sample comprised 70 males and 85 females.

Harvard Group Scale of Hypnotic Susceptibility (HGSHS)

The Harvard Group Scale of Hypnotic Susceptibility (HGSHS) is an adaptation of the SHSS by Ronald Shor and Emily Orne to permit the administration of the test to groups as opposed to individuals. It provides for self-report scoring by the subjects and enables a researcher to screen large numbers of potential hypnotic subjects rapidly. Induction and testing time for a group of any size is approximately 50 minutes, and the items are essentially those of the SHSS. A maximum total score of 12 is possible.

Norms for a variety of national populations (e.g., German, Canadian, and

Australian) for this test have been published (Bongartz, 1985; Laurence and Perry, 1982; Sheehan and McConkey, 1979).

McConkey, Sheehan, and Law (1980) have factor analyzed the structure of this instrument and found that the challenge and ideomotor factors are the most stable, while the cognitive factor was noticeably less stable across samples.

R. J. Miller (1980) has demonstrated that scores on the HGSHS relate to some degree with measures of nonhypnotic suggestibility on the Suggested Syllables Test.

Kihlstrom and Register (1984) advocate that the scoring of the amnesia item on this test take into consideration not just the number of items recalled under a suggestion of posthypnotic amnesia but also how much recovery of memory occurs after a release signal is given. Although their argument is theoretically sound (see chapter 4), the HGSHS does not take into account the restoration of memory after a release signal because it was designed to be compatible with the SHSS (E. Orne, personal communication).

Children's Hypnotic Susceptibility Scale (CHSS)

The Children's Hypnotic Susceptibility Scale (CHSS) was designed by Perry London to measure hypnotic susceptibility in children. It has two forms: one for children from 5 years through 12 years, 11 months of age, and the other for children from 13 years to 16 years, 11 months. The items on both forms are the same; the major difference is the age appropriateness of the instructions and procedures. Test items comprise the following:

Part I
1. Postural sway.
2. Eye closure.
3. Hand lowering.
4. Arm immobilization.
5. Finger lock.
6. Arm rigidity.
7. Hands moving together.
8. Verbal inhibition.
9. Auditory hallucination (fly buzzing).
10. Eye catalepsy.
11. Posthypnotic suggestion.
12. Amnesia.
Part II
13. Reinduction by posthypnotic signal.
14. Visual and auditory television hallucination.

15. Cold hallucination.
16. Anesthesia.
17. Taste hallucination.
18. Smell hallucination.
19. Visual hallucination.
20. Age regression.
21. Dream induction.
22. Awakening and posthypnotic suggestion.

Each item is scored from 0 to 3, or, if the tester prefers, the items may be scored on a dichotomous scale. Scoring criteria for the 4-point scale are given on the scoring forms that come with the test. The major value of this instrument over the ones previously described is that the instructions and procedures are designed for use with either children or adolescents.

Hypnotic Induction Profile (HIP)

The Hypnotic Induction Profile (HIP) was developed by Herbert Spiegel for clinical use. Like any clinical instrument, it is designed to be individually administered. The main advantage claimed for it is its speed of administration. It expresses hypnotic susceptibility on a 5-point scale and requires only about 5 minutes to administer. Like all of the foregoing instruments, this one is based on the induction of a hypnotic state, but the induction procedure never uses the word *hypnosis, trance,* or *sleep,* and in this sense it is an indirect procedure that might be useful with a patient fearful of being hypnotized.

Scoring criteria are based on the amount of eye roll produced in a subject requested to roll his eyes upward and then slowly close his lids, arm levitation, posthypnotic response, amnesia, and subjective reports. Although the test manual does not give either reliability or validity data, or clear scoring instructions, this information is published elsewhere by Spiegel (1977). Test-retest reliability is 0.76, and Hilgard (1975) reported that this instrument correlates positively with other standard measures of susceptibility. Most researchers have found that the eye roll test is not significantly correlated with SHSS scores or the rest of the HIP items, and it is now possible to measure an "induction" score on the HIP ignoring this subtest. This score correlates about 0.34 with the SHSS forms A and C, which Orne et al. (1979) characterize as moderate, although the present author would characterize a test that accounts for only 12% of the variance of another test as having a low relationship with the latter. Hilgard finds this relationship nonsignificant "by ordinary standards" (Frischholz et al., 1980, 1981; Hilgard, 1978–1979, 1981b, 1981c; Sheehan et al., 1979; H. Spiegel, 1977; Stern, Spiegel, and

Nee, 1978-1979). While the reliability coefficient reported by Spiegel seems too low to make this instrument a measure of choice in experimental work, it may be adequate for clinical work (for which it was designed) and for situations where a quick estimate of susceptibility is more important than obtaining an accurate or the most sensitive measure possible.

Stanford Hypnotic Arm Levitation Induction and Test (SHALIT)

Like the HIP, the SHALIT is a brief test designed for clinical usage. It scores the amount of arm levitation during a standard induction procedure. It has a stability reliability coefficient of 0.88, and it correlates 0.63 with a 10-item abbreviation of the SHSS form A. Thus, it is probably a useful scale for clinical work although not sensitive enough for experimental usage because it is limited to a single factor measurement (an ideomotor task) (Hilgard, Crawford, and Wert, 1979).

Stanford Hypnotic Clinical Scales for Adults (SHCSA) and Children (SHCSC)

This instrument is also a shortened test for clinical use but one that is longer and more varied that the SHALIT. It consists of five scales (hand moving, hypnotic dreaming, age regression, a posthypnotic suggestion, and posthypnotic amnesia), four of which are common to the SHSS form C. It provides a more varied measure of hypnotic abilities than just the ideomotor factor of the SHALIT, and Hilgard and Hilgard conclude that this test performs better than such a single-item scale (Hilgard and Hilgard, 1979; Morgan and Hilgard, 1978-1979b). A similar clinical version is available for children. There are two forms of the children's test: one for children from ages 5 to 12 and one for children from ages 13 to 16 (Cooper and London, 1978-1979; Morgan and Hilgard, 1978-1979b). These tests correlate 0.72 and 0.67 with the SHSS forms C and A respectively (Morgan and Hilgard, 1978-1979).

Barber Suggestibility Scale (BSS)

Unlike any of the foregoing instruments, the Barber Suggestibility Scale (BSS) does not depend on the induction of a hypnotic state under standardized conditions. It does not purport to be a test of hypnotic susceptibility but of *suggestibility,* the ability of a subject to produce hypnotic-like behavior whether or not previously subjected to a hypnotic induction procedure. In order to understand the need for this scale and why it was developed, it is necessary to describe Barber's theoretical orientation toward hypnosis.

Barber believes that the concept of a hypnotic state is not useful in the study of hypnotic phenomena. He advocates (as did Hull before him) that psychologists should study what precedent conditions (independent variables) are necessary and sufficient to produce responses (dependent variables), such as catalepsy, analgesia, hallucinations, and so on, that are normally labeled hypnotic behavior. For example, he notes that in most hypnotic induction procedures, at least four specific kinds of independent variables are confounded under the label *hypnotic induction:*

1. The situation is defined to the subject as hypnosis.
2. Suggestions of drowsiness, eye closure, and sleep are made.
3. The subject is told that it will be *easy* to respond to suggestions.
4. The subject is motivated to make the suggested responses.

Barber has investigated the effect of each of these factors individually in producing the kinds of behavior commonly labeled as hypnotic. Barber calls instructions including items 3 and 4 only *task motivational;* he finds that by themselves they are just as effective as hypnotic induction in eliciting hypnotic-like behavior on the BSS. Because of his theoretical and methodological orientation, Barber and his students like to put quotes around the terms *hypnosis* and *hypnotic,* leading some of his critics to conclude, unjustifiably, that his position denies the existence of hypnotic phenomena. This criticism is inaccurate; his position is not that the phenomena are not real but that the hypnotic state is not a useful explanatory concept to account for them.

Since Barber's theory holds that hypnotic phenomena are produced by some antecedent events that should be isolated, it follows that a test of hypnotic-like behavior—one that does not depend on the prior induction of a hypnotic state—is needed to test these factors. Hence, the BSS can be used to elicit hypnotic-like responses either with or without a prior induction procedure.

As a result of his research, Barber reports that in addition to task-motivational instructions, the tone of the operator's voice and the subject's attitudes and motives (due to pretest instructions and what the subject is told regarding the purpose of the study) affect results on the test. Variables that do not seem to affect suggestibility measures are whether the subject's eyes are open or closed, whether instructions are given personally or by tape recording, and the personality of the subject as measured by most standardized test instruments.

The types of items on the BSS are similar to those given on standardized tests of susceptibility; the main difference is that the instructions make no mention of hypnosis. Items tested include the following:

1. Arm lowering.
2. Arm levitation.
3. Hand lock.
4. Hallucination of thirst.
5. Verbal inhibition.
6. Body immobility.
7. "Posthypnotic-like" response.
8. Selective amnesia.

Following the test and the objective scoring, the subject is asked if he really felt the effect suggested or just went along to please the examiner. The subject is given a subjective score of 1 for each item that he says he really experienced. Thus, subjects get both objective and subjective scores on this scale, each having a maximum value of 8 (Barber and Wilson, 1978-1979).

Creative Imagination Scale (CIS)

Wilson, a student of Barber, developed in her doctoral dissertation the Creative Imagination Scale, which was designed to make suggestions calling for the usual hypnotic responses in a permissive as opposed to an authoritarian manner. Since the scale is labeled as a test of creative imagination, it is especially suitable for research in schools where the word *hypnosis* would be an effective obstacle to obtaining permission to do research. This test correlates about 0.6 with the BSS. Its split-half reliability coefficient is 0.89 (Hilgard, Sheehan, Morteiro, and MacDonald, 1981; McConkey and Sheehan, 1982a; Wilson and Barber, 1978).

Myers (1983b) published norms for this test based on a sample of 1302 children aged 8 to 17. McConkey, Sheehan, and White (1979) found that the CIS correlated 0.28 with the HGSHS form A, but that the former measures primarily imagery and imagination rather than the other factors involved in hypnotic susceptibility.

FACTORS RELATED TO HYPNOTIC SUSCEPTIBILITY

Implicit in the idea of measuring hypnotic susceptibility is the notion that it is a stable personality characteristic as opposed to a situational variable. If susceptibility is, in fact, a stable characteristic of a person, questions arise about what factors cause some people to develop a markedly greater capacity for hypnosis than others and how readily this capacity can be modified. Does repeated experience with hypnosis improve a subject's ability to achieve a deeper state, in the sense of being able to do things under hypnosis that he formerly was incapable of achieving?

These questions are not easy to answer because of the confounding of susceptibility with other variables. For example, in order to be hypnotized a subject not only has to have the trance capacity, but must also want to be hypnotized and must actively cooperate in the process. It is conceivable that a person with a lot of ability as a hypnotic subject may be afraid of being hypnotized, react negatively to the hypnotist, or be suffering from some physical or mental distraction at the time of an original attempt at hypnosis. The subject will thus appear to be a poor subject. If after repeated hypnotic sessions these fears abate, the subject's rapport with the hypnotist improves, or his motivation to be hypnotized increases, he may achieve a much deeper trance. This result may give the illusion that practice has improved the subject's basic trance capacity when in fact it has not. It is clear that the best subject cannot be hypnotized unless he wants to be. Thus, tests of hypnotic susceptibility are valid only when the tester is certain that the subject is well motivated and doing his best.

This is true on any ability or aptitude test such as an IQ or even a scholastic aptitude test; however, in the latter situation at least, motivation may safely be assumed from the circumstances of taking the test. In an IQ test this is not always true, and for a test of susceptibility to hypnosis the issue is even less certain. To avoid semantic confusion the term *hypnotic susceptibility* or *trance capacity* will be used when referring to the stable or long-term ability of a subject to be hypnotized, and the term *hypnotizability* will denote the net effect of susceptibility plus any operative situational factors affecting the hypnotic ability of a subject at a given time. Unfortunately, this distinction is not generally made in the literature, and usually the terms *susceptibility* and *hypnotizability* are used interchangeably, resulting in a great deal of confusion in research dealing with the issue of whether susceptibility is modifiable. Most studies yield a negative answer to this question, and when positive results are obtained, it may be that transient situational factors rather than underlying susceptibility are being affected (Crouse and Kurtz, 1984; Diamond, 1977*a*, 1977*b*; Reilley, Parisher, Carona, and Dobrovolsky, 1980; Wickramasekera, 1977). Saavedra and Miller (1983) found that susceptibility could be reduced but not increased by manipulating subjects' expectations, strongly suggesting that situational factors rather than underlying trance capacity is what was being affected.

On the other hand, Goldfarb and O'Brien (1985), in an investigation designed to test Salter's theory that hypnosis is a classical conditioning phenomenon, report significant and substantial increases in susceptibility scores, (attained by subjects initially scoring low on the SHSS:A) as a result of being exposed to words such as *sleep* or *heavy* used as conditioned stimuli and paired with nitrous oxide (used as an unconditioned stimulus) in a classical conditioning paradigm. Posttreatment susceptibility was measured on the SHSS:B. Control groups with subjects exposed to the stimulus words alone, nitrous oxide and neutral words, or neither were used to control for the effect of the words or chemical alone, practice effects, or the passage of time. Whether these results are viewed as reflecting an increase in hypnotic susceptibility as reported or as an increase in hypnotizability due to the improved efficacy of the particular induction procedure used due to a conditioning effect, they are supportive of the theoretical position that classical conditioning may play a role in hypnotic induction subsequent to an initial induction. They do not establish that hypnosis is exclusively a matter of conditioning, for it is obvious that in order for classical conditioning to occur there must be some unconditioned stimulus originally capable of producing hypnosis and its associated behaviors prior to conditioning.

Relaxation training prior to hypnosis, with or without electromyographic biofeedback, failed to enhance susceptibility scores (Radtke et al., 1983).

The author once treated a couple who were trying to stop smoking through hypnosis. The husband was highly motivated to be hypnotized because a close friend of his own age had recently died of lung cancer. But he was a poor hypnotic subject until it was discovered that he felt hypnosis involved giving over control of the situation to the therapist, which he was unwilling to do. He was then able to achieve a deeper state with a more permissive technique and, ultimately, self-hypnosis. The wife, on the other hand, was an excellent subject until the third visit, when she suddenly realized during induction that she did not want to stop smoking but was pressured by her husband into coming for treatment. From the moment she developed this insight into her real feelings about smoking, she would not permit herself to be hypnotized. A therapist seeing her for the first time would have rated this excellent subject as having little, if any, susceptibility. This case illustrates the need to evaluate carefully a subject's motivation to cooperate before relying on the results of any test of susceptibility. It is only when subjects can be demonstrated to be equally motivated and cooperative that differences in susceptibility scores obtained before and after some procedure can be taken to reflect a change in basic hypnotic ability.

It is a common experience that subjects exposed to repeated hypnotic sessions tend to enter the trance state more rapidly on successive sessions and often appear to develop greater depth. It is for this reason a good idea not to give up therapeutic efforts on what may seem like a poor subject without at least a few trials. (Fortunately many therapeutic applications do not require a very deep trance anyway.)

Reyher (1968) cites Moll (1958) who frequently achieved success in trance induction only after 40 attempts and Vogt who in 1896 hypnotized one subject after 700 failures!

As, Hilgard, and Weitzenhoffer (1963) found that in spite of the common clinical impression to the contrary, repeated inductions and other deepening techniques did not result in increased susceptibility scores. This represents a common situation in which the results of controlled experimentation are often in conflict with clinical findings. This does not necessarily mean that the clinical findings are inaccurate. It may simply mean that the more precise experimental procedures are so well controlled that they represent an artificial situation quite different from the more complicated situation in clinical practice. For example, it may be that repeated inductions per se do not increase hypnotic susceptibility, but when done in the context of a therapeutic setting, the degree of rapport or transference with the hypnotist does change, and it is this latter factor that enables the subject to attain a deeper trance. How much of the improvement in hypnotic performance, if any, is due to increased susceptibility and how much is due to reduction of anxiety, learning to be a subject, and other situational variables is difficult to determine, however.

Havens (1977) reports a study where scores on the Harvard Group Scale of Hypnotic Susceptibility (HGSHS) were modified in the predicted direction by subjects observing a model punished or rewarded for hypnotic behavior and also by their being exposed to positive or negative information about hypnosis. It seems probable that both of these independent variables affected the subjects' motivation and attitudes toward hypnosis rather than their basic hypnotic susceptibility.

If there is indeed a long-term, stable personality attribute over and above transient motivational and attitudinal factors that we can call hypnotic susceptibility (as would seem likely from the long-term stability of susceptibility scale scores), it would appear that one way to identify it might be by seeing if it correlates highly with such other demographic factors as age, sex, IQ, education, college major, occupation, nationality, race, religion, and childhood experiences. We will now consider each of these factors in turn.

Age

In general, very young children are poor subjects, probably because, as Hull (1968) points out, they lack the requisite language skills to be influenced by predominantly verbal induction procedures. Sternlicht and Wanderer (1963) report that a minimum mental age of 5 or 6 is required to be a good subject.

Children of age 7 and above tend to be good subjects, and their susceptibility appears to increase to a maximum by puberty (9-14 years) (London, 1965). By age 15 susceptibility begins to decrease to the adult level. It then decreases slowly throughout life, and there are fewer good subjects among the elderly than in the young adult population.

The period from ages 14 to 21 represents the best period of adult life for both speed of induction and depth of trance (the two are not necessarily correlated) and is the age of the subjects in most hypnotic studies, which, like psychological studies in general, tend to use college populations because of their ready availability.

Hull (1968) cites a study by Liébeault involving 23 subjects under age 7 and 65 subjects between 7 and 14 years of age. He had a 100% success rate in inducing hypnosis in these subjects as compared with a 10% failure rate with subjects over 14.

Barber and Calverley (1963c), measuring "hypnotic-like" suggestibility on the Barber Suggestibility Scale without trance induction, found children between 6 and 12 years of age were more suggestible than adults (children 8 to 10 were the most suggestible). There were no differences in suggestibility between age groups within the 14- to 22-year-old range.

Sex

There is a stereotype that women are better hypnotic subjects than men. This belief may have resulted from women's traditionally more passive social roles combined with the notion of the hypnotic situation as one in which a dominant hypnotist controls a passive subject. The research in general does not support this belief.

Hull found that women were more susceptible than men but only to a very small degree, and Kihlstrom and his associates (1980) reported similar results. Hilgard (1968) reports that the sex of neither the subject nor the therapist is critical. He cites a study by Weitzenhoffer and Weitzenhoffer (1958) of 160 men and women in which half of each group were hypnotized by a male hypnotist and half by a female hypnotist. Neither the sex of the subject nor of the hypnotist produced significant differences in susceptibility.

IQ

There appears to be a slight positive correlation between IQ and hypnotizability. A certain minimal amount of intelligence is required for a subject to be able to concentrate properly and follow instructions. For this reason mental defectives are difficult or impossible to hypnotize, in proportion to the amount of deficit. It is doubtful that any IQ can be specified below which hypnosis is impossible, as some writers have attempted, since IQ is measured by a composite of different abilities. Two individuals with the identical IQ can have very different patterns of specific abilities.

Education

To the extent that education and IQ are correlated, an increase in susceptibility with an increase in education would be expected. Since therapists have more in common with highly educated subjects, it may also be expected that the increase in subject-hypnotist rapport will result in a higher level of hypnotizability. Probably more important in affecting susceptibility than the amount of education is the kind of education. Thus, the nature of the educational experience must be considered.

College Major

There are small but consistent differences found between liberal arts majors (English, humanities, social sciences, and so on) and business, engineering, or science majors, with the former making better subjects than the latter. The question is whether these differences are caused by the nature of the material studied or if the nature of the material studied is influenced by preexisting personality factors that also influence susceptibility. This question could be answered by studying subjects who plan to enter these various fields before they begin college, but it is quite probable that both types of factors are at work. Although a certain type of personality tends to pursue an engineering career, the discipline itself (like any other study) affects the individual's personality. Closely related to college major is choice of occupation.

Occupation

Arons (1961) claims that people in monotonous occupations such as assembly-line workers, and people used to instantaneous obedience, like soldiers, tend to be good subjects. The same is said to be true for artists and other imaginative people, while scientists, engineers, and people used to analytic thinking tend to be poor subjects.

Athletes also are reputed to be poor subjects. As in the case of academic major, these differences may be due to underlying personality factors that lead people into different occupations rather than the effects of occupational differences. Often the evidence for intergroup differences in susceptibility is based on clinical impressions rather than experimental findings.

Nationality, Race, and Religion

Certain nationalities have stereotypes associated with them. For example, Italians or Spaniards are said to be emotional, and the English are said to be more reserved. If these stereotypes were valid characterizations, they would suggest differences in hypnotic susceptibility between groups. It seems unlikely, however, that such national stereotypes are accurate and that there is not a great deal of intragroup variability with respect to the characteristics included in these stereotypes. Nevertheless, Arons claims, without citing evidence, that the French, Spanish, and Italians make excellent subjects, while the Germans, English, and Americans are much more variable, ranging from excellent to poor. He also reports that people from torrid climates tend to make good subjects, presumably because they are more experienced in relaxation. It is not unlikely that his impressions about the susceptibility of subjects of various nationalities, while based on substantial personal experience, may have been influenced by selective perception and preconceptions.

Based on cultural differences with respect to the prevalence of various types of meditative experiences, one might theoretically expect that there would be a higher percentage of good subjects among Asians or Indians than among Western Europeans, but this is only a theoretical expectation that needs to be tested.

Balaschak and her colleagues (1972) found no significant difference in hypnotic susceptibility for white subjects when hypnotized by a white or black hypnotist. Hong, Skiba, Yepes, and O'Brien (1982) found similar results using Anglo and Chinese and Anglo and Hispanic subjects and hypnotists. No permutation of ethnicity of hypnotist and subject increased susceptibility.

With respect to religion, it would be expected that people who are capable of suspending critical judgment and accepting religious beliefs wholeheartedly should be able to use this ability to be a good subject. Probably the individual commitment of the subject rather than his or her denomination is the more important factor; that is, a born-again Christian or a person with mystical experiences would be more likely to be a good subject than Sunday churchgoers, unless, of course, their particular religious beliefs oppose permitting themselves to be subjects (Hilgard, 1965a).

Childhood Experience

Query (1981) reports finding no relationship between family size or birth order and susceptibility. Nash, Lynn, and Givens (1984) found that 16 adults who reported being physically abused prior to age 10 had higher susceptibility scores than a control group of 300 nonabused adults. Their scores were bi-

modally distributed, with 80% having high and 20% having low susceptibility.

Personality

The term *personality* is one of the broadest in psychology. As used here,
it includes every factor within an individual that affects behavior. Hypnotic
susceptibility is therefore an aspect of a personality. What will be considered
now is what, if any, other factors of a personality are correlated with hypnotic
susceptibility.

Spiegel (1977) describes three personality types with respect to cognitive
styles. The Apollonian type, named for Apollo, the Greek god of reason, is
concerned with critical thinking and ratiocination as opposed to affective activity and is oriented toward future goals. The Dionysian type is more emotional than analytical and lives more in the present. The Odyssean personality
lies between these two extremes. Spiegel believes, on clinical grounds, that
the Appollonians (engineers, scientists, and accountants) make poor hypnotic subjects, while the Dionysians make excellent subjects. The Odysseans
are average subjects.

Hilgard believes that the ability to suspend critical judgment and reality
testing is crucial to a good hypnotic subject. This belief is not very different
in essence from Spiegel's view. Thus, a person who gets totally absorbed in
a book or movie or who identifies with the hero and hates the villain is likely
to be a good subject. It is a common finding that a positive relationship exists
between the ability to become absorbed in a task or fantasy on the one hand
and susceptibility on the other (Baum and Lynn, 1981; Davis, Dawson, and
Seay, 1978; Fellows and Armstrong, 1977; Finke and MacDonald, 1978;
Myers, 1983a; O'Grady, 1980; Yanchar and Johnson, 1981.

Barber and Calverley (1965c), however, found no significant correlation
between verbal reports of fantasy or imaginative experiences and hypnotic
susceptibility in spite of intuitive expectations to the contrary.

Although the terms *imagery* and *fantasy* are often used interchangeably,
the former refers to the concrete aspects of something that can be imagined
as if it were a perception, while the latter refers to a make-believe involvement
that is not primarily sensory (Fromm and Shor, 1979; Lamb, 1982). J. R.
Hilgard (1979) discusses the relationship between imaginative capacity and
susceptibility in her book on personality and hypnosis, and Sheehan (1982)
has reviewed the recent literature on hypnosis and imagery. He concludes
that the relationship between the capacity to engage in imagery and hypnotic
susceptibility is a nonlinear one and that the absence of imagery ability is a
better predictor of poor susceptibility than its presence is in predicting high
susceptibility. In spite of the widespread clinical belief that hypnosis enhances

vividness of imagery, Coe, St. Jean, and Burger (1980) found only equivocal evidence for this belief. In some situations, it did (when hypnosis was expected and followed waking tests of imagery), and in others, it did not (when hypnosis preceded waking tests or was unexpected). This suggests a practice effect may have been operating. Even when hypnosis was effective in increasing the vividness of imagery, the effect was independent of susceptibility, which the authors interpreted as meaning it was not affected by depth of trance.

A lucid nocturnal dream is one in which the dreamer is aware that he or she is dreaming. Some people have the ability to control the content of a lucid dream, but this ability is unrelated to hypnotic susceptibility. On the other hand, the ability to awaken voluntarily from a dream is negatively correlated with susceptibility (O'Brien, 1976; unpublished study).

Hilgard and Bentler (1963) found a small but significant relationship ($r = 0.21$) between extraversion and susceptibility, but a variety of other investigators found no significant relationship between these factors (Barber, 1964a).

On intuitive grounds, self-centered, dependent, or impressionable persons would seem likely to be good subjects. With respect to common pathological conditions, they are best considered individually. There is some conflict in the literature concerning the hypnotizability of neurotics as a group, but the consensus seems to be that there is little, if any, difference between them and nonneurotics as hypnotic subjects.

There is much more conflict in the literature concerning the hypnotic ability of hysterics, probably because of the imprecise way in which most writers use the term. The term *hysteric* may be used to refer to a neurotic individual suffering from the condition variously known as conversion hysteria, the conversion reaction, or, more archaically, hysteria. This is a neurosis in which anxiety is converted into some physical symptom. Hysteria may also refer to a person having a hysterical personality type, which is very different from conversion hysteria. As a personality type, *hysterical* refers to an overly dramatic, seductive, vain woman.

Thus, good hypnotic subjects do not score higher on the (conversion) hysteria scale on the Minnesota Multiphasic Personality Inventory (MMPI), but hysterical personality types are described by many clinicians as good subjects. This may be an artifact, for the fact that the subject is a hysterical, seductive woman may affect the nature of the interaction between the subject and the hypnotist.

Regressed schizophrenics are usually regarded as poor subjects because they are difficult to contact and are unlikely to be able to concentrate properly. Obsessive-compulsive neurotics are often also poor subjects. Paranoids are generally the most difficult, if not impossible, subjects. They are not able to develop the proper relationship of confidence and trust with the therapist.

Scagnelli-Jobsis (1982, 1983) reviewed the experimental and clinical literature on the use of hypnosis with psychotic patients and concluded that many psychotics are capable of being hypnotized and that (despite fears often voiced about hypnosis precipitating further personality disintegration, withdrawal into fantasy or excessive dependency), it is a safe and often effective method of treatment when used by a therapist competent to work with such patients. Baker (1983a) goes even further and takes the position that it is well documented that psychotics are as hypnotizable as any other patient population. On the other hand, David Spiegel (1983), while conceding that some psychotics may be hypnotizable (particularly hysterical psychotics), finds that most schizophrenics have very little susceptibility. He claims that low scores on the HIP are more associated with psychopathology than low scores on the SHSS, possibly because the former instrument requires comprehension of more complex instructions.

Pettinati (1982) argues that the common clinical opinions that psychotics have reduced trance capacities and that all patients may benefit to some extent from hypnotic intervention may be incorrect. She advocates measuring susceptibility in psychotic patients prior to making decisions about the use of hypnosis with them. This appears to be a reasonable position, for the important issue in clinical work is not what percentage of a psychotic population is amenable to hypnosis (however important this may be theoretically) but whether this procedure is likely to be of value for a particular patient.

Frankel and Orne (1976) report that while normal people are better subjects than patient populations, patients with phobias, especially multiple ones, are relatively good subjects compared to patients seeking treatment to stop smoking. Kelly (1984), in a replication of this work, found 22 phobics to be more susceptible than 112 nonphobic patients on either the HIP or the SHSS. No individual phobic was low in susceptibility, but, as Kelly notes, he was not unaware of the subject's diagnosis at the time of susceptibility testing, and this may have biased the results.

PERSONALITY TESTS AS PREDICTORS
OF HYPNOTIC SUSCEPTIBILITY

There are two basic approaches used in measuring personality. The first, called a *projective technique,* involves presenting the testee with an ambiguous stimulus and requiring him or her to respond to it. Since the stimulus is ambiguous, any response to it must come from the testee and not the stimulus, and thus reflects something about his or her personality. The difficulty with this type of test is not in the theory but in figuring out how to interpret exactly what the testee's response reveals about his personality. Examples of this type of test are the Rorschach and the Thematic Apperception Test (TAT).

The second approach to measuring personality is a *personality inventory.*

The testee is required to agree or disagree with a series of statements about himself, which have been calibrated against a group of subjects in a particular diagnostic category. For example, on the MMPI, there are a series of statements with which people in different diagnostic categories tend to agree. Thus, the more statements that the testee agrees with that are commonly accepted by hypochondriacs, the more likely the testee is to be a hypochondriac. The number of agreements on this factor provides a direct index of this likelihood. In effect, a personality inventory attempts to convert personality, an essentially nominal scale, into an ordinal scale and provide a score in numbers by a process of counting responses.

Measures obtained by either approach are not highly correlated with measures of hypnotic susceptibility. Neither the Rorschach nor the TAT, two of the most popular projective techniques, predicts hypnotic susceptibility scores, except that responses to card 12-M on the TAT (the hypnotist) may provide some information about a potential subject's attitude toward hypnosis that is related to hypnotizability.

Hilgard (1968) reports a large number of personality inventories whose results are unrelated to hypnotic susceptibility. These nonpredictors include:

1. As Questionnaire (Barber and Calverley, 1965c).
2. Barber-Glass Questionnaire (Barber and Calverley, 1965a).
3. Cattell 16 Personality Factor Questionnaire.
4. Edwards Personal Preference Schedule (Barber and Calverley, 1964b).
5. Guilford-Zimmerman Temperament Survey.
6. Leary Interpersonal Check List (Barber and Calverley, 1964d).
7. Maudsley Personality Inventory (Barber and Calverley, 1965c).
8. Myers-Briggs Inventory.
9. Shor Questionnaire (Barber and Calverley, 1965c).

Some scales on the California Psychological Inventory (CPI) and some scales of the MMPI correlate to a degree with hypnotic susceptibility as measured by the SHSS.

For females, the CPI scales of dominance, self-acceptance, and communality correlate 0.23, 0.25, and 0.26, respectively, with form A of the SHSS. For males, there is a correlation of -0.19 and -0.20, respectively, with the scales measuring self-control and sense of well-being.

On the MMPI, there are significant correlations between the following scales and form C of the SHSS: lie scale ($r = -0.14$), K scale ($r = -0.12$), hypochondriasis scale ($r = 0.18$), mania scale ($r = 0.25$), and the sum of all "true" responses ($r = 0.22$).

The Motoric-Ideational Activity Preference Scale (MIAPS) shows a negative relationship between motoric interests and hypnotic susceptibility ranging from -0.02 to -0.34, which varies with the sex of the subject.

Three experience inventories—Shor's Personal Experience Questionnaire, the As Experience Inventory, and Lee's Hypnotic Characteristics Inventory—measure five areas of experience correlated with hypnotic susceptibility:

1. Ability to assume a role.
2. Conformity.
3. Trancelike experiences.
4. Impulsivity.
5. Ability to concentrate.

The correlation coefficients between these factors and susceptibility are in the area of 0.3. It should be noted that although the correlation between hypnotic susceptibility and some of these personality scales is of theoretical interest, in no case are these correlations sufficiently high to make the screening of hypnotic subjects by means of these personality tests practical. The highest correlation reported, 0.34, means that the personality scale involved accounts for only 11.6% of the variance in hypnotic susceptibility scores.

No relationship was found between the cognitive styles of field dependence versus field independence (as measured on the Embedded Figures Test and the Rod and Frame Test) and suggestibility (as measured on the BSS) (Bergerone, Cei, and Ruggieri, 1981).

In accordance with Sheldon's notion of a relationship between body type and personality, Edmonston (1977c) investigated the relationship between body type and susceptibility. He reports positive correlations in 87 male subjects between both endomorphy and ectomorphy and hypnotic capacity ($r = 0.21$ and 0.22, respectively) as measured by the HGSHS. Mesomorphy was found to be unrelated to susceptibility. No significant relationship was found between susceptibility and any component of physique in 48 female subjects.

Barber (1964a) found no relationship between "hypnotic-like" suggestibility in children from age 10 to 13 and general ratings of their personality by their teachers. He believes that the major personality characteristic of good subjects, or the "hypnotic attitude" as he calls it, is the ability to become intensely preoccupied with something. Typically if a good subject is asked what he is thinking during an induction procedure, he will either say "nothing" or describe what he was instructed to think about. In addition to this "hypnotic attitude," Barber believes that a subject needs an attitude of "basic trust," at least with regard to the particular hypnotist involved. That personality tests are poorly related to hypnotic susceptibility may be explained by the following considerations or any combination of them:

1. Present personality tests do not tap those factors important in determining susceptibility.
2. Hypnotic susceptibility may be due to a particular combination of personality factors.

3. Personality tests are not reliable or valid enough.
4. Hypnotizability is more dependent on transitory situational factors than an underlying stable personality characteristic of susceptibility.

LATERAL EYE MOVEMENTS

It has been reported that nonanalytic activities are primarily a function of the nondominant cerebral hemisphere, and hypnotic susceptibility and non-analytic attending are correlated. Spanos and Barber (1974) found a positive correlation between hypnotic susceptibility and vividness of imagination and imagery.

Spanos, Rivers, and Gottlieb (1978) reported a tendency of right-handed males to move their eyes to the left when answering questions requiring re-flection. This movement was taken as evidence of right hemisphere activity. Their research, however, failed to support the notion that left eye movements indicated a facility for nonanalytic modes of thought. While previous studies had found a positive correlation between left eye movements and hypnotic susceptibility on the SHSS form C, they failed to replicate such results with the SHSS form A in male subjects. DeWitt and Averill (1976), however, found substantial correlation between left eye movements and scores on the SHSS form A in right-handed females. Hence the relationship between lateral eye movements and hypnotic susceptibility seems to be a function of sex, the susceptibility scales used, and the type of questions asked.

Smith (1980) also suggests that the position of the questioner might play a role, though he was unable to demonstrate this. He found that under con-ditions of rest, high-susceptibility subjects made more initial eye movements to the right and spent less time looking centrally than did low-susceptibility subjects.

Taken as a whole, these results seem to indicate that so many factors are involved in lateral eye movements produced by questioning that they are unlikely to be useful as an informal estimate of hypnotic ability.

SITUATIONAL VARIABLES IN HYPNOTIZABILITY

Subject-Hypnotist Relationship

It is well documented that some people are good subjects with one hyp-notist and poor subjects with another (Barber, 1964a). The better the subject-hypnotist rapport, the higher the hypnotizability of the former. Barber sug-gests that one of the reasons for the apparent high reliability of hypnotic sus-ceptibility scale scores is the consistency of this subject-hypnotist relationship and motivation rather than the stability of an underlying trait of hypnotic susceptibility.

Fourie (1980) reports on a preliminary study relating 11 factors of subject-hypnotist interaction prior to hypnosis and subsequent measures of hypnotizability. The three factors significantly correlated with hypnotizability were direct aggression ($r = -0.70$), dependence ($r = 0.49$), and rated hypnotizability ($r = 0.48$).

Reyher, Wilson, and Hughes (1979) found that the type of interpersonal interaction between patient and therapist affected suggestibility, with a silent patient being more suggestible than one engaging in self-initiated speech.

McConkey and Sheehan (1976) found that while a collaborative as opposed to a contractual atmosphere between hypnotist and subject produced a more favorable attitude toward hypnosis, it did not affect hypnotic performance. Perry and Sheehan (1978), in following up their research, found that while high-susceptibility subjects were not affected differently by videotaped and personal induction procedures, medium-susceptibility subjects and simulators were.

Subject Motivation and Attitude

Hypnotizability is typically high if the subject is strongly motivated to be hypnotized and has a positive attitude toward hypnosis and low if the converse is true (Barber and Calverley, 1962, 1963b, 1963c). This effect can be seen when otherwise mediocre subjects are able to undergo surgical procedures under hypoanesthesia when their physical condition would not permit them to survive the use of a chemical agent. Rockey (1977) describes several such situations in which lung surgery was performed. The very powerful motivation to remain alive of an otherwise poor hypnotic subject enabled the patient to achieve a deep enough trance to have chest surgery performed with no anesthetic other than hypnosis. It is a common clinical experience that injury victims normally exhibiting low-susceptibility scores on standard tests are usually readily hypnotized for purposes of pain control.

Sensory Deprivation and Drugs

Reyher (1968) reported a modest increase in hypnotic susceptibility scale scores during sensory deprivation procedures. If induction procedures are delayed until symptoms of sensory deprivation begin to appear, however, the increase in hypnotizability becomes marked. Barabasz (1980b, 1982) found a significant increase in hypnotizability and EEG alpha activity from baseline measures following 10 months of arctic isolation.

In 1953, Weitzenhoffer asserted that no drugs have been shown to increase susceptibility. He later (1957) discussed the use of drugs in hypnotic induction.

Hull (1968) found that alcohol had a slight or negligible effect, but scopolamine (1/200 gram, injected in 3/4 cubic centimeters of water) had an effect on some subjects. An unsusceptible subject remained so, but a susceptible subject became markedly more so.

D. Spiegel (1980) reports that among 115 patients, no significant changes in HIP scores resulted from antipsychotic or antidepressant drugs or lithium. Antianxiety drugs produced higher-susceptibility scores, which he characterizes as "nearly significant." These data suggest that although these drugs are ineffective in increasing susceptibility, at least their usage does not interfere with hypnotherapy.

It was found by Kelly, Fisher, and Kelly (1978) that cannabis intoxication produced an increase in suggestibility similar to that produced by hypnosis. They speculate that the reason prior attempts to increase hypnotic susceptibility by the use of this drug failed was because subjects have a ceiling level of suggestibility, which once attained, either through the use of hypnosis or drugs, cannot be exceeded.

PREINDUCTION "TESTS" OF HYPNOTIZABILITY

In addition to formal scales of hypnotic susceptibility, informal "tests" of hypnotizability are commonly used immediately prior to hypnotic induction procedures. These "tests" generally consist of a series of waking suggestions designed to elicit the same types of behavior that are commonly elicited in the hypnotic state or in its induction. These are particularly useful if it is necessary to select good hypnotic subjects from a group of volunteers in giving demonstrations of hypnosis, but, except for this situation, these techniques have more important uses than the estimation of hypnotizability. (Volunteers tend to be better-than-average subjects. The decision to volunteer is indicative of a positive attitude and motivation toward being hypnotized [Brodsky and McNeil, 1984].)

The more important use of these prehypnosis tests is to give subjects a warm-up period and practice in the kind of concentration and uncritical thinking that they must engage in to bring about the hypnotic state. Often the operator will tell the subject "to make your mind a blank," which usually confuses the person. It is better to be more specific and tell the subject not to think critically or analytically and to try to experience the effects being suggested. In addition to providing practice in noncritical thinking, these tests provide an opportunity for the rapport between the subject and the operator to develop and for the subject to develop a "set" for following the latter's instructions.

Finally, these procedures enable the operator to select the best method of formal induction for the particular subject. For example, for a subject who displays a good response to arm levitation suggestions, this ideomotor response can be utilized for trance induction; if the subject displays a poor response, some other method of induction should be chosen.

An infinite number of ideomotor or cognitive responses to suggestions could be used for a quick estimate of hypnotizability, but only a few are commonly used. These are usually presented in a sequential order of increasing difficulty and are primarily ideomotor in nature because this makes it easier to evaluate the subject's reactions objectively. An ideomotor response refers to one obtained by a subject's imagining that some motor effect (like arm levitation or body sway) is occurring without consciously or intentionally producing this effect. Human nervous systems are "wired" is such a manner that people have the subjective impression that they are "inside" their limbs, and when they want to move them, they simply think about the movement (as opposed to controlling or even knowing which small muscle groups are being activated). It follows that even thinking about a bodily movement without intending the movement to occur produces some efferent nervous output to the area of the body in question. With concentration, this can be enough to produce gross movements that give the illusion of being autonomous.

Usually only two or three preinduction tests are given. If subjects are to be selected from a group of volunteers for demonstration purposes, the first one or two screening tests can be group procedures, and the final one may be individual.

The fact that the same type of responses that can be obtained under hypnosis can be obtained prior to formal hypnotic induction procedures, either to induce a trance state or to estimate hypnotizability, has theoretical implications. Theorists such as Barber, who do not believe that the concept of a trance state is useful, use this phenomenon to bolster their position. Theorists who think a trance state is a useful concept sometimes deal with the empirical facts by considering the question of when hypnosis is actually commenced. It has been argued that the phenomenon of waking suggestions results from the induction of a hypnotic state without a formal trance induction procedure. It is possible to get just about any type of behavior suggested on the part of a hypnotized subject, including having the person behave in a manner indistinguishable from that of a nonhypnotized person. This position is in consonance with the view of some "trance state" theorists that a subject carrying out a posthypnotic suggestion automatically reverts to a *minitrance* state. Although we will not pursue these arguments any further at this point, the author's opinion is that, whether the essence of the hypnotic experience is conceived of as the production of a trance state or some other condition precedent for responsiveness to suggestions, whatever happens to a subject begins to happen from the moment he enters the hypnotist's office (or before) and continues until he leaves. If the hypnotic session is properly managed these effects build on one another, and the subject becomes more suggestible as the experience continues. But it is neither possible nor especially desirable to be able to indicate an exact time when a subject goes from a normal or "waking" state into a hypnotic state.

We will now examine five of the most common prehypnotic tests of hypnotizability: the Chevreul pendulum, arm levitation and arm heaviness, hand clasping, hand attraction or repulsion, and postural sway and falling. The first and the last of these tests are individual ones; the others may be done with individuals or groups. Only the first requires any type of apparatus.

Chevreul Pendulum

A Chevreul pendulum consists of a small weight at the end of a piece of chain or string about a foot long. Commercial models are available using glass spheres as weights, but an effective pendulum can be improvised from a bunch of paper clips and a piece of string.

The subject holds one end of the string while concentrating on a suggested motion of the weight. Usually the motion suggested is either toward and away from the subject or from side to side. The suggested motion may also involve the weight's describing a circle in a clockwise or counterclockwise direction. The suggestibility of the subject is demonstrated by the ease with which the suggested motion is obtained and the facility with which the direction of movement can be changed by suggestion from clockwise to counterclockwise or from a to-and-fro motion to a side-to-side motion.

There are many variations of the basic method. The subject can have an elbow supported on a table, but if the pendulum is held in an unsupported outstretched arm, the natural instability of the arm will make the initiation of motion easier. If a target, consisting of a circle of about 10 inches in diameter with two mutually perpendicular diameters inscribed, is placed with the center an inch or two under the resting pendulum, it may make it easier for the subject to notice the small initial movements and facilitate the effect. It is fairly easy to obtain positive results from this test even in mediocre hypnotic subjects. Because this test requires some apparatus, is an individual test, and is relatively easy to pass, it is not particularly good for screening subjects, but it can make an interesting classroom demonstration.

Arm Levitation and Heaviness

This is a useful group screening device. Subjects are requested to extend both arms in front of them, parallel to the ground, and to close their eyes. Typically they are told to turn one hand palm up and imagine that a very heavy weight has been placed in it. It is best to make a concrete suggestion that can produce a sensory image—for example, that a heavy bowling ball has been placed in the subject's hand. Then suggestions are made that the arm is getting more and more tired, and it is harder and harder to hold up while at the same time the bowling ball is getting heavier. In addition to suggestions of heaviness of the hand holding the weight, subjects may also be told to imagine that a string attached to a helium balloon has been tied to the thumb of their other hand and is constantly pulling it up with an ever-increasing force. After a short period of time good subjects will have lowered the hand with the bowling ball and raised the hand attached to the helium balloon. Subjects can then be requested to open their eyes and notice where their hands are. This request will often serve to convince subjects of the efficacy of the operator's suggestions.

Although either of these suggestions may be made separately, there is an advantage to suggesting them at the same time. One reason is that the appearance of an arm-raising or a levitation effect is more convincing evidence of suggestibility and hypnotizability than an arm-lowering effect, for it is produced in opposition to the effects of gravity and fatigue, while the latter is augmented by these. On the other hand, since the arm-lowering effect is easier to obtain, it may be sufficient to produce a substantial enough difference between the subject's hands to give the person confidence in the operator and his own hypnotic ability. If the operator is contemplating the use of the arm leviation method of hypnotic induction, this test will show how likely this method is to succeed with the subject being tested.

One rare problem with this method of testing or induction is that occasionally some very good subjects will levitate an arm so rapidly that the operator may not have time to finish giving instructions. Stage hypnotists in particular, as well as experimenters, have to be on guard against potential subjects who fake a response—that is, make the suggested movements voluntarily—in order to be selected for the demonstration or to take part in the experiment. With a little experience, the hypnotist will learn to distinguish a voluntary from an involuntary response. The latter can be quite rapid at times, although it is usually slow, but it typically consists of a sequence of jerky motions, often picking up speed after the initial motion is begun. On rare occasions, a negativistic subject will be found who consciously resists the suggestions and ends up raising the hand with the weight and lowering the hand with the helium balloon. If such a subject is to be hypnotized for some clinical purpose, this resistance should be discussed with him and the reasons for it worked through prior to attempts at induction, if possible. Such a subject should be avoided for demonstration purposes.

Hand Clasping (Finger Lock)

Another useful group screening test is the hand clasping method. Subjects are typically requested to extend their arms directly in front of them and clasp their hands tightly. It is then variously suggested that their hands will begin to tighten all by themselves as though they had a volition of their own or that they are welded or glued together or are being pressed together in a vise, and that when the operator counts to 3, they will be so tightly joined that the subjects will be unable to separate them until the operator tells them that they can. In fact, they are told that the harder they try to separate their hands, the more solidly glued together they will be. The operator then counts to 3 and challenges the subject. It is important to include the statement that the subject will be able to separate his hands when the hypnotist says to, or there may be difficulty in terminating this test due to the subject's misunderstanding of what is expected.

This effect depends partly on the physical fact that it is mechanically difficult to separate a pair of clasped hands, and it requires that the fingers be relaxed a little before separation can occur. The tester should note the amount of difficulty that the subject experiences in opening his hands and stop the challenge promptly (by telling the subject that he can now open his hands), before it becomes apparent to the subject that he is about to be successful. A good subject may be able to open his hands but will experience various degrees of difficulty in doing so. The operator should point out this difficulty, however, slight, and try to give the potential subject the feeling of success rather than failure in this test. It is a rare subject indeed who is totally unable to open his hands after a prolonged effort, and the experienced tester looks for signs of difficulty, not total failure to separate. An inexperienced operator may give a subject with an excellent response to this test a feeling of failure because he was ultimately able to separate his hands.

Hand Attraction or Repulsion

For this test, the subject is instructed to place his hands comfortably in front of him with the palms facing each other and separated by about 6 inches. Suggestions are then made that the hands are magnets or subject to an ever-increasing powerful force tending to pull them together or force them apart. Suggestions that the hands are being drawn together can be followed up with suggestions that they are held together by a powerful vise and a challenge to the subject to separate them. Failure or difficulty in doing so is more impressive than a similar failure in the hand clasping test because no mechanical effect is aiding the operator.

In all of these tests, the results are more impressive if the failure to meet a challenge is accompanied by obvious efforts to do so as opposed to a passive failure to attempt the challenged response. As in any other type of challenge, the operator must be alert for signs that the subject is about to be successful and terminate the challenge by saying, "OK, now stop trying" or

"Now you can do it," before the subject discovers that he will be successful. Success in meeting the challenge can undermine the subject's confidence in the operator and expectations of success in the ultimate induction of hypnosis. Successful suggestions of hand attraction can also be followed up by suggestions that the direction of the force is now reversing and the hands will be pushed apart. One advantage of this test over hand clasping is that gradations of response are easier to notice and measure.

Postural Sway

This is an individual test. The subject is instructed to stand erect with arms by his side and feet together and pick a spot on the wall somewhat above his normal line of vision to fixate on. This stance has the effect of tilting the subject's head slightly backward and makes the desired effect somewhat easier to obtain. The subject may be asked to close his or her eyes and continue fixating through closed lids or may be permitted to keep them open. It is a good idea to have the subject move his feet around a little initially in accordance with the operator's directions. This is a subtle way of getting the subject used to following the hypnotist's suggestions in a very natural situation.

The subject is then told to imagine that a very powerful force is pulling him backward and that he is not to try either to help or oppose it but just let himself be pulled over. The subject must be assured that the operator is ready to catch him and will not permit him to fall. Some operators precede suggestions of falling over backward with suggestions of swaying to and fro, and some make suggestions of falling forward. The former may facilitate the effect sought; the latter is merely an alternative procedure.

If the subject shows signs of not responding after a reasonable period, the operator may gently pull him backward by the shoulders. If the subject puts one foot backward to retain balance when pulled backward, it is a sign that he is afraid that the tester will let him fall and that he requires reassurance on this point. Such reassurance may result from the hypnotist's preventing the subject from falling after tugging on his shoulders.

About one out of 100 subjects given this test will prove negativistic and may fall forward when a backward fall is suggested. For this reason, the operator should stand to one side of the subject rather than squarely in back in order to move quickly in the direction of the subject's fall. It is also important when dealing with a large or a heavy subject to position oneself so that the subject can be caught safely. A heavy subject should not be permitted to fall so far that the operator has to support the subject's full weight in stopping the fall. It is better to err on the side of safety in this regard than to try to make the test more impressive.

If the postural sway test is used as an individual follow-up to a group screening procedure or two (such as arm heaviness and levitation, and hand clasping), it is a good idea to perform this individual test in the presence of all the subjects who will be involved later. The first subject to be tried should be the best potential subject of the group (based on the group tests), because seeing a good effect will make it more likely for the other subjects to perform well. If the first subject tested fails, this may have an adverse effect on the following subjects by undermining their confidence and expectations of success.

If preinduction tests are used with clinical patients who must have hypnosis attempted in any event, the major value of the testing is to provide the subject with a warm-up or practice period. Whatever his performance on the test, the subject must always be given the impression that he performed well and in accordance with the hypnotist's expectations and that the results indicate he is likely to be a good subject.

Some hypnotists, like Kroger, do not think preinduction testing is necessary and regard it as a waste of time; others, like the author, think it is useful in easing a subject into a hypnotic situation in a nonthreatening way. In any event, these tests are primarily useful with subjects who have no previous experience with hypnosis. They are not necessary with experienced subjects who neither fear the experience nor need any practice in the noncritical type of thinking necessary for induction.

Other authors (Frankel, 1978-1979; Hilgard, 1982) take the position that formal susceptibility testing should be used to a greater extent in clinical work, both to provide a basis for scientific reporting of treatment results and because they believe that the common clinical opinion that trance depth is of minor importance in clinical work may be true in some conditions but not in others. For example, there is evidence cited by Deyoub and Wilkie (1980) that susceptibility, although unrelated to success in treating smoking, is correlated with success in wart removal, asthma relief, and pain control.

Mott (1979) argues that in spite of occasional dramatic responses to hypnosis occurring during a light trance, the literature reflects instances of a high degree of correlation between susceptibility and therapeutic responsiveness, as well as diagnoses and etiology.

On the other hand, Joseph Barber (1980) takes the position that the use of indirect and nonauthoritarian procedures produces therapeutic responsiveness independent of susceptibility, a view with which Frischholz, Spiegel, and Spiegel (1981) take sharp issue.

The present author would agree with the need for susceptibility testing if the clinician intends to publish results with a particular patient (in which case the clinician is functioning simultaneously as an investigator). In a routine case, however, it would not appear to him to be worth the time, for even if the patient turns out to be a poor subject hypnosis may still yield good results. If it does not, this will be discovered rapidly, and an alternative approach can be employed. In any event, a patient low on susceptibility cannot be traded in for a better patient as an experimental subject can. Also, as Gruenewald (1982a) points out, the applicability to clinical practice of standardized susceptibility tests (which are vital in research) or of shortened clinical versions of them is unknown. In other words, success in hypnotherapy does not necessarily depend solely on hypnotic phenomena, and the correlation between susceptibility scores and success in clinical work needs to be investigated before clinical decisions can be based on such scores. Sacerdote, while agreeing with the notion of using standardized tests of susceptibility in clinical practice, points out that the types of abilities measured on such instruments are often not those that are of major importance in clinical work, and he stresses the need for the development of more appropriate clinical instruments (Frankel, 1982; Sacerdote, 1982a, 1982b).

Although the principal objection to the use of formal tests of susceptibility in clinical work might appear to be an economic one (and this objection becomes less cogent with patients whose therapy is unlikely to be short term), there is another pitfall common to the use of all psychological tests: the tendency of many clinicians to place more reliance on the pronouncements of such instruments than they merit. It must be remembered that all psychological tests are validated for groups, and although they may make excellent predictions about group behavior (which is what they are used for in experimental work), they can be misleading when used to make predictions about individuals. In general, they are useful when looked upon as sources of additional information or possibilities about a clinical problem. At the current state of the art, even the best of these is a poor second to skilled clinical observation, experience, and judgment. In any event it seems clear that the current trend is for the increasing use of formal susceptibility testing in clinical practice.

CHAPTER 3

Induction and Deepening Procedures

This chapter presents a variety of methods for inducing and deepening what is commonly referred to as a hypnotic state or trance. It has already been noted that there are both state and nonstate theorists; the latter do not believe that the concept of a trance state is necessary to account for the type of behavior commonly referred to as hypnotic. Theorists like Barber prefer to look at the antecedents necessary to induce the hypnotic state and to account for hypnotic behavior directly in terms of these variables rather than talk about a trance state's increasing the suggestibility of a subject. Thus an impressive amount of accumulated research indicates that many of the phenomena than can be produced under hypnosis also can be produced in non-hypnotized subjects under task-motivational instructions. Although there have been methodological controversies concerning this research, even state theorists concede that to some degree at least, "hypnotic" effects can be produced in nonhypnotized subjects.

Because of his nonstate position, Barber has often inaccurately, been accused of denying the existence or utility of the hypnotic state. To say that hypnosis is not a necessary condition for hypersuggestibility is very different from saying it does not exist or is not a sufficient condition for enhanced suggestibility. The fact that hypnotic effects can be produced by means other than trance induction in no way logically establishes the ineffectiveness of a trance state. Even Barber, who does not feel a trance is necessary in hypnotic treatment, will use one if it conforms to a patient's expectations or desires. Barber, Wilson, and Scott (1980) report that a traditional trance-induction procedure increased suggestibility when measured on a scale that is "hypnotist oriented" (that is, the hypnotist suggests the effects are occurring [BSS]) but did not raise suggestibility with reference to nonhypnotized control subjects when it was measured on a "subject-centered" scale (that is, the subject is asked to imagine that effects are occurring [CIS]).

The view of a trance that will be taken in this book is that it is a series of responses to a sequence of trance-inducing suggestions. These suggestions are typically sequential and are graded from very simple to more complicated. The successful completion of each suggestion increases the probability of success with the later suggestions, and the sequence of events finally produces a subjective state in which the subject feels somewhat different than usual and, as a result of his responses to the induction procedures, becomes more likely to respond as requested to further suggestions. This state may be called an *altered state of consciousness,* a *state of heightened suggestibility,* or a *trance.* All of these terms are somewhat unfortunate, however, because they carry a connotation of something mysterious or unusual occurring. An even more unfortunate, and incorrect, connotation of the term *trance* is that it implies a state that a person is either in or out of rather than a continuum. In actuality, what is usually meant by the expression *trance depth* is the probability that a subject will respond as requested to a suggestion. This probability varies from the moment a patient enters the hypnotist's office until the moment he leaves. In the average induction procedure, it probably increases fairly rapidly at the onset but may fluctuate considerably throughout the entire session if it is a lengthy one. There is really no one point when a subject can be said to have "become hypnotized," although we colloquially use expressions like this for convenience in describing procedures.

Field, Evans, and Orne (1965) tested the common clinical notion that success with easier suggestions leads to future success, failures predispose to more failures, and therefore hypnotic suggestions should be sequenced from easier ones at the beginning of a session to more difficult ones, requiring lower probability responses, later in the session. Using the tests of the HGSHS, they found that, in general, this hypothesis was not supported. There was no significant difference between mean scores obtained if test items were presented in an easy-to-difficult order or a difficult-to-easy one. There was also no significant difference in variability between scores arrived at under these two conditions. It should be pointed out, however, that these tests were administered following an induction procedure in which subject suggestibility was presumably already maximized. The results therefore have no application to the likelihood of there being an order effect of items during induction as was suggested here.

There are a great number of ways of inducing a hypnotic trance state (Malott, 1984). Since the types of responses that a subject will make to induction suggestions are a function of the suggestions themselves and the subject's own expectations, it follows that there is an infinite number of potential "hypnotic" or "trance" states. For example, it is possible to hypnotize a person and suggest that he will appear normally awake. He may then attain a very deep hypnotic state (as inferred from responses to suggestions), which is indistinguishable from the waking state, even by an expert. Gibbons (1976), instead of using the customary suggestions of relaxation and drowsiness, makes suggestions of euphoria and a "high" state, which results in what he calls a *hyperempiric trance*. This appears to be just as effective as a conventional trance in increasing subject suggestibility.

Banyai and Hilgard (1976) report active hypnotic inductions performed while the subjects were pedaling a bicycle ergometer under load. Subjects so hypnotized performed equally well when compared with subjects hypnotized by eye fixation and standard relaxation instructions, as measured by performance on the SHSS forms A and B. Both types of subjects also reported the subjective effect of experiencing an "altered state of consciousness."

Since there are common culturally determined expectations among potential subjects and since most workers in this field have been trained in a few standard methods of induction, such as those described in this chapter, it follows that there are enough common responses to most induction procedures to be able to describe certain "signs of hypnosis." However, it is important for readers to realize that these are in no way either necessary or sufficient conditions for the hypnotic state. They simply occur in a large number of subjects because they have been suggested either directly or indirectly. For example, Orne (1962a) found that subjects led by a previous lecture to believe that catalepsy of the dominant arm was characteristic of the hypnotic state developed this reaction spontaneously under hypnosis. Control subjects, of course, developed no such atypical reaction. If a new method of induction is designed and used on a subject with no previous hypnotic experience, the responses produced may be quite different from the customary ones.

Before discussing some of the more common formal induction procedures, it is important to realize that the actual induction process begins when the subject initially enters the hypnotist's office or laboratory. Ideally the first step in the procedure should be to have a discussion with the subject about hypnosis to find out what he knows or believes about it. Usually the subject has some misconceptions, which should be corrected. The problem is that although this discussion can always be had in a clinical situation, in experimental work, because of the nature of the investigation, it is often not possible to conduct any such preinduction interview with the subject. Thus, many experimental inductions must be done under less than optimal conditions.

In a clinical situation, the patient should not only have misconceptions corrected and fears alleviated but should also be told exactly what procedures will be used and what to expect. This preinduction conference should not be rushed or perfunctory. It will often make the difference between a smooth, successful induction and a failure produced by a tense, fearful patient. The use of printed material answering common questions that subjects have about hypnosis, whether commercially prepared or written by the therapist (which will be less likely to contain statements with which he or she disagrees), may be valuable, not as a time-saving device to avoid discussing the subject's concerns but as a means of preparing the subject for such discussion and ensuring that he is less likely to forget potential questions.

Although it may not be possible in experimental work because of design considerations, all clinical subjects, regardless of how confident they are about being hypnotized or how motivated they are for hypnotic treatment, should be given a few of the preinduction tests described in Chapter 2 prior to initial formal induction procedures, if only to ease them into the situation in a non-threatening manner and to give them practice in the kind of noncritical thinking necessary to go into the hypnotic condition. Actually these so-called tests are as much a part of the induction procedure as the formal induction itself. The same is true of the preinduction discussion with the patient.

A good clinical hypnotic induction procedure is one that is uniquely tailored to the requirements of an individual subject and must take into account the purpose of the induction, as well as the personalities of both the subject and the hypnotist. Hypnosis primarily involves an interpersonal relationship between the hypnotist and the patient (Diamond, 1984: McConkey and Sheehan, 1982b; Sheehan, 1980). Sometimes in experimental work or in measuring hypnotic susceptibility, standardized methods of induction must be used, but these have no place in clinical work. What is about to be described are a half-dozen of the more common types of induction procedures. These will be described in general terms and their special advantages and disadvantages will be noted, but no attempt will be made to give word-for-word instructions for the subjects, as these must be varied in accordance with their moment-by-moment reactions. No competent psychologist would attempt to induce hypnosis by reading a script, except in an experimental or testing situation where standardization is more important than rapport with the subject.

It is important to note that prior to any hypnotic induction, subjects wearing contact lenses should be requested to remove them because some subjects will develop tearing of the eyes under hypnosis.

ARM LEVITATION METHOD

The first step in this, or any other method of induction, is to have the subject either lie down on a couch or sit in a comfortable chair. The chair may be anything from an upholstered armchair to a simple unpadded folding chair, but it should be sturdy and comfortable. The discomfort caused by a poorly designed chair can have a deleterious effect on the induction and subsequent utilization of the trance state because it will serve as a constant distraction. For this method of induction, it is preferable to use either a chair without arms or one large enough so that the chair's arms will not interfere with the free movement of the subject's arms. The subject should be instructed to settle down and get as comfortable as possible and should sit with legs uncrossed and feet squarely on the floor. The subject's hands should be placed palms down and resting on the thighs. The reason for asking the subject to uncross his legs is to prevent possible discomfort from maintaining this position for a protracted period of time while in the trance state. Hypnotized subjects are usually unlikely to make any spontaneous movements, and therefore this position, constantly maintained, is likely to produce leg cramps.

After getting into the proper position and becoming as relaxed as possible, the subject should be requested to concentrate on the sensations that he is about to experience in a specified hand. He is told that he is about to experience a very interesting phenomenon: his hand is going to become lighter and lighter until it becomes so light that it will float up in the air all by itself and touch his face. He is further told that as his hand gets lighter and lighter and rises higher and higher, he will become more and more relaxed, and by the time his hand reaches his face, he will be in a very deep, relaxed, pleasant hypnotic state.

It is important to describe the foregoing sequence of events and what is expected to happen at the onset of the formal induction, for there are some good subjects (particularly those displaying a marked response to the arm heaviness and levitation tests) whose hands float up and touch their faces before the hypnotist has a chance to finish telling them that they will be in a very deep hypnotic state when this occurs. Once the overall sequence of events has been suggested to the subject, the hypnotist's task is simply to make suggestions to help the process along. The most difficult part of the operation for some subjects is to get the motion of the hand started. Once it begins it usually proceeds quite readily and can easily be speeded up by suggestions that the hand is getting lighter much more rapidly now and is beginning to move faster and faster. Suggestions may also be made to the effect that there is a powerful force, like a magnet, pulling the hand faster and faster toward the face and that the closer the hand gets, the more powerful the force becomes. During the motion of the hand the hypnotist may begin to make suggestions of deeper and deeper relaxation, slower and deeper breathing and the eyes' becoming heavier and heavier until they are impossible to keep open. These suggestions have the effect of reinforcing the original implied suggestion that the entrance into hypnosis will occur gradually as the hand rises. For some subjects these are not necessary; the original suggestion having been made, the subject will carry it out even if the operator remains silent as the hand is levitating. For other subjects, these suggestions may be helpful or even necessary, and it probably never hurts to make them.

Most subjects who require help need it in getting the hand motion started. This help can be provided if the hand does not respond within about a minute by focusing attention on the hand with suggestions that soon it may feel a little numb or develop peculiar or interesting sensations, and the subject should be sure to notice these early signs. Sometimes he is told the movement may be preceded by little twitching motions of the fingers (which will usually occur spontaneously). The hypnotist should watch the subject's hand carefully and note the slightest amount of movement and point it out to the subject as it occurs. After a minute or two if no overt motion is visible, it should be suggested that the hand is beginning to feel a little numb, and it is already resting more lightly on the subject's leg. What the operator is really doing is watching for the beginning of a sequence of normally occurring responses and pointing them out to the subject just as they occur or sometimes a little before they occur. The subject therefore is given the illusion that these spontaneously occurring events are somehow being caused by the hypnotist's suggestions, thus increasing the subject's confidence and expectations concerning a successful induction. This illusion, in turn, makes it more likely that he can imagine and therefore make the kind of ideomotor response necessary to produce arm levitation. When the levitation does occur the subject experiences his arm floating up without apparent effort on his part, and this unusual event greatly increases his confidence in success and therefore his suggestibility. A good hypnotist constantly observes all of the subject's spontaneously occurring responses (such as eye fluttering and closure, slowing the deepening of the breath) and includes them in the induction patter to give the subject the impression that the operator is producing these responses and that they are all signs that he is becoming hypnotized.

Often as a hand starts to levitate, the subject appears startled or frightened. It is important, therefore, to offer reassurance by telling him not to be afraid and neither to help nor hinder the movement of the hand but simply experience it. The hypnotic state should be described as very pleasant and secure. Sometimes the imminence of the hypnotic state so frightens a subject that he may suddenly awaken. The inexperienced hypnotist may be upset by this, but the awakening is a good sign that the subject is beginning to experience an effect. He should be reassured and told that he has not spoiled anything and can pick up right where he left off. If he is properly reassured, induction is usually quite rapid following this interruption. If, in spite of all attempts to suggest the hand into motion, the subject is still unsuccessful, the hypnotist may suggest that the hand is already so light that if the operator were to lift it a little, it would keep traveling upward all by itself. If this suggestion is followed by a gentle lifting of the hand, imparting a small upward movement, often it will continue to float up all by itself. This necessity for moving his hand should never be presented to the subject as being required by his poor response but rather as a matter of freeing his hand from its constricted position so that it is free to move. If the subject was not positioned properly prior to the start of induction suggestions, the constricted position of his arm may in fact be the real reason for the initial failure of his hand to levitate.

Other methods of helping to start a hand levitation that do not involve physical intervention include such goal-directed fantasies as suggesting that a helium-filled balloon is tied to the hand and is getting bigger and bigger, thus exerting a more and more powerful upward pull on the hand, or that a very powerful force is pushing the hand up off the leg.

In the initial instructions to the subject, many hypnotists will direct him to look at the hand to be levitated as a way of focusing attention on it and cutting down on distracting visual stimuli. If the subject has been shown to have good ideomotor responses to an arm levitation preinduction test, this is a good idea; but if this response was equivocal or such a test was not performed, it is preferable to ask the subject to fixate his eyes on a point that he selects either on the ceiling or high on the opposite wall. This may weaken the concentration of the subject on his hand somewhat, but it is often not much of a drawback. It has the advantage that if the subject does not respond well to hand levitation suggestions, the operator can easily shift the focus of suggestions to another method of induction (such as Braidism), usually without the subject's ever being aware of the change and thus without experiencing any feelings of failure or of being a poor subject.

As in any other method of induction, there are endless variations of this basic technique. Instead of suggestions of arm levitation, suggestions of arm heaviness and the lowering of an extended arm can be used. In fact, any ideomotor response such as hand attraction or repulsion can be used in the same manner.

The arm levitation method of induction is one of the author's favorites, not primarily because it was the method he was originally trained in but because it has many advantages. One critic of the method has said that it has little to recommend it because the effect of arm levitation has to be produced against gravity and is thus quite difficult to attain. This observation is certainly true, but it appears to be one of the strengths of this method. It is not a response likely to be made by a poor subject, and the mere production of an arm levitation is often quite impressive to the patient. It is a good idea to make this even more impressive by telling the subject in advance that the method of induction to be used is a difficult one, but the operator is sure the subject will be good enough to succeed with it, and it will result in the induction of a deeper trance than other methods. Whether this statement concerning the superiority of this method for inducing a deeper trance is true or not is problematical, and there is some evidence that there is little difference in trance effectiveness as a function of method of induction. However, telling a subject that he is likely to be a good enough subject to respond to a difficult method of induction often helps him to do well in the induction. Although logically this may seem to be a difficult method of induction and patients will certainly think it is if it is suggested to be, it really is not. A person with good ideomotor responses can perform an arm levitation quite readily if the suggestions are properly timed and worded. Describing it as difficult but well within the subject's capabilities is not likely to decrease the probability of success, but in the event of a failure, it gives the hypnotist a chance at a later session to try a "much easier" method.

The real advantage of the arm levitation method is that the position and movement of the subject's arm provide the operator with a continuous index of the state of transition from the subject's normal "waking" state to a fairly "deep" state of hypnosis. When working with a single patient, this index is not essential because there are many signs that the operator can use to gauge the subject's progress into hypnosis, such as, respiration rate and depth, eye blink and closure, and facial and bodily muscle relaxation. In experimental or demonstration situations when several subjects must be hypnotized simultaneously, however, an index becomes extremely valuable, since there will generally be large individual differences in the rate of hypnotic induction, and the operator has a limited amount of time to observe each subject.

One of the difficulties in doing a group hypnotic induction is that since individual subjects will be in different stages and thus making different responses at the same time, the operator must either use only suggestions that are equally applicable to all subjects or must make it clear to the subjects to which one of them a given suggestion is directed—perhaps by the use of a name if it is known or by some other signal, such as prefacing a suggestion with the phrase, "You whose shoulder I am touching . . ." This latter device should be used only if a subject's name is forgotten in the middle of a group procedure. Referring to a person as "you" is impersonal and offensive, whether the person is hypnotized or not. (An operator who cannot remember names should write them on cards if necessary to avoid this situation.) Because group suggestions must apply equally to all subjects in the group, there can be a general loss of control. For this reason, a hypnotist should limit group inductions done for demonstration purposes before a professional audience to about three subjects. If subjects have been prescreened for susceptibility, anything that has to be demonstrated probably can be observed in at least one of three good subjects.

Another, more subtle, difficulty in doing group inductions is that if suggestions have to be made to an individual subject—for example, to speed up an arm levitation—this will often cue the subject to the fact that he or she is not performing as well as the other subjects.

Group inductions performed on professional audiences to permit them to experience the subjective effects of hypnosis are less demanding because the trance state is unlikely to be utilized for any specific effects. Whenever a subject is hypnotized before an audience the operator needs to exercise caution, for it is not uncommon for some of the more susceptible members of the audience to experience inadvertently some degree of hypnotic effect. Group inductions of a therapy group will be less difficult since the patients are familiar to the therapist, and he or she is unlikely to forget their names if he or she suddenly has to refer to them individually.

BRAIDISM

A method of induction called Braidism because it was originally devised by James Braid was based on the erroneous idea that hypnosis is a physiological response produced by the fatigue of the eye musculature. Braid had subjects fixate on a bright object held about 10 inches away and somewhat above their normal field of vision to produce eye fatigue. It is now known that fixation of the eye muscles without expectations of hypnotic induction induces not a trance but merely eye fatigue. What produces the hypnotic state in this method, as in all others, is the subject's acceptance of the suggestions sequentially made and his confidence in and expectations of hypnosis. (Kirsch, Council, and Vickery [1984] found that subjects' prehypnotic expectancies were not correlated with suggestibility in subjects subjected to a conventional hypnotic induction, but they were correlated in subjects subjected to a "skill induction," a procedure emphasizing the role of the subject's imagination and control over his responses, and training the subjects to respond effectively [Council, Kirsch, Vickery, and Carlson, 1983; Diamond, 1982; Katz, 1978]. Frischholz, Blumstein, and Spiegel [1982] agree with Katz that social-learning training significantly increases hypnotic responsiveness, but they maintain this is because it trains subjects to be active responders rather than increasing susceptibility.)

It is not necessary to hold a bright object over the subject's eyes to use this method. It is much easier for the hypnotist to have the subject fixate either on a prearranged target point or to let him pick out his own target point in the form of a smudge on the ceiling or high on the opposite wall. The author has even used this method successfully by having the subject fixate on the ace of diamonds held in his hand, a method that produces minimal eye fatigue, if any. The fixation of the eyes eliminates visual distractions, causes fatigue of the eye muscles, and produces a desire on the part of the subject to rest his eyes by closing them. The hypnotist takes advantage of this normal physiological response by suggesting to the subject that his eyes are getting heavier and heavier, and it is becoming harder and harder to keep them open. Soon, he is told, it will be impossible to keep them open, and they will close by themselves, and he will be in a very deep, pleasant, hypnotic state. As the eyes fatigue, the lids will begin to flutter involuntarily, and the hypnotist will point this out to the subject as evidence that it is soon going to be impossible to keep them open. If, after a prolonged period of time, the subject's eyes still fail to close, the operator may say that they are so tired the subject should stop trying to keep them open (in effect, he tells the subject to close his eyes voluntarily, without saying so directly) and go into a deep hypnotic state.

Whatever method of induction is used, most subjects, with the exception of children, will close their eyes at some point during the induction procedure; and if a rare subject fails to show any signs of eye fluttering or fatigue, he can simply be instructed to close his eyes and "go deeper" into the trance.

During any type of induction, and particularly with this method, some hypnotists suggest to subjects following eye closure that their lids are stuck together, and they can no longer open their eyes. Some will go a step further by challenging subjects to try to open their eyes and telling them that the harder they try, the more their eyes will be stuck. If such a challenge is made and a subject tries and fails to open his eyes, it will enhance or deepen the trance state; the subject will take it as evidence that the effect is real. The author believes, however, that such challenges should be avoided or at least restricted to situations where there is a reasonable certainty that they will be effective. If the subject can perform the behavior that the operator says he cannot, the trance state will be weakened. If a subject's ability to open his eyes must be challenged to test the amount of eye catalepsy present, suggestions should first be made of relaxation of the facial and eye muscles, for the eyelids cannot be opened if these muscles are fully relaxed. Also, challenges should not be prolonged for more than a few moments, as this increases the likelihood that the subject will successfully meet the challenge. If the operator waits too long, and it is obvious that the subject is about to open his eyes, he or she should say: "OK, now you can open them. Now close them again and go down even deeper." If this maneuver is timely made, the subject may not realize that his success was not due to the suggestion, and instead of weakening the trance, the net effect may be to enhance it.

During the period while the eyes are building up fatigue, the same kind of suggestions concerning relaxation, drowsiness, and breathing that are made during the arm levitation method are made in this (and all other usual) methods of induction.

There are many variations of this method. A small pocket flashlight or a flickering candle can function as a fixation point. One book on stage hypnotism even advocates the ill-advised idea of having the subject concentrate on an after-image produced by an intense light source. Another variation of this method reported by Hunchak (1980) is to have the subject close his eyes and concentrate on the self-illumination of the retina or phosphenes.

If a small black dot is used as a fixation point, many subjects will develop the illusion that this dot is beginning to rotate, and suggestions to this effect made after a minute or so will cause the subject to assume that this effect is a sign that he is becoming hypnotized. An archaic variation of this method is to have the subject stare directly at the hypnotist's eyes instead of a fixation point. Most modern hypnotists scorn this method because of its associations to primitive beliefs about the "hypnotic powers" of the operator or his or her "hypnotic eye." Also it is extremely fatiguing to the operator, who must keep his or her eyes immobile during the procedure. A trick of the old-time hypnotists who used this method was to stare at the bridge of the subject's nose instead of his eyes. This is easier to do both physiologically and psychologically, and it still gives the subject the illusion that the hypnotist is looking directly into his eyes. Another variation is to put either a small coin or a finger on the subject's forehead and ask him to rotate his eyes upward and fixate on it through his head. This method will produce a great deal of eye fatigue rapidly.

The advantages of Braid's method, particularly if the operator does not hold the fixation object by hand, is that it is simple and easy for the operator and the subject. The operator has a better idea of the subject's subjective feelings in this method than in any other one, since he or she knows that the eye muscles are being fatigued and hence can determine precisely what suggestions to make and when to make them.

COGNITIVE INDUCTIONS

Cognitive inductions involve having the subject concentrate attention on imagery generated by the hypnotist's suggestions as opposed to concentrating on ideomotor reactions (as in the arm levitation technique) or on some external stimulus (as in Braidism). In effect the hypnotist tries to paint what English teachers like to call a vivid "word picture." Although this picture may be predominantly visual, a skillful hypnotist will try to maximize the vividness of the image by bringing as many of the sense modalities as possible into play. For example, if as a result of a preinduction conference with the subject, the hypnotist learns that the subject enjoys sunbathing on the beach, he or she may decide to induce hypnosis by having the subject concentrate on a beach scene. The operator will not only describe the sand, sky, clouds, water, and other visual stimuli but will also instruct the subject to imagine the feeling of pleasant warmth produced by the sun shining on his skin, feel the cooling breeze, and listen to the monotonous and soothing sound of the waves breaking on the shore. In short, the hypnotist tries to describe the scene so realistically and so vividly to the subject that the latter becomes completely absorbed in it to the exclusion of all the external stimuli around him. When the subject is so absorbed, the conventional suggestions of deep relaxation and responsiveness to the hypnotist's suggestions are then made. Kroger and Fezler (1976) give numerous verbatim descriptions of such scenes, each designed to produce a somewhat different effect.

This can be an interesting method of induction for the subject (particularly for children who normally have a rich fantasy life) and is especially useful for subjects with a highly developed capacity for imagery. Its unique utility is for applications where it is desirable to manipulate the emotional state or mood of a patient under hypnosis, for this can often be controlled quite directly by the choice of the induction scene. It is important, however, to establish the meaning of a particular setting and its effect upon the individual subject in advance. In general, a seascape is a restful and relaxing setting for most subjects, but it may produce a different effect on a subject with past traumatic experiences in such a setting.

PROGRESSIVE RELAXATION METHOD

The method of progressive relaxation is probably the most time-consuming and tedious of all induction methods. It consists essentially of suggesting relaxation to the subject and shifting the focus of such suggestions from one region of the body to the next. After being comfortably settled in a chair, the subject may be told to concentrate his attention on his arms and let them grow limp and heavy. He may then be told to imagine all of the tension being drained from his arms as if it were being soaked up by a sponge, leaving each little fiber completely and wonderfully relaxed. The operator will then go on and suggest relaxation of the legs, feet, abdomen, chest, neck, and face. Some hypnotists prefer to work their way down the body; others start from the feet and work up. The sequence of bodily areas is actually quite unimportant. Some hypnotists use Jacobson's (1938, 1962) technique of having the subject tense up each muscle group prior to relaxing them as a means of focusing attention on the subjective feelings coming from the muscles.

Another variation of the progressive relaxation method, the spiral technique, is reported by Venn (1984). It differs from progressive relaxation in that the subject is focused successively on the joints and viscera in various regions of the body as opposed to the striated muscles.

The author's view of this method is that it is unduly lengthy and boring to the subject and occasionally runs the risk of inducing a state of sleep rather than hypnosis. It takes an unusually skilled hypnotist to be able to pace this kind of induction to avoid these pitfalls.

The method does have at least one unique advantage. A certain number of subjects will be found who could benefit from hypnotic treatment but who fear being put into a trance and resist all attempts at reassurance. Such a subject can be hypnotized without ever using the words *hypnosis* or *sleep* by simply referring to what the operator is trying to attain as a "deep state of relaxation." This can be done with any method of induction, but it would seem that because of its nature, the method of progressive relaxation is the most appropriate for such a subject.

It is possible to get into the pseudo-ethical problem of the right of a therapist to do something to a patient that the patient is unwilling to have done to him. This is referred to as a pseudo-problem because in this case the operator is not doing anything that the patient did not consent to. The subject is willing to be put into a deep state of relaxation, and that is all the hypnotist has done. The patient does not know what hypnosis means, but the term has enough upsetting connotations that he does not want to experience it. He knows perfectly well what deep relaxation means, and since he is willing to experience this, he does. Also, the operator has not placed the subject in this state; the subject himself has done so. He is the only person who can. Whether the operator refers to the product of an induction procedure as hypnosis, a deeply relaxed state, a state of meditation, or anything else, it should always be made clear to the subject that he, not the hypnotist, produces this effect. The role of a hypnotist is simply to guide the subject's own thinking and thereby help him to attain this goal. Not only is this statement the truth, but it has practical significance as well. Some subjects will resist hypnotism because they fear or resent giving control over themselves to another person. If such a subject is made to understand that he will never relinquish control over himself and that it is he, not the operator, who produces all of the effects sought, this resistance may be overcome in many cases. Also in the event of a failure in the initial attempts at induction, the subject will not lose confidence in the hypnotist but place the "blame" for the failure where it belongs—on himself. Hence at a later time, he may be told that as a result of his past training, his ability to be hypnotized may have increased or that a different method to be used will prove easier for him, and subsequent attempts at hypnosis may prove more successful.

FLOWER'S METHOD

This method of induction is probably one of the most stereotyped. The subject is seated and told to look at the opposite wall but not to fixate on any point. He is then told to close his eyes and that the operator is about to start counting slowly up to some number. Each time a number is counted, he is to open his eyes for a moment and then close them again. It is suggested that each time he does this, his eyes will become heavier and more tired, and it will be harder and harder for him to open them. Also, he will become more and more relaxed until finally he will be unable to open his eyes and will be in a very deep and pleasant hypnotic (or relaxed) state.

The operator starts the count and observes that the subject is following instructions correctly. During the counting, no suggestions are made, because they would interfere with the rhythm of the count. In this method, all suggestions about what will happen in the hypnotic state are made prior to the beginning of the count. Once the eyes remain closed, the subject is assumed to be in some level of hypnosis, and, as in all other methods, suggestions are begun to "deepen" the trance. If the specified number is reached and the subject is still able to open his eyes but appears to be affected, the count can be continued by starting over at one. If the subject continues to be able to open his eyes or shows no signs of being affected after a repetition of the count, the hypnotist can shift to another method of induction without the subject's being aware of the failure in most cases.

Many variations are possible with this method. Instead of counting, the hypnotist can request the subject to open and close his or her eyes in time to the beat of a mechanical metronome. The subject may or may not be requested to count to himself with each beat. With or without a metronome, this method can be used without specifying the number to be counted to. Not specifying a number minimizes the risk that a subject will pick up the repetition of the count as a sign of failure. The real value of specifying a number is that it communicates indirectly to the subject information concerning approximately how soon he is expected to go into hypnosis. The number 20 is a realistic expectation for most subjects. It should be made clear to the subject, however, that he does not have to wait for the completion of the full count to go into a trance. If the operator lacks the confidence to specify a number, then he or she can say something like, "In a very short time, your eyes will become so heavy that you will be unable to open them."

Using a mechanical device like a metronome ensures a steady rhythmic beat and is easier for the hypnotist, but it deprives the operator of the opportunity to communicate suggestions of tiredness by voice tone. There does not appear to be much difference in results obtained between hypnotists who are quite dramatic in their approach and intonation (as many stage hypnotists are, primarily for the benefit of their audience) and hypnotists who talk in a more matter-of-fact tone (as most professionals tend to). Some renowned hypnotists have either poor diction or marked accents. Furthermore, studies have shown little difference in induction results from audiotape recordings as opposed to a physically present operator, in spite of the loss of the nonverbal communication components in the former case (Barber and Calverley, 1964g).

A possible reason for the seeming lack of effect of such nonverbal communication made by a physically present hypnotist is that such communication is usually in consonance with verbal suggestions, which are generally enough to communicate the message. It seems likely that if the nonverbal communication were opposed to the verbal message (as, for example, signs of lack of assurance of success unwittingly conveyed by an inexperienced operator), it could be quite disruptive. Also, once the subject closes his or her eyes, gesturing becomes ineffective and tone of voice can be as varied on a tape as in a person-to-person situation.

Videotapes have also been used to induce hypnosis, and these usually produce the same distribution of trance depth as personal induction does (Ulett, Akpinar, and Itil, 1972), although Johnson and Wiese (1979) report that live hypnosis is more effective than taped inductions in analgesia research with clinical populations. This effect may be due to the interpersonal relationship or transference possible with a human therapist rather than a deeper trance. Orne (1964) reports that a patient of his was inadvertently hypnotized while watching him demonstrate a brief induction procedure on television. The television networks' concern that on-the-air hypnotic inductions could inadvertently hypnotize members of the audience is probably well founded. It is paradoxical that although the subject's own thought processes produce hypnosis, he does not always have to be aware that this result will occur. Advantage is taken of this state of affairs in the so-called chaperone method of induction, where hypnosis is induced in a patient who fears trance induction while ostensibly witnessing an induction of another.

TRANCE INDUCTION BY POETRY

Eventually most hypnotists come to realize that what they actually say during hypnotic induction and deepening procedures is less important than their manner of delivery and the subject's expectations. Orne (1982) reports a hypnotic induction occurring when a subject was inadvertently left to listen to a record of a Swiss yodeler instead of the recorded induction procedure intended. The lack of importance of the literal meaning of the words used in hypnotic pattern may be the reason that Denver, Grove, DeVarennes, and Gagnon (1979) found that subjects not very proficient in a second language could be readily hypnotized with it.

It has been reported that certain poetry has a trance-inducing effect, while other poems do not (Snyder and Shor, 1983; Silber, 1980). The factors favoring induction ability seem to be freedom from abruptness, soothing rhythms, frequent repetition, attention-fixing ability, and vagueness of imagery.

MECHANICAL AIDS

There are a host of devices on the market that can be adapted to induce hypnosis or have been specifically designed for that purpose. All are primarily attention-capturing devices and all are effective if used properly. They are also unnecessary unless the hypnotist is engaged in research on the effects of different methods of inducing hypnosis or just wants to do something different for variety's sake.

The use of a metronome has already been mentioned in conjunction with Flower's method. Some metronomes also have flashing lights, which can be used as an interesting fixation point. Indeed the most common use of a mechanical hypnotic aid is to provide a fixation target. There are hypnodiscs that provide a fixation point in the form of a small button with a spiral pattern. A bright coin can serve as well. Rotating mirrors or larger spiral discs and other patterns come with motors to rotate them and provide compelling visual effects. These devices are usually priced far in excess of what they are worth; and although they may have a placebo effect on some subjects because of their associations with hypnosis, they are equally likely to frighten other subjects for the same reason. Chevreul pendulums consisting of a glass globe suspended from a chain can be purchased, and their associations with a crystal ball and magic might make them useful with some subjects, but any small weight on a chain or string would do just as well, as would many small amulets and pendants. Hypnotists of an earlier generation who wore vest pocket watches found that their watch and chain made an ideal fixation point for an eye fixation technique and doubled as a Chevreul pendulum.

Under the topic of mechanical aids should be included many commercially available tapes containing induction procedures. Except possibly in experimental work, where standardization of procedure is important, the hypnotist would be better advised to do his or her own inductions. No tape can ever be as responsive to the reactions of an individual subject as a physically present hypnotist can. Furthermore, the use of a tape during induction diminishes the opportunity for the hypnotist to develop the proper therapeutic relationship needed ultimately to utilize the resultant trance state. If a cognitive induction is to be used, a tape read from a script might be practical because it is often difficult to draw a multisense image extemporaneously. Even in such a case, however, there is no reason why the therapist could not record the tape. Using a personal tape will make it easier for the hypnotist to take over from the tape at its conclusion and to utilize the trance because the voices and personalities of the speakers will be unchanged. The real value of a tape-recorded hypnotic induction is to give a hypnotist an example of the techniques used by a colleague and a chance to learn new methods or variations on old ones. One exception would seem to be the case of inducing hypnosis in connection with a test of susceptibility. In this case, a standardized induction could be ensured by the use of a prerecorded tape, but this might require a revision of most standardized tests, which normally include some change in wording dependent on subject response. Group tests like the HGSHS have been successfully recorded. The announcer who recorded one such version reports having been inadvertently hypnotized by listening to his own recorded voice (Dumas, 1964).

One type of tape recording that has occasionally been used as a hypnotic aid, and probably should be used more often in psychotherapy in appropriate cases because of its mood-affecting potential, is recorded mood music. A patient who is having difficulty relaxing because he does not know how to and finds that trying to relax tenses him even more could be helped by a soft, relaxing musical background, which can produce some relaxation involuntarily. This medium is occasionally used in hypnotic induction but rarely, if ever, in psychotherapy, probably because of the mechanical difficulties of introducing it at the right level and time and preventing it from distracting the patient. It is an area worthy of much more research attention.

Gardner and Tarnow (1980) used music in therapy with a 16-year-old boy with a severe personality disorder who loved music.

The major use of music by psychotherapists today is as a noise-generating device in their waiting rooms to ensure privacy if the walls are not soundproof enough. But a patient who hears the music from the waiting room will recognize that the wall is not soundproof and may be inhibited in presenting material. The proper remedy for this situation is to soundproof the wall or find another office more appropriate for the practice of psychotherapy.

Kline (1978) reports a case where background music used in an induction procedure in a dentist's office was alleged to have been heard inadvertently over a car radio, reinducing a trance and causing an accident. If, in fact, such a spontaneously induced trance state did cause an accident, it appears more likely to have done so by the trance acting as a conditioned stimulus to reactivate feelings of detachment suggested in the original trance rather than because of the effects of hypnosis per se.

NEW METHODS AND COMBINATIONS
OF METHODS

People seem to have a need to classify and pigeonhole things into categories, probably because such classification provides some sense of order in what would otherwise be a confusing array of unrelated facts. Also classifying and naming things, such as clinical syndromes, provides the comforting illusion that we know what we are talking about. Hence, we commonly classify into groups mental illnesses, methods of psychotherapy, and methods of hypnotic induction. Most of these methods of classification are quite arbitrary and often misleading. (A prime example of this is the Diagnostic and Statistical Manual [DMS III], an atheoretical listing of diagnostic categories whose prime purpose seems to be placating insurance companies by giving names to collections of symptoms that are rarely, if ever, seen in isolation in clinical practice and treating them as if they were distinct disease entities.) We talk about such methods of psychotherapy as classical psychoanalysis, Rogerian therapy, behavior therapy, and so on as though they really existed as separate entities. No therapist actually practices any of these methods exclusively in its pure form. The same is true of methods of hypnotic induction. Like a good therapist, a competent hypnotist borrows .a little from many different methods to come up with a combination that is best suited for a particular subject and his or her own capabilities and limitations. Although each therapist may have a favorite method of induction, often it will be contraindicated for a particular subject. Furthermore, a so-called arm levitation method of induction will be done somewhat differently by every hypnotist who uses it. Indeed, it will and should be different for each patient he or she works with. The author does not believe that he has ever hypnotized two different subjects in the same manner, except when two or more subjects were being hypnotized simultaneously. Even in such a case, specific suggestions must frequently be addressed only to certain subjects.

If a specific technique is not working, it is a mistake to stop and then try another method. The subject will have a feeling of failure, and the second attempt will be more difficult. The proper technique is to change strategy and go on to the other method as though it were what was originally intended. If this also fails, the "confusion technique" is worth a try before giving up. This technique is to make a rapid-fire sequence of contradictory suggestions that so confuse or overwhelm the subject that he uses going into hypnosis as an escape from the untenable situation. For example, he can be told to concentrate exclusively on his hand and his eye muscles at the same time or, along with a suggestion of arm levitation and numbness, be given the suggestion that his arms are heavy as lead.

If in spite of all the operator's skill and persistence he or she should fail to hypnotize a particular patient, the session should never be terminated by telling the patient that the latter failed. The patient should be told that he did very well for his first efforts, and the hypnotist is confident that he will do even better the next time. This type of optimistic statement is entirely justified because one will rarely have a patient who cannot attain at least a very light hypnotic state, and for many therapeutic applications a deeper state is not needed. Even poor experimental or demonstration subjects should be sent away with some positive feelings about their performance, but usually working further with such subjects will not be productive.

Once practitioners observe a number of hypnotic inductions by different methods and perform a number of them themselves, they will notice the common elements of these varied techniques and can begin to devise a personal repertoire. This can be a useful pastime as it prevents boredom and tends to keep a therapist sharper. Ritualistic and stereotyped inductions are useful in research and in testing susceptibility but have no particular advantage in clinical practice. What, then, are the essential elements that seem to be present in all of the techniques described?

First, the subject is made comfortable, and distracting stimuli are minimized. Some people like to work with subdued lighting and in a quiet room, but a good subject who can concentrate on what he is asked to can be hypnotized in a brightly lighted room with all kinds of distracting noises and even a large audience staring at him.

Second, he is told to concentrate his attention on one specific thing, such as a spot on the wall, the sensation of his hand rising, or an imagined scene, further taking him away from his immediate environment. Some hypnotists think that this type of "monoideism" is the essential element in inducing hypnosis. Whether that is true or not, it seems to be important. Conventionally, suggestion's of drowsiness and relaxation are made that further detach the subject from the environment, but these are clearly not necessary, and hypnosis may be produced with the opposite type of suggestions.

What the hypnotist really does, having initiated this process, is to suggest to the subject what he is expected to experience in the trance state (such as relaxation or pleasant floating sensations). Then having defined what a trance is like, the hypnotist suggests certain events and feelings that he or she either knows will occur or that are observed happening or about to happen (for example, "Your eyes are getting tired; your eyelids are blinking"). When these suggested effects occur, the subject interprets them as being caused by the operator's suggestions and accepts this as evidence that something is happening. This evidence increases his expectations of future effects and thus renders him more suggestible. It may sound as if the hypnotist is performing a sort of magic act, fooling the subject into thinking a real effect is present when it is not. At the beginning of an induction procedure, this is often true. But as a result of this original bit of deception, the subject is set up to produce responses to further suggestions that are real in the sense that they would not have occurred without the suggestion. That is, they are not physiological responses caused by the experimental situation.

Any method that will cause a subject to concentrate all of his attention on something (and thus detach himself from his environment) and that is followed up with a graded series of suggestions within the subject's immediate response capability (and which capitalize on his spontaneous feelings and responses) is as likely to produce hypnosis as any more established method. Although some hypnotists think that the monotony and the rhythm of their suggestions are important, this does not seem to be universally true. The important thing seems to be getting the subject to focus attention on one thing to the exclusion of everything else.

It is customary during hypnotic induction to suggest to a subject that no matter how deep he goes, he will always be able to hear the hypnotist's voice and respond to any suggestion made unless he does not desire to comply with the suggestion. Some operators tell a subject: "You can hear only the sound of my voice." This is a poor suggestion to make because the hypnotic subject can hear everything else and this suggestion, contrary to his own experience, will tend to weaken the effect. Rather, the subject should be told, "You will ignore everything but the sound of my voice." Subjects can do this quite well. One can induce hypnosis in a good subject in the presence of a great deal of noise and other distracting stimuli. One case was reported where a subject was hypnotized utilizing the noise of hammering in the adjacent apartment as a metronome (Kroger, 1977b).

Also, if a patient is so distracted by pain that he is unable to concentrate on some external stimulus, he may be successfully hypnotized by directing his attention and concentration to the pain itself (London and Forman, 1977). Some hypnotists try to take advantage of external distractions by suggesting to the subject that when these things occur, they will be a signal for the subject to go under even deeper.

HYPNOTIC *PASSES* AND *STROKING*

Passing the fingers over the limbs of the patient or by his face and particularly his eyes dates back to the mesmerists' theory of magnetism and the application of the magnetic fluid. The early magnetists wrote detailed instructions about how these passes should be made and the effects of different directions of movement. Professional hypnotists generally shun these practices because they are too theatrical, but stage hypnotists use them for that very reason. When they are used today by a therapist, it usually amounts to an attempt at nonverbal communication. The therapist is trying too hard to induce an effect and is therefore talking with his or her hands. The use of these passes has no effect other than as nonverbal communication to the subject, although Arons (1961) claims that moving the hands over the eyes can produce a helpful blinking effect of the light passing through the closed lids. In this connection, it should be noted that flickering lights of the correct frequency (as from an improperly working television set) have been reported to have triggered epileptic seizures in susceptible individuals. Although such a result from a hypnotic pass is of very low probability, it can hardly be looked upon as an advantage of the technique. The communicative effects of hypnotic passes are so slight that their use or nonuse is a matter of no practical consequence. However, from these passes developed the practice of some hypnotists of stroking a subject with the fingertips, usually along the arm, particularly in connection with suggestions of lightness in arm levitation, numbness, or relaxation. Such strokings can have a relaxing effect but are probably of limited utility. They can also have an erotic effect or can be misinterpreted by a patient. For this reason, the author believes they should not be used in induction. Hypnosis, like all other psychotherapy is basically a verbal interaction between two people, and physical contact is contraindicated except in very circumscribed situations. For example, it is necessary to move a subject's arm to test arm catalepsy; some posthypnotic suggestions for reinduction may require a touching of the forehead or shoulder as a signal; and the HIP test requires the stroking of a patient's forearm. Thus it is inaccurate to say that no physical contact between a hypnotist and a subject is ever necessary, but it ought to be kept to a minimum.

"INSTANT" HYPNOSIS

Enough has been written, mostly by stage hypnotists, on the subject of so-called instant hypnosis to justify some discussion of this topic. The only true method of instant hypnosis is to give a previously hypnotized subject the post-hypnotic suggestion that on a given signal he will instantly go back into the hypnotic state. This suggestion, like any other posthypnotic suggestion, may be effective for variable periods of time and may produce anything from a light hypnoidal state to a very deep trance in seconds. It would appear to be a poor practice to leave a subject between sessions with such a suggestion. Its principal utility would be in cases where a subject has to be constantly hypnotized and dehypnotized in a single session, either for demonstration purposes or in certain deepening procedures. If such a signal is to be used on a subject in hypnotic therapy to prevent the necessity of a separate induction procedure at each session, the signal should be carefully chosen so that it is not likely to occur inadvertently between sessions (for example, the hypnotist touching the patient on the forehead). Second, it should be made clear to the subject that this signal must be given by the hypnotist and no one else, and it will be effective only when the patient is in the hypnotist's office and wants to be hypnotized.

Actually a better practice is to rehypnotize the subject in each session, for with practice, a reinduction often will take no more time than would normally be spent in deepening the trance after reinduction by signal. One can experiment a little initially by using a different method of induction for each session and letting the subject decide which one is the easiest and quickest for him. Should a posthypnotic signal for reinduction be used and it proves ineffective or almost so, the operator should act as though the subject reacted as expected and go on to reinduce hypnosis under the guise of deepening the trance. If the posthypnotic signal produces a very shallow trance, one simply proceeds to make deepening suggestions, as is usually done following any type of induction. The same can be done at all subsequent sessions, or, if preferred, the use of the signal can be stopped and hypnosis formally reinduced at each session.

If a subject is to be hypnotized repeatedly, whether at the same or subsequent sessions, the initial session at least should be followed by a discussion with the patient concerning his subjective feelings and reactions. This discussion will give the hypnotist first-hand information on how this subject reacts, and this feedback can be used in framing suggestions for future inductions, which will make them easier. For example, if the subject reports experiencing a floating sensation under hypnosis, at the next session suggestions of a floating feeling during induction may speed up the process. Such discussions need not be limited to the initial hypnotic session and are useful learning devices for the hypnotist, who will soon develop an appreciation of both the common subjective experiences under hypnosis and the wide range of individual differences.

It is possible to induce hypnosis over the telephone by means of a verbal signal or by a letter utilizing a written signal, but the utility of such an induction except for demonstration purposes is questionable (Gravitz, 1983). If it became necessary to hypnotize a patient over the telephone in an emergency, such a signal would not be necessary, and the induction could be made by standard verbal means with an experienced subject. It would not be a good idea for a patient who had not been previously hypnotized by the operator, since the hypnotist is deprived of all visual feedback concerning the subject's responses to suggestions. Also if such an induction is to be attempted, a responsible person should be with the patient to be sure that he does not let the telephone slip out of his hand and thus lose contact with the therapist. Such a person can advise the hypnotist of any problems that may develop.

Cooperman and Schafer (1983) report the successful use of the telephone for hypnotherapy with a former patient physically unable to come to the therapist's office. The patient did not feel that a sense of closeness and rapport depended on personal contact, and the therapist, who was blind, did not feel at a disadvantage by working over the telephone. On the other hand, Stanton (1978a) reported on successful hypnotherapy by telephone with both a former patient and one whom he had not previously met. Interestingly, he found work with the former patient by telephone personally less satisfying than work with the strange patient, who was perceived as more of a challenge. Although face-to-face contact may not be essential for the development of rapport with a patient, it seems to the author to be a major advantage, and in view of the importance of both rapprochement and nonverbal communication in psychotherapy, it is his view that any kind of telephone therapy would be best limited to emergency situations or those in which there is no viable alternative.

There are other techniques of hypnotic induction that give the illusion of being instantaneous because an untrained observer incorrectly assumes that the hypnosis begins when the operator suddenly looks at the subject and forcibly commands him to "sleep." For example, in any of the preinduction tests (such as the hand clasping test), if a subject appears to have an unusually strong response, often he will close his eyes and go into some level of hypnosis if suddenly given a command to do so. A stage hypnotist can follow up with deepening suggestions, and the audience gets the impression that the trance produced was both instantaneous and deep. Actually hypnosis was begun with the hypnotist's initial remarks and was continuing through all of the tests performed. This method is a derivative of a method used by some stage hypnotists of inducing a trance in some subjects by literally shouting commands at them to sleep and generally intimidating them. How much hypnosis and how much role playing this produces is problematical, but such a method is contraindicated in a clinical situation. The former method is also contraindicated, not because a little showmanship might not be useful in helping a patient into hypnosis, but because it sets up a situation where, if the method fails, it will clearly be perceived as a failure by the patient and will make subsequent efforts more difficult.

Some hypnotists try to get instant or rapid induction of a trance by telling the subject that they are going to apply pressure to certain "hypnotic nerve centers." There are, of course, no such centers, and in most cases what is sought is a placebo effect. A psychologist ought to be cautious in using this technique because it may give the impression that he or she is practicing medicine and also because few subjects are naive enough for this technique to work on anyway. A technique that sounds similar to this is referred to as the *carotid artery pressure method*. Nobody, whether medically trained or not, should ever use this technique. This method is dangerous and if used on a person with a sensitive Hering reflex may cause cardiac arrest or death. It involves putting pressure on the common carotid arteries in the neck. What happens is that the subject's (or rather the victim's) blood supply to the brain is interrupted, and he begins to faint. On rare occasions the shock of this trauma may trigger a trance state, but more commonly a stage hypnotist using this method will pass off the faint as a trance state to the audience. The danger in this method concerns a blood-pressure-regulating servomechanism, with receptors sensitive to the pressure of the blood located in the carotid sinuses. These send signals back to the brainstem and cause the heart to accelerate or decelerate as the blood pressure gets too low or too high, respectively. As a result of pressure on these arteries, the receptors start signaling a rise in blood pressure, and the heart is commanded to slow down. In some cases, it may stop, and a life-threatening emergency ensues. There is no conceivable circumstance under which this technique is ever justified, and its use ought to be regarded as prima facie evidence of professional incompetence. The fact that a hypnotist may be a physician and be adequately equipped to deal with a sudden cardiac arrest does not justify exposing a patient to a method of induction involving such a risk, especially since its probability of success is small and there is a wide variety of safe alternatives available.

Matheson and Grehan (1979) and Wicks (1982) report a method of rapid induction based on arm catalepsy. The patient's arm is lifted and released after an indirect suggestion such as, "Would you like to go into hypnosis rapidly today?" In most cases, these authors assert, the arm will become cataleptic, and the patient will go rapidly into hypnosis. Their method gives the illusion of a rapid induction because a witness assumes that hypnosis is begun when the arm is moved rather than at its real inception, the start of the hypnotist-subject relationship.

It has been the author's personal experience that hypnotic induction is so easy and rapid in a properly prepared and well-motivated patient that so-called rapid induction techniques are of little utility in clinical work.

HYPNOTIC INDUCTION DURING SLEEP

There is some literature suggesting that it is possible to convert normal sleep into a hypnotic state by talking to a sleeping person. If suggestions are made to a sleeping person he generally will not follow them. Talking may awaken the subject. If a trance state is obtained, what probably happens is that the subject is awakened first, and then the trance is induced. That this is possible probably results from the fact that in this type of research, subjects must be informed in advance of what is going to happen, and hence they go to sleep expecting to be awakened and hypnotized. Barber (1956a) reports that some sleeping subjects who were told in advance that suggestions were to be made to them during sleep acted as though they were in the second stage of hypnosis as measured by the Davis-Husband Scale, in that they were completely unable to separate their clasped hands. Some acted as though they were in stage 3 with complete amnesia for the suggestions, or they followed a posthypnotic suggestion to awaken in 5 minutes and drink a glass of water. With respect to the amnesia produced, it is not clear how long the subject was permitted to sleep following this procedure. This is of importance in establishing whether the amnesia produced was really post-hypnotic, since more recent research indicates that memory of dreams drops linearly to about zero in 10 minutes. If a dreaming subject is not awakened within 10 minutes of having a dream, he will generally remember nothing about it. Barber reported at a proseminar lecture in 1978 that if this type of study is performed without informing the subjects in advance, their general reaction to such suggestions is to awaken in an agitated or frightened state.

AUTHORITATIVE VERSUS PERMISSIVE DIMENSION

One issue related to induction techniques has to do with whether hypnosis should be presented to the subject as something that is imposed on him by the hypnotist or as something that he himself produces, with the hypnotist merely guiding the subject's own efforts. There are numerous gradations of hypnotist behaviors between the two approaches. A skilled hypnotist may be able to use either very authoritative or very permissive inductions with different patients depending on the needs of the patient, but most hypnotists are probably most comfortable with whatever level of authoritativeness best fits in with their own personalities. The more modern approach is a permissive one, and this is particularly helpful with patients who are fearful of losing control under hypnosis or who resent being ordered around. A permissive way of making a suggestion might be, "You can do such and such if you really want to," or "It is your concentration and imagination that make everything happen."

Permissive suggestions seem more appropriate for use with modern subjects who, unlike the ignorant peasants once treated by the highly educated authoritative hypnotists of the nineteenth century, are generally well-educated and of the same social class as the therapist.

An authoritative approach may still be indicated with a patient who has a need for a magical cure or a placebo effect. Deciding which approach is best for a particular patient is largely a matter of clinical judgment and is one of the decisions that must be based on the preinduction interview with a patient. In the case of an experimental subject, this decision is a matter of experimental design and will usually have nothing to do with the requirements of an individual subject.

SIGNS OF HYPNOSIS

The responses of a subject to induction suggestions are what we collectively refer to as a *trance*. These responses are a function of what suggestions are made and the subject's own preconceptions of what a hypnotic state is like. These suggestions and preconceptions in turn are usually similar enough, even in nominally different methods of hypnosis, to produce common reactions in different subjects, which are usually taken as evidence of hypnotic induction. Indeed, hypnotic induction proceedings are often stereotyped enough so that what is really remarkable is not the similarity of reactions among different subjects but the fact that there is so much variability.

With respect to an individual subject, the initial induction is a very important event. Although little has been written on this topic, it appears likely that the reactions obtained in this session will determine the subject's personal expectations concerning the hypnotic state and will tend to reappear in all subsequent sessions. Thus, individual reactions to hypnotic inductions tend to remain similar from session to session unless specific suggestions are made to vary them.

The signs of hypnotic induction can be divided into objective signs that the hypnotist can observe directly and subjective signs that the subject must be asked to describe. Some of the more common objective signs of hypnosis are the following:

1. Initial eyelid fluttering followed by eye closure.
2. Deep relaxation as evidenced by limpness of the limbs, lack of facial expression, and marked disinclination to move or talk spontaneously. If the subject is asked a question, there is often a long pause preceding the response, and he may have to be told firmly that he is able to answer. The subject's speech is often markedly slow and effortful. Some subjects tend to slump in their chairs or let their heads slump over; some do not. Few, if any, subjects will relax enough to fall out of their chairs, but if one looks as though he might, this situation should be countersuggested (Benson, Arns, and Hoffman, 1981).
3. Literalness in the understanding and following of suggestions. Often hypnotic subjects behave as though their understanding of language is more primitive; metaphoric expressions or idioms may be given their literal meanings. A subject told to raise his hand, for example, may simply raise the hand alone while leaving the arm unmoved, or a subject told to "Write your name" may literally write "your name." For this reason, it is important to word suggestions carefully and, if necessary, repeat them in somewhat different words to ensure that the subject interprets the suggestion as intended. A subject may be asked by a hypnotist if he understands what the latter is saying and this is a good practice, but it will only detect situations in which the operator has confused the subject. It will not detect the situation where the subject has misinterpreted a suggestion but is not confused.
4. In some subjects, there may be excessive salivation and swallowing or excessive tearing of the eyes.
5. If a subject is connected to a galvanic skin response (GSR) apparatus (a device to measure the amount of sweating indirectly by measuring the electrical resistance of the skin), skin resistance will increase with hypnosis. This is not a measure of hypnosis but of the associated relaxation. During the induction procedure, such commands as "Go deeper" may awaken fears in the subject, as can his own responses to suggestions, and this may be punctuated on a GSR record as a sudden decrease in skin resistance. Also, emotion-creating suggestions made under hypnosis may lower skin resistance (a sign of increased sweat gland activity).
6. Other physiological responses that reflect emotional states or relaxation and that are commonly recorded on a polygraph (such as respiration rate, heart rate, or blood pressure) may reflect the subject's state of physical relaxation and hence be used to infer hypnosis. For example,

the same vasodilation response and increase in skin temperature obtained in relaxed subjects are also obtained in hypnotized subjects (Peters and Stern, 1973).

7. Even without instrumentation, the subject's respiration rate can usually be observed to become slower and deeper.

8. One of the major characteristics of the hypnotized subject, which must be tested rather than directly observed, is increased suggestibility. This is used not only to test the presence of hypnosis but also to estimate the depth of the state produced. In general, when it is said that a subject is in a deeper state, it means that the probability of his carrying out a suggestion is higher than it would be for the same suggestion in a lighter state. If a subject performs a suggested response that he would be much less likely to perform in the waking state, this is generally taken as evidence of some degree of hypnosis. In testing suggestibility under hypnosis, the distinction between a *suggestion* and a *command* must be clearly made. For example, an arm levitation suggestion involves getting the subject to imagine that his arm is becoming lighter and levitating without any conscious effort on his part. The statement "Raise your arm" will generally be interpreted by a subject not as a suggestion to let his arm rise but as a command to raise it voluntarily. Any phrase likely to be interpreted by a subject as a command is, of course, no test either of the presence of hypnosis or its depth. (Spanos and DeGroh, 1983)

9. A characteristic of a hypnotized subject that some would call a defining feature of hypnosis is the tolerance of the subject for inconsistencies or anomalies in experience or perception, that is, trance logic (Perry and Walsh, 1978; Ryan and Sheehan, 1977; Sheehan, 1977).

These signs of hypnosis, while common, are all highly individual. One subject may display most of these responses and be only in a very shallow state, as measured by his responsiveness to suggestions. Another may not show any of these signs and yet be in a very deep state. After working with an individual subject often enough, the hypnotist will be able to gauge this subject's trance depth from his objective responses.

The subjective feelings accompanying hypnotic induction are even more variable. They often include one or more of the following:

1. Feelings of deep relaxation and disinclination to expend any kind of effort.
2. Feelings of bodily heaviness, particularly in the limbs.
3. Feelings of numbness, tingling, or dullness in the limbs or hands.
4. Feelings of floating or lightness.

5. Feelings of detachment and being out of touch with the environment, which appears to be distant. (This effect is enhanced by eye closure, shutting out all patterned visual stimuli.)

6. Noticing of commonly ignored distracting stimuli, such as development of itching sensations. (This can be distracting and probably results from the ignoring of most stimuli that would normally distract the subject from these feelings.)

A common phenomenon in hypnotic sessions is the development of what is usually called *rapport* between the subject and the operator. This means that the subject reacts only to suggestions made by the hypnotist and treats suggestions made by anyone else as part of the background stimuli or noise, which he ignores. Some operators believe that this is an essential aspect of hypnosis, but, like all other characteristics of a trance, it probably results from either an explicit or an implicit suggestion. For example, if the hypnotist tells the patient, "Attend only to the sound of my voice," as is commonly done during induction to help the subject concentrate and ignore distractions, he or she is in effect specifically telling the subject in a literal manner not to respond to the suggestions of any other person. If a subject is not so instructed and has no expectation that such rapport will occur, it usually will not. If, for whatever reason, this rapport does occur, and it becomes necessary for another person to take over the hypnotist's role, the original hypnotist can *transfer control* to the other person by suggesting to the patient that the next voice he will hear will be that of Dr. X, and he is to follow all of his or her suggestions. If a patient is to be in a situation where it is desired that more than one person be able to make suggestions to her (such as a woman undergoing childbirth under hypnosis where both the hypnotist and the obstetrician, if they are different people, might have occasion to make suggestions), she should be instructed accordingly before the necessity for the suggestion occurs.

Often following an initial hypnotic induction a patient who was in even a fairly deep hypnotic state will deny being hypnotized because he remembers everything or because he was not unconscious. If it is important for the operator to convince the subject that he was in fact hypnotized, to take advantage of the placebo effect intrinsic in the use of such a dramatic procedure as hypnosis, it becomes doubly important to explain to the subject beforehand that he will not become unconscious during hypnosis. This preparation will not only allay whatever fears about hypnosis that the subject may have, but, coupled with the therapist's prestige in the eyes of the patient, will reduce the likelihood of the subject's erroneously concluding that he was not hypnotized when in fact he was. Goldstein (1981) reports that women in a hypnotic treatment group for obesity lost more weight when the reality of hypnosis was demonstrated to them by means of an arm levitation suggestion.

In experimental work, the subject's doubt that hypnosis occurred is usually irrelevant to the study. If it is important to convince a patient of the reality of trance induction and the preceding steps leave him unconvinced, then hypnosis should be reinduced and the subject given some posthypnotic suggestions to perform, such as developing an amnesia for the number 5. This will usually convince a skeptical subject.

DEEPENING TECHNIQUES

Except in situations in experimental work where a standard method of induction is required, it is common practice to give trance-deepening suggestions following induction and prior to the utilization of the trance state. Basically there is no difference between the induction procedure and the deepening procedure except possibly in the mind of the hypnotist. Deepening suggestions are simply a continuation of the induction procedure and are commonly given until the subject appears to be as deep as he is capable of getting. The principal value of referring to these latter suggestions as deepening ones is the implication to the subject that he is already hypnotized and everything has gone successfully and as expected to this point. The exact point in the procedure when the hypnotist tells a subject that he is now in a hypnotic state and changes over suggestions from those of going into hypnosis to those of going deeper, will vary from one operator to another, although sometimes a particular induction procedure will define this point. For example, if the subject is given the suggestion that when it becomes impossible to keep his eyes open any longer, he will close them and go into a deep, relaxed, hypnotic state, then a few moments after the eye closure, the suggestions should change to exhortations to go even deeper. Some hypnotists dislike defining the exact point that hypnosis is to ensue to avoid having the subject feel that the induction is a failure if he does not suddenly feel different at that point, and they imperceptibly will change over from suggestions of hypnosis or sleep to suggestions of greater depth in accordance with the subject's reactions. In other words, the subject is never made aware of the transition from waking to hypnosis until he has been feeling different for some time.

Just as the successive suggestion of more and more difficult or low-probability responses during induction will increase the subject's suggestibility, so too will his performance of suggestions after a trance state is attained. Hence the same test suggestions made to estimate the depth of a trance will also serve to deepen it further.

Besides observing the subject's objective appearance and behavior, trance depth can be estimated by the same types of scales used to estimate hypnotic susceptibility. The difference is that the use of a standardized method of induction prior to the test is eliminated and the hypnotist tries to get the deepest state possible. Although the scales described in Chapter 2 could be used for this purpose, certain older scales, such as the Davis-Husband or the LeCron-Bordeaux modification of this scale, are more appropriate for the estimation of trance depth because they are designed to categorize depth of trance into five or six levels respectively that are more convenient to talk about than an arbitrary numerical score. Indeed, since there is no standardized induction procedure for use with these tests, it would seem more appropriate to call them tests of trance depth rather than susceptibility, and this is, in fact, how the latter test is labeled.

The Davis-Husband Scale describes five levels of trance depth: insusceptible, hypnoidal, light trance, medium trance, and deep trance or somnambulism. Scale items are listed in order of difficulty like a Guttman-type scale, and the score and category of hypnotic depth are thus determined by the most difficult item successfully achieved. A score of 0 is categorized as insusceptible, 2–5 as hypnoidal, 6–11 as a light trance, 13–20 as a medium trance, and 21–30 as somnambulistic.

The types of items produced in the lightest or hypnoidal state include varying degrees of relaxation, eyelid flutter, and closure. In a light trance state, catalepsy of the eyes and limbs and anesthesia are obtained. A medium trance is characterized by partial amnesia, simple posthypnotic suggestions (including anesthesia), personality changes, and complete amnesia. In a somnambulistic trance, the subject can open his eyes without breaking the trance, will accept bizarre posthypnotic suggestions, and can experience visual and auditory hallucinations, both positive and negative.

In a sample of 55 college students, 9% were insusceptible, 29% hypnoidal, 18% in light trance, 15% in medium trance, and 29% were somnambulistic (Hilgard, 1968).

LeCron and Bordeaux modified this scale by increasing the number of graded test items to 50. In recognition of the fact that the order of difficulty is based on group data and hence the scale is not a true Guttman type, they arrive at a total score by crediting 2 points for each item passed. They also include a sixth category of depth called a planary trance, one that is even deeper than a somnambulist state, in which all spontaneous activity is eliminated.

There are differences in the ordinal position of some items common to the Davis-Husband and the LeCron-Bordeaux scales. For example, LeCron and Bordeaux believe that analgesia is more characteristic of a medium than a light trance.

There have been many other schemes to categorize the various stages or depths of hypnosis. Liébeault proposed a six-stage system and Bernheim a nine-stage one that are cited in Hilgard (1968), but the Davis-Husband Scale is probably the most convenient in that the categories correspond to the usual terms used to describe trance depth. All of these systems are completely arbitrary; their principal value is in making the work of various investigators comparable. In clinical work they are relatively unimportant.

Another way of estimating the depth of a trance is to utilize a *state report,* or the subjective impressions of the subject by asking him to estimate how deep he is "on a scale of from 1 to 10, where 1 is fully awake and 10 is as deep as possible" (Tart, 1978-1979). Subjects can make ratings on such a scale, but the ratings made are relative. In other words, a subject can meaningfully say how much deeper or shallower he is now than he was at some other time, but his absolute rating without such a reference point is probably subject to great individual differences. For example, two subjects may be in the same subjective state, but one will say that he is deeply hypnotized because he feels so relaxed, while the other will say that he is in a very shallow state because he is aware of everything that is happening. While such a subjective estimate of trance depth by subjects may lead to large within-subjects error terms in experimental work, in clinical work it may be the most important measure of trance depth, for it reflects the subject's belief in the success of the induction procedure. This belief is probably the most important factor in predicting the success of the subsequent utilization of the trance state.

Hilgard (1973a), Tart (1970), Wedemeyer and Coe, (1981), and Perry and Laurence (1980) report that subjective or state reports correlate positively and significantly with objective or behavioral measures of depth. Barber and his colleagues (1968, 1972) and Radtke and Spanos (1981a, 1982) have shown that subjective reports concerning the existence or depth of hypnosis made after hypnosis is terminated are a function of how the question is worded. They are also displaced in the direction suggested by any estimate of depth of hypnosis that the experimenter may communicate to the subject. These studies are not directly applicable to the accuracy of subjective state reports, which, by definition, are made during hypnosis and not subsequent to it. (See also Jupp, Collins, and McCabe, 1985.)

In addition to such common suggestions as arm catalepsy, rigidity, levitation, or heaviness, which are often made early in hypnosis to test trance depth and which tend to have deepening effects, certain deepening suggestions often made do not involve the testing of depth or the challenging of the subject.

One of the most common of these techniques is to have the subject count forward to some number or backward from some number with the suggestion that with each number counted, he will go deeper and deeper into sleep or hypnosis. Some operators tell the subject that he will go twice as deep with each number, but this is not a good practice because most subjects will not experience so dramatic an effect, and any suggestion made that is not effectuated may tend to weaken a trance.

Cognitive suggestions can be used to deepen a trance either by themselves or in combination with counting techniques. For example, a subject may be asked to imagine that he is at the top of a long escalator and with each count he descends deeper and deeper into hypnosis. Scenes of the subject floating on a cloud may also be used. These, like cognitive induction techniques, are examples of communicating symbolically with the subject. The descent of the escalator is symbolic of his descent into deeper levels of a trance. Although there is not any real descent or deeper levels of a trance literally but, simply, an increase in the subject's probability of responding to certain suggestions, as long as the subject conceptualizes the trance in such terms, these suggestions enable him to use his own ability to generate imagery to achieve the desired state. It is important to take individual characteristics of a subject into account in making cognitive suggestions. While a descending escalator may be a good metaphor of increased trance depth for most subjects, it could upset one with a fear of heights. In such a case, a descending elevator might be in order.

Another method sometimes useful in increasing the depth of a trance is called *fractionation*. The subject is hypnotized and dehypnotized successively with the suggestion that on each subsequent hypnosis, he will go "even deeper than now." The subsequent hypnosis may be induced by a posthypnotic signal or by a separate induction procedure using subject feedback.

Since most hypnotic subjects tend to breathe more slowly and deeply as they relax, it is often useful to point this out to them and to suggest that with each breath they take, they will go deeper and deeper.

Music has been used as both an induction and a deepening aid (Channon, 1982; Walker and Diment, 1979). In addition to its attention-focusing qualities and its ability to mask distractions, music has a unique ability to create or intensify a variety of emotional responses.

During the utilization phase of the trance, deepening suggestions should occasionally be made, because in the absence of any suggestions, subjects may begin to move into lighter stages unless they have been actively engaged in making deepening suggestions to themselves. Many hypnotists will interpose deepening suggestions between all suggestions made for any other specific purpose.

Related to deepening suggestions is the suggestion that is often given that the subject will not awaken until the hypnotist tells him to. Such a suggestion is designed to minimize the likelihood of a spontaneous awakening, which sometimes happens, and is particularly important in such situations as hypoanesthesia. Because of the literalness of hypnotized subjects, the suggestions should be clearly worded to indicate that when the hypnotist instructs him to, he will awaken.

TERMINATING A TRANCE

A trance can be terminated by suggesting to the subject that he is to open his eyes and be wide awake. A more usual practice is to count to 3 or 5 and instruct the subject that as you count, he will begin to awaken gradually, and by the number designated, he will open his eyes and be fully awake. This practice provides the subject with a more comfortable, gradual transition from a deeply relaxed hypnotic state to the more active waking condition.

A small percentage of subjects on awakening may report a headache, a feeling of numbness, or a muscle cramp. These may be readily suggested away by the operator, in some cases without even the necessity for reinduction. Some subjects experiencing such effects may not report them, and for this reason the hypnotist should always inquire how the subject is feeling. Although these reactions can be easily dealt with, it is better to prevent their occurrence by including in the waking instructions suggestions that the subject will feel relaxed and well on awakening. Some hypnotists prefer to limit these suggestions to positive statements of well-being and not specifically counter-suggest such problems as headaches or numbness because they fear the mention of such reactions might give the subject the idea that they might occur and hence cause them. This is as much a misconception as the fear of some therapists that questioning a depressed patient concerning the presence of suicidal ideation may put such ideas into his head. In addition to making positive suggestions of well-being, the author always specifically tells patients that they will have no headache, feelings of numbness, muscle cramps, or any other discomfort. He has never had any of these reactions develop in the face of such instructions, although, uncommonly, some of them will occur if such specific instructions are omitted and only general suggestions of well-being and feeling rested are made. Such reactions, when they occur, are probably due to the deep relaxation of the subject and his disinclination to spontaneous movement while in the trance state. Some people will awaken with a headache if they sleep unusually late on a weekend, and sitting immobile in a chair for a protracted period of time can produce muscular discomfort. A common subject reaction on awakening is to stretch.

Rarely, a subject may refuse to awaken when so requested. One possible reason for this situation is the fact that the hypnotist may have suggested that he will not awaken without including the qualifying phrase "until I tell you to." Another common reason for difficulty in getting a person out of a trance is that the subject finds the condition pleasant and relaxing. If difficulty is experienced in ending a trance and a firm repetition of the request to awaken is ineffective, the operator should ask the subject why he will not awaken. He will usually give the reason, and if it is the result of a misunderstanding of the instructions, the hypnotist can clarify them. One reluctant subject who was enjoying the tranquility of the hypnotic state was awakened by being told that if he did not awaken, he would no longer be able to be hypnotized. The hypnotist may try telling a patient who is reluctant to awaken that if he wants to continue to "sleep" for a while he may, but since he is tying up the hypnotist's office, he will have to be charged for the additional time at the therapist's usual rates.

If the difficulty cannot be overcome by the operator, there is no need for panic. The patient can simply be watched until he either falls into a natural sleep (from which he will awaken normally) or awakes spontaneously. He will invariably do one or the other.

Unless the therapist intends to have a suggestion made under hypnosis continue to have an effect or has suggested some posthypnotic response, it is important to remove all suggestions made under hypnosis, even those that the subject appears not to have accepted. If, in testing for depth, the hypnotist has suggested that the subject would be unable to remember the number 5 and then had him count to 10 and discovered that he did indeed remember it, he should still be told, "Now you can remember the number 5." This is a good practice, to guard against a remotely possible future difficulty in remembering the number. Not only should all suggestions be removed specifically prior to awakening, but a general statement to the effect that the subject will be just as he was before hypnosis (except for any therapeutic suggestions made) is a good practice. On awakening, the subject should be checked to make sure that there are no unwanted residual effects. If amnesia for a number was suggested, whether successfully or not, the subject should be checked to ensure he has no difficulty remembering the number when awake.

CHAPTER 4

Hypnotic Phenomena

In this chapter, some of the phenomena commonly elicited under hypnosis and usually associated with it will be discussed, and their nature and limitations will be described. These phenomena are part of the body of data that any theory of hypnosis must account for, and they are also the kinds of behavioral responses that can be used in the practical applications of hypnosis that will be discussed in Chapter 5.

Some of the effects to be described are relatively easy to produce on a statistical basis, while others are much more difficult to demonstrate and can be obtained only in a small proportion of subjects. This situation is accounted for theoretically in one of two ways. Investigators like Erickson would say that the more difficult phenomena require a much deeper trance state to elicit. Investigators like Barber, who feel that hypnotized subjects do only the kinds of activities under hypnosis that they are ordinarily capable of doing without the hypnosis, would say that they require a better subject. In some respects, these two positions are quite similar because a better subject is more likely to attain a deeper trance. The former view, however, implies that the same subject might succeed or fail to produce an effect at different times, depending on the depth of trance. The latter view would hold that a subject capable of producing an effect like a hallucination would do it regardless of trance depth if properly motivated.

The specific effects and the research relating to them described in this chapter are not arranged in their order of difficulty but in as logical a manner as possible. Although in general research clusters centering around a specific type of effect will be grouped together, this is not always possible when the studies cited deal with more than one type of effect.

Since the suggestions made by the hypnotist are such important factors in the elicitation of hypnotic phenomena, some remarks concerning them are in order. Suggestions can be made directly and in an authoritarian manner: "Your arm is as rigid as a steel bar"; or directly in a permissive manner: "If you really want to, you can experience your arm as a rigid steel bar," or "Think, feel, and imagine that your arm is a rigid steel bar." Suggestions may also be made indirectly as typified by Erickson's approach to hypnotic suggestion. If it is suggested to a subject that his arm is feeling cold or numb, it is implied that it is also becoming anesthetic. With subjects who resent relinquishing control, permissive and indirect suggestions are more likely to be effective than authoritarian ones. The latter may be more effective for people with a need to be dominated or who, like soldiers, are used to obeying commands. Yapko (1983), in discussing the advantages and disadvantages of direct and indirect suggestions, claims that by approaching a problem indirectly a suggestion is less likely to activate resistance. In an experimental context, McConkey (1984) found that real subjects were more heterogeneous in their responses to indirect suggestions than simulators, with only 50% of them responding positively to an indirectly suggested visual hallucination (although all had previously responded to a direct suggestion of a visual hallucination).

Matthews, Bennett, Bean, and Gallagher (1985) report that in a three-way factorial study (sex x order x methods of induction), there were no significant differences in objective behavioral responses between subjects hypnotized by direct or indirect suggestions. Subjectively, however, indirectly hypnotized subjects reported feeling more deeply hypnotized than when they were hypnotized by direct suggestions regardless of the order of these treatments.

When suggesting effects, it is often useful to specify a time at which the suggestion is to go into effect. For example, instead of saying, "Your arm will become as rigid as a steel bar, and you will be unable to bend it," the hypnotist might say, "When I reach the count of three your arm will become as rigid as a steel bar." The latter method may be less confusing to the subject; the former will prevent the subject from perceiving the failure of the arm to become rigid on cue as a failure and thus permit the hypnotist to continue making suggestions to produce the effect sought. Suggestions of limb rigidity, catalepsy, or paralysis may be tested with challenges to try to move the limb as a measure of trance depth, but these are better omitted in any practical applications of a trance; because if the subject successfully meets the challenge, his conviction of the reality of the hypnotic state will be weakened, and trance depth will be lost.

Goal-directed fantasies may be useful in making hypnotic suggestions more effective (Spanos, 1971). A goal-directed fantasy is the imagination of conditions that, if they existed in reality, would tend to make the hypnotic suggestion occur. For example, in an arm levitation suggestion, a goal-directed fantasy would be for the subject to imagine that a helium balloon is attached to his hand, pulling it upward (Coe, Allen, Krug, and Wurzmann, 1974). Spanos and McPeake (1977) point out that in assessing the effectiveness of suggestions incorporating goal-directed fantasies, it is necessary to determine whether the subject developed the fantasy suggested and also whether control subjects, not given such instructions, have employed a goal-directed fantasy on their own.

PHYSIOLOGICAL EFFECTS OF HYPNOSIS

In Chapter 3, a number of common effects of hypnotic induction were described under the rubric of signs of hypnosis. If conventional methods of induction, utilizing suggestions of relaxation and sleep are used, these effects commonly include slight to profound muscular relaxation, with consequent alterations in facial expression and posture, eye closure, and lack of spontaneous movement or speech. Other usual concomitants of the hypnotic state include a literalness and specificity in the understanding of suggestions (making it imperative that the operator carefully phrase suggestions) and in some cases the development of *rapport*, a condition in which the subject ignores all suggestions except those made by the operator. It is tempting to describe reactions that result from the induction of the hypnotic state per se, or so-called neutral hypnosis, as general responses to distinguish them from those made only in response to specific instructions. This, however, would be misleading; these reactions, like any other obtained under hypnosis, are most likely made in response to suggestions. In the case of these general responses, the suggestions are being made explicitly or implicitly in the suggestions used for trance induction. If an individual subject interprets the hypnotist's exhortation to "respond only to the sound of my voice" as meaning the institution of a state of rapport, he will develop one; if not, he will not. Thus, although the present author agrees with Edmonston (1977b) that relaxation is a common concomitant of hypnosis, he disagrees with his thesis that it is the equivalent of neutral hypnosis. It results simply because of the usual way in which hypnosis is induced—by suggestions of drowsiness and relaxation—and is not essential to hypnosis, as demonstrated by the work of Gibbons (1974, 1976, 1979). The equating of relaxation and neutral hypnosis is another common misconception and was the reason that Swartz (1982), in a review of the first edition of this book, took exception to the author's statement that, by itself, hypnosis is neither helpful nor harmful, since he (as the author), believes relaxation is valuable in tension-related conditions.

In this section we consider what physiological reactions can be modified by suggestions, direct or indirect. Responses involving the autonomic nervous system (ANS) are of special interest since such responses are normally not under voluntary control and hence cannot be produced directly. However, they can probably be altered by the mediating action of thoughts, ideation, or goal-directed fantasies.

Crasilneck and Hall (1959), Gorton (1949a, 1949b), and Barber (1961b, 1965d) have reviewed the literature on the physiological effects of hypnosis. This literature is often in conflict because of the absence of adequate controls, especially in the earlier studies. Thus several studies have reported a decrease in heart rate in neutral hypnosis, while others have reported a rise. Probably both effects occur. Heart deceleration may result from the relaxation instructions used to induce hypnosis and heart acceleration from the idiosyncratic reactions of subjects to the subjective feelings aroused by trance-induction procedures. If the subject is frightened by the prospect of hypnosis, heart rate may increase. Gorton (1949a, 1949b) reports that except for a slight lowering due to relaxation, cardiac activity is about the same for subjects under hypnosis as it is when they are awake. Cardiac rate is much lower during sleep than in either hypnosis or waking.

Bauer and McCanne (1980b) found no significant differences in decrease in heart rate, alpha activity, skin conductivity, or respiratory rate between six hypnotized female subjects and six female simulators.

Barber (1961b, 1965d) reports that hypnotized and waking subjects can increase or decrease their heart rate in response to specific suggestions to do so, but hypnosis does not enhance this effect. It is not possible to determine whether direct suggestions to vary the heart rate are effective without the help of mediating ideation because it is not possible to control what the subject is thinking. Since the autonomic nervous system (ANS) is not under direct voluntary control, if heart rate is to be controlled by a subject, it probably must be done indirectly by an emotional response to ideation produced by suggestions. Barber also points out that alterations in respiration rate, which can be made voluntarily, can affect heart rate. However, it is difficult to distinguish the direct effects of suggestions, if any, from the emotional concomitants of mediating ideation, goal-directed fantasies, or simply relaxation.

Barber cites a study by Van Pelt in which the latter appears to have produced cardiac acceleration in a calm subject while controlling for the level of adrenaline in the blood. Raginsky (1959) produced a cardiac block for a brief period by hypnotic suggestion. He also produced extra systoles in labile subjects (Raginsky, 1953). Linton and colleagues (1977) found no evidence of concordance of heart rate between subject and hypnotist based on empathy, as some have suggested, but found some concordance during induction. Morgan and coworkers (1976) reported that suggestions of heavy work produced no alteration in cardiac rate in either hypnotized or waking subjects, but they were effective in producing an increase in ventilation. Barber found that in neutral hypnosis, muscle tension, measured by electromyograph (EMG), was significantly lower, but pulse rate was unchanged. Hilgard and colleagues (1974) reported a significant difference in heart rate following suggestions of analgesia that was unrelated to the amount of subjective pain reduction but no significant rise in heart rate with hypnotically hallucinated pain. Electrocardiogram changes have been reported following emotion-producing suggestions (Bennett and Scott, 1949; Berman, Simonson, and Heron, 1954).

Blood pressure is affected by both cardiac rate and the peripheral resistance in the arterioles produced by the activity of sphincter muscles under the control of the ANS. As in the case of heart rate, neutral hypnosis usually neither raises nor lowers blood pressure, but the relaxation effect may reduce the systolic pressure slightly, and any apprehensions that the subject has may raise it. On the other hand, suggestions can produce marked changes of up to 40 millimeters of mercury systolic pressure and 20 millimeters of mercury in diastolic. Suggestions of relaxation and well-being typically have a greater effect on the systolic pressure, and suggestions of temperature change primarily affect the diastolic pressure. Suggestions of warmth lower the diastolic pressure, and suggestions of cold raise it. Holroyd, Nuechterlein, and Shapiro (1982) found that hypnosis reduced systolic blood pressure when biofeedback did not, but biofeedback was superior to hypnosis in reducing forehead muscle tension. These effects were independent of subjects' hypnotic susceptibility.

A large number of clinical reports are cited by Crasilneck and Hall (1959) to the effect that bleeding can be increased or decreased by hypnotic suggestion, although they report a failure to demonstrate such a relationship experimentally. Some clinical sources describe reduction in bleeding as a concomitant of hypnoanesthesia even in the absence of specific suggestions to this effect. Arons believes that only capillary bleeding can be controlled hypnotically because veins have no sphincter muscles. A research difficulty results from the fact that venous, and certainly arterial, bleeding requires immediate control, so anything less than immediate and total control over them produced by hypnosis is not likely to be experimentally measurable.

The limited supply of blood in the body is normally differentially routed to the various viscera and skeletal muscles as needed by the action of the ANS on the sphincter muscles of the arterioles. The vascularization of the skin is under the exclusive control of the sympathetic division of the ANS. To the extent that both divisions of the ANS are represented in the other regions of the body, they function as antagonists. The effect of the sympathetic system is to put blood into skeletal muscle, while the action of the parasympathetic system is to route it into the viscera.

Although there is conflict in the literature over the issue of whether neutral hypnosis produces any change in the peripheral distribution of blood, the evidence seems consistent that hypnotic suggestions can influence the distribution of blood to the skin and other structures. Many of the effects reported on skin temperature, galvanic skin response (GSR), mammary gland development, and the production and alleviation of skin eruptions are probably explainable in terms of alteration of blood flow to these areas (Barber, 1978c). Timney and Barber (1969) replicated earlier findings that subjects in neutral hypnosis developed a significant increase in oral temperature, while Jackson and Hastings (1981) found no significant difference in oral temperature between hypnotic and simulating subjects. In a second study, they found a marginally greater decrease in oral temperature in high-susceptibility female subjects. By imagining that their hands are in cold or hot water, subjects are able to produce temperature differences of up to 20°F between their two hands. Maslach, Marshall, and Zimbardo (1972) have found that while hypnotized subjects were able to change the skin temperature in their two hands in the opposite direction simultaneously, waking controls were unable to do so. Similar effects have been produced using biofeedback. Piedmont (1981) and Crosson (1980) confirmed that skin temperature is alterable by suggestion under hypnosis, and Raynaud and her colleagues (1984) found that neutral hypnosis did not affect rectal or skin temperature, but the suggestion of the sensation of heat decreased rectal temperature and raised mean skin temperature.

McDowell (1953) reported vasodilation in a subject's leg following suggestions of the leg being immersed in warm water, and Nallapa (1952) reported increasing circulation in a case of Buerger's disease (thromboangiitis obliterans) by hypnotic suggestion. Reiter (1956) reported that suggestions of increasing blood flow to the thyroid gland increased the basal metabolism rate (BMR) to 110, resulting in body weight being reduced to normal in an obese patient.

Hypnosis itself does not affect BMR, but emotions produced by hypnotic suggestions may increase or decrease it (Wallis, 1951; Whitehorn et al., 1932). Posthypnotic suggestions have induced body temperature elevation, but Kline (1957, 1958c) believes that direct suggestions are ineffective and that emotive or hallucinatory suggestions are needed.

Contrary to Pavlov's theory that hypnosis involved vasoconstriction in the cerebrum, Nygard found no difference in cerebral circulation in waking or hypnotized subjects.

The GSR refers to the electrical resistance of the surface of the skin. Skin resistance is lowered by the activity of the sweat glands, which secrete an electrolyte onto the surface of the skin. Crasilneck and Hall (1959) report conflicting studies concerning the effects of neutral hypnosis and suggestions of anesthesia on GSR. Using six subjects, Barber and Coules (1959) found no change in skin resistance during induction and a gradual increase of resistance throughout the remainder of the experiment, which was punctuated by responses to individual suggestions. Since sweating is a response to stress produced by the sympathetic division of the ANS, it is likely that what happens is a function of an individual subject's reactions to suggestions. If the subject views the induction procedure as a relaxing event, he will probably respond with lowered sweat gland activity and a higher skin resistance. If he is apprehensive, either about the procedure in general or about some specific suggestion, he is likely to sweat more and thus have a lowered skin resistance. Often the subject's subjective feeling that he is about to go into an unusual state of consciousness may be enough to frighten him into producing a sudden change in GSR level.

A large variety of skin conditions appear to be affected by hypnotic suggestions. Congenital ichthyosiform erythroderma, a scalelike eruption, has been improved by hypnotic suggestion, and in some cases, results have been reported that were limited to the specific areas of the body to which suggestions were directed (Mason, 1952; Schneck, 1954). Large nevi and warts have been reported successfully treated by hypnotic suggestion (Asher, 1956; Fernandez, 1955; McDowell, 1949). Asher reported 15 out of 25 susceptible patients cured of warts. Barber (1978b) reported a rapid cure in 3 out of 11 patients, but an attempt to limit a cure to warts on only one hand by suggesting an alteration of the blood supply to the warts and "feeling them tingle and dry up" was unsuccessful. Both hands cleared up.

In 1941, Pattie reviewed the literature on blister formation. In a typical experiment of the time, blister development was attempted by telling a subject that he was being touched with a hot iron. Results were mainly negative, and, since many of the cases reported were poorly documented or controlled, there is conflict in the reports. The issue of whether a blister can be produced is still unresolved, but the weight of the evidence is negative. On occasion, erythema or a welt may be produced in a susceptible subject, and these may have been reported as blisters in some studies.

Johnson and Barber (1976) were unable to produce a blister in 40 subjects, although two developed a localized inflammation. One of these reactions was attributed to self-injury, a problem that Pattie noted in this type of research. Evidently some good subjects are so anxious to produce the effect the hypnotist seeks, they will actually injure themselves to produce it. The researcher must be able to observe subjects constantly or make the skin area in question inaccessible to them from the time of the suggestion until the time of observation of effects. Spanos, McNeil, and Stam (1982) age regressed 17 previously burned subjects to the time of their injuries and suggested that a blister was forming. None showed evidence of blister formation or even skin discoloration, but one did develop an elevated skin temperature at the site of the injury compared to the contralateral site.

Barber (1961b) reports that cold sores can be produced in susceptible subjects by suggestion, and probably even without hypnosis.

Ikemi and Nakagawa (1962), using high school students in Japan who were sensitive to a poisonous plant (similar to poison ivy), had both hypnotized and control subjects touch this plant. Both groups were told that it was not the plant they were allergic to. The vast majority of both groups developed no dermatitis. The study was then reversed; both hypnotized and control subjects were instructed to touch a nonpoisonous plant they were told was poisonous. All subjects in both groups developed a dermatitis from slight to marked. Thus, psychological factors have been demonstrated to affect the course of allergic reactions both with and without hypnosis.

A number of studies suggest that breast size may be increased by hypnotic suggestion. Williams (1974), employing controls for weight gain, phase of the menstrual cycle, and measurement position, reported an average increase of 2 inches in bust size in 13 subjects after 12 weekly treatments involving suggestions of warmth, blood flow, tingling, and so on. Home practice sessions were also employed. Willard (1977) replicated this experiment and reported an average gain of 1.5 inches in nine sessions. Staib and Logan (1977) found these gains were retained after 7 months. Erickson (1977b) reported successful hypnotic breast development in a clinical setting.

Respiration rate can be changed by direct or indirect emotion-producing suggestions (Crasilneck and Hall, 1959). Hypnosis per se probably lowers the respiration rate. Reiter (1956) reports that suggestions of pain, anxiety, and grief increase both the depth and frequency of respiration.

Arterial oxygen level is increased by the induction of a pleasant emotion under hypnosis and decreased by the induction of an unpleasant one (Lovett, 1953a, 1953b). Hypnosis per se decreased the waking levels of oxygen saturation. The blood glucose level is closely related to the level of arousal and can be varied by hypnotic suggestion (Barber, 1961b). Olness and Conroy (1985) found that nine out of eleven children between the ages of seven and seventeen were able to increase tissue oxygen in response to taped suggestions. Eight children were experienced in self-hypnosis; three were not. Of the children successful in this task, only one had no previous self-hypnosis training; two children without this training were unable to increase their tissue oxygen.

Hypnosis has often been reported as a treatment for an asthmatic attack (Franklin, 1957; Solovey and Milechnin, 1957; Van Pelt, 1953). Thorne and Fisher (1978) found that high- and medium-susceptibility subjects who were given hypnotic suggestions of experiencing an asthmatic attack were convinced that they had experienced one, though physiological measures failed to reveal a typical asthmatic pattern. Low-susceptibility subjects were unconvinced of the effect.

In a book published in 1953, the same year that Aserinsky and Kleitman published their paper on rapid eye movements (REMs) in sleeping infants that was to revolutionize concepts concerning the stages of sleep and dream research, Weitzenhoffer concluded that hypnosis resembled a stage of light sleep more than either deep sleep or the waking state. In an early article, Barber (1956a) came to the same conclusion. More recent evidence indicates that EEG records obtained during hypnosis are about the same as are obtained in the waking state or in stage 1 sleep (the lightest stage). The EEG record in stage 1 sleep is identical to a waking EEG record except for the appearance of periodic REMs, which is why this stage is sometimes referred to as paradoxical sleep.

No change in a preexisting alpha level is noted on induction (Dynes, 1947). On the other hand, alpha waves were inhibited in nine out of eleven subjects who were given suggestions for visual hallucinations while under deep hypnosis with their eyes closed. Such disruption in an alpha pattern would normally be produced by a subject either thinking or opening his eyes and permitting a visual pattern to stimulate his occipital cortex.

In addition to being capable of producing deep relaxation of the voluntary muscles, hypnosis may be capable of increasing the capability of muscle. Weitzenhoffer (1951) concluded that hypnotic transcendence of voluntary muscular capability is a valid phenomenon. Mead and Roush (1949) noted a significant increase in strength during hypnosis when measured by an arm dynamometer but not when measured with a hand dynamometer. Watkins (1949) suggests that this enhanced muscular ability may be due to the anesthetic effect of hypnosis on pain and fatigue.

Barber and Calverley (1964e), using 60 female volunteers, found that strength of grip was not increased by hypnotic suggestion or by task-motivational instructions. On the other hand, hypnosis per se depressed weight-holding endurance, but task-motivational instructions, with or without a preceding hypnotic induction, increased endurance. In a review of the literature on the subject in 1966, Barber concluded that hypnosis by itself does not increase either strength or endurance, but motivational instructions increase both—with or without hypnosis. Albert and Williams (1975) examined the effects of posthypnotic suggestions on physical endurance. Endurance was found to be lowered with posthypnotic suggestions of fatigue but not increased with facilitating instructions. Nonhypnotized control subjects were not affected by either suggestion. The Borge ratings of perceived exertion indicated that the subjects subjectively perceived the effects suggested.

In a study of maximum endurance on a treadmill running task, Jackson, Gass, and Camp (1979) compared groups exposed to hypnosis alone, to hypnosis plus motivating suggestions for both high- and low-susceptibility subjects, and a control group. When tested posthypnotically, high-suscepti-bility subjects given motivating suggestions under hypnosis and subjects given waking motivating suggestions performed equally well and better than control subjects. Low-susceptibility subjects given motivational suggestions under hypnosis and subjects exposed to neutral hypnosis did not improve their per-formance.

Performance on a pursuit rotor task was significantly improved equally by posthypnotic or waking suggestions (Pearson, 1982).

Abramson and Heron (1950) found a significant reduction in labor time with hypnotic analgesia during childbirth, suggesting that hypnosis may pro-duce a more effective contraction of the uterine muscles, a more effective cervical dilation, or both.

Neutral hypnosis depresses gastric secretion, while emotion-producing suggestions under hypnosis may alter it in either direction (Crasilneck and Hall, 1959). Suggestions of eating a delicious meal increased gastric acidity and secretion in 34 of 36 subjects.

Barber (1965d) makes the point that in most of the studies investigating the physiological effects of hypnosis or hypnotic suggestions, no evaluation was made of the relative effects of the specific suggestions, the positive mo-tivation on the part of the subjects, general suggestions of relaxation, or de-fining the situation as hypnosis. In cases where these parameters are inves-tigated, he asserts, it is usually found that direct, indirect, or even waking suggestions are effective.

HYPNOTICALLY INDUCED EMOTIONAL STATES

Since an emotion is generally regarded as a combination of the activities of the ANS, the subjective perception of these activities, and the accompa-nying ideation, it follows that hypnotically suggested emotional states are closely related to the physiological effects of hypnosis. Because the ANS is generally not under voluntary control, many of the physiological effects pro-ducible under hypnosis may in fact be mediated by emotional states that are more directly produced by hypnotic suggestion.

Hodge and Wagner (1964) cited a collection of studies that utilized hyp-notically induced emotional states to test the validity of the Rorschach test by inducing various emotional states in subjects and seeing if the resultant Ror-schach protocol was changed in the predicted direction (Bergmann, Graham, and Leavitt, 1947; Counts and Mensh, 1950; Lane, 1948; Levine, Grassi, and Gerson, 1943; Mercer and Gibson, 1950; Sarbin, 1939). They then embarked on a line of inverse research designed not to demonstrate the va-lidity of a projective technique but to show the reality of hypnotically sug-gested emotional states by demonstrating that these states produced appropriate changes in responses to a projective test assumed to be valid. For this purpose, the Hands Test, which consists of nine pictures of a pair of hands in ambiguous positions, was used. The subject was required to describe the activities the hands were engaged in. For a tenth card, which was blank, the subject was required to imagine a set of hands and describe their activities. In the first study, a middle-aged patient was used as the only subject. She was tested in the normal waking condition to establish a baseline and was diagnosed as a passive-dependent personality type. She was then given the test under neutral hypnosis, with remarkably similar results. She was subsequently administered this test under five different hypnotically induced emotional states (with instructions after each testing to forget the test). The five emotional states suggested were:

1. Dwelling on a happy thought.
2. Anticipating a pleasant sexual experience.
3. Unhappiness over her husband leaving her.
4. Anger over unjust criticism.
5. Falling in love.

Hodge found that in each state, the patient's basic personality features were reflected in test results, but the effects of the suggested emotional state were also apparent.

In a follow-up study, seven subjects were tested to permit a statistical analysis of results. Only two induced emotional states, affection and aggression, were used. Responses to the Hands Test obtained in these states were compared to the results obtained from the administration of the test in the waking and neutral hypnosis conditions. In both emotions, it was found that the number of test responses appropriate to the suggested emotion increased from the baseline condition. It was also noted that responses appropriate to the noninduced emotion were lower than in the baseline condition (Hodge, Wagner, and Schreiner, 1966a). Hodge, Wagner, and Schreiner (1966b) concluded that a hypnotically induced emotion can be considered similar to a naturally occurring one, provided it can be demonstrated that the behavior and test responses of subjects are similar (under the hypnotically induced emotion) to their behavior and test responses under the naturally occurring emotion. They also found that the subject's behavior was different from that in the control state, that each test situation was perceived by the subject as a new experience, and that the effects of acting could be eliminated.

Hodge and Wagner (1969a) found differences in Rorschach protocols obtained from three subjects under waking, medium-trance, and deep-trance conditions. They report that as trance depth increases, ego functions (such as reality testing) and secondary processes diminish, and primary processes predominate. While these results are cast in terms of psychoanalytic concepts, the essential point is that the protocols obtained were sufficiently different so that 17 graduate students were consistent in ranking the protocols in terms of the depth of hypnosis under which they were measured. Only two students made the mistake of confusing the waking and medium-trance state.

In a study designed to compare the responses of simulators with those of hypnotized subjects to emotion-generating suggestions, Gaunitz, Nystrom-Bonnier, and Skalin (1980) suggested that a signal light would cause a sense of discomfort posthypnotically, which could be terminated by the subject's pressing a switch. They found that both hypnotized and simulating subjects behaved similarly with respect to shortened reaction times, increased heart rate, and electrodermal responses. However, the two groups differed sharply in their verbal reports of their subjective experiences. Hypnotized subjects reported experiencing the discomfort suggested and its relief on pressing the switch; simulators reported not having these experiences.

Wilcox and Dawson (1977) reported that hypnotized subjects simulating paranoia on the MMPI were not detectable by that instrument's validity scales, but Lundy, Geselowitz, and Shertzer (1985) were unable to replicate these results.

HALLUCINATIONS

A hallucination is defined as a perception in the absence of a real external stimulus. Usually the occurrence of a hallucination is a symptom of a psychotic disorder, but under certain circumstances, normal people may hallucinate. These situations include conditions of sensory deprivation, extreme hunger or thirst, fever, drugs, REM sleep (nocturnal dreams), and, in some cases, scrying (crystal ball gazing). Normal people may also hallucinate under the influence of suggestions, hypnotic or otherwise.

Psychotic hallucinations in general have both a characteristic sensory modality and a characteristic content that vary between diagnostic categories. For example, schizophrenic hallucinations are predominantly auditory and have a characteristic obscene or self-critical content. Most psychotic hallucinations are accompanied by a delusional belief in their objective reality that is often absent in the hallucinations of normal people. This phenomenon is not intrinsically unreasonable, for psychotic hallucinations tend to be consistent with past experience. For example, a hallucinated image will usually obscure parts of real images lying in back of it in the visual field, and it will cast a reflection in a mirror. All of his life the patient has been correct in believing the information his sense organs have communicated to him about the external world, and there is no reason why he should not believe in the veridicality of these images when they are hallucinated.

In the case of a hypnotically suggested hallucination, the modality and the content of the hallucination are functions of the suggestions made. Hallucinations can be suggested in any sense modality; the ones most commonly used are vision, audition, olfaction, gustation, touch, heat, and cold.

Positive hypnotic hallucinations may be suggested in specific modalities or in general terms that may produce multimodality effects. For example, the hallucinated fly in the Stanford test (SHSS:A) may produce visual, auditory, and even tactile effects. In addition to positive hallucinations, negative hallucinations, where the subject fails to perceive some real external stimulus, may also be suggested. These are analogous, if not identical, to the everyday situation where a person is looking directly at an object that he is searching for but fails to notice it. Those portions of the external environment that are not altered by hypnotic suggestions are generally perceived accurately if noticed by the subject (Orne, 1962d).

Hallucinations in general are difficult to elicit under hypnosis, and there is a differential difficulty between the various sensory modalities. Tactile hallucinations are comparatively easy to produce. Suggesting to a group of nonhypnotized subjects that they should notice that their noses are beginning to itch will produce an effect in many of them. So will reading a paragraph describing the wording that might be used in making such a suggestion. The relatively vague senses of olfaction and gustation are also more amenable to suggestion than the more highly developed senses of audition and vision (Hilgard, 1968).

There is much conflict in the literature when it comes to specifying how difficult it is to produce a given type of hallucination. With unselected subjects, Faw and Wilcox (1958) reported that only 4% of subjects reported seeing a visual hallucination, and none reported believing in its objective reality ($N = 80$). Weitzenhoffer and Hilgard (1962) found that only 9% of unselected subjects experienced a suggested auditory hallucination ($N = 203$).

On the other hand, Spanos and Barber (1968) and Barber and Calverley (1964k) have found that the baseline for auditory and visual hallucinations in nonhypnotized, randomly selected subjects was surprisingly high, ranging from 48 to 54% for auditory and 27 to 33% for visual hallucinations. Either hypnotic suggestions or task-motivational instructions were found to increase the percentage of subjects developing both types of hallucinations. However, when subjects were told specifically to be honest in their reports and not to say things just to please the experimenter, this demand for honesty showed that no increase over the baseline for visual hallucinations was produced by either hypnosis or task-motivational instructions. No increase over the baseline for auditory hallucinations was produced by task-motivational instructions, but one was produced by hypnotic suggestion. One of the reasons for the conflict noted in the data is that different researchers use different criteria for the occurrence of a hallucination.

Orne (1962d) points out that when a visual hallucination is suggested to a subject he may react in a variety of ways. He may act as though he sees what has been suggested or seem disturbed because he does not experience it. In the former case, if he is questioned after the experience, he may say that (1) he saw nothing but felt compelled to act as if he did; (2) he experienced a visual image but knew it was unreal; (3) he experienced a real external image but it had illogical aspects to it (e.g., he could see a chair through a hallucinated person); or (4) he experienced an image indistinguishable from reality. Thus Orne categorized the subject's subjective experience into one of four categories. He considers only the last two as true hallucinations. In actuality, there is probably an infinite series of gradations of subject responses, and individual investigators differ in what they define as a positive response to a suggested hallucination.

Another point needs to be made: there is no way for an experimenter to observe the subject's hallucination directly. Hence he or she must rely on the subject's verbal report of his or her experiences. Thus it is possible, and indeed probable, that one subject who experiences a hallucination more vividly than another may report it as less vivid because of individual differences in the use of language and subjective standards of what the term *vivid* means. This is the same problem experienced by dream researchers who purport to be studying dreams but are actually studying verbal reports of dreams. The only hallucinations that an investigator can observe directly are his or her own, and these are necessarily individual and atypical. The question about the relative subjective experiences of two different subjects reporting their own hallucinations, no matter how similar or different their verbal descriptions, is as unanswerable by observation as is the question of whether two subjects describing the same stimulus as blue are having the same or radically different subjective experiences. Such questions are philosophical, not scientific, ones.

Although the degree of the apparent reality of a hallucination can only be estimated by a verbal report, Orne (1962d) attempts to distinguish effects that are actually experienced from those that are simulated by subjects motivated to produce what the experimenter wants them to by the use of stimulating subjects. These are subjects who have not been hypnotized but have been instructed to act as if they have been and to attempt to deceive the experimenter making the behavioral observations (who is not told which subjects are actually hypnotized). Simulators are usually informed that if the experimenter discovers that they are simulating, he or she will halt the procedure; hence, its continuation lets the simulator know he is successful in efforts at deception. The logic behind the use of simulating subjects is that both hypnotized subjects and simulators are equally motivated to produce the suggested behavior, but if only the hypnotic subjects actually experience the effects suggested, their behavior may be different to some degree from that of the subjects who are faking an effect. The lack of knowledge on the part of the experimenter of the real or simulating status of a subject eliminates experimenter bias and prevents any unconscious systematic differential treatment of the two types of subjects.

There are behavioral differences between real subjects and simulators. If a subject is told to hallucinate the experimenter sitting in a chair and is then told to turn around and look at where the experimenter really is, he will often appear surprised and report seeing him twice. He may not know which image is real. (Some subjects will distinguish the real from the hallucinated image by having the hallucinated one raise his hand.) Simulating subjects will usually deny seeing the experimenter when looking at him because they believe they are not supposed to.

If a negative hallucination is suggested so that the subject is told he can no longer see a chair and then is asked to walk in a direct line with the chair, hypnotized subjects will avoid bumping into the chair, while simulators will usually walk into it.

Spanos, Churchill, and McPeake (1976) found that a cooperative attitude toward hypnosis and involvement in everyday fantasy were each positively correlated with the ability of a subject to experience visual and auditory hallucinations. Visual hallucinations were more difficult to produce than auditory hallucinations, but they found that the abilities to produce these two types of hallucinations were correlated. They reported no sex difference in the ability to hallucinate. A large majority of their subjects reported their experiences as imagined rather than seen or heard.

Ham and Spanos (1974) report that with 60 male and female subjects equally assigned to hypnotic and task-motivational groups, the task-motivated subjects performed better in response to suggestions of visual or auditory hallucination. Spanos, Mullens, and Rivers (1979) in a 2 x 3 factorial study compared hypnotic and task-motivated subjects in performance of visual and auditory hallucinations in response to brief suggestions, long suggestions, and suggestions providing an imaginary context. Task-motivated subjects performed better than hypnotic subjects on auditory hallucinations, and the authors report a "trend toward significance" in this direction on visual hallucinations. Both long and image-involving suggestions were equally more effective than short suggestions for auditory hallucinations but were not significantly different for visual hallucinations.

Barber (1964e) concluded that the research failed to demonstrate that hypnosis produces auditory or visual hallucinations that are the same as perceptions or different from imagination. Erickson (1938a; 1938b), on the other hand, took the position that often hallucinations are quite real and reported that suggestions of negative auditory hallucinations, or deafness, could not be distinguished from organic deafness by ordinary means. His subjects displayed no startle response to an unexpected loud sound, failed to raise their voices in speaking when background noise was increased, or failed to blush to auditory stimuli that would normally produce such a response in a particular subject. He also found that a conditioned finger withdrawal response to an auditory-conditioned stimulus disappeared during hypnotically suggested deafness and reappeared after the hypnosis. Black and Wigan (Barber, 1964c) found a similar result with an autonomic nervous system response not under conscious control as a finger flexion is. Pattie (1935) reported the failure to produce uniocular blindness in a small group of subjects as disclosed by stereoscopes, filter, and Flees box tests. To reconcile these conflicting views, it will be necessary to sample a number of lines of research.

Barber and Calverley (1964j) report that suggestions of deafness were effective in 15 hypnotized and 15 nonhypnotized subjects. However, if these subjects were subjected to delayed auditory feedback where the sound of their own voices was delayed slightly, they reacted as do typical subjects with normal hearing by stuttering, mispronouncing words, increasing vocal intensity, and talking more slowly.

Barber (1964c) reports that in hypnotically suggested deafness in one ear, subjects who display positive results still report hearing a beat note if stimulated with slightly different frequencies in each ear. Weitzenhoffer criticized this study on the grounds that the frequency applied to the "deaf" ear could have reached the other by bone conduction, but it is interesting to note that the one subject who did not experience the beat note was a physics major presumably familiar with the phenomenon of beat notes.

In a study providing results analogous to the common finding that hypnotic pain control has little effect on physiological measures correlated with pain, Sabourin, Brisson, and Deschambault (1980) found that hypnotically induced deafness did not influence a conditioned heart rate response or the response time in a key-pressing task to an auditory stimulus in subjects reporting a positive subjective effect.

Spanos, Jones, and Malfara (1982) found that high-susceptibility subjects reported greater deafness than low-susceptibility subjects in response to suggestions of unilateral deafness but did not differ objectively in impairment from the latter as measured by responses to words presented in dichotic pairs. Crawford, MacDonald, and Hilgard (1979) found that reduction in hearing in response to hypnotic suggestion correlated 0.59 with hypnotic susceptibility but the "hidden observer" technique (see p. 116) disclosed that covert hearing was at least 20% greater than reported overtly by the subjects.

Subjects who are instructed to hallucinate a background (which normally produces an optical illusion effect) over a figure do experience such an illusion but not as strongly as they would with a real picture of the background added and no more than nonhypnotized subjects instructed to imagine the background (Barber, 1964e). Miller, Hennessy, and Leibowitz (1973) found that if such an illusion-producing background was negatively hallucinated away, the Ponzo illusion did not disappear.

Hypnotic subjects capable of negatively hallucinating portions of visual stimuli showed varying degrees of ability to attenuate the Tatchner-Ebbinghaus circles illusion posthypnotically (Blum, Nash, Jansen, and Barbour, 1981). Miller and Leibowitz (1976) found that a hypnotically produced restriction of the visual field produced behavior no different from that obtained from a group of simulators. Similar results were reported by Leibowitz, Lundy, and Guez (1980). Leibowitz, Post, Rodemer, Wadlington, and Lundy (1980) found that the amount of visual field narrowing occurring in response to instructions to simulate such narrowing was a function of the method of measurement, with direct measurement by perimetry yielding the most effect.

Dorcus (1937) found no pupillary reflex in response to suggestions of light intensity change. He also found that the postrotational eye movement (nystagmus) produced in four subjects after hypnotic suggestions that the subject was rotating in a chair were voluntary and not the same as the eye movement produced by the same subjects when actually rotated. Also, falling responses

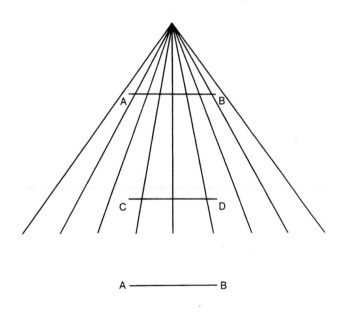

Figure 4-1. Ponzo Illusion.

following rotation suggestions did not appear unless the subjects had prior experience actually being rotated, and when produced under these circumstances, they were in the wrong direction for the rotation direction suggested.

Wallace (1980) reports that perceived autokinetic movement of a hypnotically hallucinated light was a function of hypnotic susceptibility as measured by the HGSHS. Since the subjects were all psychology students, it is not possible to confirm the present author's opinion that performance was also a function of the subject's knowledge of psychology. The suggestion of a hallucinated light in a dark room is an indirect suggestion to produce autokinetic motion to a knowledgeable subject.

Erickson (1939b), using very deeply hypnotized subjects, produced some degree of color blindness as measured by the Ishihara plates. Barber and Deeley (1961) report producing color-blind responses in nonhypnotized subjects by instructing them to "concentrate away from red and green." Cunningham and Blum (1982) and Harvey and Sipprelle (1978) found significant differences between the subjective experience reported by subjects successfully experiencing hypnotically suggested color blindness and the behavior of people with congenital defects in color vision.

Some subjects who are instructed to hallucinate colors either under hypnosis or task-motivational instructions report the occurrence of negative afterimages. Barber (1964c, 1959b) suggests that such reports do not occur in subjects who are naive concerning the phenomena of negative color afterimages, but if they do occur, the afterimage colors reported are those commonly described in elementary psychology texts—that is, the complementary color of the one hallucinated (e.g., red-green, blue-yellow) instead of the somewhat different (more pastel) colors usually reported in actual negative afterimages. Similarly, if an actual color was shown and the subject was told it was different, the actual color, not the hallucinated one, determined the nature of the afterimage (Barber, 1964d).

In view of the foregoing studies, the question arises about which viewpoint, Barber's or Erickson's, is correct concerning the reality or validity of positive and negative hypnotic hallucinations. In the view of the author, both are correct. Erickson is right that these are real experiences; Barber is right that hallucinations are different from ordinary sensations. Hypnotic blindness or deafness is not the same as organic blindness or deafness any more than hysterical blindness or deafness is.

Of course, negative afterimages do not occur in subjects not familiar with this phenomenon. How could they? A negative afterimage produced by a real external stimulus is a retinal phenomenon produced by the differential fatigue of different visual receptors. A hallucinated color does not result from retinal activity but from suggestions reaching the cerebral cortex. Sensations or physiological responses in sense organs are not modified in hypnotic hallucinations; perceptions or higher-level mental processes are. An afterimage produced to a hallucinated color is as much a suggested effect as the color itself. It is an excellent example of an indirect suggestion. This does not mean that it is not experienced.

The real question asked when we inquire about the reality of a hypnotically induced hallucination is, How vivid is it, or How similarly does the subject experience it to a real external stimulus? This is an unanswerable question. Trying to render the question answerable by equating "real" with similarity to a sensory experience in a physiological sense only introduces confusion.

In spite of their rather divergent views, the work of Barber (1958d) and Erickson (1944) seems to support the general conclusion that subjects given hypnotic suggestions of deafness or blindness for a particular person or object behave as though they are trying to avoid perceiving that person or object. Subjects try to avoid focusing or looking at the subject of the negative hallucination or report perceiving it vaguely. A similar result is reported by Hilgard and colleagues for negative hallucinations of pain in that a subject able to ignore the suffering aspects of pain will still report experiencing the sensations in some manner if he is instructed that there is a hidden observer who can report these sensations (Hilgard, Morgan, MacDonald, 1975). Barber claims that to get a subject not to experience the object of a negative hallucination, it is necessary to convince him of the objective truth of the experimenter's statement that the object is no longer present. Thus, if a subject is told that a chair is no longer present, he will try to look away from it but will not bump into it if it is directly in his path of travel. If, on the other hand, noises are made simulating the removal of the chair while the subject's eyes are shut, he will act as though he really does not see it at some level and will walk directly into it. Erickson reported a similar effect when a subject acted as though he really did not see one negatively hallucinated person but did show some signs of perceiving another for whom the suggestions were made more recently. He ascribed this difference in reactions, in accordance with his characteristic view that a very deep trance is required for this effect, to the fact that it takes time for the suggestions to become fully effective.

Although it seems clear that a positive hallucination of a complex sense modality like vision originates in the cortex, not in a sense organ, some of the easier-to-elicit tactile hallucinations may, partially at least, involve paying attention to a certain amount of dermal stimulation normally present and customarily ignored.

In the case of a negative hallucination there are several alternative mechanisms that are possible and not necessarily mutually exclusive. The classic study, in which afferent impulses traveling on a cat's auditory nerve in response to the ticking of a clock were terminated by the cat's focusing its attention on a mouse moved into its visual field, suggests that the cortex's responses to hypnotic suggestions may generate inhibitory neural impulses that travel down to the sense organs. This does not appear likely with respect to hypnotically induced deafness, for the subject who responds well to this suggestion and appears to be deaf will readily respond to auditory suggestions made by the hypnotist, particularly suggestions that his hearing is now restored. It seems probable, in view of most of the studies reported, that the mechanism of negative hallucinations is similar to that of positive ones and involves the cortical rather than the peripheral aspects of perception. Some subjects may be quite frightened or upset when experiencing hypnotic blindness or deafness, which suggests that they are experiencing a real effect and not just role playing, but there is no way of proving that the emotional reaction is not also being role played.

Stage hypnotists in demonstrating hallucinations will usually use the relatively easier-to-elicit gustatory or olfactory hallucinations. For example, they will tell a subject that a lemon he is sucking is very sweet or a bottle of ammonia contains a pleasant perfume. A stage hypnotist who tries to demonstrate a visual hallucination will usually tell a group of subjects that they are watching a funny or sad television program. How much of the subject's laughter or other emotional reaction is due to a real hallucination as opposed to the effect of the responses of the other subjects and the presence of the audience is hard to estimate, but the effect of these factors is probably considerable.

TRANCE LOGIC

Trance logic is a term coined by Orne (1959) and is often regarded by state theorists as one of the unique characteristics of a deep trance state (Perry and Walsh, 1978). It refers to the ability of a deeply hypnotized subject to tolerate, without apparent disturbance, the coexistence of two or more logically inconsistent perceptions or ideas. In examples of trance logic, two perceptions are usually involved: one hypnotically suggested and one purely sensory. Orne regards the double hallucination effect, where the subject sees a hallucinated person or object in one location and the real person or object in its actual location simultaneously, as a prime example of trance logic. The common description of a hallucinated object as transparent is another example of a hypnotized subject's accepting a perception at odds with all his previous experience and is therefore also an example of trance logic. The essence of this phenomenon seems to be the suspension of critical thinking. It is clearly different from the notion of "logic-tight compartments" in the mind where most people harbor totally inconsistent ideas (such as the pacifist who is prepared to demonstrate violently for peace), because in trance logic, the inconsistent perceptions are not kept isolated but appear in juxtaposition. It does appear quite similar to the common phenomenon of people accepting as reasonable all kinds of experiences during nocturnal dreams that they would be dumbfounded by in waking life (e.g., one dream character turning into another).

Sheehan (1977), Sheehan, Obstoj, and McConkey (1976), and Mc-Donald and Smith (1975) have experimentally investigated this phenomenon in studies with hypnotic and simulating subjects. In general, the results of these studies are not clear-cut. Subjects who are good enough to develop difficult visual hallucinations often but not invariably report double hallucinations. Simulators also often report double hallucinations to the extent that it would be difficult to distinguish hypnotized subjects from simulators on this basis. This, however, does not justify a conclusion that trance logic occurs in nonhypnotized subjects and hence is not an important index of hypnosis. Whether reports of double hallucinations are obtained often depends on the experimental manipulations. For example, under "high-cue" conditions, subjects who report experiencing the suggested hallucinations are asked to look directly at the real objects and describe what they see. This command directs the subject's attention to the object and may imply what the experimenter expects. It is more likely to result in a report of a double hallucination, therefore, than the "low-cue" condition in which the subject is merely asked to look around the room and report what he sees.

All that can be learned from the use of simulating subjects is whether a hypnotized subject's behavior can be accounted for solely in terms of motivation or role playing. It does not permit the inference that because role playing and hypnotized subjects behave similarly, their subjective states of mind are similar or that the causes of their objective behavior are identical. Clearly those simulating subjects who responded with a report of a double hallucination did so because they thought that was what was expected of them. Those who did not report a double hallucination failed to do so for the same reason. There was nothing at all incongruous about this situation to them. Hypnotized subjects, on the other hand, who report double hallucinations often report themselves confused by this state of affairs and cannot account for it, as simulators often do, by saying glibly, "It is because I am hypnotized." With respect to hypnotic subjects who do not report double hallucinations, it may be that this is because of their unique interpretation of the experimental instructions. In other words, the suggestion to hallucinate a person seated in a chair may also carry the implied or indirect suggestion to some subjects to negatively hallucinate the real person.

HYPNOTIC ANALGESIA AND ANESTHESIA

Pain is a complex and poorly understood subjective experience that involves more than the physiological reactions of pain receptors and their afferent pathways terminating in the cerebral cortex. This physiological component of the total experience of pain is usually referred to as pain sensation. The second major component of the total pain experience is generally referred to as suffering, and often this component is more distressing to a patient than the pain sensations themselves. All pain sensations are accompanied by, or occur in the context of, certain mental and physiological concomitants. The most common mental correlates of pain are the emotional responses of anxiety, fear, and apprehension. Physiological effects of either the pain sensations or the accompanying emotions may include blood pressure elevation, altered pulse or respiration rates, and possibly EKG and EEG changes. Increased muscular tension, facial grimacing, and withdrawal responses may also be noted. Some of these physiological responses, such as facial grimacing, are more subject to voluntary modification than others. Galvanic skin response (GSR) is also subject to variation with painful stimulation but is probably the least reliable index of perceived pain.

There is much conflict among studies that try to verify the analgesic effect of hypnotic suggestions by measuring these physiological analogues of pain, with some studies showing these indexes eliminated, reduced, or unaffected. Usually the more voluntary physiological components of a pain response are diminished, while the involuntary ones remain (Hilgard, 1975, 1977). As Orne (1976) points out, it is a mistake to evaluate the effectiveness of hypnotic pain control by the effect it has on physiological responses to pain. Pain and suffering are subjective experiences and can be quite different from what these more objective measures may indicate.

There are often great differences between what the clinical and experimental literature indicate with respect to the issue of hypnotic pain control. An important reason for these seeming discrepancies is the fact that clinical pain usually results from some organic or at least functional pathology and thus carries with it considerably more threat and anxiety than laboratory-induced pain, which the subject is aware is innocuous and will terminate with the experimental manipulation.

Beecher (1946) reported that soldiers suffering severe wounds in combat suffered surprisingly little from pain in comparison to comparable civilian injuries. Only about one-fourth of them requested a painkiller. That this lack of sensitivity to the suffering aspect of pain was not due to shock was demonstrated by the fact that these men complained about the pain of inept venous punctures. The suggestion is that the comparative freedom from suffering was due to the fact that the wound removed them from a highly traumatic combat situation in an honorable and face-saving manner, whereas a similar injury to a civilian involved in an auto accident would simply be a disaster with no positive aspects.

Barber (1959a, 1960a, 1963) has taken the view that pain is a complex phenomenon and that not all aspects of it are abolished by hypnosis. He notes that in patients who achieve pain control after a prefontal lobotomy, the sensation of pain is usually still present, but the patient is no longer bothered by it. He therefore takes the view that what hypnosis does is eliminate not the sensation of pain but the accompanying anxiety, worry, and concern and the readiness of the patient to concentrate on and respond to the pain. In other words, he believes that the suffering rather than the pain is what is controlled. Only about 5% to 25% of the population are capable of experiencing such classic hypnotic effects as age regression, hallucinations, analgesia, and amnesia. He believes that persons who are able to achieve these effects under hypnosis are capable of achieving similar effects without an induction procedure, and thus there is no need for the concept of a trance state. At the time of these writings, he claimed that there was no evidence that hypnosis gave better pain relief than a placebo, although Orne's (1976) later work would appear to establish that it does.

Other factors in the apparent control of pain that Barber considers are amnesia for the pain experienced or the reluctance of patients to tell the physician that they have experienced pain (and hence his or her efforts were a failure). Barber claimed that the essential factors in the success of hypnotic pain relief are not the trance state but (1) suggestions of pain control made within the context of (2) a close, personal relationship with the therapist. He also found the common clinical observation of no relationship between the depth of the trance as ordinarily measured and pain relief.

In more recent research, Barber (1974) measured the pain responses of waking subjects to heavy weights on their fingers and to immersion of their hands in ice water as a baseline measure. These procedures were then repeated with half of the subjects hypnotized and half awake. The hypnotic and control subjects were further subdivided; some received no suggestions, while others, on a random basis, were either instructed to think of something pleasant or to imagine that the area stimulated was numb and insensitive. He found that all groups given suggestions, whether hypnotized or not, reported reduced pain, and he concluded that this was due to their employment of a "cognitive strategy." Spanos, Horton, and Chaves (1975) reported similar results using unhypnotized subjects.

With respect to the use of hypnoanesthesia in surgical procedures, Chaves and Barber (1976) are equally skeptical and point out that most of the internal viscera are not sensitive to cutting pain (although they are sensitive to stretching), and the major pain sensations from most surgery arise from the skin incision. They also cite numerous instances of physiological signs that patients under hypnoanesthesia may indeed by experiencing pain. In their view, at least six factors are commonly involved in hypnotic surgical pain control:

1. Careful patient selection (probably less than 10% of the population is suitable for this type of anesthesia).
2. The patient-physician relationship.
3. Preoperative education and "walking the patient through" all of the procedures to reduce uncertainty and apprehension.

4. Adjunctive use of drugs, including local anesthetics to control skin pain and anti-anxiety and relaxing agents.
5. Suggestions of analgesia.
6. Procedures to distract the patient from his pain.

They believe that these same factors also account for the success of acupuncture.

In 1964, Barber and Hahn did an inverse study to measure the ability of hypnosis to produce rather than alleviate pain. After establishing waking baselines for subjective reports of pain and physiological reactions to it by having subjects immerse a hand in 2°C water without pain-reducing suggestions, subjects were divided into one hypnosis and three control groups. One control group and the hypnosis group were told to imagine that they were again experiencing hand immersion in the cold water while inserting their hands in water at room temperature. A second control group was reexposed to the cold water, and the third control group was exposed to the room-temperature water. They found that the suggestion to imagine the painful stimulation was more effective with the hypnotic than the control group with respect to eliciting subjective reports of pain and discomfort, but the physiological effects produced were the same for both groups: increased heart rate, frontalis muscle tension, and reduced skin resistance. These responses were similar to those of the second group (cold water) and different from those of the third control group (room temperature water). Spanos, Radtke-Bodrik, Ferguson, and Jones (1979), in an attempt to assess strategies used by subjects to control cold pressor pain, assigned subjects, stratified for hypnotic susceptibility, into four treatment groups: hypnosis plus suggestions of analgesia, hypnosis alone, suggestions alone, and no hypnosis and no suggestions. They found that high susceptibles reported the use of more cognitive strategies and achieved greater pain control whether or not they were given suggestions, provided they were "noncatastrophizers" (i.e., did not dwell on the unpleasantness of the pain situation). The variable of hypnosis failed to affect either strategy use or pain control.

In a study involving high-susceptibility subjects and cold pressor pain, Stam and Spanos (1980) found that the relative effectiveness of hypnotic analgesia, waking suggestions, or no suggestions was a function of subject expectations produced by varying the order of these treatments. Similarly Spanos, Kennedy, and Gwynn (1984) report that when suggestions of control of cold pressor pain were preceded by a hypnotic induction procedure, hypnotic susceptibility was positively correlated with success in pain control, whereas with the same suggestions given in the absence of an induction ritual success was unrelated to susceptibility, although pain reduction was as great as in the hypnosis group and greater than in a control group given no suggestions or hypnosis. They interpret these results as indicating that the relationship between hypnotic susceptibility and hypnotic analgesia is modified by the subject's attitude and expectancies in situations defined as hypnosis.

In a study not involving hypnotic induction, Spanos, McNeil, Gwynn, and Stam (1984) found that while suggestions for analgesia were more successful for high- than low-susceptibility subjects, the use of a shadowing task (a distraction procedure) was equally effective as suggestion in pain control for both high- and low-susceptibility subjects. Furthermore, combining distraction and suggestion was no more effective than either technique alone. The authors interpret these results as speaking against a dissociation view of pain control. Similar results were reported by Farthing, Venturino, and Brown (1984).

Orne (1976), while recognizing the difficulty imposed on research by the subjective nature of the pain experience and the absence of any objective indexes of pain, nevertheless believes in the reality of hypnotic control, not just of suffering but of pain sensation itself. He believes that this is so in spite of the research involving automatic writing or Hilgard's method of getting subjective reports from a *hidden observer* within a subject, which indicates that, under hypnoanalgesia, pain sensation does arrive at the cerebral cortex. Evidently the effect of hypnosis is to alter the normal cognitive processing of these impulses so that the subject is not aware of them to the usual extent.

In order to demonstrate that hypnoanalgesia was more than a mere placebo effect, he designed a study with a hypnotic group of 12 highly susceptible subjects and a control group of 12 low-susceptibility subjects to demonstrate that any effect produced by the nonhypnotized group was unlikely to have been produced by inadvertent hypnosis. The study was a double-blind design, with the experimenter unaware of which subjects were high or low in hypnotic susceptibility. To prevent the low-susceptibility subjects themselves from finding out about their status, they were subjected to a session of relaxation suggestions that produced a deep state of relaxation and were given suggestions that one of their hands would become analgesic. They were then given electric shocks in each hand, and by a surreptitious manipulation of voltage, were made to believe that they had produced a marked analgesia in the suggested hand. All subjects were then given baseline measurements of their tolerance for ischemic pain by means of a pumping task, while blood flow to their arms was occluded with a blood pressure cuff inflated to 200 millimeters of mercury. All subjects were then subjected to a relaxation method of hypnotic induction, and analgesia was suggested in one arm. Tolerance for pain was then reassessed.

In a third session, subjects were given what they were told was a powerful new drug to control ischemic pain. Results showed that both hypnotized and nonhypnotized subjects produced elevated ischemic pain thresholds, but the effect was much greater for hypnotic subjects. The responses of both groups to the placebo were identical. These results strongly suggest that there is a different mechanism at work in hypnosis than in a placebo in spite of the widespread impression to the contrary (Kihlstrom, 1979). Orne takes the view that these two effects are probably additive. Recent pharmacological research has cast some light on the probable mechanism of a placebo effect. The fact that a chemical that counteracts the effect of morphine also counteracts a placebo effect suggests that morphine-like endorphins are produced in the brain in response to a placebo, and the ultimate mechanism of a placebo may thus be a chemical one.

Sternbach (1982) reports on a pilot study attempting to investigate the chemical mechanism for hypnotic analgesia. The hypothesis that this might be mediated by acetylcholine in the brain was not supported since atropine (an inhibitor of acetylcholine) did not significantly reduce hypnotic analgesia. Frid and Singer (1979) report that naloxone (an opiate antagonist) inhibits hypnotic analgesia of ischemic pain in the presence of stress much more than under conditions of no stress. The present author believes this indicates the potential of stress per se to generate endorphins rather than to suggest their presence is involved in the mechanism of hypnotic pain control.

The fact that about 90% of the population shows an increase in pain threshold with hypnotic suggestion while only about 20% of the population is capable of attaining a deep trance is cited as further evidence of the different processes involved in hypnotic pain control. Orne (1976) thinks that hypnotic analgesia is best viewed as a negative hallucination for pain and, like all other hallucination phenomena, requires a very good subject. Although he does not believe it is often indicated in the treatment of functional pain, where it is important to understand the meaning of pain, he believes it is useful for temporary physician-induced pain or for chronic organic pain of known etiology. Hypnoanalgesia, where indicated, is safe, nonaddictive, and produces no dangerous side effects.

West, Niell, and Hardy (1952), using seven subjects as their own controls, reported hypnotic suggestions were effective in elevating pain thresholds for noxious thermal stimuli. These suggestions also reduced the subjects' ability to discriminate among stimuli of different intensities. GSR to noxious stimulation was diminished and sometimes eliminated. They also reported some correlation between depth of hypnosis and the degree of pain modification obtained.

Stacher and his associates (1975) demonstrated that while relaxation instructions given either in the waking state or under hypnosis were effective in raising pain threshold and tolerance to an electric stimulus, suggestions of both relaxation and analgesia resulted in greater increase in threshold and tolerance when given under hypnosis. This study is in opposition to the sometimes reported view that a pain threshold is relatively more subject to physiological variables, while pain tolerance (as suggested by Barber) is more subject to psychological factors. Here there was considerable interdependence shown between these two dependent measures.

Wallace and his colleagues have demonstrated that with hypnoanalgesia suggested in an arm, proprioceptors in the joints were also affected, and the lack of proprioceptive feedback produced a decrement in the ability of a subject to touch his nose with his eyes closed, to draw, or to compensate for visual distortions produced by perceiving arm motion through prisms (Garrett and Wallace, 1975; Wallace, 1976; Wallace and Garrett, 1975; Wallace and Hoyenga, 1980, 1981).

Spanos and his associates failed to replicate the findings of Wallace and Fisher (1979) and Wallace and Garrett (1975) that high-susceptibility subjects with hypnotically induced arm anesthesia fail to develop a reduction in pointing accuracy following the removal of displacing prisms from the eyes (Spanos, Gorassini, and Petrusic, 1981; Spanos, Dubreuil, Saad, and Gorassini, 1983). They found that highly susceptible hypnotic subjects, low-susceptible simulators, and control subjects given no special instructions all displayed a large aftereffect and speculate that the results of Wallace and his associates may have been due to the inadvertent cueing of subjects of the expectations of the experimenters. Wallace and Fisher (1982, 1984), on the other hand, defend their findings by pointing out differences in procedure between their research and the attempted replication. This controversy points up a common problem in research: the failure to distinguish between a replication study and a study designed to correct perceived shortcomings in the design of a previous study.

The function of a replication study is to increase confidence in previous findings. Thus if statistical tests show an effect to be significant at the 0.01 level (which means the results would not be obtained by chance alone more than one time in 100), then replicating this study and getting results again significant at the 0.01 level means that the real significance level is $0.01 \times 0.01 = 0.0001$; that is, the result would not occur by chance alone more than one time in 10,000. Thus replication provides a measure of significance that would require uneconomically large samples to demonstrate in a single study. Unfortunately, replication studies are rare since most journals are reluctant to publish them, preferring original research. There is a real need for journals that will publish replicating studies.

If a study is designed to demonstrate a defect in a previous study or demonstrate that the results would have been different under different circumstances, the preferable procedure would be to replicate the original study exactly and then rerun it with the appropriate changes. This may be impossible to do because the original procedure may not be reported in enough detail due to space restrictions in journals. However, since this was not done in the present situation, it is possible for the kind of controversy reported to go on indefinitely, with no way of conclusively resolving the issue.

Hilgard (1977a) investigated the question of how a subject's ability to control pain hypnotically was related to measured hypnotic susceptibility. Subjects were rated on form A of the Stanford Hypnotic Susceptibility Scale (SHSS) and were exposed to cold pressor pain of the hand using water of 0°, 5°, and 10°C. Although some subjects were able to reduce their pain completely, most did not. Two-thirds of the most susceptible group (scores on SHSS of 8-12) were able to reduce their pain by one-third or more to a readily tolerable level. Only one-eighth of the least susceptible group (score on SHSS of 0-3) were able to do this well. The correlation between hypnotic susceptibility and success in pain reduction was 0.5, which demonstrated a positive relationship between these two factors. While cold pressor tests permit the subject to give verbal subjective reports of pain intensity on a scale of 1 to 10, the pain intensity increases so rapidly there is no time to get relative reports on the pain and suffering components separately during stimulation. Hence Hilgard also utilized ischemic pain, which may take as much as 20 minutes to reach its maximum (as opposed to 60 seconds in cold pressor pain). He was able to get subjective reports on both sensory pain and suffering during exposure to the pain-producing stimulus. Ischemic pain control is related to hypnotic susceptibility in the same manner as cold pressor pain control.

The results showed that, unlike the situation in lobotomies, hypnotic analgesia reduced both pain and distress, not just the latter. Hilgard agrees with Orne that the effect of hypnosis is not accounted for in terms of either a placebo effect or anxiety reduction, although these variables are involved. He cites a 1973 study by Chapman and Feather, which showed that while anxiety was being reduced by Valium, pain could continue to increase.

Hilgard also investigated the paradoxical situation of subjects who reported satisfactory subjective pain control but still displayed the same physiological responses to pain as subjects normally experiencing the pain would have, such as increased heart rate and blood pressure. Voluntary responses such as grimacing, muscle tension, and verbal exclamations tended to diminish (Hilgard and Morgan, 1975).

This puzzle was resolved by Hilgard's discovery, through the agency of automatic writing, that some pain was still being experienced at a covert level. This pain was generally greater than reported overtly under hypnotic analgesia but of a lower level than would normally be expected (Hilgard, 1978). Kline (1978) described a clinical patient having thyroid surgery performed painlessly under hypnoanesthesia whose arm, under instructions for automatic writing, wrote: "You SOB, you are killing me!"

Hilgard (1978) and his associates developed the technique of *automatic talking* in lieu of the automatic writing method. Subjects were instructed that when the experimenter touched their shoulder, "a hidden part of you that knows things that are going on in your body, things that are unknown to the part of you to which I am now talking" would talk to the experimenter. Subjects were told that they would not know what the other part was saying or even that it was talking. This other part of the subject was dubbed the *hidden observer*.

Knox, Morgan, and Hilgard (1974) subjected eight highly susceptible subjects to ischemic pain under conditions of waking, neutral hypnosis, and hypnosis with suggestions of analgesia. They found that subjects were able to distinguish and report on felt pain sensations and concomitant suffering on subjective numerical scales. Suggestions of analgesia reduced both pain sensations and suffering in the "open" reports for 90% of the subjects. The hidden observer reports of pain and suffering, however, obtained through automatic talking were not significantly different from open reports obtained under neutral hypnosis.

Hilgard, Morgan, and MacDonald (1975), using 20 highly susceptible subjects exposed to a cold pressor test, again attempted to verify that pain blocked by hypnoanalgesia can be perceived at some level. Three reports were obtained from subjects: the usual open, subjective verbal report on a numerical scale, a manual report by automatic key pressing, and a retrospective verbal report by the hidden observer technique. Nine subjects who were amnesic for both key pressing and automatic talking reported more pain in the automatic reports than in the open verbal reports. Eight of the nine, after release from amnesia, had a clear perception of the two levels of awareness of pain: the usual hypnotic experience of pain attenuation and the knowledge at another level of a more severe pain. Unlike the foregoing study, however, no subject gave a report of covert suffering.

These data required Hilgard to propose a two-component theory of hypnotic pain reduction that assumes the existence of two cognitive systems processing information at dissociated levels of awareness. It does not, however, cast doubt on the clinical effectiveness of hypnosis in pain control. Thus, the first component of pain reduction includes the effects of distraction of attention, relaxation, and anxiety control. It is available to patients with little hypnotic susceptibility and may account for the common observation that there is little relationship between trance depth and trance productivity in clinical practice.

The second component requires a deeper level of hypnosis because dissociation and amnesic reactions appear to be involved. This component permits a subject to process information about pain at a hidden level where it does not disturb him. This covert experience becomes available to consciousness only when special techniques such as the hidden observer or automatic writing are used to uncover it.

The implication of this line of research is that hypnosis affects the perception of pain by its action on cortical processes involved rather than by interrupting or blocking pain pathways. Hence, the fact that physiological responses to pain are present in subjects claiming not to experience the pain is neither paradoxical nor an indication that the subject is role playing or lying to avoid offending the hypnotist.

A *hidden observer* effect is not noted among all highly susceptible subjects given pain-reducing suggestions, with various studies reporting an incidence of from 87% of eight subjects to 39% of 23 subjects (Hilgard, Morgan, and MacDonald, 1975; Hilgard et al., 1978; Knox, Morgan, and Hilgard, 1974; Laurence and Perry, 1981). Laurence and Perry (1981) found that subjects who displayed a *hidden observer* effect also displayed a "duality" effect in response to age-regression suggestions. When regressed to age 5, they wrote and correctly spelled words well beyond the capacity of a 5-year-old as though part of their ego was regressed to the age of 5 and part retained its adult status. This adult part seems quite similar to an observing ego. Their work suggests that Hilgard's *hidden observer* may simply be a new name for an observing ego. Thus, although the term *hidden observer* is associated primarily with work in hypnoanalgesia, where it was coined, similar phenomena are observable in many research areas, such as hypnotic deafness and age regression (Williams, 1984). Subjects who did not display a *hidden observer* effect did not even attempt the writing task under age-regression suggestions.

Spanos and Hewitt (1980) took a social role rather than a dissociation view of the *hidden observer* effect and demonstrated that by manipulating subjects' expectations, *hidden observer* reports of less rather than more pain could be elicited. Hence they view this effect as an experimental artifact rather than a reflection of an unconscious level of processing sensory inputs. In response to criticism of their methodology by Laurence, Perry, and Kihlstrom (1983), Spanos (1983) noted that in many previous studies a *hidden observer* effect was not deemed to be present unless covert reports of greater pain than reported directly under hypnosis were made.

Laurence, Perry, and Kihlstrom (1983) point out that the fact that covert reports may be modifiable by suggestion does not demonstrate that they may not also reflect unconscious sensory processes.

The conclusions relating to the relative importance of the specific effects of hypnotic suggestions versus the general effects of relaxation and anxiety reduction of a placebo effect are based on research with the nonthreatening type of pain produced in the laboratory. In clinical practice, it is possible and even likely that the importance of these components may be reversed, and much more of the efficacy of hypnotic pain alleviation may be based on anxiety control rather than on hypnotic suggestion and dissociation. This may account for the fact that hypnoanalgesia and hypnoanesthesia are effective in such a relatively high percentage of patients. It may also explain why motivation is often capable of making a normally poor subject able to undergo surgery under hypnosis when chemical agents would be too dangerous.

In consonance with Hilgard's work with the *hidden observer,* Chertok, Michaux, and Droin (1977) reported on two patients who underwent surgery successfully under hypnoanesthesia and who were able to recall details of their experience under subsequent hypnotic recall. Both patients were able to recall experiencing the pain at different levels but did not report suffering. One of the patients described the pain as though it were happening to someone else. When asked how the other woman felt, she replied, "It hurt her." An interesting sidelight of this work is the citation of studies indicating that even under chemical anesthesia, where the patient is assumed to be unconscious, patients can, under subsequent hypnosis, recall details of the conversation between the surgeons during the operation. The fact that emotional responses are evoked by these memories suggests that surgeons ought to be aware of this phenomenon and be careful of offhand remarks made in the presence of anesthetized patients, for these may elicit undesirable emotional reactions in patients and impede recovery, even if the patient is not consciously aware of the source of these reactions (Cheek, 1959, 1964, 1965, 1966).

Joseph Barber (1977) reports what he refers to as a *rapid induction analgesia (RIA)*, which is essentially a permissive induction procedure with suggestions of deep relaxation, a reinterpretation of experiences, and amnesia. He claims success rates of 27 out of 27 and 99 out of 100 subjects in producing dental analgesia for a wide variety of dental procedures without the need for chemical agents. The procedure takes from 11 to 20 minutes. The induction procedure itself does not appear to contain anything unusual enough to account for the atypically high success rate, unless the fact that the author was called in as an outside expert to induce the hypnosis enhanced his status with the subjects. Also, the procedure employs the novel step of developing the dental analgesia as a posthypnotic response instead of the more common practice of performing the work while the patient is in the trance state. If these success rates prove to be replicable, it would suggest the need for additional research to determine both the essential element that produces this high success rate and the limits of applicability of this technique in other areas.

Some subsequent studies have failed to replicate these findings, however. Gillett and Coe (1984), using J. Barber's procedure in its usual and a shortened form, found only a 52% success rate in 60 unselected dental patients. Success in pain control appeared unrelated to hypnotic susceptibility. Barber's procedure was modified in this study, however, in that tape-recorded rather than personal inductions were used, and no preoperative testing of analgesia was performed. Also, the standards for failure of analgesia were different and more stringent in Gillett and Coe's study. A request by the patient for additional posthypnotic cue presentation was regarded as a failure of pain control.

Using a cold pressor test rather than clinical dental work as a source of pain, Van Gorp, Meyer, and Dunbar (1985) found that RIA did not control pain when compared with a control group, while traditional hypnosis did.

Similarly, Skiba (1983) compared RIA with traditional hypnosis in the control of cold pressor pain. Using a 2 between, 1 within variable, 3 x 2 x 2 factorial design (susceptibility x order x treatment), with order of treatment counterbalanced, he found that traditional hypnosis decreased pain sensation and increased pain tolerance more effectively than RIA for all levels of susceptibility.   .

On the other hand, Fricton and Roth (1985), measuring threshold to electrical stimulation of tooth pulp as an indication of pain control, found that indirect hypnotic induction by Barber's method was superior to a direct induction technique in that it raised pain thresholds independently of the subject's hypnotic susceptibility. Direct induction techniques were found to be effective only in high-susceptibility subjects.

Melzack and Perry (1975), using patients suffering from chronic organic pain, found that alpha feedback training combined with hypnosis reduced pain, as measured by the McGill Pain Questionnaire, by 33% in 58% of the patients. Both the sensory and affective dimensions of the pain were diminished. Patients who received alpha feedback training alone increased their alpha output (as did subjects treated with hypnosis alone) but did not experience pain reduction. Subjects treated with hypnosis alone showed "substantial" but not significant pain decrease. The authors see the role of alpha production not as beneficial per se but as providing a distraction to the pain. They also speculate on the role of relaxation, ego strengthening, suggestion, and the development of a sense of control over the pain as contributing to the success of the combined treatment.

Ahlberg and colleagues (1975) compared the effects of hypnosis, placebo acupuncture, and acupuncture in the control of pain produced by electrical stimulation near the supraorbital nerve in 14 subjects. As the stimulus intensity was increased, the levels necessary to produce a minimum sensation, a minimum pain, and the maximum tolerable pain were successively noted. With hypnotic suggestions of analgesia, the intensities of stimulation needed to produce all of these effects were increased. Neither acupuncture nor placebo acupuncture produced any raising of these thresholds. In line with the previously described studies, neither hypnosis nor acupuncture consistently changed such physiological indexes as blood pressure, pulse rate, EKG, EEG, or respiratory rates.

Saletu and coworkers (1975) also compared hypnosis and acupuncture with each other and with analgesic drugs (morphine and ketamine). Pain, induced by electrical stimulation on the wrist, was evaluated by subjective and physiological measures. It was significantly reduced by both hypnosis and the drugs, but acupuncture was effective only when applied to the specific loci described in the literature and the needles were electrically activated. EEG changes in hypnosis varied with the wording of suggestions but were characterized in general by an increase in fast waves. Acupuncture produced just the opposite EEG changes. Evoked potential studies suggested that ketamine attenuates pain in the thalamocortical pathways while hypnosis, acupuncture, and morphine work on the higher-level pathways in the cortex.

Stern, Brown, Ulett, and Sletten (1977) found that ischemic and cold pressor pain control by hypnosis or morphine was related to hypnotic susceptibility, but the effectiveness of acupuncture was independent of susceptibility. Frost (1978) and Knox, Gekoski, Shum, and McLaughlin (1981) also discuss differences between hypnosis and acupuncture. MacHovec and Man (1978) report that correct-site acupuncture or hypnosis was more effective in treating smoking than placebo acupuncture or a placebo control condition, and individual hypnosis was more effective than acupuncture or group hypnosis. These studies taken together suggest that contrary to popular belief, hypnosis and acupuncture are likely to be two different phenomena in spite of their superficial similarities or the presence of implied suggestion in the acupuncture procedures. Also, both mechanisms are likely to be different from a mere placebo effect, although such an effect may be a concomitant of clinical procedures utilizing either technique.

Several authors have discussed similarities between meditation and hypnosis, and here the evidence that these are different phenomena is less convincing (Delmonte, 1984; Morse et al., 1977). It was found that success in reducing anxiety by meditation was predictable to some degree from hypnotic susceptibility (Heide, Wadlington, and Lundy, 1980).

POSTHYPNOTIC AMNESIA

Posthypnotic amnesia is a condition that occurs when, with or without explicit or implicit suggestions to do so, a subject is unable to remember some or all of the events that occurred in the hypnotic state when he is subsequently awakened. Typically these unavailable memories can be restored suddenly and without any intervening opportunity for relearning by means of a prearranged release signal. These memories are also freely retrievable in a subsequent hypnotic session. It is this property of reversibility or retrievability that differentiates true posthypnotic amnesia from some types of pseudo-amnesia, which may be caused by simple forgetting or by the failure to attend to or learn material while in the hypnotic state. The material lost as a result of this kind of pseudo-amnesia is not recoverable posthypnotically; the loss is permanent. The phenomenon of reversibility also demonstrates that posthypnotic amnesia is not caused by a failure to record material in the hypnotic state but by an interference with the normal retrieval or playback mechanism for gaining access to material in memory (Kihlstrom, 1977; Kihlstrom and Evans, 1976; Nace, Orne, and Hammer, 1974; Orne, 1966b; Spanos and Bodorik, 1977). This conflicts with Hilgard's hypothesis that posthypnotic amnesia occurs because subjects under hypnosis suffer from a reduced ability to retain memories just as sleeping subjects do. This is particularly so in view of the findings of Nace, Orne, and Hammer (1974) that there were no significant differences between high- and low-susceptibility subjects in total recall of events experienced under hypnosis. Furthermore, Orne (1966b) demonstrated that the suggestion made to subjects in stage 1 sleep that their noses would itch when a cue word was spoken elicited scratching behavior in subsequent stage 1 sleep. This suggestion was also effective on the following night, even though the subjects were amnesic for the suggestion during the waking interval between the two laboratory sessions. This suggests that even sleeping subjects may have more capacity to retain memories than is generally indicated (by studies showing that nocturnal dreams are usually forgotten if a subject is not awakened within 10 minutes of the REM period during which the dream occurred). Perhaps it was the active response of the subject to the suggestion that enabled the memory trace to be recorded.

While spontaneous posthypnotic amnesia is commonly regarded as a sign of somnambulism and is thought by some to be one of the signs of a deep hypnotic state, the experimental literature is in agreement that this phenomenon rarely occurs in the laboratory (Barber and Calverley, 1966c; Kihlstrom, 1977; Kihlstrom and Evans, 1977).

Kihlstrom and Twersky (1978) found that not only is posthypnotic amnesia not caused by poor waking memory but subjects displaying marked posthypnotic amnesia actually had superior long-term retention of intentionally learned material in the waking state.

Young and Cooper (1972) demonstrated the effect of implicit suggestion on the development of posthypnotic amnesia in subjects whose expectancies concerning the development of amnesia following hypnosis were manipulated. Half of their subjects were exposed to a prehypnotic lecture on hypnosis stating that posthypnotic amnesia invariably follows hypnosis, and the other half were told that it never occurs spontaneously. A significantly greater number of subjects expecting to develop posthypnotic amnesia developed it spontaneously.

In a study involving suggested rather that spontaneous posthypnotic amnesia, Ashford and Hammer (1978) found a nonsignificant relationship between inferred subject expectancies of posthypnotic amnesia and its subsequent development following its suggestion on the HGSHS:A. Simon and Salzberg (1985) also found that manipulating subjects' expectations had no effect on the occurrence of posthypnotic amnesia on the SHSS form A but hypnotic suggestion did. Hypnotic subjects given no specific suggestion for amnesia had less memory than nonhypnotized control groups, which suggests the possibility of self-suggestion. Perhaps the reason for the apparent conflict between this study and the findings of Young and Cooper was that in the present study subjects' expectancies were manipulated by having some of them read a paragraph denying the spontaneous occurrence of posthypnotic amnesia. None was cued to expect this phenomenon, and since the initial expectancy of posthypnotic amnesia in these subjects seemed to have been low to begin with, this "manipulation" may not have produced two groups differing in expectancies. Orne (1966b), on the other hand, cites the cross-cultural occurrence of spontaneously developed posthypnotic amnesia, particularly in hypnotic-like religious and mystic experiences. He believes that this phenomenon deserves more attention than a glib dismissal of it as being due to implicit suggestion. Orne further notes that emotionally charged material relived by patients during hypnosis is usually forgotten spontaneously on awakening. This material is often related in language appropriate to an earlier stage of life, and he suggests that part of the difficulty in memory may involve the need to translate this material into adult patterns of thought. He reports that patients have difficulty in integrating this type of material into present consciousness even after they have the opportunity to listen to a tape recording of their hypnotic session while awake. Kline (1966) also notes that amnesia is more common following hypnotherapy than other types of hypnosis, and its extent seems to be related more to the material brought up under hypnosis than to the depth of the trance.

As in many other areas of controversy in hypnosis, perhaps both sides in this conflict are right. Although the development of spontaneous amnesia is rare in the laboratory, typical hypnotic research does not deal with affect-laden events, and there is no dynamic need for subjects to display an unsuggested amnesia. In clinical practice, however, where affect-laden material is routinely dealt with under hypnosis, spontaneous amnesia may be more common. Indeed, under these circumstances, the amnesia may be caused by the same dynamic factors that produced the original repression rather than by any special properties of the hypnotic state. Thus, as Orne suggests, there may be two different mechanisms involved in the production of posthypnotic amnesia: one based on suggestions in experimental work and one based on repression in clinical phenomena. His idea that dissociation may result from essential differences between the hypnotic and waking thought processes is more difficult to square with the apparent lack of spontaneous amnesia in experimental work, unless it is realized that clinical investigations typically deal with personal memories as opposed to material learned under hypnosis. Suggested posthypnotic amnesia has many subclassifications. Generally it is not an all-or-none phenomenon and can vary in degree from complete to slight. This is indeed fortunate, for the occurrence of partial posthypnotic amnesia makes it possible to study the effects of hypnotic suggestions on the mechanisms of memory retrieval. This would not be possible if amnesia were complete (Evans and Kilhstrom, 1973).

Suggested posthypnotic amnesia can be general—all memories of the hypnotic experience are interfered with—or specific—only certain memories (either acquired under hypnosis or previous to it) are inhibited. In the former case, the subject may develop pseudo-memories and fill in the gaps with confabulations, as sometimes happens with patients having organic memory defects (Orne, 1966b). If a specific amnesia is suggested for a familiar name or a number, there will be marked differences in both the subjective experience and objective behaviors of subjects responding to such a suggestion. Some subjects will report totally forgetting the name or number, while others will report remembering it but be unable to pronounce it when challenged to do so. It is quite common for such a suggestion made to a group of subjects to be interpreted differently by individual subjects. Hence these differences in responses are not due merely to the wording of the suggestions but also to the individual interpretations of these words made by each subject (and possibly to individual differences in hypnotic depth and the resulting literalness of understanding).

There was a time when it was widely believed that in order for a posthypnotic suggestion to be effective it was necessary at the time of making the suggestion also to suggest a specific posthypnotic amnesia for it. Although this is no longer regarded as essential, Orne (1966b) believes that posthypnotic suggestions made with suggestions of amnesia tend to last longer. In any event, subjects carrying out posthypnotic suggestions without awareness of the source of their behavior tend to justify their seemingly odd conduct with rationalizations. Subjects aware of the cause of their behavior tend to experience a compulsion to carry out the suggested actions (Estabrooks, 1957; Orne, 1966b).

Posthypnotic amnesia may be divided into source amnesia or content amnesia. *Source amnesia* is commonly produced when a hypnotized subject is given some obscure bit of information that he would have been unlikely to be aware of prior to hypnosis. Following a suggestion for a general posthypnotic amnesia, it is found that he is immediately aware of this information on waking but is unaware of its source. This reaction, like most other hypnotic alterations of memory, is similar to the normal waking characteristics of memory. Most people retain factual information of the type learned in school in isolation from the context in which it was learned. Thus the average adult will be unable to tell the circumstances under which he learned the date of the discovery of America or the Pythagorean theorem. Source amnesia can be a source of torment for an author who remembers an appropriate quotation but cannot remember who said it. Memory that includes the contextual situation surrounding the information recalled is referred to as redintegration. It usually is related to personal experiences rather than factual or theoretical data. Unlike content amnesia, source amnesia is not often suggested explicitly under hypnosis and usually occurs spontaneously (Kilhstrom, 1977; Nace, Orne, and Hammer, 1974; Orne, 1966b; Thorne, 1969).

Evans (1979) found that source amnesia occurred in 31% and 33% of

29 and 12 deeply hypnotized subjects, respectively, who displayed a total recall amnesia for all other events under hypnosis, but it did not occur in 15 simulating subjects. Hence he concluded that it resulted from a dissociative phenomenon rather than the demand characteristics of the hypnotic situation or subtle cues given concerning the expectations of the experimenter (who was blind as to the hypnotic or simulating status of the subject).

Like all other posthypnotic phenomena, a posthypnotic amnesia can last for a variable period of time following termination of hypnosis. In some subjects, this period can be quite lengthy. A posthypnotic suggestion that a subject will not develop a posthypnotic amnesia or that one developed will terminate is usually effective in preventing any spontaneous amnesia. Besides being terminated suddenly by a posthypnotic release cue or the reinduction of hypnosis with suggestions that the subject will now be able to regain all memories from the previous hypnotic experience, hypnotic amnesia can be permitted to dissipate with the passage of time.

A 1949 film, *Unconscious Motivation,* was designed to demonstrate the effect of unconscious ideation on behavior. A male and a female college student were given the suggestion under hypnosis that as children they had failed to return a pocketbook they had found containing two coins and had used the coins to buy candy. The subjects were given a suggestion of posthypnotic amnesia for this fantasy, and it was found to produce an unpleasant affective state in them, although they were unable to assign a reason for their feelings. In spite of their lack of conscious awareness of this ideation, it affected their responses on TAT-like and Rorschach-like tests, as well as word association responses. The amnesia was broken down without a prearranged release signal by the kinds of associations used in psychotherapy. Often incomplete memories obtainable under conditions of posthypnotic amnesia can be used as a starting point for associations to break the amnesia, and sometimes total recall can be obtained soon after the first breakthrough is attained.

Orne (1966*b*) believes that memories retained during a suggested posthypnotic amnesia relate to events during relatively light periods of the trance. Thus, he believes that the effectiveness of a suggestion for posthypnotic amnesia is determined not by the overall depth of the trance but by its depth immediately preceding the suggestion of amnesia. A subject's failure to respond to suggestions early in the trance may not interfere with the development of the suggested amnesia, provided that he is given suggestions that he can respond to just prior to the suggestion for amnesia. The converse is also true; failed suggestions just prior to suggesting amnesia may interfere with its being developed in spite of previous successful tests of trance depth. This was demonstrated by giving the Harvard Group Scale of Hypnotic Susceptibility (HGSHS) to two groups of subjects. Test items were given to one group in ascending order of difficulty and to the other in descending order of difficulty. Although mean scores for the two groups did not differ, subjects getting the easier items last developed significantly more posthypnotic amnesia than the group getting the more difficult items last. Based on these results, Orne says that to facilitate the production of a posthypnotic amnesia, it should be linked with some suggestion that the subject has demonstrated he is capable of effectuating. For example, a subject who has developed a good response of arm catalepsy may be told that when he is awakened his arm will remain rigid, and he will not know why.

Orne further notes that there are clusters of hypnotic tasks for which performance tends to be highly correlated. Subjects who perform well on one item in the cluster generally perform well on others. He delineates these clusters as ideomotor behaviors, challenge items (such as arm catalepsy), and hallucination, posthypnotic suggestions, and amnesia. Thus, performance of some items within a cluster may serve as predictors of performance on other items in the cluster. He believes that posthypnotic amnesia is rare in subjects who fail challenge suggestions or fail to hallucinate.

Kilhstrom and Evans (1977) replicated Hilgard and Hommel's (1961) earlier finding that there is a residual deficit of memory remaining in subjects displaying suggested posthypnotic amnesia even after a prearranged release cue is given. Thus the reversibility of the memory deficit is not complete. Unlike Hilgard and Hommel, Kilhstrom and Evans tried to eliminate the effect of pseudo-amnesia by eliminating subjects low on hypnotic susceptibility and by considering the amount of memory retrieval by high-susceptibility subjects who displayed a true, reversible posthypnotic amnesia. Compared with equally high-susceptibility subjects not subjected to suggested amnesia, these subjects still displayed a smaller amount of total recall following the release signal. Although it is possible that some of the memory loss of these subjects may have been due to pseudo-amnesia, it does not seem likely that they would be more subject to this effect than the control subjects not given amnesia suggestions. Hence, Kihlstrom and Evans conclude this effect is real, and they speculate that it may be that posthypnotic amnesia takes more time to dissipate totally after a release cue than has previously been assumed.

In 1965 Williamsen, Johnson, and Eriksen reported on an experiment designed to investigate differences in posthypnotic behavior as a function of hypnotic susceptibility of subjects. Subjects were given the Stanford Hypnotic Susceptibility Scale (SHSS), trained on a list of six words under hypnosis, and given instructions for posthypnotic amnesia. A second group (simulators) was not hypnotized but given the list to learn and instructed to act as though hypnotized and made to forget these words. A third group (control) was given the list to learn with no instructions concerning amnesia. All subjects were then tested for direct recall of these words, recognition of partial critical words interspersed with neutral ones, and responses to a word association test that contained first associates to the critical words along with other stimuli. The third group was designed to provide a reference against which to measure the magnitude of the amnesia effect suggested to the first group. The second, or simulation, group was designed to test the authenticity of the amnesia produced by the first group to see if it could be accounted for simply in terms of role playing or by a tendency on the part of subjects to behave in the manner they perceived the experimenter expected. The investigators found that posthypnotic amnesia was a function of both the susceptibility of the subjects and the kind of test used to measure it.

Control subjects recalled more words than hypnotized subjects, and simulating subjects "recalled" no words. High-susceptibility hypnotic subjects recalled fewer words than low-susceptibility hypnotic subjects. Following the release signal, there were no significant differences in recall among the three groups.

Simulators recognized significantly fewer of the critical words when presented partially than did either the control or hypnotized subjects, who did not differ significantly from each other in this regard. There were no significant differences among any of the three groups with regard to recognition of distorted neutral words, but both hypnotic and control groups recognized more critical words than neutral ones. The simulation subjects did not. There were no significant differences among the three groups on the word association tests with respect to number of critical words elicited or latencies of response.

This study demonstrated that although posthypnotic amnesia did impair recall of words learned under hypnosis, it did not diminish recognition of distorted words nor reduce availability of these critical words as responses on a word association test. It also demonstrated that there are substantial differences in behavior between subjects to whom posthypnotic amnesia is suggested and simulators, who in general overplay their role.

Barber and Calverley (1966c) pointed out that in the foregoing study, simulation instructions were confounded with a waking condition, and suggestions for amnesia were confounded with a hypnotic state. Hence, it was not clear to what extent differences in behavior among these groups should be attributed to differences in suggestions as opposed to differences between the hypnotic and waking states. They also concerned themselves with the issues of whether authoritarian suggestions as used in the foregoing study might not be more appropriate and effective in the hypnotic state than in the waking state, and with the experimenter's difficulties in using identical intonations with waking and hypnotized subjects. To resolve these issues they designed a 16-group, 2 x 2 x 4 factorial study with three independent variables:

1. Method of presentation of suggestions (spoken versus tape recorded).
2. State of subject (waking versus hypnosis).
3. Suggestions made:
   a. Authoritative suggestion of amnesia.

    b. Permissive suggestion of amnesia.
    c. Instructions to simulate amnesia.
    d. No instructions concerning amnesia.

    Each of the 16 groups received a different permutation of these three var-
iables. Three of these groups received treatments identical to the three groups
in the study by Williamsen and associates, and the results of that study were
completely replicated. However, the results for the remaining 13 experimental groups prevented Barber and Calverley from accepting the implied conclusion of that study that the presence or absence of hypnosis was an important variable in the production of amnesia. They found that with respect
to direct recall of words, waking groups did not differ significantly from hypnotized groups when both were given authoritative suggestions for amnesia.
However, when permissive suggestions were used, hypnotic subjects displayed less amnesia than waking subjects. As found by Williamsen, Johnson,
and Eriksen (1965), simulators overplayed their roles and verbalized fewer
words than nonsimulating subjects. Groups that differed in the dimension of
permissive versus authoritarian instructions for amnesia did not differ significantly from each other, and both verbalized fewer words than control groups
given no instructions about amnesia.
    With respect to the recognition of partial or complete critical words, sim-
ulators recognized significantly fewer words than all the other groups, which
did not differ significantly from each other. With respect to neutral words, no
significant differences were produced among any groups. All groups recognized more critical than neutral words. Finally, there were no significant differences in memory among groups when told that the experiment was over.
    Neither hypnotic nor waking control subjects developed any amnesia, fur-
ther evidence for the proposition that spontaneous posthypnotic amnesia is
rare in experimental settings. Hypnotic and waking simulators did not differ
on tests of amnesia, and both groups showed apparent amnesia for partial
or whole critical words. Barber and Calverley note that "amnesia" subjects
in all groups recognized more critical words than neutral ones, and they appear to regard this as a sign that the amnesia was in fact unreal, reported
merely to please the experimenter. In support of this viewpoint, they note
that few experimental subjects questioned after the study reported that they
completely forgot the critical words during the period of amnesia. Rather,
they simply did not think about them. They may have been making an effort
to comply with the desires of the experimenters by a deliberate attempt not
to think of the critical words. This view would appear to overlook the different
performance characteristics of subjects given amnesic instructions and simulation instructions.
    A large body of research confirms the paradoxical observation that the
amount of posthypnotic amnesia present is a function of the test used to

measure this amnesia. Findings from the research in ordinary waking memory suggest a more interesting and tenable explanation of this seeming anomaly.

Kihlstrom (1977) considers four models of suggested posthypnotic amnesia that integrate and explain some of these apparently conflicting findings from a number of alternative theoretical points of view.

Although it is clear that posthypnotic amnesia is not a problem of information recording but of retrieval, many of the principles derived from the study of general memory and forgetting find important application in this area. Hence the model of posthypnotic amnesia as forgetting is useful. In commenting on the Williamsen study reported above, Kihlstrom points out that it should cause no consternation, that in that study, recognition measures disclosed more memory than recall measures. This is consistent with the general finding that recognition is a more sensitive measure of retention than recall. Kihlstrom and Shor (1978) note that the greater amount of memory demonstrated by recognition testing over recall testing is relative and is still less than the memory displayed after a release signal to terminate the amnesia. An even more sensitive measure of memory that will disclose its presence when tests of recall or recognition are negative is Ebbinghaus' savings or relearning method.

In a typical memory study, a list of nonsense syllables is learned to some criterion of performance, such as one perfect recitation. Following an interval of time during which forgetting occurs, the list is relearned. The savings score is taken as the difference between the number of trials to criterion in the original learning situation and the number of trials required to relearn the material to the same criterion of performance. This is expressed as a ratio of the difference to the original number of learning trials in accordance with the following formula:

$$\text{Savings score} = \left[\frac{\begin{array}{c}\text{Number of original} \\ \text{trials}\end{array} - \begin{array}{c}\text{Number relearning} \\ \text{trials}\end{array}}{\begin{array}{c}\text{Number of original} \\ \text{trials}\end{array}}\right] \times 100$$

This score is a direct measure of the retained effect of the original learning. Kihlstrom cites a study by Strickler in Hull's laboratory in which subjects were trained on a paired associates list of nonsense syllables during hypnosis and then given a suggestion of posthypnotic amnesia for this list. On an initial test, subjects recalled only 3% of this list as opposed to 86% recall in waking trials. However, when instructed to relearn the material while awake and amnesic, the group showed a 48% savings score on relearning. (The waking control group had a 98% savings score.)

Another basic paradigm in memory research is that of retroactive inhibition. This is based on the theory that forgetting is caused not by the passive decay of memory traces but by an active interference with material subsequently learned. This theory explains why normal people can forget comparatively recent memories while retaining much older ones intact. A fairly common example of this mechanism can be seen in the destructive effects on retention of a previously learned foreign language caused by learning a new language.

The standard paradigm for research in retroactive inhibition is the following:

Experimental
Group: Learn task A → Learn task B → Test task A

Control
Group: Learn task A → Rest → Test task A

The logic of this design is that any passive deterioration in memory traces due to the passage of time will affect both groups equally. Hence any differences in the final test of task A must be due to the effect of the interspersed learning, task B. Graham and Patton (1968) had subjects learn a list of adjectives (task A) in the waking state. A second list (task B) was learned under hypnosis followed by suggestions for posthypnotic amnesia. Despite a high degree of amnesia for the second list, these subjects displayed the same amount of retroactive inhibition for the first list as did control subjects who learned both lists but were given no suggestions of amnesia.

Coe, Basden, Basden, and Graham (1976) reported a similar study using a free recall test (as opposed to a paired associates or serial list). In a free response list, the order of the recalled items is immaterial. Essentially the results of Graham and Patton were replicated. There were no significant differences between amnesic and nonamnesic subjects in hypnotic susceptibility or in initial levels of learning either list. There was also no difference between groups in the recall of list one either before or after the amnesia was removed. Recall on the second list was, of course, improved for the amnesic subjects following the removal of amnesia. An interesting result noted was that when amnesic subjects had their amnesia for list two removed, they had a significant improvement of performance on list one. The authors suggested that this effect was caused by the distracting effect of the effort required to avoid recalling list two. They support this view with evidence given in support of the neodissociation theory, which holds that when subjects are given two tasks to perform simultaneously (one on a conscious level and the other on an unconscious level) by hypnotic dissociation, performance on the conscious task deteriorates due to the effort necessary to dissociate, or keep out of awareness, the unconscious task (Hilgard, 1974a, 1975). This situation can be seen in automatic writing or automatic talking, as in the case of Hilgard's *hidden observer*. Coe and associates speculate that the reason the hidden observer may notice more pain than is ordinarily experienced in consciousness is that the reporting of the hidden observer represents a second task that interferes with the first task of pain suppression. In a proactive inhibition study (where the effect of previously learned material on the subsequent learning of new material is evaluated), Dillon and Spanos (1983) found that posthypnotic amnesia of a previously learned word list did not eliminate interference with the learning of a second, similar word list. The paradigm for a study in proactive inhibition is as follows:

Experimental
Group: Learn task A → Learn task B

Control
Group: Rest→ Learn task B

    The foregoing evidence that the extent of posthypnotic amnesia is a function of the memory test used to measure it can be interpreted in a variety of ways. If posthypnotic amnesia is accepted as a real phenomenon, this foregoing research is further evidence that it is related to an inhibiting effect on the retrieval rather than on the recording mechanism in memory. Thus, the suggested amnesia primarily affects the less sensitive recall mechanism, while recognition and relearning memory are considerably less impaired.
    The interfering power of the amnesic material is also undiminished, as shown by retroactive and proactive inhibition studies. Kihlstrom (1977) notes that posthypnotic amnesia may have a selective effect since only certain aspects of the critical material can be remembered. This selectivity itself is likely to result from expressed or implied suggestions as, for example, the subject who remembers to perform a posthypnotic suggestion but has amnesia for the source of the behavior. Indeed this situation is often used as an example of the motivating effect of unconscious ideation.
    If the validity of posthypnotic amnesia is questioned, these same facts can be looked at as an example of what Kihlstrom (1977) called "amnesia as the keeping of secrets" or what· Barber has called the "neglect hypothesis." In other words, the subject has no difficulty in remembering but either tries to avoid remembering or actually deceives the experimenter in an effort to comply with the latter's desires. Since it is more difficult to fake indirect measures,

they reveal the presence of the memory. When given the release signal, the subject believes that it is now legitimate to report the critical memories, and this gives the appearance of reversibility. As Kihlstrom points out, this view overlooks a great deal of the findings from research on waking memory. It also overlooks substantial differences found in the behavior of hypnotized and simulation subjects. Simulators do remember the material and seek actively to deceive an experimenter who is unaware of their true status. Thus they typically display greater deficits in recall than subjects with a real posthypnotic amnesia, and they respond with fewer solutions on partial word recognition tasks. When real hypnotic subjects and simulators are led to believe that an experiment is over, simulators typically display full memory recovery, while only half of hypnotic subjects do. Furthermore, posthypnotic amnesia is not usually breached by imploring hypnotic subjects to make a greater effort to recall or to be completely honest in their reports.

A third way of reconciling the data that Kihlstrom considers is to regard posthypnotic amnesia as a form of repression. The fact that the material subject to amnesia is indirectly subject to access presents no problem to this point of view; one of the basic tenets of Freudian psychology is that repressed material expresses itself indirectly in the form of symptoms, dreams, or slips of the tongue.

The problem is that in repression, the patient is not normally aware of the existence of the repressed material, while in posthypnotic amnesia he usually is. Only rarely will a subject displaying a good amnesic response have the subjective impression that he simply closed and immediately opened his eyes. Subjects are usually aware of the passage of time between induction and awakening. Also, the motive for naturally occurring repression is the disturbing nature of the material repressed. It does not appear likely that this need is adequately replicated by the experimenter's suggestion, although the work of Milgram (1963, 1969) suggests that the desire to please an authority figure may be a powerful motive.

Kihlstrom speculates that if posthypnotic amnesia is a form of repression, then subjects most likely to achieve it should be those most likely to employ the defense of repression in everyday life. Studies show more tendency toward repression in these subjects than in those who do not develop posthypnotic amnesia.

Nace, Orne, and Hammer (1974) found that high-susceptibility subjects recall fewer items following a suggested posthypnotic amnesia than low-susceptibility subjects and also retrieve a higher percentage of the items following an appropriate signal to remember. Therefore they also concluded that hypnotic amnesia was an active process interfering with memory retrieval as opposed to a passive one involving a recording difficulty. They point out that to test for posthypnotic amnesia one must notice not only what is not recalled during the amnesia but also what is recovered on cue. They also note that the ability of a hypnotized subject to keep material out of conscious awareness is analogous to the mechanism of repression. Thus the ability of hypnosis to lift this amnesia suggests its clinical usefulness in dealing with naturally occurring repression. They suggest the untested hypothesis that those who show the most striking reversal of posthypnotic amnesia are the most likely to recover significant emotionally charged material under hypnotic treatment.

Coe, Baugher, Krimm, and Smith (1976) investigated a finding by Hilgard and Hommel (1961) that hypnotic subjects, especially medium or poor ones, tended to remember a higher percentage of passed than of failed items under a suggested posthypnotic amnesia. Pettinati and Evans (1978) found that this effect was independent of hypnotic susceptibility, while Pettinati, Evans, Orne, and Orne (1981) found it was limited to subjects not high in susceptibility and regarded its absence in high-susceptibility subjects as supporting the view of Evans and Kihlstrom (1973) that posthypnotic amnesia results from disruption of memory retrieval cues and organization. These results could be accounted for either in terms of the repression of failed items or an enchancement effect produced by success. Recognizing that subjects may have a different impression of whether they passed or failed a hypnotic suggestion than the experimenter has, subjects in the Coe et al. study were asked for their opinions about whether they successfully passed each suggestion. They were also asked for their feelings for the item. The results failed to support either theory, and the investigators found that there was not enough emotional response to the average hypnotic suggestion used in research to test the hypotheses.

Finally, Kihlstrom likens the effect of posthypnotic amnesia to the everyday experience of forgetting a name or fact that the person feels is "on the tip of his tongue." It is a temporary and selective disruption of certain routes to remembered material.

Thorne (1969), following up on the line of research of Williamsen, Johnson, and Eriksen (1965) and Barber and Calverley (1966c), compared three groups of subjects matched for hypnotic·susceptibility but differing in motivational instructions for amnesia. One group received task-motivational instructions under hypnosis, the second task-motivational instructions while awake, and the third nonmotivational instructions while awake. Instead of using free recall testing as did the earlier studies, Thorne used a paired associates task and measured the effect of the amnesia·by a word association test to minimize the effects of subjects' deliberately withholding memories. The theory behind this technique is similar to the theory behind a retroactive inhibition paradigm. A paired associates list consists of pairs of words. The first word of each pair functions as a stimulus to which the subject must learn the second word as a response. Ordinarily these stimulus words will elicit a response from an untrained subject instructed to say the first word that comes to mind upon hearing the stimulus word. These naturally occurring responses for each word have been rated for their probability of occurrence on standardized word lists.

By training a subject to respond with a low-probability response word, an interference effect will be set up that should prevent the higher-probability response from being made on subsequent testing during amnesia if the amnesia is not totally effective.

Thorne found no significant differences among the three groups with respect to neutral words (those not used as stimuli on the paired associate learning task), but there were differences on the critical words. The hypnotic task-motivational group showed less amnesia than the other two. Since the instructions used were permissive, he regarded this finding as a cross-validation of Barber and Calverley's results. More important, it was again demonstrated that suggestions for amnesia do not effectively block access to learned material when this access is tapped indirectly rather than by direct recall. In a follow-up study, Thorne and Hall (1974) reported that there was little effect of suggestions of amnesia when measured by a word association test, but the crucial variable was not hypnosis versus waking but task-motivational instructions versus nonmotivating instructions. Highly susceptible subjects responded more to suggestions of amnesia. They also found that paired associates memory performance was not affected by the authoritarian or permissive nature of the suggestions. Kihlstrom (1980) found that even high-susceptibility subjects who developed a marked suggested amnesia for a word list learned under hypnosis, when measured directly ("episodic" memory), had the critical words elicited by a word association test ("semantic" memory). He finds that the fact that response latencies are not inhibited in word association tests speaks against a repression view of posthypnotic amnesia. He believes suggestions of posthypnotic amnesia produce a temporary dissociation of the contextual features of a memory trace. Spanos, Radtke, and Dubreuil (1982), on the other hand, argue that differences between episodic and semantic memory improvement result from a strategic social behavior that depends on the subject's perception of how he is expected to act in the hypnotic situation.

Evans and Kihlstrom (1973) investigated the mechanism behind the well-established paradox that posthypnotic amnesic subjects who cannot recall events that transpired under hypnosis nevertheless show evidence of the presence of these unavailable memories. Some investigators regard these findings as evidence of the lack of validity of posthypnotic amnesia and thus regard it as role playing. Evans and Kihlstrom find that this viewpoint neglects important aspects of the data. They note the significant differences between hypnotized subjects and simulators and the common observation that simulators never develop source amnesia. Based on subjective reports of subjects following experiments in suggested posthypnotic amnesia, they conclude that more was involved than the subjects' merely trying not to recall the material. Orne (1966b) reported that when amnesic subjects were questioned on awakening by an experimenter other than the one who induced the hypnosis, some said that they always had the memory available but were unable to verbalize it to the original experimenter. Others reported that they were unable to recall when speaking to the original experimenter, but the memory came back in whole or part with the passage of time. Still others were unable to recall even when urged to remember. Since an essential characteristic of suggested posthypnotic amnesia is its reversibility on a prearranged signal, it is clearly a disturbance in memory retrieval rather than one of memory formation. Hence Evans and Kihlstrom reasoned that a study of those subjects displaying less than complete failure of recall might shed some light on the mechanism underlying this disturbance.

Studies of ordinary memory show that when no constraints are placed on the order of item recall, subjects tend to use various organizational schemes to recover material recorded in memory. Most of these devices take advantage of associations among the items filed in memory. These organizational schemes may be based on conceptual categories, structural similarity, or spatial-temporal context.

Evans and Kihlstrom (1973) found that hypnotized subjects under posthypnotic amnesia who were able to recall some items did so in a random order, as compared to the sequential order in which insusceptible subjects recalled the material. Kihlstrom and Wilson (1984) also found that highly hypnotizable subjects under suggestions of posthypnotic amnesia displayed a breakdown in temporal organization of the material recalled. The organization returned following a release signal. Geiselman, Bjork, and Fishman (1983) found that retrieval inhibition plays a role in nonhypnotic directed forgetting as well. These studies indicated that the effect of suggested posthypnotic amnesia on recall is to disrupt the normal organization of the recall process. This effect would account for the findings that the recognition or associative processes that do not depend on this kind of organization are left relatively intact. Wagstaff (1977a) reports a study giving role-playing instructions to unhypnotized subjects that suggested that the disruption of retrieval behavior displayed in posthypnotically amnesic subjects may be accounted for in terms of role playing and demand characteristics.

Coe and his associates (1973) attempted to extend the findings on disrupted retrieval by studying the effects of posthypnotic amnesia on the semantic organization of recall of a previously learned 35-word list. The list consisted of five different classifications of words with seven items in each classification. The dependent variable was the amount of clustering of similar items during recall. The researchers found no differences in clustering between subjects with suggested posthypnotic amnesia and those not given this suggestion.

Spanos and Bodorik (1977) thought that this negative result may have been due to the fact that there were only three learning trials given in the preceding study, and hence the amount of preamnesic organization may have been too small for any effect to be noted. They therefore used a nine-word list with three examples in each of three categories: birds, flowers, and alcoholic drinks. Subjects were trained on this list until they reached the criterion of two successive correct trials, ensuring a more adequate opportunity for preamnesic, semantic organization of list items to occur.

Since most studies have shown that hypnotic and task-motivated subjects tend to respond similarly to suggestions of amnesia, Spanos and Bodorik also investigated the breakdown in categorical organization in both types of subjects. Using 27 posthypnotic amnesia subjects and 25 exposed to task-motivational instructions for amnesia while awake, they found that seven subjects displayed total nonrecall, and seven displayed partial nonrecall.

Clustering of list items in the partial amnesia group was negatively related to nonrecall ($r = -0.67$). In other words, subjects with the largest memory defects displayed the least clustering, as predicted by the notion that posthypnotic amnesia functions by disrupting the organizational strategy of memory retrieval.

Hypnotic subjects did not show a different amount of clustering before or after amnesia than task-motivated waking subjects, but they did show less than them during the amnesia period. Contrary to Barber's findings, task-motivated waking subjects did not develop amnesia as well as hypnotized subjects. These results were replicated in a number of subsequent studies (Radtke-Bodorik, Planas, and Spanos, 1980; Radtke-Bodorik, Spanos, and Haddad, 1979; Radtke and Spanos, 1981a; Spanos and D'Eon, 1980; Spanos, Radtke-Bodorik, and Stam, 1980; Spanos et al., 1980b). Spanos and co-workers (1980c) found that the amount of posthypnotic amnesia displayed by subjects not highly susceptible could be manipulated by changing preliminary instructions that affected the subjects' interpretation of the hypnotic situation. Spanos, Radtke, Bentrand, Addie, and Drummond (1982) found that simulators did not display disordered recall during feigned amnesia and hence concluded that this strategy was not suggested to subjects by the experimental situation. Thus, it was unlikely to result from subjects faking an amnesia. Spanos and Bodorik (1977) think it likely that the amount of amnesia in past research is overestimated; they believe that measures of amnesia should be based on subjective reports of subjects in addition to the usual measures of temporary nonrecall followed by reversibility of amnesia.

The diversity of categories into which Spanos and Bodorik classified post experimental subjective reports of subjects is interesting. (They point out that the following subcategories are neither mutually exclusive nor exhaustive.) The subject:

1. Remembered but chose not to verbalize. ⎫
2. Remembered but was unable to verbalize. ⎬ no amnesia

3. Tried to force words out of awareness. ⎫
4. Tried to distract himself from the word. ⎬ effortful
5. Use goal-directed fantasies. ⎭
6. Was relaxed and unmotivated to try to recall. ⎫ effortless
7. Did nothing to achieve or maintain nonrecall. ⎭

The theoretical implications that these investigators derived from the foregoing results were that in normally aroused individuals, the retrieval process for a newly formed list of words goes on automatically, and this process is experienced subjectively by the subjects as the words "popping" into their minds in an organized manner. These automatic processes function less efficiently during low arousal (relaxed state). Thus, subjects relaxed under amnesic instructions could have retrieved the word if they made the effort to do so, but they did not. Less relaxed subjects tended to experience the words inadvertently and in order to forget consciously had to direct and sustain attention away from these words. This process is an effortful one.

In comparing recognition with the usual recall measure of posthypnotic amnesia, St. Jean and Coe (1981) found that only 50% of posthypnotically amnesic subjects displayed temporal disorganized recognition of items and that the disorganization effect on recall was weak and inconsistent. They thus questioned the utility of the disrupted search hypothesis to account for posthypnotic amnesia. Spanos, Radtke-Bodorik, and Shabinsky (1980), using hypnotized and task-motivated subjects to learn a list of unrelated nouns (as opposed to a categorized list) and then to develop a suggested amnesia for the list, found that both hypnotic and task-motivated subjects showed an equivalent breakdown in subjective organization following suggestions for amnesia. However, subjects who were able to recall the list fully developed as much breakdown in subjective organization as did subjects displaying partial amnesia. Hence, the authors concluded that the disruption of subjective organization accompanied but did not cause the amnesia.

Contrary to Evans and Kihlstrom (1973), they found no relationship between susceptibility and subjective disorganization but note that the amount of subjective organization employed prior to suggestions of amnesia was quite low in this study due to the easy list used. They also found that hypnotic subjects learned the list more slowly than did task-motivated subjects but developed more amnesia. While nonrecall subjects were higher in susceptibility than full recall subjects in the hypnosis group, full and nonrecall task-motivated subjects did not differ in susceptibility.

Interestingly some nonrecall subjects were verbal inhibitors (44% of the total nonrecall subjects), and the authors take this to indicate that previous studies that did not inquire into the subjective states of subjects have substantially overestimated the amount of total amnesia displayed.

Kihlstrom and Evans (1976) note that while reversibility of amnesia is not scored as part of the amnesia items on standardized tests of hypnotic susceptibility, it is essential in distinguishing real posthypnotic amnesia from pseudo-amnesia. It should be recognized, however, that although reversibility will distinguish posthypnotic amnesia from pseudo-amnesia involving a failure to learn the material or an ordinary failure of memory, it may not distinguish it from a pseudo-amnesia due to nonreporting of memory by the subject or the lack of effort to recall.

The problem in measuring reversibility is that more-susceptible subjects tend to display a higher amount of posthypnotic amnesia. This may give rise to a spuriously high measure of reversibility because there are more items available for good subjects to recover (due to their initial poor memory for the list), when compared with poor subjects who remembered most of the list under suggestions of amnesia.

Nace, Orne, and Hammer (1974) tried to make reversibility measures independent of a subject's initial recall of a list by expressing it as the ratio of items recalled after a release signal to the total number of items potentially recoverable. Kihlstrom and Evans accomplished the same result by using enough subjects so that hypnotizable and nonhypnotizable subjects could be matched for recall during initial amnesia testing. At virtually every point along the distribution of the initial amnesia response, they found that hypnotized subjects were able to recapture more previously blocked memories than were insusceptible subjects.

Generic recall is a situation analogous to a person's having information on the tip of his tongue but being unable to recall it fully. In other words, the person has some idea about the general nature of the information but cannot gain access to the specific memory sought. Kihlstrom and Evans (1978) had *blind* raters inspect memory reports of 725 hypnotized subjects for instances of generic recall. They found that during periods of suggested posthypnotic amnesia, generic recall occurred significantly more often in reports of hypnotizable than in reports of insusceptible subjects. Generic recall was found to be inversely related to the number of critical items recalled. Finally, there was a marked shift from generic to particular recall after the posthypnotic amnesia was removed.

Howard and Coe (1980) and Schuyler and Coe (1981) investigated factors influencing the breakdown of posthypnotic amnesia prior to a release signal in order to contrast theoretical views of posthypnotic amnesia. They reasoned that theories such as Hilgard's (1973b, 1974a, 1977b) neodissociation view or Kihlstrom and Evans's (1973) disrupted retrieval theory would imply that posthypnotic amnesia is a "happening" that subjects have no control over, and hence it cannot be voluntarily breached, while Coe's (1978) contextual view, which regards it as a "doing," implies that, if motivated, subjects could breach it.

They found that some subjects experienced posthypnotic amnesia as involuntary, while others perceived it as voluntary and hence requiring effort on their part to maintain. It was found that posthypnotic amnesia was initially equal for both voluntary and involuntary subjects, but it could be breached only in the voluntary subgroup by exhortations for honesty or telling subjects that their withholding of information could be detected by lie detection apparatus. While Coe and his associates interpret these results in terms of the coercive power of these manipulations, a more interesting issue (not discussed) is why subjects subjectively experience the results of suggestions for posthypnotic amnesia differently.

Kihlstrom, Evans, Orne, and Orne (1980) found that attempts to breach a posthypnotic amnesia with highly susceptible subjects capable of dissociation of memories, by means of instructions to try harder or be honest, were no more effective than retesting. Kihlstrom, Easton, and Shor (1983) found that some memory returns prior to a release signal due to the passage of time rather than to the effect of retesting. Spanos and his colleagues found that although hypnotic amnesia typically decreased on successive tests, it did not decay passively with time, as suggested by Kihlstrom and his associates. In accordance with Spanos's view that posthypnotic amnesia resulted from an active strategic action on the part of the subject to conform to the social demands of the hypnotic situation, Spanos believes it could be manipulated by changing the subject's expectation of how a deeply hypnotized subject would behave (Bertrand, Spanos, and Parkinson, 1983; Dubreuil, Spanos, and Bertrand, 1982-1983; Spanos and Radtke, 1982; Spanos, Tkachyk, Bertrand, and Weekes, 1984). Thus, if led to believe that good subjects normally increased instead of decreased posthypnotic amnesia on subsequent tests, subjects would display an increase in amnesia in order to present themselves as good subjects.

Kihlstrom (1978) compares Coe's contextualist view (which he equates with the belief that a posthypnotic amnesia is not real but is due to the subject's actively trying to avoid remembering the material to meet social expectations), with his own cognitive view (that the amnesia is real and the material is unavailable even though recorded in memory and subject to retrieval at a later time). In support of this viewpoint, he relies on evidence from the research on nonhypnotic memory loss and recovery.

In an interesting set of studies, McConkey, Sheehan, and Cross (1980) and McConkey and Sheehan (1981) investigated the capacity of a high-cue situation (the viewing of the events of hypnosis on a videotape) to break down a posthypnotic amnesia prior to a release signal. Both amnesic and nonamnesic subjects showed greater recall for critical items following viewing of the tape, but the results showed posthypnotic amnesia to be a robust phenomenon. Only 50% of the amnesic subjects showed a substantial increment of recall, and, as the authors note, they may have been remembering the events of the tape rather than the hypnotic session. Some amnesic subjects were unable to remember the events of the tape, in addition to not being able to remember the events of the hypnosis, and some made a distinction between remembering the occurrence of events. (which they could) and remembering the experiencing of these events (which they could not).

Geiselman and his associates (1983), comparing hypnotically induced amnesia with nonhypnotic directed forgetting, concluded that the demand characteristics associated with hypnosis are not apparent in the nonhypnotic situation, and hence it is not likely that hypnotic amnesia is entirely the result of subjects responding to the demand characteristics of the situation. Similarly Simon and Salzberg (1985) found that manipulating subjects' expectations had no effect on the occurrence of posthypnotic amnesia on the SHSS form A.

In a 1973 study, Evans, Kihlstrom, and Orne reported that blind ratings of subjects' hypnotic susceptibility could be reliably made from written reports of their responses to the amnesia item on the HGSHS:A. These ratings were not based on the number of items recalled or even the relatively random order of the items listed but on the tendency of good hypnotic subjects to describe experiences unrelated to specific items suggested on the test about 50% of the time (such as subjective distortions in body size or cognitive changes in the visual field associated with the induction procedure). These findings indicated that a suggestion for posthypnotic amnesia may have other demonstrable effects on subjects' behavior beyond producing a deficit in the ability to remember the details of experience while in the hypnotic state.

HYPNOTIC HYPERMNESIA AND EFFECTS ON LEARNING

The use of hypnosis to augment recall, or to produce *hypermnesia,* is the opposite of its usage in producing a posthypnotic amnesia. A large clinical and anecdotal literature attests to the remarkable powers of hypnosis to improve memory for forgotten, crucial, personal incidents or details of a crime witnessed. By and large, the experimental literature offers little support for such claims, at least with respect to the kind of materials used to test recall in experimental work.

Basically there are two major types of studies in this area: studies of the effect of hypnosis or hypnotic suggestions on learning (the *memory recording function*) and studies of the effect of hypnosis or hypnotic suggestions on the recall of previously learned material (the *retrieval function*). In the first type of study, the subject learns material while in a hypnotic state and is typically tested for recall while awake. In the second type, the subject learns the material in the waking state and is tested for recall under hypnosis. A number of investigators have provided reviews of the recent and older literature in this area (Barber, 1965c; Cooper and London, 1973; Dhanens and Lundy, 1975; Relinger, 1984; Swiercinsky and Coe, 1971).

In 1925 Young reported no differences in acquisition or recall of meaningful words or adjective-noun paired associates lists among subjects who were hypnotized, waking, or simulating hypnosis. He did find that hypnosis produced an improvement in the recall of meaningful childhood events.

In 1930 Huse found no significant difference, 24 hours after learning, between waking recall and recall under neutral hypnosis of a list of symbols paired with nonsense syllables. Each subject was his own control, and the order of waking and hypnotic recall trials was counterbalanced. Mitchell (1932) also found no improvement produced by hypnosis in the recall of nonsense syllables.

Stalnaker and Riddle (1932) compared the recall of prose and poetry learned at least a year earlier under conditions of hypnosis plus suggestions of heightened recall or waking with no such suggestions. The order of waking or hypnotic memory testing was counterbalanced. They found that hypnosis plus suggestion significantly improved recall.

In consonance with the foregoing results, White, Fox, and Harris (1940) compared waking and hypnotic recall after 24 hours, using paired nonsense syllables, poetry, or visual scenes as the material to be recalled. They found that hypnosis did not improve recall for nonsense material or visual material but significantly improved recall for the meaningful poetry.

Rosenthal (1944) also found, by using material of varied meaningfulness or of varied capacity to evoke anxiety, that hypnotic hypermnesia occurs with meaningful or anxiety-producing material, while single innocuous words that are not organized or meaningful are not subject to such an effect. He speculated that the calm, relaxed state produced by hypnosis counteracted the anxiety that was interfering with memory and thus permitted the free flow of the meaningful material into awareness.

True (1949) found better recall than would be expected in waking subjects by using the technique of age regression instead of suggestions of improved powers of recall. Subjects were asked the day of the week for their birthdays and Christmas in the year that they were regressed to.

Hammer (1954) found that the learning of a variety of cognitive tasks, except for meaningful prose, can be increased with appropriate posthypnotic suggestions of increased confidence, motivation and ability. Similarly, Sears (1955) found that subjects who were hypnotized and given suggestions that they would learn easily and remember well learned Morse code more proficiently than did control subjects. Sears (1954) also found that neutral hypnotic recall was superior to waking recall of a large number of items scattered on a table top and observed for 30 seconds. Recall was tested immediately and at subsequent intervals of 1 and 3 weeks. However, since waking recall always preceded hypnotic recall, the advantage reported for hypnotic recall may be due, in whole or in part, to a practice effect.

Crawford and Allen (1983) reported that high-susceptibility subjects under hypnosis displayed more visual memory than low-susceptibility subjects or waking controls as measured by a task requiring them to notice changes in detail on successively presented pictures. High-susceptibility subjects changed cognitive strategies from a waking emphasis on memorizing details to a more holistic strategy; low-susceptibility subjects did not.

Das (1961) found no differences in either acquisition or recall of a list of meaningful paired associates between hypnosis and the waking state.

Salzberg (1960) gave suggestions for enhanced performance to subjects performing under hypnosis. Some subjects who performed under hypnosis were also given posthypnotic suggestions. Tasks involved simple counting, memorization of nouns, and abstract reasoning. The suggestions facilitated performance on all tasks for both hypnotic groups but not for the control subjects. However, hypnotic subjects were high in hypnotic susceptibility, whereas control subjects were unselected on this factor.

A number of studies reported that hypnotic suggestion of enhanced performance was effective in improving concentration or study habits and in aiding acquisition or retention (Eisele and Higgins, 1962; Krippner, 1963; McCord, 1956). However, as Barber (1965b) points out, none of these studies utilized a control group that was given the same motivating instructions in the waking state.

When As (1962) age regressed subjects to a time when they spoke a foreign language, he found better recall of the former language under hypnosis than in the waking state. However, since hypnotic recall was always tested after waking recall, it is not possible to say how much of this improvement was due to the hypnosis and how much due to a practice or warm-up effect. As in the True study, age-regression suggestions were not given to a control group of waking subjects.

De Zulueta (1984) cited two cases in which hypnotic age regression enabled subjects, aged 18 and 28, to recover substantial amounts of facility with languages not spoken since ages 6 and 4, respectively.

Rosenhan and London (1963) found that learning a list of nonsense syllables under neutral hypnosis (without suggestions for enhanced performance) produced a slight decrement in learning for high-susceptibility subjects and a significant improvement for low-susceptibility subjects. This result was replicated by London, Convant, and Davison (1966). Schulman and London (1963), using poetry and nonsense syllables (as did Das), found no improvement in acquisition or recall under conditions of neutral hypnosis.

They found no difference in performance between high- and low-suscepti- bility subjects. Cooper and London (1973), taking all of these results into account, concluded that hypnosis used without suggestions for improved per- formance improves neither learning nor recall.

Illovsky (1963) found that hypnosis plus suggestions of improved reading ability was more effective in improving reading test scores for poor readers than a control condition without such suggestions.

Fowler (1961) found that suggestions of intense concentration, increased comprehension, and better memory were equally effective with waking sub- jects and hypnotized ones and increased reading scores for both groups.

Brabender and Dickhaus (1978) report that hypnosis hindered compre- hension of auditory verbal material in comparison to waking motivational in- structions. They account for this result in terms of the relaxation and low tension level that neutral hypnosis produces. Sweeney, Lynn, and Bellezza (1985) also found that neutral hypnosis may decrease subject motivation and performance. Specifically they found that hypnosis did not improve perfor- mance in learning an imagery-mediated paired associate list, but this study appears to have confounded hypnosis with motivating instructions.

Parker and Barber (1964) pretested subjects on a digit-symbol substitution task, memory for meaningful nouns, and an abstract reasoning task. They then divided highly susceptible subjects into one of three experimental groups. One group received task-motivational instructions in the waking state, the second group received the same instructions in the hypnotic state, and the third group received neither the instructions nor the hypnotic treatment. A fourth group, which served as a control for susceptibility, was made up of low-susceptibility subjects who received task-motivational instructions in the waking state. They found that task-motivational instructions, whether given under waking conditions or in the hypnotic state, were ineffective in increas- ing the performance of any subject on the noun memory or abstract reasoning tasks. However, task motivation was effective (with or without hypnosis) in increasing performance of both high- and low-susceptibility subjects on the simpler digit-symbol substitution task.

Barber (1965c) critically reviewed and classified much of the foregoing literature into three major categories:

1. Studies that confounded the hypnotic state with suggestions for im- proved performance (Eisele and Higgins, 1962; Hammer, 1954; Il- lovsky, 1963; Krippner, 1963; McCord, 1956; Sears, 1955; Stalnaker and Riddle, 1932).
2. Studies that investigated the effects of hypnosis per se in the absence of specific suggestions (Das, 1961; Huse, 1930; Rosenhan and Lon- don, 1963; Sears, 1954; Schulman and London, 1963; Young, 1925).

3. Studies that investigated the relative effectiveness of hypnotic versus waking suggestions (Fowler, 1961; Parker and Barber, 1964; Rosenthal, 1944; Salzberg, 1960; White, Fox, and Harris, 1940).

He concluded from these studies that the weight of the evidence shows that waking suggestions are no less effective in enhancing learning or recall than the same instructions given under hypnosis. He further concluded that in studies purporting to find hypnotic suggestions more effective than waking suggestions (Rosenthal, 1944; White, Fox, and Harris, 1940), the hypnotic state was always confounded with some other variable that may have affected recall. For example, hypnotic subjects were tested with their eyes closed while waking controls were tested with their eyes open; the implicit suggestion of enhanced performance was incidental to the induction of hypnosis; or experimenter bias was produced by differences in the experimenter's intonation and manner when addressing hypnotized or waking subjects. He concluded that neutral hypnosis in the absence of suggestions of high performance enhances neither learning nor recall.

Barber and Calverley (1966b) undertook a study to correct what they considered to be some of the design deficiencies in the prior research, such as the confounding of the hypnotic state with motivational suggestions, subject susceptibility, or eye closure; the lack of waking controls in age regression studies; and the effects of experimenter bias. They used a 3 x 3 factorial design in which 90 subjects were randomly assigned to each experimental group. The first independent variable (condition of subject) consisted of three levels: hypnotic induction with eye closure, no hypnotic induction with eye closure, and no hypnotic induction with eyes opened. The second independent variable (conditions of recall) was also divided into three levels: no suggestions, task-motivational suggestions, and suggestions of age regression to the period of the original learning.

All subjects learned a list of 12 nonsense syllables in a 5-minute period and were immediately given a 3-minute recall trial to establish a baseline. Two months later, they were individually tested under the various experimental permutations for recall of the nonsense syllables. Instructions for all groups were given by tape recorder to eliminate experimenter bias. The mean recall for all groups was extremely low (less than one nonsense syllable), and no significant differences were found due to any experimental condition or interaction between the independent variables. While the age-regression condition was not found to improve recall significantly, subjects exposed to this condition met criteria for its establishment whether in the waking or hypnotic state. Subsequent to the study, subjects were measured on the Barber Scale of Suggestibility (BSS); no relationship was found between suggestibility and recall scores.

As Dhanens and Lundy (1975) point out, this was not a very fair test of hypnotic hypermnesia. Nonsense syllables rather than meaningful material were used, and the prior literature indicates that little hypermnesia would be expected under such conditions. (For an atypical contradictory finding, see Augustynek, 1978.) Also, the amount of retention was so small that it seems likely there was not enough memory recorded for any method to retrieve it. There is ample evidence in the literature of learning that memories require a period of time to set before becoming permanent. During this time, either the rehearsal of rote memory materials or the subject's ruminations over meaningful material may play a role in the creation of a permanent memory. In this case, the subjects had no motive to review this material subsequent to the initial learning, and the various experimental manipulations may have been ineffective in enhancing recall because there were not any memory traces formed to be recalled (i.e., a "basement effect" was operating).

Swiercinsky and Coe (1970, 1971) reviewed the literature and concluded that most studies show that the learning and recall of the kinds of test material studied in short-term verbal memory research are not improved by hypnotic suggestions when compared with control conditions. Using a reading comprehension task, they divided subjects into three groups. One group received an "alert" hypnotic treatment (to avoid suggestions of relaxation or sleep) plus posthypnotic suggestions of enhanced recall. A second group was not hypnotized but merely given task-motivational instructions to concentrate. Another control group was neither hypnotized nor given any special instructions designed to enhance performance. No differences in reading comprehension scores were found among the three groups. However, in view of clinical reports, the authors do not rule out the possibility of long-term hypnotic training increasing verbal recall.

Gilbert and Barber (1972) report substantially negative results in measuring the effects of duration of hypnotic induction, subject susceptibility, and presence or absence of task-motivational suggestions (arranged in a 3 x 2 x 2 factorial study) on the subsequent performance of subjects on three out of four cognitive tasks.

Cooper and London (1973), using a 513-word article on the characteristics of a rare chemical, found that neither the condition of being awake or hypnotized nor the susceptibility of the subject produced a difference in the amount of material recalled after a 2-week period. They point out, however, that this result should be limited to highly factual material having little emotional impact. They note that the type of material dramatically recovered in clinical reports is usually highly emotionally charged.

Dhanens and Lundy (1975) reviewed the literature on hypnotic recall and concluded that the kind of material to be recalled is a crucial variable. Studies with meaningless materials such as nonsense syllables invariably produced negative results, while studies with meaningful material sometimes produced positive findings. In a complicated 2 x 6 factorial design, they investigated the effects of five factors on hypnotic recall:

1. Task-motivating instructions.
2. Attempts to age regress subjects to the time of the original learning.
3. Relaxation instructions.
4. Eye closure.
5. Susceptibility of subjects.

All 122 subjects were required to learn a 184-word biographical article and a list of 13 nonsense syllables. All experimental instructions were given via tape recorder to eliminate experimenter bias. Subjects chosen had scored either high or low on form A of the HGSHS and were assigned to one of six treatment groups:

1. Hypnosis plus task-motivating instructions.
2. Waking plus task-motivating instructions.
3. Hypnosis plus age-regression suggestions.
4. Waking plus age-regression suggestions.
5. Waking plus relaxation instructions.
6. Waking plus no special instructions.

Half of the last (control) group were instructed to keep their eyes open, and half were instructed to close their eyes. Recall trials were held a week after the original learning. All groups were first tested for waking recall to establish a baseline before being tested for recall under the experimental condition to which they were assigned.

Consistent with the prior literature, no significant effects were found for any of the variables with respect to recall of the nonsense syllables. For the meaningful material, significant differences were found between high- and low-susceptibility subjects in the hypnosis plus motivational instructions condition. High-susceptibility subjects displayed higher recall gains under the hypnosis plus motivational condition than under the relaxation instruction condition, while low-susceptibility subjects did not. Contrary to Barber's general findings, motivational instructions without hypnosis were not effective in enhancing recall, nor was any other experimental condition. Thus the results of this study, like those of the rest of the literature in general, were mixed. The only treatment that improved recall was hypnosis plus task-motivating instructions and this only for highly susceptible subjects being tested on meaningful material. Neither Barber and Calverley's (1966b) totally negative results nor Sears's (1954) totally positive results were replicated. Rosenthal's (1944) speculation concerning the role of relaxation in hypnotic recall was not confirmed either, but it should be noted that the meaningful material in this study was not of an anxiety-producing type. This may also account for the ineffectiveness of the age-regression techniques employed in this study.

Wall and Lieberman (1976) employed a questionnaire of early memories concerning such items of early experience as teachers' names, color of family car, and old addresses. They found no difference in recall improvement from a waking baseline measure among a hypnotic group, a waking task-motivational group, and a control group. All three groups displayed *hypermnesia* in that their memory improved about the same amount on the second measurement. It is not clear from the report of this experiment just how (if at all) responses of subjects were verified for accuracy, and it may well be that what was measured was not an increase in memory but an increase in propensity to make responses to the questionnaire.

Stager and Lundy (1985) found that recall of details of a short entertaining film after a delay of 1 week was greater for hypnotized than waking subjects, but this effect was limited to highly susceptible subjects. More interesting, and in contradiction to previous studies, was the fact that the increase in accuracy of answers to questions was not accompanied by an increase in inaccurate material. They note that this may have been due to the absence of misleading cues and the particular questions used, which required short specific answers and did not provide the opportunity for confabulation that free recall does. Hence, these results may not be generalizable to such real life situations as forensic investigations. While hypnosis was found to increase recall in this study, no difference in learning was observed between hypnotized and waking subjects.

Baker, Haynes, and Patrick (1983) found that hypnosis did not enhance recollection of nonsense syllables studied or incidental memory of photographs of varied neutral objects displayed during learning of these syllables.

Sheehan and his associates, in a study finding no evidence of hypnotic memory enhancement of slides when measured by structured testing, found that both hypnotic and simulating subjects incorporated misleading information given them into memory reports. If the information was given prior to hypnotic induction, both groups showed similar distortion, but hypnotic subjects showed more distortion if the misleading information was given following hypnotic induction. This held true for both structured and unstructured recall. More ominously for forensic applications of hypnotic memory refreshment was the observation that hypnotic subjects displayed greater confidence in the correctness of their inaccurate reports (Sheehan, Grigg, and McCann, 1984; Sheehan and Tilden, 1983, 1984).

Wagstaff and Sykes (1984) found that a waking control group was superior to a hypnosis group in recalling details of a 3-minute tape recorded story about a car accident (emotionally charged material). They produced more accurate information without an increase in erroneous intrusions. Klatzky and

Erdelyi (1985) argue that the foregoing type of studies fail to ascertain the effects of hypnosis on hypermnesia because they do not discriminate between the amount of material retrievable from memory and the criteria adopted by subjects for reporting their memories.

The foregoing research seems to show little support in the experimental literature for many of the clinical claims made for the power of hypnosis to provide a subject with total eidetic imagery-like recall of past events, particularly through the utilization of age-regression techniques. Unquestionably many such clinical reports result from the uncontrolled conditions under which clinical observations are made, a lack of appreciation on the part of the clinician of the ability of an unhypnotized subject to recall, and occasionally, an overenthusiastic reporter. On the other hand, some of the negative results in studies attempting hypnotic memory retrieval may simply be due to the fact that no memory was recorded to be retrieved in the first place. Memory research has indicated the need for a certain amount of rehearsal for memories of rote materials to be set. In many of the foregoing studies, particularly those involving the rote memorization of nonsense materials, subjects had no reason to rehearse this material subsequent to the learning session. They were neither instructed to do so nor was the material of such a nature as to stimulate rehearsal on the part of the subjects. The ability of a person to forget meaningless material and not record it in the nervous system is probably as important as the ability not to attend to irrelevant stimuli. Life would be chaotic indeed if every important memory had to be searched out from a file containing every irrelevant stimulus that ever impinged on us from the time of birth. Also, if a memory has been recorded in the nervous system, the ordinary process of memory retrieval, in the absence of any impediment to its operation, may be efficient enough to retrieve it with maximum effectiveness so that it cannot be augmented by hypnosis or any other means.

Thus the kind of memory that hypnosis could logically be expected to improve would be the kind of memory, typically reported in the clinical literature, that involves affect-laden material that the subject has repressed because of the discomfort that its recollection would cause. This material is typically both meaningful and anxiety producing, such as forgotten memories by a witness to a crime or traumatic early experiences. The experimental literature does not preclude the possibility that hypnosis may enhance the recall of this type of material because of its ability to lower the anxiety associated with it. This may be accomplished by producing effects that are incompatible with anxiety, such as relaxation, heightened self-confidence, and a transference relationship with a hypnotist. The studies on posthypnotic amnesia provide clear-cut evidence that hypnosis can be effective in the recovery of a memory temporarily unavailable to conscious awareness for psychological reasons.

In a study designed to test the effects of arousal level on hypnotic hypermnesia, DePiano and Salzberg (1981) showed subjects three films designed to induce traumatic arousal (a surgical operation), sexual arousal, or low arousal. Subjective reports of subjects and physiological measures confirmed that the arousal manipulation was effective. However, while memory enhancement of hypnotic subjects given task-motivating instructions for incidental auditory learning was greater than for waking subjects, the effect was independent of arousal conditions. The authors note the possibility of differences in magnitude of the emotional responses obtained in this study from those occurring in actual situations as a limit on the generalizability of these results.

There is another point worthy of consideration with respect to the clinical recovery of inaccessible memories by hypnotic means. Unlike an experimental situation, in clinical practice the usefulness of the material elicited is of more practical importance than its accuracy. This is similar to the situation in clinical dream interpretation. It is not important that the interpretation of a dream be correct but only that it be useful to the therapy. This is fortunate since it is impossible to determine if a dream interpretation is correct. The fact that a patient accepts or rejects an interpretation is no evidence either way. If, however, an interpretation results in the patient's attaining a new insight or the introduction of important new material into the analysis, it is a useful one. If it fails to accomplish this, the effort is a total waste of time, no matter how correct the interpretation may be. Similarly, a memory retrieved under hypnotic age regression in therapy may be quite useful to the therapeutic process even if it is distorted, inaccurate, or a total fantasy as opposed to a real memory.

HYPNOSIS AND CREATIVITY

Creativity is a psychological term that has different meanings to different investigators. Getzels and Jackson (1962) used a battery of tests to measure it. These ranged from measuring unique responses to a word association test, through requiring subjects to devise unusual uses for common objects, finding hidden shapes in geometric patterns, making up problems concerning common activities, and ending a fable in a humorous, sad, or moralistic manner. Wallach and Kogan (1965) were critical of this battery because of the low degree of correlation between the subtests and the absence of any common creative factor that corresponded to g in intelligence. This criticism seems based on the notion that g is a basic factor common to all intelligent behavior, when in fact it is simply a measure of the inability to design a test that taps only one specific ability. (For example, tests of arithmetic ability correlate somewhat with tests of rote memory because the latter is necessarily involved in the former.) They devised a battery that included tests of the number of instances of a class concept that the subject could think of, unusual uses of common objects, line and pattern meanings, and similarities. All of these items were scored for the number and the uniqueness of the responses. Like an IQ score, scores obtained on a typical creativity battery are composite scores, and people with the identical score do not necessarily have the same pattern of creative abilities.

Often different types of abilities are measured on specific tests of creativity. As a result, different studies of creativity deal with different human abilities. One of the problems with research in this area is the lack of agreement on what types of behavior should be subsumed by the term *creativity*. For example, a unique response to a stimulus word in a word association test may, in a sense, be considered creative. It may also be considered bizarre in some circumstances. There are also questions (reminiscent of Thorndike's views on intelligence) about whether there are many different types of creativity and how they may be related to each other. Is the type of creativity exhibited by an engineer in creating a new design the same type of creativity involved in writing poetry or painting a picture?

It seems to the author that the term *creativity* ought to be restricted to the area of problem solving. Thus, the solution of problems when the means for the solution are available is an example of intelligent behavior. The solution of problems when the means of solution do not exist but have to be created by the problem solver is an example of creative behavior.

While creativity is a separate ability from intelligence and children can be selected who score high on one of these attributes and low on the other, there is a certain amount of correlation between the two measures, probably because of the problem-oriented nature of creative ability. In other words, it takes a certain amount of intelligence to be able to demonstrate creative ability.

Creativity, like intelligence, is regarded positively in our culture but probably is much rarer. Whether the comparative rarity of creativity is due to the fact that it is not reinforced in our mass-production educational system, where it can be a source of problems for teachers, is a question that remains to be answered. There is little, if any, well-controlled research concerning the effects of hypnosis on creativity because of the immature state of the art with respect to studies on creative behavior.

In theory, hypnosis would not be expected to improve creative behavior unless there were some psychological factors at work that prevented the full expression of a subject's creative abilities that could be removed by hypnotic suggestion. An example of this type of factor can be seen in the theoretical foundation for a method of group problem solving called brainstorming. A common difficulty in problem solving is that many problems require the skills and knowledge of more than one person for solution. Hence these problems must be solved at meetings. In an ordinary meeting, many ideas may not be presented because their originator fears group rejection or criticism. Not only may workable solutions be lost in this manner, but some suggestions not practical in themselves, which may, however, suggest other more feasible solutions, will also be lost to the group. Brainstorming tries to get these ideas expressed by establishing the ground rule that all ideas, however inane they may seem, will be presented and accepted uncritically until they are all on the table. They will then be evaluated and accepted or rejected. Although the theory seems reasonable, the research does not indicate that groups using brainstorming techniques solve problems any better than groups using conventional techniques.

To extrapolate from brainstorming, if creative ability is being inhibited by fear of ridicule or criticism, then hypnosis may be able to increase creativity under these circumstances. Sanders (1976) discusses factors believed to facilitate or inhibit creative behavior and reports results that suggest group hypnosis may be effective in improving the ability of subjects to solve real-life problems more creatively. Gur and Reyher (1976) report that hypnotized subjects performed significantly better than simulators and waking controls on the figural and overall creativity scores of the Torrance Test of Creativity but not on verbal creativity. Using highly susceptible female subjects, Ashton and McDonald (1985) found that hypnosis did not generally improve creative performance as measured by the Torrance Test of Creative Thinking or the Sounds and Images Test when compared to the performance of simulators or a waking relaxed control group. However, hypnotic subjects were significantly higher in verbal flexibility and figural elaborations. The differences between these results and those of Gur and Reyher may relate to the use of all female subjects, since sex is a factor thought to mediate the relationship between hypnosis and creativity. Straus (1980) found no enhancement of scores on the Creative Imagination Scale produced by a clinical induction procedure administered to subjects in therapy for weight control treatment, although these results can hardly be taken as an indication that hypnosis is incapable of modifying scores on that instrument since no specific suggestions of better performance seem to have been made.

In addition to removing factors that inhibit creative expression, hypnosis may be useful in encouraging the imagery and imagination that are often involved in creative thinking. Gur and Reyher (1976) suggest that the psychoanalytic concept of "regression in the service of the ego" may be an appropriate description of how hypnosis may aid creativity. In other words, a person is regressed to permit a more primitive type of pictorial imagery in thinking, which may be better for solving some problems creatively than the usual adult pattern of verbal thought. Simon (1977) and Khatami (1978) speculate on the role of altered states of consciousness in the genesis of creative thinking and compare this type of thought process with conventional logical thinking.

Hong (1982) reviewed the literature suggesting that hypnosis can enhance divergent or creative thinking by a combination of relaxation, suspension of critical thinking, elimination of distraction, and the fostering of self-confidence and noted that most of the studies cited used one of two methodological approaches: either direct suggestions of improved creativity or image-generating suggestions. Hong contrasted the effectiveness of these two treatments in improving creative behavior as measured by an abbreviated version of the Torrance Test of Creative Thinking. For each treatment group, there were two control groups made up of high- or low-susceptibility simulators. He found that both types of suggestions improved overall verbal and figural creativity scores, although a predicted differential effect on these two measures did not occur.

Since persons with a good imagination and the ability to generate imagery are typically good hypnotic subjects, it would appear likely that future research may disclose a relationship between hypnotic susceptibility and creativity. This is also suggested by Patricia Bower's (1978) work, in which she found that highly creative people and good hypnotic subjects report their creative behavior or hypnotic responses as occurring effortlessly. She thus investigated the possibility that the capacity for "effortless experiencing" might be a common denominator between creativity and hypnosis. She found a high degree of correlation between susceptibility and both effortless experiencing and creativity.

HYPNOTIC AGE REGRESSION AND REVIVIFICATION

The phenomenon of hypnotic age regression is demonstrated when it is suggested to a hypnotic subject that he is going back in time to an earlier period of his life. Good subjects given suggestions that they are getting younger typically display immature behavior characteristic of an earlier period of life. The issue investigated by a large body of research deals with the reality of this age regression. Orne (1951) viewed the issue as a choice between two alternative explanations for the subject's observed behavior. One explanation is that in an age regression, all experiences subsequent to the time period suggested have been ablated from the subject's memory, and he has returned to the characteristic patterns of thought and behavior of the age level suggested; that is, he experiences a revivification. The other explanation is that the subject is engaged in role playing or trying to comply with the experimenter's suggestion by acting out the part. Barber (1962a) pointed out the semantic difficulties with casting the problem in these terms. A hypnotically regressed subject is probably not engaged in role playing if that term is taken to mean trying to deceive the experimenter. Typically, good hypnotic subjects given age-regression suggestions imagine that they are younger and act appropriately. The issue usually investigated is how closely the behavior of such subjects approaches the behavior of children of the suggested age or, when information is available, the behavior of the same subject at the younger age.

To answer this question, age-regressed subjects have been subjected to such tasks as psychological tests (Rorschach, figure drawing, Bender-Gestalt, IQ tests, and tests of moral development), tests of hypermnesia, and optical illusions. They have also had physiological measurements, including EEG recordings and Babinski tests, made on them, and they have been tested for the presence of conditioned responses to stimuli when regressed to a time prior to the conditioning (or subsequent to conditioning but prior to extinction).

Orne (1951) age regressed ten students to age 6 and then administered a Rorschach test, took a handwriting sample, and had the subjects draw a man, a house, and a boat. The same measures were later taken with the subjects awake and, finally, with instructions to the waking subjects to simulate the responses of a 6-year-old. A real effect was produced by age-regression suggestions, but this effect was clearly not a revivification. Characteristically the response of subjects showed some childlike features and some adult features. For example, the subjects wrote in a childlike scrawl but had no apparent difficulty in either spelling or understanding words well beyond the ken of an average 6-year-old (such as *hypochondriac*). The simulated drawings of some subjects were similar to their productions when age regressed. An actual Rorschach was available from one subject, taken at age 6, and an actual drawing, drawn by another at the same age. Their productions when age regressed were very different from these historical records, again suggesting that under age-regression instructions, subjects do not relive their past but simply imagine themselves younger and act more immaturely.

McConkey and Sheehan (1980) found differences in performance between hypnotic subjects and simulators when cued by the experimenter to behave logically or illogically in response to age regression suggestions. Some subjects were told that they were able to spell key words in a sentence, which they were asked to write under age regression (illogical behavior); others were told that a 7-year-old could not spell these words. Nine out of 39 hypnotized subjects and only 2 out of 39 simulators ignored the cue to misspell the words (i.e., act logically). The authors concluded that although hypnotized subjects are influenced by experimenter-supplied cues, they are also controlled by their subjective interpretation of the situation.

Sarbin and Farberow (1952) regressed six adults to ages 18, 13, 6, and 3. As in Orne's study, they found both adult and childlike responses to the Rorschach test, and drawings tended to be superior to those produced by children at the suggested age level.

The studies are in good agreement that drawings produced by age-regressed subjects generally contain both mature and immature features and that they are usually somewhat superior to drawings produced by children actually at the age in question. Often there is little difference in drawings between hypnotically age-regressed subjects and subjects told to simulate by making the type of drawing that a child of a certain age would.

Barber (1961c) reviewed several lines of research investigating the issue of the reality of hypnotic age regression. The first of these relates to evidence reported in 1948 by Gidro and Bowersbuch, who noted that subjects regressed to less than 5 months of age developed a Babinski sign in response to stimulation of the sole of the foot. Many neurology textbooks regarded this reaction, which is abnormal in adults, as characteristic of infants, and hence this finding was taken as physiological evidence of the reality of age regression. This finding was replicated by True and Stephenson (1951) and McCranie, Crasilneck, and Teter (1955). Barber cited a 1941 study of 75 infants by McGraw, who found that contrary to some neurology texts, young infants did not characteristically display a Babinski sign. The usual response to plantar stimulation in infants up to 3 months was leg withdrawal, and this reaction was shown in 70% of the infants up to 7 months of age. Barber speculates that the Babinski signs elicited in age-regression research may have been due to a loss of tonicity due to the "assumption of the infantile sleeping posture" or a realization of what the experimenter wanted and the voluntary making of the response.

Raikov (1983–1984) reports the alteration of EEG recordings in four out of five highly susceptible subjects under hypnotic age regression to infancy with the production of high-amplitude theta and delta waves. No similar changes were noted in the same subjects when given waking age-regression suggestions. Raikov also reports a variety of age-specific behaviors appearing in deeply hypnotized subjects regressed to early infancy, such as reflexive sucking, crying without tears, disassociated eye movements, and grasping reflex (Raikov, 1980, 1982). None of these subjects displayed these behaviors prior or subsequent to the age regression, nor did they or professional actors perform these neonatal responses as frequently when instructed to act like an infant. Interestingly, Raikov does not report any instance of a deeply hypnotized subject age regressed to the neonatal period losing toilet training.

Another type of research is exemplified by a case reported by Kupper (1945) involving a patient who, since the age of 18, had been subject to epileptic seizures related to problems with his father. On age regressing the patient to age 12, the EEG record became normal and remained so as the patient was gradually brought back toward his current age, until he reached the age of 18. Barber points out that in this case, the hypnotic age regression was not necessary, for Kupper reported that only the patient's emotional state centered on his problem could trigger a seizure.

In a similar vein, Ford and Yeager (1948) reported that a patient who was cured of a visual problem (homologous hemianopia) by the surgical removal of a cyst in his third ventricle had the visual problem return when age regressed to a time prior to the operation. Barber notes that an objective visual test was either not made or not reported, so that the issue of whether this effect was real (in the sense that it was physiological) was not resolved. This argument seems spurious. If by the reality of hypnotic age regression we mean that it is a physiological process, it would appear unlikely that it could meet this requirement. If the subject was subjectively blind in part of his visual field, it would seem that this is a real effect, whether or not an objective test of the optical pathways disclosed that they were functioning normally and that the difficulty in vision was psychological. No one disputes the reality of hysterical blindness or paralysis in the absence of an organic lesion.

True (1949) reported that when adults were regressed to Christmas day or their birthdays at ages 10, 7, and 4, a high percentage of them could name the correct day of the week on which these occasions fell. Numerous attempts to replicate these studies were unsuccessful (Barber, 1961c; Best and Michaels, 1954; Reiff and Scheerer, 1959). In addition, Barber found that children 4 years of age generally do not differentiate the days of the week.

Barber (1961c, 1962d) reviewed a series of studies utilizing age-appropriate performance on tests of intelligence as evidence of age regression. In 1933, Platonow found that two out of three subjects, age regressed to 10, 6, and 4, respectively, closely approximated the appropriate mental age of the Stanford-Binet Test but performed somewhat better than the age level suggested. The subject regressed to age 4 passed all of the items for a mental age level of 7.

Young (1940) regressed five subjects to age 3 and gave them items from the 1916 Stanford-Binet Test. All subjects attained a change in mental age levels, but their measured mental age was somewhat higher than the level suggested. The mean mental age measured for the group was 4 years, 8 months. He then age regressed nine subjects to age 3 and at the same time instructed seven unsusceptible subjects to try to respond to test items as a 3-year-old would. He found that unhypnotized simulators did as well as age-regressed hypnotic subjects. Mean mental age of the groups were 5 years, 5 months and 5 years, 11 months, respectively.

Spiegel, Shor, and Fishman (1945) gave the Stanford-Binet Test to a 23-year-old subject under normal waking conditions and under hypnotic age regression to 12 different ages ranging from 1.5 to 20. The subject's waking IQ was 123; under age regression, it varied from 95 to 134. Since IQ was obtained at that time by dividing a subject's mental age by his chronological age and multiplying by 100, it followed that if a subject responded appropriately at each suggested chronological age level for a person with his own basic intellectual ability, his IQ would remain constant. To the extent his responses at an earlier age are too mature, his IQ score would rise. The apparent problem in administering the same test to the same subject 12 times is ameliorated to some extent since, on the Binet test, different items are asked at different age levels, although with 12 increments some overlap was inevitable.

Sarbin (1950a) found nine adults for whom the results of a Binet test administered between ages 8 and 9 were available. He hypnotized and age regressed these subjects to the exact day of taking the test and readministered it. The same subjects were also given the test when awake with instructions to simulate the performance of an 8- or 9-year-old. All scores were higher under age regression than under the original testing, again confirming the common finding that age-regressed subjects act more immaturely than usual but less immaturely than the age level selected. The average overestimation of the suggested mental age (MA) under hypnosis was 3.5 years. This was a better performance than obtained from the same subjects when simulating an age regression; then they overestimated the MA by 5.25 years on average. Kline (1950), on the other hand, age regressed ten college students to ages 15, 10, and 8 and used equivalent forms of the Otis Self-Administering Test of Mental Ability at each age level and under normal waking conditions. He found that, at all levels, the subjects' IQs remained practically constant; that is, their measured mental ages were appropriate to the suggested age.

Barber (1961c) found that unhypnotized simulating subjects were able to give as convincing a performance of age regression as hypnotized subjects and in fact were slightly more accurate in their approximation of the behavior of a 10-year-old. Crasilneck and Michael (1957) had ten student nurses copy the geometric patterns of the Bender-Gestalt Test under normal waking conditions, under waking instructions to simulate the behavior of a 4-year-old, under hypnotic suggestions to simulate the behavior of a 4-year-old, and under hypnotic age regression to 4 years. Three clinical psychologists rated the maturity level of the drawings blind and found the mean maturational levels of the groups to be 11.2, 9.9, 7.8, and 7.3 respectively. Again, age-regressed subjects acted less maturely when rated on a psychological test but still more maturely than the age level suggested. In this case, the hypnotic subjects were more successful in their regressed behavior than simulating subjects, but the fact that the raters found the mean maturity level of the student nurses to be 11.2 under normal waking conditions suggests that the test is not a particularly good one for estimating ages of subjects.

Gard and Kurtz (1979) report that simulators show less mature performance in cognitive tasks than hypnotically age-regressed subjects but that the latter report experiencing profound changes in memory and feelings that simulators do not.

LeCron (1952) conditioned a hand withdrawal and an eye blink reflex and found that both ceased to be elicited by the conditioned stimulus when the subject was hypnotically age regressed to a time prior to the conditioning. McCranie and Crasilneck (1955) replicated this effect for a hand withdrawal but not for an eye blink. Barber (1961c) criticized these experiments on the ground that these conditioned responses are not involuntary and can be simulated or inhibited voluntarily. Actually, conditioning research with eye blinks has indicated that there are several types that must be distinguished, some of which are involuntary and some of which are not.

Edmonston (1960) conditioned an eye blink response and subsequently extinguished it. He found that the eye blink was reinstated when the subject was age regressed to a time subsequent to the conditioning but prior to the extinction. Aside from the issue of the involuntary nature of this reflex, another interesting question is whether the reinstatement of the conditioned response might be the result of the relaxed hypnotic state's facilitating the normal process of spontaneous recovery of an extinguished conditioned response. This might be expected by some theorists (such as Hull) who regard reactive inhibition or fatigue as partially responsible for some of the loss in reactive potential during extinction. It is this part of the extinguished habit that is thought to be recovered during spontaneous recovery following a period of rest.

In an interesting study, Reiff and Scheerer (1959) discovered that simulating subjects were reluctant to accept a lollipop when their hands were covered with mud after playing in a sandbox. Subjects under hypnotic age regression to age 4, however, in accordance with the experimenters' expectations, were not reluctant to accept the lollipop under these conditions. O'Connell, Shor, and Orne (1970), possibly because they had no such expectations to convey subtly to their subjects, were unable to replicate this result and found no significant difference between hypnotically age-regressed and simulating subjects with respect to propensity to accept a lollipop while their hands were muddy.

Parrish, Lundy, and Leibowitz (1969) found that the magnitude of the effects of the Ponzo and Poggendorff optical illusions obtained from ten age-regressed subjects was in accordance with the normative data for young children. Perry and Chisholm (1973), using low- and medium-susceptibility subjects as simulators, were unable to replicate these findings in hypnotic or simulating groups. They found that the performance of hypnotically age-regressed subjects can be matched by nonhypnotized control subjects.

Walker, Garrett, and Wallace (1976) tried to demonstrate the reality of hypnotic age regression utilizing the phenomenon of eidetic imagery. Eidetic imagery (a photographic memory) is found, according to these authors, in from 8% to 20% of young children but is essentially nonexistent in adults. They were able to produce eidetic imagery in two of 20 subjects by hypnotic age regression as measured by the recognition of a correct figure in three 10,000-dot stereograms. No subject correctly identified the figure while awake (Wallace, 1978). Spanos, Ansari, and Stam (1979) were unable to replicate this effect in any of 24 subjects who described themselves as having been "eidetiken" as children. In view of the low level of the effect reported by Wallace and his associates, this failure is not particularly surprising nor does it demonstrate that the earlier results were not valid.

O'Brien and associates (1977) presented five.moral dilemma problems to subjects given task-motivational instructions to act like first-grade students and to hypnotically age-regressed subjects. Their purpose was to ascertain subjects' level of moral development in terms of Kohlberg's stage theory of moral development. A control group was given the same items without age regression. Both treatment groups were found to react as if at a significantly lower level of moral development than the control group, but there was no significant difference between them. As is typical in this type of study, actual first graders were at a much lower level of moral development than either the hypnotically age-regressed or task-motivated subjects.

Nash, Johnson, and Tipton (1979) found that although hypnotically age-regressed subjects and simulators behave quite similarly with respect to objective cognitive behavior, if the dependent variable involves affective processes, such as responses involving a "transitional object" (the child's first

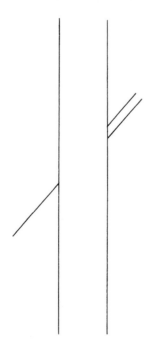

Figure 4-2. Poggendorff Illusion.

treasured possession, such as a teddy bear or other toy), then the two groups act quite differently in the presence of threat (an absent mother). Nash, Lynn, Stanley, Frauman, and Rhue (1985) confirmed and expanded upon this finding to nonthreatening situations when the mother is present.

In a typical clinical study, Twerski and Naar (1976) reported the cases of two women suffering from depression as the result of feelings of guilt about the childhood deaths of a sister and playmate, respectively. They were benefited in therapy by a revivification and abreaction of the original traumatic experience under hypnotic age regression. The importance of these cases and other cases like them does not depend on whether age regression is real (in the sense that the person is actually returned to his mental status as a child) or whether he merely imagines he is a child again. The essential question in a clinical application is whether the technique is useful. Does it benefit a patient who was not helped by alternative procedures? In these cases, the answer would appear to be that it does.

To summarize a great deal of research, it would appear that good hypnotic subjects given age-regression suggestions imagine themselves to be younger and typically display behavior more appropriate to an earlier age but still more mature than the age specified. It appears extremely unlikely that a hypnotic age regression is capable of producing physiological responses characteristic of an earlier period of life. This does not mean that age regression is any less real. It simply means that, like all other hypnotic phenomena, it is a psychological effect produced by the subject's imagination and thought processes. As further evidence of this position, it is well known that, besides being age regressed, subjects can be given age-progression instructions, and under these conditions they typically act as they imagine older people would. Obviously age progression cannot be real in the sense that a person is transported to a future state of being, but it is psychologically as real a form of subjective reality to the subject as age regression is. The same can be said of studies that purport to age regress a subject to a previous life. This experience may be subjectively real to the subject, although objectively such results appear to be totally invalid. Baker (1982) showed that the production of reports of regression to previous lives was a function of previous statements made to subjects that were positive, neutral, or negative with respect to the issue of reincarnation.

HYPNOTIC DISTORTION OF SUBJECTIVE TIME

Another commonly reported hypnotic effect is the subjective distortion of time. Under hypnosis, good subjects generally report that suggestions that time is passing more slowly or quickly are effective in altering their perception of time. Subjects' estimates of the duration of an interval of time are typically displaced in the predicted direction. In the absence of specific suggestions of time speeding up or slowing, it is a common finding that hypnotic subjects tend to underestimate time spent in a trance by an average of 40% (Bowers, 1979a; K. S. Bowers and Brenneman, 1979; St. Jean, MacLeod, Coe, and Howard, 1982; Swartz, 1982). This effect is unrelated to susceptibility. It is generally accounted for by assuming it is due to the high degree of absorption of subjects under hypnosis or is related to posthypnotic amnesia, the theory being that the fewer events a subject is able to recall, the shorter he assumes the interval to have been. St. Jean and coworkers (1982) found no relationship between the extent of posthypnotic amnesia and the shortening of the estimate of hypnotic duration. This confirms similar findings by Bowers (1979b) and disconfirms the hypothesis that posthypnotic amnesia accounts for subjective time shortening. Furthermore, not all subjects report a shorter duration of subjective time. St. Jean and McLeod (1983) note that some subjects overestimate elapsed time, and under some circumstances, time estimation may be quite accurate. The length and type of activity occurring under hypnosis appear to be major determinants of the accuracy and direction of the reported duration of hypnosis.

Cooper and Erickson (1954) suggested to deeply hypnotized subjects that time would go slowly, and seconds would seem like minutes or hours. The subjective reports of their subjects confirmed that time seemed to go more slowly for them. Individual subjects reported imagining performing very complex activities such as watching an entire basketball game in a real-time interval of 1 second or individually counting 9,200 BBs in a 5-second interval.

These reports are reminiscent of the fallacious ideas concerning nocturnal dreams that were prevalent prior to dream studies involving EEG measurement during sleep. It was formerly thought that long, involved dreams could take place in a few seconds of real time. When the correlation between REM patterns on the EEG and dreaming was discovered, it provided a means for measuring the real-time interval during which a dream occurred. It was found that the thought process was not speeded up during nocturnal dreams, and, in fact, it took, about as long to dream of an event as the event would have taken to occur in waking life.

One thought behind time distortion research was that by slowing down subjective time, the thought processes could be speeded up. To demonstrate that the subjects were not just verbally agreeing with the experimenters because of social pressure to develop the effect sought, investigators tried to demonstrate that this alteration of time perception could produce objective as well as subjective effects. In other words, the slowing down of subjective time should result in a relative speeding up of the thought processes and hence make possible an increased amount of learning in a given interval of real time. No effect of hypnotic time slowing was found on a motor task involving learning to write with the nondominant hand. However, Cooper and Erickson found in a one-subject study that this markedly increased the subject's ability to learn a list of nonsense syllables.

Barber and Calverley (1964*i*) sought to answer three questions raised by this study:

1. Does hypnotic time distortion produce reliable objective effects such as facilitating verbal learning?
2. Is it possible to produce hypnotic time distortion without spending up to 20 hours in training the subject to product this effect (as thought necessary by Cooper and Erickson)?
3. Is hypnosis necessary to produce this type of time distortion?

They pretested 48 subjects on a 12-item list of nonsense syllables in a free recall situation. Subjects were then divided into one of three experimental groups. Group one was composed of 16 high-susceptibility subjects given suggestions of time distortion under hypnosis. The remaining two groups had subjects randomly assigned to them without regard to susceptibility. Group two was given time distortion suggestions under waking conditions, and group three was a waking control group given no special instructions. The dependent variables measured were the subject's subjective reports and learning performance on a list of 12 nonsense syllables. Ninety-five percent of the hypnosis group and 81% of the waking-time distortion group experienced some degree of time distortion as opposed to only 12% of the control group. Both experimental groups differed significantly from the control group with respect to estimated duration of a 5-minute interval but did not differ significantly from each other. The control group's average estimate of the 5-minute interval was 4.2 minutes, while the means for the hypnotic and waking-time distortion groups were 89.1 and 46.9 minutes, respectively.

With respect to performance on the learning task, none of the three groups differed significantly from any other, nor did any hypnotic subject display a marked increase in performance on the learning task. Barber and Calverley speculated that neutral hypnosis by itself may reduce performance on a learning task simply by virtue of its relaxing effect, which makes the subject less active. There is much evidence that the more active the learning process, the better the retention of the material. It should be noted that when the effects of hypnotic instructions on learning and retention were previously considered, instructions were given to enhance motivation and confidence in an effort to increase learning. Here the instructions tested for their effect on learning were instructions to slow time down, and this study suggests that such instructions are ineffective. It also demonstrated that extensive training was not necessary to produce a subjective time-distorting effect in hypnotic subjects, and, in fact, hypnosis itself was unnecessary to produce such an effect.

In 1974, Krauss, Katzell, and Krauss reported that in a free recall learning task, learning could be improved by the suggestion that 3 minutes of real study time would seem like 10 minutes. They reported that subjects given these instructions learned as much as did control subjects given 10 minutes of study time. They speculated on the potential value of this phenomenon in speeding up the educational process and increasing the amount of learning possible in a human lifetime.

Johnson (1976) and Wagstaff and Ovenden (1979) were unable to replicate these results, however. Johnson used five different treatment groups. The first three groups were given 3-minute study periods under conditions of hypnotic time distortion, task-motivational instructions, or no special instructions. The remaining two groups were given 10-minute study periods under task-motivational instructions or no special instructions. Johnson found that regardless of the subject's treatment group, the number of items learned on a 60-item list was solely a function of the amount of study time. For 3 minutes of study time, from 15 to 20 words were learned; with 10 minutes of study time, from 28 to 31 items were retained.

St. Jean (1980) found that no combination of hypnotic susceptibility and type of time-distorting suggestions improved subject performance on a verbal learning task compared to waking and hypnotic control group performance but that highly susceptible subjects reported convincing changes in experienced time duration following time-distorting suggestions.

While the weight of the evidence suggests that time-slowing suggestions do not improve verbal learning performance, Baer (1979, 1980) provides evidence that they may produce objective effects in perceptual motor tasks. Subjects displayed increased performance on a video ball-hitting game when it was suggested that the speed of the ball was decreasing. Also, the rate of response to a button-pressing task learned on a variable interval schedule was decreased in response to time-slowing suggestions. Since subject reinforcement was based on the number of responses in the latter study, Baer thinks it unlikely that the lower response rate was made to please the experimenter.

It should be pointed out that while the subjective slowing down of time under hypnosis does not speed up or otherwise improve the learning process for verbal material, the subjective effect may be quite real. Thus, when hypnotic suggestions are made to immobile patients or patients in pain that time is speeding up and hours seem like minutes or seconds, these may be effective in reducing the patient's suffering, which is, after all, a subjective, not an objective, event.

Like most other hypnotic phenomena, hypnotic time distortion is a special instance of a normal psychological effect. Examples of common nonhypnotic distortions of subjective time are the feeling that time is flying by when one is enjoying oneself or dragging during a dull lecture (McCue, 1982).

POSTHYPNOTIC SUGGESTIONS

A *posthypnotic suggestion* is generally defined as a suggestion made during hypnosis that is intended to be carried out in the subsequent waking state, usually in response to some cue. It is also possible to have a type of posthypnotic suggestion for which the response is not to be made to some posthypnotic cue but is merely a continuation into the waking state of a response originally made under hypnosis. For example, arm catalepsy may be produced under hypnosis and the subject told that it will continue when he is awakened. In this type of posthypnotic behavior, it is customary to use a release signal to terminate the effect in the waking state. Most of the research to be reported here, however, involves the first type of situation.

In 1941 Erickson and Erickson published a paper critical of much of the previous research in posthypnotic behavior because it concentrated on the overt behavior of the subject and ignored his mental condition at the time of the behavior. They claimed that close observation disclosed that a special mental state invariably develops when a cue for the performance of a posthypnotic behavior is given, and this special mental state disrupts the subject's ordinary waking behavior. This state persists until the posthypnotic suggestion is effectuated. In effect, the hypnotic trance is involuntarily reinstated, and this reinstatement requires neither suggestion nor instruction to occur. This minitrance state was said to be in no way different from the original trance. The manifestations of this reinstated trance include a slight pause in the subject's immediate activity, a facial expression of distraction and detachment, glassiness of the eyes and dilation of the pupils, and a marked loss of contact with the general external environment. The completion of the posthypnotic act was said to terminate this trance, but its termination was punctuated by a brief interval of confusion and disorientation.

To demonstrate this trance, these authors advocated either making a suggestion to the subject or interfering with the posthypnotic act at the time the cue for its execution is given. Typically, they claim, the subject will pause and is obviously in a trance state awaiting instructions. Upon completing the posthypnotic act, there will be a spontaneous awakening from the reinstated trance, with amnesia for both the act and the trance state, although some subjects may have a hazy awareness of the act.

The authors report the performance of posthypnotic acts after periods of from months to 4 or 5 years from the hypnotic session. They claim that apparent exceptions to the invariability of the spontaneous posthypnotic trance arise from any of the following:

1. The failure to develop amnesia for the posthypnotic suggestion (In this case the act is performed voluntarily, as opposed to the usual way without knowledge of the cause or motivation behind the behavior.)
2. The ambiguity or uncertainty of the posthypnotic suggestion.
3. The unwillingness of the subject to perform the suggested act.
4. Failure of amnesia for the trance.

Thus, to Erickson and Erickson, the revivification of the original trance state was an integral part of the execution of a posthypnotic suggestion, and the spontaneous development of this trance while executing such suggestions was evidence of the validity of the original trance. Unhypnotized, simulating subjects who voluntarily perform "posthypnotic" acts do not develop a spontaneous trance. Erickson and Erickson regarded the posthypnotic trance and act as a form of dissociative behavior and thus a useful tool to determine the capacity of a subject to carry out two tasks at the same time: one on a conscious level and one on an unconscious level. Upon completion of the posthypnotic act, the subject may resume his waking activity where he left off or appear confused, depending on how disruptive the posthypnotic act was of ongoing behavior at the time it was elicited.

Barber (1958c) takes the position that there is no essential difference between a subject's hypnotic and posthypnotic behavior. He says that a hypnotic subject behaves differently because he conceives of himself and his environment differently. Thus, suggestions are accepted by the subject in the posthypnotic period if he believes that the relationship of hypnotist and subject still exists between himself and the experimenter. They are not accepted if he believes that this relationship is over. It is this conception of a continuing relationship rather than a spontaneously reinstated trance that produces the subject's posthypnotic hypersuggestibility. Barber notes the common observation that subjects immediately on awakening from hypnosis usually accept any suggestions made to them that they would have accepted had they remained hypnotized. This is so even before any cue for posthypnotic behavior is given. Also, they display the same hypersuggestibility even after the performance of the posthypnotic act.

Contrary to Erickson and Erickson, Barber says that amnesic and nonamnesic subjects carry out posthypnotic suggestions in an identical manner. If amnesia is not suggested, subjects carry out posthypnotic suggestions with complete awareness of the cause of their actions. Even when amnesia is suggested, subjects typically are either aware that a cue has some significance for them or that the behavior elicited was suggested under hypnosis (possibly because the behavior would otherwise be inexplicable to them).

If a posthypnotic suggestion fits into a subject's normal pattern of behavior (e.g., scratching his head while talking), Barber says that he does not "go deeper" into a trance when he carries it out; that is, a reinstatement of the trance is not an inevitable concomitant of a posthypnotic act. However, if the behavior cannot be carried out without "going deeper" into a trance—that is, becoming relatively inattentive to himself and his environment—then he will go into the type of trance described by Erickson and Erickson. For example, a posthypnotic suggestion to hallucinate a cat would require considerable detachment from the subject's surroundings. In short, Barber claims that a subject executing a posthypnotic suggestion behaves essentially the same way he would if during hypnosis he were told to open his eyes and pretend he is awake.

Barber, in a 1962(b) review of the literature cited a variety of early studies reporting that waking subjects given task-motivational instructions perform posthypnotic like behaviors on cue as often as hypnotized subjects given posthypnotic suggestions (Barber and Calverley, 1962; Barber and Glass, 1962; Fogelman and Crasilneck, 1956; Kellogg, 1929; Patten, 1930; Wells, 1940). Fisher (1953) comparing the results of giving posthypnotic suggestions to dream versus giving waking suggestions to the same effect to his friends, concluded that the relationship between the experimenter and the subject is the crucial factor in predicting the acceptance of the suggestion to dream.

Barber goes on to consider the evidence for five widely held views concerning how the carrying out of posthypnotic suggestions differs from the carrying out of ordinary waking suggestions. The first common view, as expressed by LeCron and Bordeaux (1949), is that if the subject is amnesic for the posthypnotic suggestion, then it is carried out under a strong compulsion. On the other hand, there is much evidence that if the posthypnotic suggestion is in conflict with the subject's standards of proper behavior, good subjects either refuse to execute the suggestion or modify it so that the result is acceptable to their personal standards. Indeed, one of the common ways of using hypnosis to generate a conflict in studies of symptom formation is to suggest just such unacceptable behavior.

The second common view is that a subject reenters a trance when performing a posthypnotic act. This is also not universally true according to Barber. Thus, a subject told to hallucinate a cat posthypnotically did go into a spontaneous trance on the signal for the hallucination, but a subject instructed to scratch his head on cue did not.

Therefore the notion that a subject becomes hypersuggestible while performing a posthypnotic suggestion because of the reinstatement of the trance state sometimes conflicts with the data. Furthermore, all subjects are somewhat hypersuggestible on awakening from the trance state, whether or not a posthypnotic suggestion has been made. Barber noted in one study that all subjects accepted a suggestion of foot immobility on awakening from a trance and before any cue for posthypnotic behavior that might reactivate the trance state was given. Barber would account for this by saying that the subject responds in this manner because he conceives the hypnotist-subject relationship as still in effect.

The view that subjects performing posthypnotic suggestions are not conscious of the motivation for their behavior would also appear not to be universally true, but it is common to suggest amnesia for posthypnotic suggestions on the theory that suggestions are more likely to be followed under these conditions. Fisher (1955) found that both amnesic and nonamnesic subjects performed suggestions to cough and hallucinate the smell of Noxema equally well. Barber found similar results with ten somnambulists instructed to stand up and walk around when the experimenter lit a cigarette. On the other hand, Sheehan and Orne (1968) found that of eight subjects who performed a posthypnotic suggestion well (both inside and outside the experimental situation), six had complete amnesia for the entire hypnotic situation and one had amnesia for the posthypnotic suggestion. Thus, although posthypnotic suggestions can be effective without amnesia, they concluded that amnesia may enhance the effect.

Last, the view that subjects performing posthypnotic suggestions invariably have amnesia for both the act and events occurring at the same time is not accurate. Indeed, it is not uncommon for a subject performing an incongruous posthypnotic act, the cause of which he is unaware of, to rationalize reasons for his actions (Reyher and Smyth, 1971). Sheehan and Orne (1968) conclude that amnesia is neither a necessary nor a sufficient condition for posthypnotic behavior to occur.

Sheehan and Orne distinguish the situation in which amnesia for the posthypnotic suggestion is not suggested from the case where it is suggested but breaks down. They speculate there may be less of an effect due to the lack of amnesia in the former case than in the latter because it does not involve the failure to follow the suggestions of the experimenter. Even when the subject is aware of the posthypnotic suggestion, there appears to be an element of compulsion in its execution that is reminiscent of a Zeigarnik effect: there appears to be a motive to complete an uncompleted task. Like Barber, Sheehan and Orne found that only unusual posthypnotic tasks or those frequently tested had a tendency to disrupt the subject's waking stream of consciousness. They also found that a posthypnotic cue can elicit the suggested behavior on some occasions and not on others. The subject had to be aware at some level that the signal was indeed a cue. On the other hand, if the subject failed to respond to a signal for a posthypnotic response in an unambiguous situation, the response was never reinstated in real hypnotic subjects, although it might be with simulating subjects. It was also found that hypnotic subjects are just as likely to respond to cue words when they are embedded in a sentence as when they are presented alone, but simulators responded less frequently to words embedded in sentences.

When hypnotized and simulating subjects were given instructions to touch their foreheads whenever the word *experiment* was spoken posthypnotically, it was found that five of 17 hypnotic subjects made this response when the word *experiment* was uttered by a secretary away from the experimental area, but no simulators did so (Orne, Sheehan, and Evans, 1968). This suggests that role playing, or the notion that the subject conceives the experimental relationship to remain in effect, may not be an adequate explanation for this phenomenon. On the other hand, as Coe (1976b) points out, the fact that the experimenter is not physically present when a subject carries out a posthypnotic suggestion does not demonstrate that no relationship between the hypnotist and the subject is operating. Out of sight is not necessarily out of mind.

St. Jean (1978), comparing rates of responding to posthypnotic suggestions between hypnotic and task-motivational subjects as a function of experimenter surveillance, found, as predicted, that posthypnotic responding was markedly greater with the experimenter present (71%) than in his absence (21%). He notes that this difference supports Sarbin and Coe's (1972) role theory of hypnosis, but the fact that there are subjects who respond at all under the condition of the experimenter's absence supports Orne's state theory (Orne, Sheehan, and Evans, 1968). A strong positive association was found between posthypnotic responding and suggestibility as measured by a modified BSS test regardless of surveillance conditions. No significant difference in nonsurveillance responding was found between hypnotic and task-motivational subjects, although the number of subjects involved was too low to permit a sensitive test of this question. Based on the subjective reports of one task-motivation subject, St. Jean considers the possibility that the procedure may have inadvertently produced a "trance-like" state in this subject.

As in the case of posthypnotic amnesia, itself a special type of posthypnotic suggestion, the depth of the trance at the time of the giving of the posthypnotic suggestion seems to determine the subject's likelihood to respond posthypnotically.

With respect to the time duration of posthypnotic effects, Sheehan and Orne report studies showing effects lasting in excess of 3 months, which is considerably shorter than (but not inconsistent with) the effects reported by Erickson and Erickson. In Sheehan and Orne's study it was found that of 16 subjects who responded posthypnotically on the first day, only ten responded on the second day and only five on the third. This suggests that in ordinary experimental work, where the posthypnotic suggestions are of simple behavior having little significance to the subject, long-term effects may be rare. On the other hand, the authors speculate that in a therapeutic context involving a stronger personal relationship with the therapist and expectations of lasting results, and where the suggestions touch on important issues, posthypnotic suggestions may last much longer. Sheehan and Orne believe that it may be possible to have posthypnotic behavior, once established, continue independent of the therapist. Indeed, it would appear that this is a major goal of any method of psychotherapy.

Another often noted difference between experimental posthypnotic suggestions and therapeutic ones is that the latter are much less dependent on the depth of trance than the former (Kline, 1978). Kline uses the term *trance productivity* as opposed to *trance depth* and notes that therapeutic effects are often possible in what are otherwise light trance states. Possibly the motivation of the subject rather than the depth of trance is the controlling factor. This conclusion would appear to be supported by Barber's work with task-motivational instructions to waking subjects.

Nace and Orne (1970) did a study of the effects of posthypnotic suggestions on subjects who fail to carry out the suggested behavior on cue. Subjects were given the posthypnotic suggestion to take a blue pencil from an assortment of colored pencils and play with it. Subjects of medium hypnotic susceptibility were selected to ensure that there would be enough subjects who failed to carry out the posthypnotic suggestions to be studied. They found that some subjects who failed to respond to the posthypnotic signal did respond to the cue later, in the absence of the experimenter. They also found that subjects who failed to respond to the cue but who did respond later had a higher degree of susceptibility than those who never responded. They concluded that since responses were made in the absence of the experimenter, they could not be due to a face-to-face relationship with him. This conclusion is supportive of a special state or trance theory of hypnosis. They also believed that the subsequent performance of the suggested behavior in the absence of the experimenter is a justification for the warnings frequently made by clinicians that all suggestions made to experimental subjects should be removed prior to the termination of a hypnotic session.

Coe (1973a, 1976b) attempted to test the generality of these findings. He used both real subjects and simulating subjects who were instructed to try to deceive the experimenter observing them (which they all did successfully). He found no clear relationship between the tendency to complete an uncompleted posthypnotic suggestion and hypnotic susceptibility. In one of two studies, hypnotic and waking subjects were found to be equally likely to complete the posthypnotic behavior. In the second study, hypnotic subjects were more likely to do so than waking subjects. However, in the second study the results were the same for subjects simulating the hypnotic and waking conditions, and Coe regards this as some evidence that the demand characteristics of the situation may have played a role in these results. He claims that his data do not support the common assumption that an unperformed posthypnotic suggestion generates a psychic need to carry it out because the subjects who did perform the posthypnotic suggestion on cue also showed a tendency to carry it out later. However, the fact that a behavior is performed as requested does not imply that the motive for its future performance is totally dissipated, particularly if the subject interprets the experimental situation as requiring the continued elicitation of the response.

The present author recalls giving a hypnosis demonstration to a class and telling one of the subjects that she would feel so good on awakening that she would smile. She performed this suggestion, but about halfway through the remaining lecture, the author noticed that she was still smiling in spite of the fact that he had not said anything particularly humorous. The subject had misinterpreted the posthypnotic suggestion to mean "smile and continue smiling."

Closely related to the phenomenon of posthypnotic suggestion is the question of the effect of uncanceled suggestions made under hypnosis. This question was investigated in a series of five experiments by Perry (1977b, 1977c) and Duncan and Perry (1977). They found that only one of 18 subjects given the hypnotic suggestion of a number ceasing to exist had this idea persist beyond the hypnotic state. No subject was affected posthypnotically by an uncanceled suggestion of paralysis from the waist down, and only three of 30 reported the persistence of suggestions of arm and hand analgesia. All of the subjects reporting persistence of hypnotic suggestions were highly susceptible. The authors concluded that part of the persistence of these effects may be due to the hypnotist's implicitly cueing the subjects that he expects the results to persist indefinitely. Whether this was so or not, it seems highly likely that the subjects believed that this was the case. The most common finding was that subjects themselves canceled the instructions when the experimenter failed to do so. Perry believes that only the top 2% or 3% of highly susceptible subjects produce this persistence, but its existence in any subject would seem ample reason for hypnotists to be careful to cancel all instructions given and to guard against this kind of misunderstanding.

Barrios (1973) takes the position that hypnosis facilitates the process of higher-order conditioning: words act as conditioned stimuli to elicit responses. By putting words into a sentence, higher-order conditioning can occur, and words contiguously paired with conditioned stimuli can thus become conditioned stimuli themselves. To demonstrate this theory, he compared the results of subjects being told to hallucinate the sour taste of a lemon in response to a verbal cue, while awake or under hypnosis, and used resistance to extinction and spontaneous recovery as measures of the amount of conditioning produced. He found, as predicted, an increase in conditioning for the hypnotic group as opposed to the control group, and the amount of increase was related to the depth of hypnosis. Although the results of this study do not require the acceptance of the theoretical position taken, the paper is a fascinating one and well worth reading in its entirety for its discussion of common design deficiencies in hypnotic studies. Barrios considers many of the design problems raised by Barber and Calverley (1966b) and describes how these problems are overcome in his study. For example:

1. In many studies, there are no nonhypnotized control groups. In the present study, each subject was his own waking control.
2. Hypnotic subjects are usually preselected for high susceptibility and control subjects either unselected or selected for low susceptibility, thereby confounding hypnosis and susceptibility. In this study, subjects were not preselected.
3. In some studies using subjects as their own control, it may be quite obvious to the subjects what the control condition is. In the present study, hypnosis was not mentioned until the control condition was measured.
4. Experimenter bias may be introduced by the investigator's tone of voice. Here identical instructions were given to all subjects by tape recorder.
5. Many dependent measures in posthypnotic phenomena are subject to voluntary control or faking. In this study, salivation (an involuntary response) was measured by the increased weight of a cotton roll inserted in the subject's mouth.

One of the more interesting points made by Barrios is that a common mistake in the interpretation of studies comparing task-motivational instructions with a standard 15-minute hypnotic induction procedure is to overgeneralize and assume that the results attributed to the specific induction procedure used apply to all hypnotic inductions. Indeed, he points out that it is also an error to assume that a hypnotic induction must involve suggestions of sleep and relaxation. Barrios concludes that Barber's task-motivational instructions are really a specific type of hypnotic induction, and his results, generally showing this procedure to be as effective as a standard induction technique in producing many common hypnotic phenomena, really demonstrate that these two specific induction methods are equally effective.

O'Brien (1977) compared hypnotized and waking task-motivated subjects given the posthypnotic suggestion to feel something sticky on the sole of their shoe and inspect it on hearing the cue word *elevator*. The cue word was presented at the end of the experimental session and by friends of the subject at intervals of 1 and 3 hours after the experimental session and the following morning. Unlike the simulators used in Sheehan and Orne's (1968) study, the task-motivated subjects did not perform significantly differently from the hypnotized subjects. This is further evidence for the equal effectiveness of these kinds of treatment and suggests a reason why clinicians commonly report that light trance states are therapeutically productive. It may be that in clinical situations, the task-motivational aspects are the controlling factor.

Reyher and Smyth (1971) noted that posthypnotic suggestions are often accompanied by a compulsive urge for their completion as opposed to the passive manner in which the same suggestions are executed in a trance state. Furthermore, they note the frequent occurrence of symptoms when anxiety-producing, posthypnotic suggestions are not executed. Reyher (1968) found little support for Erickson and Erickson's reinstatement of the trance hypothesis. He concluded that a posthypnotic suggestion can be carried out in a variety of mental states, and the intrinsic difficulty of the behavior and its anxiety-producing propensity determine the state selected. Reyher and Smyth cite several unpublished studies in which subjects were trained to make some response immediately on entering the hypnotic state, such as scratching the back of their hand or feeling cold and shivering. Subjects were then given various posthypnotic suggestions, and in no case did the signal indicating the presence of a hypnotic state occur. However, the types of suggestions used (e.g., the removal of a shoe, laughing, or examining objects on a tabletop) were neither very difficult nor anxiety producing.

Sommerschield and Reyher (1973) and Burns and Reyher (1976) utilized the fact that subjects will spontaneously inhibit the expression of posthypnotic suggestions that they find morally unacceptable to generate inner conflicts and study the role of these conflicts in symptom formation. In the first study, 12 hypnotized males were given posthypnotic suggestions involving sexual or aggressive impulses toward an attractive older woman. These impulses were to be activated by a cue word. Five susceptible subjects were told to simulate the reactions of the hypnotized subjects. The hypnotic group produced significantly more symptoms and GSRs than the simulation group. There were no differences produced by the nature of the sexual or aggressive conflicts. The second study found that under conditions of hypnotically induced conflict, the number of symptoms developed is a function of the subject's ability to repress. Poor repressors produced more symptoms and larger GSRs. Matthews, Kirsch, and Allen (1984) note that Reyher and his colleagues' work has been cited by some as evidence for the psychoanalytic concept of symptom formation by the stimulation of unconscious Oedipal concepts. They investigated this question by using groups given oedipal paramnesias (involving an older woman) under hypnosis, nonoedipal paramnesias (involving a woman 1 year younger than the subject), no paramnesia, and a simulation group. There was no difference in the number of symptoms produced by the first three groups, causing the authors to conclude that a suggestion to express intense sexual feelings on cue to a stranger is stressful enough to account for symptom formation without the need of an oedipally related paramnesia.

Alman and Carney (1980) report that an indirect induction procedure (based on a modification of J. Barber's rapid induction analgesia) was more effective than a direct induction procedure in producing the posthypnotic response of neck scratching to a posthypnotic cue. They also found that there was less correlation between this response and susceptibility in the indirect induction group than in the direct induction group. They go on to speculate as to the possibility of making hypnotherapy available to lower-susceptibility subjects by the utilization of indirect techniques and question the utility of standard tests of susceptibility in predicting the value of hypnosis to such patients.

HYPNOTIC DISSOCIATION

Hypnotic dissociation refers to the situation in which a hypnotized or posthypnotic subject carries out two tasks independently, one on a conscious and the other on an unconscious level of awareness. A classic example of this type of study is one that involves automatic writing. In such studies, the subject's hand is instructed to write without his conscious awareness of what the hand is writing or even doing. Although the term *dissociation* is often used to describe such hypnotic phenomena as analgesia or amnesia, automatic writing is a difficult behavior to elicit and requires an excellent subject. Knox, Crutchfield, and Hilgard (1975) note that, except in connection with cases of multiple personality, dynamic psychology has shown little interest in the phenomenon, and much of the research in the area dates back to the nineteenth century.

Hilgard and his associates have proposed a neodissociative theory of hypnosis to explain some hypnotic and related cognitive behavior (Hilgard (1973a, 1973b, 1974a; Knox, Morgan, and Hilgard, 1974). According to Stevenson (1976), the classic view of dissociation was that it could reduce the interference between two different tasks simultaneously performed by rendering one of the tasks unconscious or out of the scope of conscious awareness. The neodissociation view was suggested by Stevenson's work in 1972 that demonstrated that two kinds of interference result when two tasks are simultaneously performed, one on a conscious level and the other on an unconscious one. The first type of interference results from the expenditures of effort or psychic energy necessary to keep one of the two tasks out of awareness; the second is the ordinary interference that would exist between the two tasks if they were simultaneously performed consciously.

Thus, when two tasks are performed under conditions of dissociation, these interfering tendencies add, and both tasks are performed less efficiently than they would be if simultaneously performed while conscious of both. Under the old view of dissociation, when Hull's associates found impaired performance of tasks performed in a dissociated state, they took it as evidence that dissociation was not attained.

Knox, Crutchfield, and Hilgard (1975) did a follow-up study on Stevenson's 1972 dissertation. They used a task of alternately pressing one of two keys three times and a task of color naming. The color-naming task was always consciously performed, while the key pressing was performed both consciously and unconsciously. Subjects were scored on the tasks when performed singly or simultaneously. Key pressing was performed (either consciously or unconsciously) in response to a posthypnotic cue. The results were supportive of the neodissociative view and the dual sources of interference alluded to previously. Subjects in this study were carefully preselected to ensure that they could perform the key-tapping task automatically and without conscious awareness.

Stevenson (1976) reported results of a similar study using an easy or a more difficult arithmetic task (counting or cumulative addition) against a conscious color-naming task. The results were clearly supportive of the neodissociative theory. Task performance on an unconscious level was inferior to conscious performance even when executed singly, demonstrating the effort required to keep the task out of awareness or "repressed." He reports a more recent study by Bowers involving dichotic listening. While a verbal message was channeled into one ear, a posthypnotic signal was occasionally presented to the other to call for a posthypnotic response of touching the nose with a finger. Subjects showed less interference between tasks when the signal for nose touching was given posthypnotically on an unconscious level than when given in an ordinary waking condition. This finding is in accordance with the predictions of classical dissociation theory, and Stevenson speculates that these results may be due to the fact that the response of nose touching is simple and may require less effort to automate than counting, the easier of his two arithmetic tasks (Bowers and Brennenman, 1981).

Zamansky (1977) investigated the common belief that hypnotic suggestions are effective because the subject becomes absorbed in them to the exclusion of incompatible thoughts by having good hypnotic and task-motivated subjects exposed to countersuggestions (ideas incompatible with the response suggested). He found that these did not interfere with performance of suggested responses, at least in good subjects (who scored 8 or higher on form A of the SHSS). What seemed perfectly related to subject performance was the belief of the subject as to how the experimenter expected him to behave. Zamansky interpreted these results in terms of the subject's capacity to dissociate two incompatible ideas and his ability to suppress actions without having to suppress thoughts, the antithesis of absorption theory.

The phenomenon of dissociation, usually in the form of automatic writing, has been used by clinicians in an effort to "talk directly to a patient's unconscious" and in experimental work by such devices as Hilgard's *hidden ob-*

server technique. An interesting question, which is not easily answered, is whether the clinical use of such techniques makes it possible to tap material not freely available to the patient's conscious awareness or whether it merely gives him an opportunity to verbalize such material under conditions that subjectively reduce his responsibility for what he is saying. It may also be that these two possibilities are not mutually exclusive and that the ultimate answer involves the operation of both factors. From a clinical point of view, the answer to this question is far less important than the therapeutic value of the material elicited. This is perhaps the real reason that clinicians have failed to investigate this issue. Experimentalists, who are more concerned with questions of this kind for theoretical reasons, are not usually able to work with the type of affect-laden material commonly thought to be the subject of repression unless they create the conflict-producing material themselves by posthypnotic suggestions. In such cases, however, the ethical standards for research set forth by the American Psychological Association create serious impediments to such studies.

Norgrady and her associates (1983) in a study designed to investigate the issue of whether the *hidden observer* effect was an experimental artifact, as claimed by Spanos, examined it in a nondirective fashion. They found that their procedures did not cue simulating subjects, and neither they nor medium-susceptibility hypnotized subjects produced a *hidden observer* effect, whereas 50% of high-susceptibility hypnotic subjects did. The criterion for the presence of a *hidden observer* effect in this study was the report of different levels of experience rather than the more common increase of reported pain (although that effect was noted in analgesia portions of the study). All subjects displaying a *hidden observer* effect also reported a duality effect in age-regression studies. Perhaps most interesting in accounting for the heterogeneity of high-susceptibility subjects with respect to hidden observer phenomena were the comments of many subjects who reported this effect, that these dissociative experiences were common in their waking lives, and they tended to self-monitor their social behavior. Again this suggests that hypnotic behavior, like abnormal behavior, is usually an exaggeration of normal behavior.

In line with this notion, Beahrs (1983) advances the thesis that co-consciousness and dissociation are not just features of altered or pathological states like hypnosis or multiple personality but are common occurrences in normal people. Ludwig (1983) describes what he considers to be the survival value of the common ability to dissociate in everyday life as well as in a variety of altered states of consciousness. This includes the automatization of habitual behaviors (like driving a car) with the resultant economy of effort, the resolution of conflicts, escape from the constraints of reality, and the isolation of catastrophic experiences, among other advantages.

Zamansky and Bartis (1984) note that most studies of hypnotic dissociation are descriptive in nature, and none has utilized dissociation as an independent variable. They sought to conceptualize dissociation in "experimentally verifiable terms independently of hypnosis" and proposed that three criteria must be met in defining an instance of dissociation:

1. Two or more cognitive processes must be engaged in concurrently.
2. These processes must occur simultaneously, not by alternation.
3. The subject must perceive one of these processes as unconscious (that is, autonomous or nonvolitional).

They report methodology to operationalize the first two requirements. They found that waking, highly susceptible subjects are significantly better able to attend to two auditory inputs simultaneously than are moderately susceptible subjects. These results were reported as suggesting that dissociative ability assessed independently of hypnosis may be a predictor of hypnotic ability.

Williams (1984), in a paper reviewing modern theoretical positions on the concepts of neodissociation and co-consciousness, makes the observation that although hypnotized subjects tend to talk more slowly (and effortfully) than when awake, their basic linguistic usage remains unchanged. During dissociated states, however, linguistic usage varies with the particular affective set involved. He claims that linguistic deficits in patients whose problems result from an early arrest in development can make therapy difficult.

HYPNOTICALLY INDUCED DREAMS

Hypnotically induced dreams can be generated either under hypnosis or subsequent to it, in which case they are just a specific type of posthypnotic phenomenon. The subject may simply be told to have and remember a dream, or the theme of the dream can be suggested with varying degrees of specificity. If the dream is produced under hypnosis, the subject can be asked to describe it as he is experiencing it. However, since dreams are predominantly visual experiences and one picture will take much more than the proverbial 1,000 words to describe it in all of its details, such simultaneous verbal reports must of necessity be gross abstractions and therefore distortions of the ongoing dream process. What will be reported is a function of the subject's expectations and mental set and what he perceives the experimenter expects. There is general agreement that hypnotic and posthypnotic dreams, especially the former, tend to differ from naturally occurring nocturnal dreams. Specifically, they tend to be shorter, more verbal, less bizarre, and contain less symbolism. Barber (1962b) says that they are often difficult to distinguish from simple verbal associations to the dream topic suggested. They resemble non-REM (NREM) nocturnal dreams, which are often described by subjects in dream studies as thinking rather than dreaming.

In a review of the literature on hypnotic and posthypnotic dreams Barber (1962*a*) concluded that:

1. Hypnotic dreams typically contain very little evidence of the operation of the dream work; that is, they are not distorted or symbolic representations and good hypnotic subjects often describe their imaginative products as dreams in order to comply with the expectations of the experimenter.
2. When hypnotic dreams are reported involving predominantly pictorial images and a high degree of symbolic material, they do not differ significantly from reports of some nonhypnotized subjects instructed to make up symbolic dreamlike material.
3. Some subjects who report dreaming about the hypnotic situation the following night in response to a posthypnotic suggestion might have done so without the suggestion since the interesting experimental situation could have functioned as an ordinary day residue.
4. Evidence was found in some studies that both hypnotic and control subjects given posthypnotic suggestions to dream at night did not sleep normally and actually awakened during the night and purposely created dreams that they were motivated to produce.
5. The notion that subjects are better able to interpret dreams under hypnosis in the absence of any familiarity with psychology has not been demonstrated.

Barrett (1979), on the other hand, in comparing the hypnotic dreams of 16 medium- to high-susceptibility male and female subjects with the nonhypnotic nocturnal dreams and daydreams of the same subjects (by content analysis of characters, emotions and themes), found a clear relationship between depth of trance and the characteristics of hypnotic dreams. She found that the hypnotic dreams of deeply hypnotized subjects were quite similar to nocturnal dreams and concluded that it was therefore appropriate to use them in therapy as though they were nocturnal dreams; but for medium-susceptibility subjects, content differences were found between hypnotic and nocturnal dreams.

The present author has difficulty with the concept that the usefulness of a hypnotic dream in therapy is a function of its similarity to a nocturnal dream. Its usefulness is a function of the fact that, like any other behavior of a patient, it reflects something about him or her without regard to its relationship to any other behavior.

Dave (1979) reports a study demonstrating the value of hypnotically induced dreams, not in psychotherapy but to aid in the development of creative solutions to problems of an academic, vocational, avocational, or personal nature about which subjects were at an impasse prior to dream manipulation.

Six out of eight subjects in the hypnotic dream group were successful in solving their problem, as compared to one out of eight in a rational-cognitive treatment group and none out of eight in a control group given only a personal interview.

Hall (1953) has noted that a large number of waking subjects without training in psychology seem to be able to interpret dreams adequately. Indeed, his theory of the cognitive functions of dreams (that the function of symbolization in dreams is not to conceal a latent meaning, as Freud had said, but to express a meaning as concisely as possible in the more primitive picture language of the sleeping mind) is based on this and similar phenomena. Hall believes that the same symbols used in everyday slang are used in dreams and that anyone who can understand slang can understand the meaning of a dream.

Torda (1975) used posthypnotic suggestions creating emotional states (anxiety and anger) to study the effects of these emotions on naturally occurring nocturnal dreams in subjects sleeping in her laboratory. Subjects were awakened after each REM period with instructions to verbalize their dreams. The effectiveness of the posthypnotic suggestions in generating the emotional states was confirmed by various physiological measures made on the subjects. This study, although more typical of ordinary dream research than research on hypnotically induced dreams, suggests that future hypnotic dream studies ought to adopt the methodology of monitoring sleep continuously with an EEG and waking subjects for dream reports after each REM period. In addition to answering Barber's questions concerning the reality of the reported dream experience, EEG research is capable of producing a greater yield of dreams and hence could pick up dreams compliant with posthypnotic suggestions that were forgotten in spite of suggestions to remember them. Most research on posthypnotic dreams relies on the memory of the subjects the following morning.

Albert and Boone (1975) used posthypnotic suggestions to inhibit and facilitate dreaming. Five subjects were given suggestions to make an effort not to dream, eight were given suggestions to facilitate dreaming, and four were given a posthypnotic suggestion unrelated to sleep or dreaming. Suggestions to inhibit or facilitate dreaming had a marked effect in the expected direction, based on subjective reports of the subjects the following morning. In addition, EEG tracings made on the subjects throughout the night showed that two of the five dream-inhibition subjects had a dramatic reduction in REM sleep. This reduction demonstrated that there was more than the demand characteristics of the experimental situation involved in the subjective effects. No increase in REM sleep was found for the dream-facilitation subjects, and subjects in the three groups did not differ significantly in NREM sleep.

Spanos and Ham (1975) analyzed and rated the hypnotic dreams of 49 female nursing students for their degree of involvement in imagining, the implausibility of the imaginings, fearfulness, and fragmentation. They found that the majority of hypnotic dreams were plausible, nonfearful, and non-fragmentary. Some subjects, however, did report implausible, fearful, and/or fragmentary dreams. They concluded that individual differences in hypnotic dream protocols were a function of the extent to which subjects became involved in their imagining and that the term *hypnotic dream* encompasses a multidimensional set of experiences worthy of further study.

Noting previous work indicating that correlations between cognitive skills, creativity or imagery, and hypnotic susceptibility are often a function of sex, Spanos, Nightingale, Radtke, and Stam (1980a) performed a similar study using 48 female and 42 male subjects. As predicted, sex differences were found. For females, hypnotic susceptibility and absorption scores correlated with judges' ratings of dream involvement, but for males neither susceptibility nor absorption scores correlated with dream involvement. In line with their belief that in certain tasks (e.g., amnesia) hypnotic subjects consistently outperform task-motivated subjects, while on other tasks (e.g., visual hallucinations) the reverse is true, they found that subjects given hypnotic or relaxation treatments performed equally well but task-motivated subjects had more diversified dreams and were more absorbed in them.

O'Brien and Rabuck (1977), in an effort to demonstrate objectively the reality of a posthypnotic dream independently of the subjective report of subjects, suggested to three young male subjects that they would have an erotic dream followed by a nocturnal emission. Subjects slept in the laboratory for two successive nights so that their bed clothes could be inspected for physical evidence of compliance with the suggestion. Results were negative. In addition to the small samples used, it should be noted that nocturnal emissions are an extremely rare phenomenon in ordinary dream research where subjects sleep in the investigator's laboratory for constant EEG monitoring. In thousands of such vigils, Hall has failed to report a single case of such an occurrence, probably because of the inhibition produced by the surroundings.

Sheehan and Dolby (1979) investigated the relationship between the subject and hypnotist as reflected in hypnotically suggested or task-motivated dreams or control imaginings. Hypnotic subjects generally had dreams reflecting a more positive rapport with the hypnotist than waking subjects and tended to see the hypnotist as an authority figure and guide or helper. They tended to be more self-involved in their dreams, although there were marked individual thematic differences. These results are generally supportive of psychoanalytic theory that all dreams contain references to the analyst and the state of the transference. Of interest here is the fact that these were experimental subjects not involved in therapy with the hypnotist and yet the experimenter appeared in the dreams of all three treatment groups from 63% to 81% of the time with no significant difference between groups.

This chapter has examined the literature of the more important types of hypnotic phenomena and provided a factual anchoring for some of the applications of hypnosis to be considered in the next chapter. This literature is too vast to permit it to be more than sampled here, but it is hoped that the material presented has given readers some insight into the major issues, methodology, and areas of investigation. The literature contains a curious mixture of old wives' tales, speculation, and poorly designed studies sprinkled among some well-designed investigations and interesting theoretical views. There are those who tend to resent studies that contradict some well-established myths and magical beliefs about the powers of hypnosis, such as its supposed ability to revive previous experiences with perceptual clarity or to enhance human abilities without limit. To them it should be pointed out that the capacity of the human imagination to transcend the reality of the immediate situation as demonstrated in the foregoing studies is remarkable enough not to need any artificial enhancement.

The failure of experimental work to replicate many remarkable clinical reports has often been taken to indicate that clinicians as a group are either poor observers or too inadequately trained in research to recognize the need for effective controls. In some cases, this may be true, but there is an alternative explanation, which is not taken into account often enough. Many of the apparent contradictions between clinical findings and experimentation arise from the fundamental error made in assuming that the results obtained in the clinical application of hypnosis are primarily due to the hypnosis rather than to the relationship between the therapist and patient. Hypnosis used in clinical work is very much like an analyst's couch. It is merely a vehicle for the therapist, which by itself, without the transference relationship, produces no benefits. This analogy is made with full knowledge that some psychoanalysts believe that a couch has magical power to produce regression all by itself, but such analysts are in the minority. It is the vital relationship between a patient and therapist that produces the results of hypnotherapy, and this is typically absent in experimental work.

CHAPTER 5

Practical Applications
of Hypnosis

The major phenomena commonly elicited under hypnosis were described in the preceding chapter. This chapter will concern itself with some of the practical uses to which these phenomena may be put. Observant readers will note that in many clinical applications of hypnosis, the techniques used are not necessarily limited to those that have been experimentally validated. Also, clinicians sometimes employ techniques beyond the limits of their demonstrated effectiveness—for example, using an age regression as though it were capable of producing a revivification of earlier experiences, an assumption which the experimental literature fails to support. This seemingly incompetent behavior on the part of therapists is not necessarily due to ignorance. Often it can be justified for at least two reasons.

First, there are sufficient differences between contrived, affect-free, experimental settings and emotion-laden, clinical situations so that the results of experimentation may not only be inapplicable to clinical situations but may even be directly opposite to what would be found in clinical practice (Sheehan, 1979). Second, the goal in clinical work is not to advance human knowledge but to help a specific patient. Thus, the test of a therapeutic technique is not whether it is right or wrong in theory but whether it is clinically useful. There are many purely empirical techniques, such as electroshock therapy, that can be shown to be useful but for which no theoretical justification can be demonstrated. If a patient believes in voodoo, and a therapist is successful in convincing him that he has removed a curse, this may prove useful clinically without committing the therapist to the theoretical position that one person can inflict a curse on another. Also, the fact that research has disclosed that many "hypnotic" effects can be produced without a trance does not diminish the clinical usefulness of hypnosis (Starker, 1975).

Another important difference between theoretical and applied hypnosis, particularly in clinical situations, is that the standard tests of hypnotic susceptibility, so important in the control of experiments, are of less practical value in applied work. This is because a therapist has to work with a particular patient, whatever his susceptibility, and cannot replace him with a better subject, as is often done in research. Susceptibility scores are not always of value in predicting who is likely to benefit from hypnotherapy, and it is a common clinical observation that even a very light trance can be clinically productive in a well-motivated patient, at least for some conditions such as nicotine addiction (for a contrary view, see Butler, 1954; Frankel, 1978-1979; Hilgard, 1982; Schafer, 1975). Also the fact that a patient is a good hypnotic subject is, by itself, no indication that hypnotherapy is the treatment of choice for him without regard to the genesis or dynamics of his problem. This appears to be one of the more clear-cut differences between clinical and experimental work. There are numerous clinical reports of essentially nonsusceptible subjects having major surgery performed solely under hypnoanesthesia, when chemical agents were either unavailable or would have proved fatal to the patient (Kline, 1978; Rockey, 1977).

Although measurement of hypnotic susceptibility may not always be particularly useful in clinical practice, some therapists, including the author, like to use a few of the preinduction tests described in Chapter 2 prior to an initial formal induction. These serve to warm up a patient, give him practice in the unfamiliar mode of noncritical thinking required to be hypnotized, and ease him into the induction situation in a nonthreatening manner. Used in this way, these "tests" are really an integral part of the total induction procedure.

This chapter considers some of the applications of hypnosis in psychotherapy, medicine, dentistry, research, law enforcement, advertising, and sports.

HYPNOSIS IN PSYCHOTHERAPY

Hypnotherapy in one form or another has reportedly been employed in the treatment of an extremely wide variety of psychological disorders, as the following sampling of the current literature attests. Its applications have included, but not been limited to, the treatment of:

Acting out (Balaam, 1984; Benson, 1984a)
Affective instability (Gruber, 1983)

Alcoholism and addictive behavior (Byers, 1975; Copemann, 1977; Katz, 1980; Manganiello, 1984; Montgomery and Crowder, 1972; Wadden and Penrod, 1981)

Amnesia and fugue (Garver, Fuselier, and Booth, 1981; MacHovec, 1981a)

Anorexia nervosa (Gross, 1984)

Blushing (Welsh, 1978)

Cervical headache (Carasso et al., 1985)

Children's night terrors (Taboada, 1975)

Conversion headache (Stein, 1975)

Crisis intervention (Baldwin, 1978)

Delayed stress reaction (Brende and Benedict, 1980; D. Spiegel, 1981)

Delusions (Berwick and Douglas, 1977)

Depression (Greene, 1973; Matheson, 1979a; Sexton and Maddock, 1979)

Enuresis and encopresis (Montgomery and Crowder, 1972; Olness, 1975; Stanton, 1979a, 1981, 1982; Tilton, 1980)

Frigidity (Cheek, 1976a, 1976b; Wijesinghe, 1977)

Hypochondriasis (Deiker and Counts, 1980; Montgomery and Crowder, 1972)

Hypnopompic hallucinations (Ortega, 1984)

Hysteria (Giacalone, 1981; Kaplan and Deabler, 1975; Patterson, 1980; Pelletier, 1977; Roden, 1979; Trenerry and Jackson, 1983; Wallace and Rothstein, 1975)

Impotence (Crasilneck, 1982; Deabler, 1976)

Insomnia (Bauer and McCanne, 1980; Graham, Wright, Toman and Mark, 1975; Levine, 1980)

Migraine (Anderson, Basker, and Dalton, 1975; Ansel, 1977; Daniels, 1976a, 1977; Friedman, Taub, and Syracuse Veterans Administration Medical Center, 1982; Friedman and Taub, 1984, 1985; Howard, Reardon, and Tosi, 1982; Stambaugh II and House, 1977)

Multiple personality (Bliss, 1980; Brassfield, 1983; Braun, 1983a, 1983b; Herzog, 1984; Horevitz, 1983; Howland, 1975; Kline, 1984; Kluft, 1982, 1983, 1985a, 1985b; Wilbur, 1984)

Nail biting (Bornstein et al., 1980; Channon, 1982; Daniels, 1974)

Nightmares (Seif, 1985)

Obsessions (Johnson and Hallenbeck, 1985; Kellerman, 1981; Taylor, 1985)

Overeating (Aja, 1977; Andersen, 1985; Bolocofsky, Spinler, and Coulthard-Morris, 1985; Bornstein and Devine, 1980; Channon, 1979; Deyoub and Wilkie, 1980; Goldstein, 1981; Mott, Jr., and Roberts, 1979; Stanton, 1975a, 1975b, 1976b; Wadden and Flaxman, 1981; Walker, Collins, and Krass, 1982)

Parents' reaction to children's tantrums (Petty, 1976)

Pathological grief (Turco, 1981)

Personality disorders

  Alexithymia (Schraa and Dirks, 1981)

  Schizoid personality (Lewis, 1979)

Phobias (Daniels, 1976c; Deiker and Pollock, 1975; Kluft, 1986; Lamb, 1985; McGuinness, 1984)

  Agoraphobia (Tilton, 1983)

  Fear of bovine sounds (Cohen, 1981)

  Choking phobia (Epstein and Deyoub, 1981)

  Contamination phobia (Scrignar, 1981)

  Dead bird phobia (Van Der Hart, 1981)

  Dental phobia (Baker and Boaz, 1983; Kelly, 1980)

  Food phobia (Van Dyke and Harris, 1982)

  Flying phobia (Bakal, 1981; Deyoub and Epstein, 1977; Spiegel, Frischholz, Maruffi, and Spiegel, 1981)

  Injection phobia (Dash, 1981; Nugent, Carden, and Montgomery, 1984)

  Nyctophobia (Williams, 1985)

  Penetration phobia (Frutiger, 1981)

  Slug phobia (Gustavson and Weight, 1981)

  Snake phobia (O'Brien, Cooley, Ciotti, and Henninger, 1981)

  Test anxiety (Boutin, 1978; Hebert, 1984; Spies, 1979)

  Voiding in public facility phobia (Seif, 1982)

  Vomiting phobia (Ritow, 1979)

Premature ejaculation (De Shazer, 1978)

Psychogenic seizures (Caldwell and Stewart, 1981; Lindner, 1973; H. R. Miller, 1983; Ravitz, 1982)

Psychogenic tremors (Fogel, 1976)

Psychogenic urinary retention (Mozdzierz, 1985)

Psychosomatic disorders (Daniels, 1975)

Reactions to incest (Miller, 1986)

Reading disorders (Van Rooyen, 1981; Wagenfeld and Carlson, 1979)

Retarded ejaculation (Pettitt, 1982)

Schizophrenia and borderline conditions (Baker, 1983a, 1983b, 1983c; D. P. Brown, 1985; Glenn and Simonds, 1977; Murray-Jobsis, 1985; Scagnelli-Jobsis, 1982, 1983; Plapp, 1976; Scagnelli, 1976, 1977, 1980; D. Spiegel, 1983)

Sexual dysfunctions (Araoz, 1983; Brown and Chaves, 1980; Brumley, 1979; Dennerstein and Burrows, 1979a, 1979b; Fabbri, 1976; Frutiger, 1981; Koadlow, 1979; Stricherz, 1982)

Sexual perversions (Epstein and Deyoub, 1983; Mutter, 1981; Polk, 1983; Stava, 1984)

Sleep paralysis (Schneck, 1977b)

Smoking Barkley, Hastings, and Jackson, 1977; Cox, 1978; Frischholz and Spiegel, 1986; Gaston and Hutzell, 1976; Glad, Tyre, and Adesso, 1976; Holroyd, 1980; Jeffrey, Jeffrey, Greuling and Gentry, 1985; London and Forman, 1977; Pederson, Scrimgeour, and Lefcoe, 1975, 1979; Perry and Mullen, 1975; Powell, 1980; Sanders, 1977a; Stanton, 1978b)

Somnambulism (Eliseo, 1975; Nugent, Carden, and Montgomery, 1984; Reid, 1975)

Speech disorders of children (Silber, 1973)

Stuttering (Dempsey and Granich, 1978)

Suicidal tendencies (Hodge, 1972; Newman, 1974)

Tics (Spithill, 1974)

Trichotillomania (Galski, 1981; Hynes, 1982; Rowen, 1981)

Vaginismus (Degun and Degun, 1982; Gottesfeld, 1978)

Thus, the list of specific applications of hypnosis in therapy is extensive. Just as varied are the methods by which hypnosis can be used to intervene in the course of a psychological disorder and the specific techniques that may be employed.

One of the least effective uses of hypnosis in psychotherapy, and the one most commonly employed by lay hypnotists treating patients for smoking or overeating problems, is the direct suggestion of symptom removal. On occasion, with a patient who has a need for a magical, face-saving cure, dramatic results are obtained, but in general results are poor and of the most transitory nature. The most effective use of hypnosis is as an adjunct to other established methods of psychotherapy. Analytically-oriented psychotherapists take the position that it is not the hypnosis but the transference, or the therapeutic relationship, that cures. In any event, it is not possible to use hypnosis effectively in psychotherapy unless the hypnotist is well trained as a psychotherapist (Mott, Jr., 1982). Because competent psychotherapists disagree on many basic theoretical issues, it will be useful to review briefly some of the major methods of psychotherapy in vogue and their objectives and methods. Then consideration will be given to the role that hypnosis can play in each.

Major Types of Psychotherapy

While it is not possible in a brief summary to cover all of the major types of psychotherapy in current use, or even to describe those to be discussed in any detail, it is hoped that enough of the ideas underlying psychoanalysis, Rogerian therapy, Gestalt therapy, Rational-Emotive therapy, and Behavior Modification can be presented so that some of their major similarities and differences can be appreciated, and the possible applications of hypnosis to their practice can be better understood.

Psychoanalysis. Sigmund Freud devised psychoanalysis at the end of the nineteenth century. Historically, it was the first major method of analytic psychotherapy and was originally developed for the treatment of neurotics, particularly hysterics. It antedated all modern knowledge of learning principles and was based primarily on Freud's clinical observations and his own lifelong self-analysis. To provide a theoretical underpinning for his method of treatment, Freud developed a theory of personality which in essence assumed the following:

1. A human personality is structured into three major components: an id, or biological component, which contains all of the person's innate biological drives (id instincts); an ego, or psychological component, concerned among other things with observing the external real world through the sense organs; and a superego, or social aspect. The latter contains the person's internalized ideas of right and wrong as taught by his or her parents and is subdivided into the conscience and ego ideal. The conscience is a negative type of introject, which causes the person to avoid behavior taught to be immoral. The ego ideal is a positive introject, which motivates him to behave in the perfect manner that he was taught he is supposed to act.

2. All persons go through similar stages of psychosexual development in which the ego develops out of the innate matrix of the id, and later the superego differentiates from the ego. These stages correspond to the libido, or the energy behind the life instincts (eros), passing from one region of the body to the other. The principal stages of psychosexual development are the oral (first year of life); the anal (at age 2); the phallic (ages 3-5), which is followed by a latency period until the final or genital stage (at puberty). Persons who leave too much psychic energy behind at the earlier stages of development (fixation) develop adult personality types characteristic of these earlier stages. Persons who in reaction to stress return to behavior patterns characteristic of earlier stages of development (regression) develop symptoms characteristic of these periods of life.

3. Both the id and the superego are irrational systems in the sense that they are completely out of contact with external reality. It is the function of the ego to mediate between the often-conflicting demands of these two systems and the real world and work out compromise behaviors acceptable to all three.

4. All human thoughts are precisely determined, just as all external events in the real world are subject to the laws of cause and effect. This is called the principle of *psychic determinism,* and it holds that every thought is caused either by the thought that preceded it or by some event from the outside world affecting the sense organs. In effect, this

principle denies the existence of free will (which it regards as an illusion) and states that there is a necessary psychic connection between the elements in a train of thought.

5. Much human ideation occurs below the level of conscious awareness, in the preconscious or unconscious. Material recorded in the preconscious, although not currently conscious, is freely accessible to consciousness. Material in the unconscious is not.

6. When an idea is upsetting to a person, it is forced into the unconscious and kept there by a process called *repression.* Since these ideas often reflect id drives (sex or aggression) that are offensive to the superego and since repressing a drive ensures that it will not be gratified, these drives get stronger, and the repression begins to break down. When this happens, the patient begins to experience the fear associated with these drives (but not the ideation, which is still repressed) as a free-floating or objectless fear, which Freud called *neurotic anxiety.*

7. Anxiety is a form of psychic pain that motivates the ego to develop compromise behaviors, unconsciously, that permit enough symbolic gratification of the repressed id drive to keep anxiety within tolerable limits. If the ego is strong enough to do this effectively, these compromises are called *defense mechanisms,* and the person stays mentally healthy. If the ego resorts to extreme behaviors that themselves become a problem to the patient, they are called *symptoms,* and the patient is said to be mentally ill.

Thus, to Freud a symptom was more than a mere maladaptive behavior pattern. It had a symbolic meaning in the sense that it was a compromise reaction to an internal conflict, and effective psychotherapy had to help identify and resolve this underlying conflict. Since a symptom was needed by the patient to control his anxiety, any direct attack on or removal of a symptom would be likely to be followed by a return of anxiety, which would motivate the acquisition of a new, and possibly worse, symptom.

The method of treatment called psychoanalysis had as its original goal the uncovering of the unconscious conflicts that Freud believed always dated back to early childhood and were the root cause of the patient's symptoms. Later Freud discovered that insight did not always help a patient; sometimes more was needed. In addition to recognizing a problem, it must also be solved.

The problem with psychoanalysis as a theory of personality is that since it is capable of accounting for all possible behaviors after they occur, it is incapable of predicting behavior in advance. Hence, it cannot be proved because it cannot be disproved and must be accepted or rejected on faith. Like any religious doctrine, the practice of psychoanalysis has become quite ritualized, at least in its classical form, which is rarely practiced today, if at all.

Classical psychoanalysis requires that the patient lie on a couch and the therapist sit behind him, out of his line of vision. Many analysts believe that a couch is a vital tool in producing the regression they think necessary to develop the primary process thinking (imagery) needed to get at the unconscious causes of their patients' problems. It is probable that, in some patients at least, a couch may generate feelings of helplessness or dependency, which the therapist may seek to utilize. However, the principal reason that Freud employed a couch was that he could not bear to have patients staring at him throughout their sessions. It is considerably easier for the analyst to work with a couch as opposed to having a face-to-face session with a patient since he or she need not be constantly on guard against inadvertently communicating to the patient by facial expressions or body language.

A psychoanalytic session lasts from 45 to 50 minutes. For the treatment to be considered psychoanalysis, a patient must be seen a minimum of three sessions a week, preferably five. The length of the period is purely arbitrary; the foreshortened hour probably resulted from Freud's need to make notes between sessions with patients. He did not take notes during the sessions, as he felt that this would be too disruptive.

The prime method by which psychoanalysis proceeds is for the patient to free associate—that is, to verbalize everything that comes to mind without censorship of any kind. Freud called this the "patient's work," and the analyst must train the patient to do this. It is totally at variance with all of the patient's previous experience, which has taught him to think before speaking. Now he is required to speak without thinking. (As one of the author's clinical supervisors put it, by the time a patient learns to free associate, the analysis is usually over.) The idea behind free association is to capitalize on the principle of psychic determinism and try to get at the unconscious material causing the patient's symptoms by working backward through its psychic connections with material in consciousness. Dreams and slips of the tongue are also interpreted using the method of free association to make the patient aware of the conflicting conscious and unconscious tendencies within himself that give rise to these forms of compromise behavior.

During the course of psychoanalysis, the patient begins to develop what analysts call resistances: behaviors that seem unconsciously designed to defeat the therapy, such as engaging in intellectual quibbles with the analyst, talking about trivia, and missing appointments. The psychoanalytic explanation of these behaviors relates to the fact that the material the patient is trying to retrieve is painful or it would not have been repressed. Hence, part of the patient's ego is trying to spare him this psychic pain or anxiety. The therapist must work through each resistance with the patient so that the latter gets insight into the psychic mechanisms at work. Typically, as soon as one resistance is worked through, a new one appears. Psychoanalysis has been compared to peeling an onion, layer by layer.

Freud regarded as essential for the success of an analysis the development on the part of the patient of strong but inappropriate emotional feelings directed toward the therapist. He referred to these feelings as transference. Today the term *transference* is often misused colloquially to mean any kind of emotional reaction on the part of a patient toward the therapist. The essential characteristic of a real transference reaction is that it is completely inappropriate to the objective situation between the patient and the analyst. If an analyst does something to make a patient hate or love him, that is not a transference but an appropriate response, which is better labeled a positive or negative rapport. The theory of transference in psychoanalysis is that the emotion felt is not caused by the therapist but by a more significant person in the patient's early life, and it is now being transferred to the analyst. The therapist must notice this emotional response, recognize that it is not appropriate to the objective patient-therapist situation, and determine from what source this emotion originated. The patient must then be made aware of the true origin of this emotion. This process is called "working through the transference" and is vital because the patient may be expressing unconscious ideas and attitudes that he is unable to verbalize, possibly because they date back to his preverbal infancy (Dollard and Miller, 1950).

More important is the fact that working through the transference with the therapist permits the patient to resolve previously unresolved past conflicts in the present by reliving the past through the symbolic interaction with the therapist. These conflicts cannot be dealt with in any way other than reliving them in the present, for the past is unchangeable.

Harry Stack Sullivan once defined psychotherapy as a process by which two people, one called a patient and one called a therapist, sit and talk and as a result of their talk one of these people, hopefully the one called the patient, is benefited. Aside from the possibility that this statement may well have pinpointed the essence of the therapeutic situation, it reminds us that a therapist is also a person, and if the patient can form a transference directed at the therapist, the latter may also form a transference toward the patient. The transferences developed by the therapist are called *countertransferences,* (as opposed to patient-induced emotions) and are disruptive to an analysis because they arise from the therapist's, not the patient's, needs. It is for this reason, among others, that all psychoanalytic institutes preparing therapists in the subspecialty of psychoanalysis require candidates to undergo a training, or personal, analysis to aid them in recognizing and working through those feelings that might predispose them to develop countertransferences. (Most modern analytic institutes require a training analysis of at least 350 hours; Freud's disciples, the first generation of analysts, typically had a training analysis of only about 200 hours.)

Patient-induced emotional responses are not really countertransferences (although they are often carelessly referred to as such), because they are brought about by the realities of the patient-therapist interaction. These may be useful, however, because the patient may generate the same feelings in others that he creates in the analyst. Thus, these feelings may provide the analyst with a clue to understanding the patient's interpersonal relationships.

Classical psychoanalysis is probably neither more nor less effective than any other method of psychotherapy. The statement is often made that all methods of psychotherapy produce about the same cure rate, and Eysenck (1961) has suggested that this is about the same as the spontaneous remission rate for the neuroses. Unfortunately, since there are neither adequate criteria for, nor universal agreement about, what constitutes a cure, such statements are not very meaningful. Furthermore, even if a particular method of psychotherapy could be demonstrated to produce a cure rate no better than the spontaneous remission rate, it might still be valuable if it substantially reduced the duration of a psychological condition capable of producing as much suffering as a neurosis. The real point to be made is that even if classical psychoanalysis had a 100% cure rate, it would still be totally valueless for the vast majority of patients, who could not possibly afford it.

Psychoanalysis has developed a great deal since Freud's time. Most of his original disciples broke away from classical psychoanalysis and developed variations of their own. These new approaches have had varying degrees of influence. Today, many analytically oriented therapists see patients only once a week, have face-to-face interviews with the patient seated in a chair instead of lying on a couch, and use a variety of techniques in addition to free association. Also, the range of disorders treated analytically is much broader than envisioned by Freud and includes character disorders such as maladaptive personality types or narcissism. In terms of Freudian theory, these conditions are caused by fixations at much earlier stages of psychosexual development than neurotic symptoms. Psychotic disorders that Freud felt were untreatable by psychoanalysis (because of the inability of a psychotic to form a transference relationship) are also treated analytically by some modern analysts.

In general, analysts working with character disorders view them as egosyntonic, as opposed to neurotic symptoms, which are ego alien. In other words, the maladaptive behavior in a character disorder is an integral part of the patient's personality and is not symbolic as a neurotic symptom is. Since character disorder patients are regarded by analysts as fixated at very early (preoedipal) levels of ego development, therapy is directed at *ego-building* experiences until the patient attains the same stage of psychosexual development as a neurotic. He is then deemed capable of conventional psychoanalysis.

The essential characteristics of psychoanalytic therapy are its concern with early, unconscious causes of abnormal behavior and its notion of the symbolic significance of neurotic symptoms. It relies on both insight (enhanced self-understanding on the part of the patient) and abreaction (the emotional reexperiencing of prior traumatic events) to effect cures. Therapies with these major characteristics are often referred to as analytic whether or not they derive principally from psychoanalysis. They may also be referred to as insight therapies because the patient's development of insight into the meaning of his symptoms is crucial. Freud's theory derived from his medical practice rather than from psychological research (in contrast to behavior modification therapies). Since he brought many concepts developed in medical practice into the area of psychotherapy (such as the idea that maladaptive behavior reflects an underlying "mental illness" analogous to a fever's reflecting an underlying physical illness), this approach to the treatment of psychological disorders is often referred to as the *medical model*. Sometimes it is referred to as a dynamic approach because it is concerned with the underlying psychodynamics, or interactions between the major systems of the psyche, in the development of symptoms.

Rogerian or Client-Centered Therapy.   Rogerian therapy approaches the problems of the neurotic with a perspective different from the Freudian view. In this therapy, the principal cause of the neurotic's unhappiness is viewed as his poor self-image, caused by a dissonance between the patient's perceived self and his idealized self-image. The latter is quite similar to Freud's ego ideal and represents the patient's view of the perfect person that he believes he should be, but is not. The goal behind this method of psychotherapy is to bring these conflicting self-systems into consonance by enhancing the perceived self—that is, getting the patient to recognize and appreciate his own strengths while whittling away at the idealized self to make it more realistic and attainable. (Rogers prefers to use the term *client* instead of *patient* to avoid the medical model, which he believes damages the client's self-esteem by suggesting that he is ill and dependent on the therapist.) The principal method for accomplishing this end is for the therapist to listen to and try to understand the patient and to communicate an unconditional positive regard for him.

Since our self-image, or system of beliefs about ourselves, tends to be learned from what Sullivan called "significant others" in our lives (persons whose opinions about us we tend to accept), the therapist's positive feelings toward the patient are likely to produce a change in the latter's own negative opinions. As in psychoanalysis, the principal therapeutic change occurs as a result of the relationship established with the therapist, although the mechanism postulated for the working of this relationship is quite different in nature. Rogerian therapists have a great deal of confidence in the ability of the patient to improve his own condition. Hence the patient, not the therapist, directs the course and pace of the therapy.

Unlike Freudians, Rogerians do not ask probing questions, seek to direct the patient's thinking, or make any interpretations. The only intervention made, beyond active listening, is the use of reflection, a technique in which the therapist repeats what the patient has said in somewhat different words, on the theory that sometimes hearing our own statements coming from someone else can help us to look at them in another light and perhaps recognize that certain of our ideas may be inappropriate. One of the major advantages of a passive therapy such as this is that the patient, rather than the therapist, controls how much anxiety he is exposed to in the course of psychotherapy. Hence, he is less likely to be driven out of therapy by an undue amount of anxiety produced by a premature interpretation.

Gestalt Therapy.   Gestalt therapy was developed by Frederick (Fritz) Perls, who became disenchanted with psychoanalysis and sought to devise a shorter-term group therapy that would be appropriate not only for neurotics but also for normal people who desire to attain greater fulfillment in living. It is founded on the notion that people's problems are caused by their rejection of certain aspects of their own personality, which they "alienate," or place outside their perceived ego boundaries, and refuse to recognize as part of themselves. The goal behind this method of psychotherapy is to get the patient to accept and reintegrate this alienated or missing part of himself into the rest of his personality and thus complete the whole (Gestalt) of the individual. Gestaltists are less concerned with investigating the roots of a symptom in early childhood than in investigating the value of a symptom to a patient in "the here and now."

Gestalt therapy is generally done in groups and tends to be a gimmicky type of therapy in that the ratio of techniques to theory tends to be high. For example, if one member of a group feels that another is failing to meet his obligation to be open and honest with the group, he may enact the role of his *alter ego* by standing in back of him and speaking what he believes the other person is really thinking instead of what he actually said. The Gestalt method of dream analysis is an illustration of the encounter method used to discover inner conflicts within a person. Perls believed that every element in a dream, whether person, animal, or inanimate object, represents some aspect of the dreamer's personality. His method of dream interpretation was to have the dreamer describe the dream in the present tense (so that he could reexperience the emotions involved) and then assume the role of each character in the dream and talk for them. When two dream characters get into a dispute, this is taken as an indication of an internal conflict. Perls felt that such an encounter would often result in one character (topdog) putting down the other (underdog). In such a situation, the character being put down represents the alienated part of the dreamer's personality that has to be identified and reintegrated. Role-playing or role-reversal techniques are also important in this approach and, as in psychodrama, give patients both the opportunity to relive significant emotional events and to express themselves indirectly and often nonverbally.

Social Learning Theory Approach. All of the foregoing types of psychotherapy and many others like them implicitly treat symptomatic behavior as a learned phenomenon but are completely silent concerning the learning processes involved, either because the therapy was created before much was known about the principles of learning (like Freud's theory) or because of the personal tastes of the founder of the method. In 1950 John Dollard and Neal Miller published a fascinating book entitled *Personality and Psychotherapy,* which attempted to form a bridge between the apparently unrelated areas of analytic psychotherapy and modern learning theory by accounting for the efficacy of the former in terms of the latter. Their approach has been labeled social learning theory.

Their major contribution appears to have been filling in the learning mechanisms omitted in Freud's theory. The basic learning principle they rely on is operant or instrumental conditioning, in which a response that occurs in the presence of a stimulus is rendered more likely to occur in the presence of the same stimulus in the future if the response is immediately followed by a reinforcement or reward. Thus, to Dollard and Miller, repression is learned because the response of not thinking about an anxiety-producing idea is reinforced by a reduction in anxiety. In a similar manner, a symptom is learned because it also produces a reinforcing reduction in anxiety level.

Extremely maladaptive behavior, as seen in neurotics or psychotics, can be learned through reinforcement because of the time contingencies involved. The reduction of anxiety produced by the symptom may be immediate, while the long-term suffering caused by it may be delayed. Dollard and Miller assert that the neurotic's principal problem is his "stupidity," which is produced by repression. Not being aware of the nature of his repressed problem, he cannot set his higher mental processes to work toward its solution. This is the reason that insight helps a patient; it liberates his higher mental processes to work out more adaptive behaviors. This also accounts for why Freud's original goal in psychoanalysis—to render the unconscious conscious—proved inadequate. Later, Freud discovered that this did not always benefit a patient. Besides being made aware of a problem, the patient had to resolve it (through the transference). The only time insight alone would be expected to cure a patient would be in cases in which the solution of a problem (which had overwhelmed the patient as a child) would be immediately obvious to an adult once he or she became aware of the problem.

Dollard and Miller regard a transference as a special example of the learning phenomenon of generalization, a process in which a response learned to one stimulus comes under the evocation control of similar but different generalized stimuli. For example, a patient may react toward a therapist in the same manner that he formerly reacted toward his father because in some ways the therapist and his father resemble each other.

Free association is effective in getting at unconscious material, in this view, because the patient interprets the therapist's acceptance of his verbalizations as forgiveness, and thus the fear associated with these ideas extinguishes. By generalization, the patient becomes able to talk about more and more anxiety-producing thoughts—first, conscious ones and later the more anxiety-laden, unconscious ones.

In summary, Dollard and Miller regard a symptom as a case of maladaptive learning and psychotherapy as a process by which maladaptive behavior may be extinguished and more adaptive behavior learned in its place. In effect, psychotherapy is a safe, artificial situation in which new behaviors may be experimented with. If they are successful in therapy, they can then be tried out in real-life situations. In a very real sense, a patient is a student and a therapist a teacher.

Following the landmark work of Dollard and Miller, it became inevitable that many psychologists, acutely aware of the shortcomings of existing methods of therapy, would be interested nor merely in explaining old methods of treatment in terms of modern learning principles but in developing new, and more effective, treatments based on these scientifically validated principles. It was in this scientific climate that the approaches collectively labeled behavior modification developed.

Behavior Modification.   The term *behavior modification* is a generic one that covers an ever-increasing variety of specific techniques. What they all have in common is that they were developed out of experimentally validated principles of learning rather than from clinical or medical practice. Thus, they are related to principles of psychology intimately, not peripherally as are many analytical therapies. The development of behavior modification therapies is one of the first significant examples of what might be termed psychological engineering or applied psychology.

All behavior modification methods are based on the notion that, contrary to the medical model, a symptom does not reflect an underlying illness; the symptom *is* the illness. If a symptom is removed, it does not make sense to refer to the patient as being "mentally ill." All behavior therapists further subscribe to the view that since symptoms are learned and represent a maladaptive type of behavior, they must be extinguished and more adaptive behavior learned in their place. This extinction and relearning process follows the same principles of learning discovered in laboratory research with rats learning to run mazes or press the bars in Skinner boxes. Characteristically, behavior modification therapists are not concerned with tracing the development of a symptom to early childhood experiences because they consider the origin of the symptom to be irrelevant. Whatever the particular reinforcement contingencies that caused the symptoms to be learned, the treatment is concerned with extinguishing the present maladaptive behavior. Analytic therapy attempts to change intrapsychic events and assumes that this will change behavior. Behavior modification seeks to change behavior and assumes that this will change subjective attitudes and feelings (Moss and Bremer, 1973).

Unlike the situation in analytic therapy where the techniques of treatment are basically similar regardless of the patient's diagnosis (and hence a diagnosis may be continuously changed during the course of therapy), most behavior therapies are individually designed and tailored to the specific problems of the individual patient. Hence, they are based on an initial detailed history that seeks to pinpoint the exact stimuli that have gained evocation control over the patient's maladaptive behavior patterns.

A few of the more common behavior therapies will be described briefly.

Rational-Emotive Therapy (RET). This method of psychotherapy developed by Albert Ellis (1962) is better classified as a cognitive therapy with emphasis on changing a patient's frame of reference or philosophical ideas rather than the development of insight. It is included here because of its interesting relationship to Wolpe's views of phobic behavior. Wolpe takes the position that in many phobias, the phobic object is a stimulus that has developed direct evocation control over the response of fear, as shown in the following paradigm:

$$S \longrightarrow R$$

phobic object   fear
(e.g., cat)

In such a situation, all the insight in the world will not help the patient. He needs to extinguish the direct control of this stimulus over the fear response. Ellis, on the other hand, believes that the response of fear is not under the direct control of the phobic object but is mediated by covert responses, which he calls "irrational ideas," as follows:

$$S \longrightarrow \underset{s}{r} \longrightarrow R$$

phobic object   fear
(e.g., cat)
       "irrational idea"
       (e.g., This cat is dangerous.)

His method of therapy is aimed at reeducating the patient to understand that these ideas are "irrational." The types of ideas that Ellis finds produce fear responses are somewhat reminiscent of what Adler called "fictional finalisms"—ideas that are taught in our culture, such as "Honesty is always the best policy," or "In the end, virtue will be rewarded." Although these ideas are expressive of culturally acceptable standards, they are generalities that are often not true. Persons whose lives are governed by them often set up extensive lists of "shoulds" for their own behavior, which generate many needless problems for themselves. The situation is analogous to what Freudians would describe as a severe superego out of touch with the realities of adult life.

An example of this type of treatment would be to get the patient to recognize that life is not always fair and that it is not rational to expect it to be. The patient must also be taught that it is not necessary to be a perfect person to be worthy and that, in fact, the patient is as good a person as it is possible for him to be, and he ought to accept himself as being of value. The philosophy espoused by this school of therapy is that every person has a basic human worth simply by virtue of being a human being and that nothing he can do is capable of either enhancing or detracting from this basic human value. This is both an attractive personal philosophy and one that is useful clinically if a patient can be helped to accept it because it has the potential to free him from self-destructive feelings of guilt or failure.

Assertiveness Training.   Assertiveness training is a specific treatment for a patient with a phobic-like reaction producing fear in interpersonal situations. It is useful for patients who are unable to stand up for themselves in interpersonal situations and who tend to be "walked on" by other people. Wolpe (1982) regards this condition as the result of childhood training that emphasized that the rights and feelings of other people were always to be considered first. He regards this type of orientation to others as just as maladaptive as the orientation that the patient always comes first and other people do not have to be considered at all. A more adaptive view in Wolpe's opinion is, "I come first, but others also have rights that must be respected." Treatment consists first of reeducating the patient so that he agrees with the reasonableness and propriety of standing up for his own rights and then providing him with practice (in role-playing situations) in asserting himself through firm but socially acceptable ways. To learn these new behaviors, the patient must ultimately try them in actual situations and be appropriately reinforced for their employment. Often a patient will be so deficient in his repertoire of assertive behaviors that the therapist may have to supply him with a group of stock phrases to be used in appropriate situations. Wolpe includes samples of such assertive phrases in his book. Assertiveness training reduces the response of fear in social situations by training the patient to develop the incompatible response of self-assertion.

Systematic Desensitization. Systematic desensitization is a treatment designed primarily for use with phobias in which the phobic object is not another person. In such a case, there is no one with whom the patient can be assertive. The treatment is based, as is assertiveness training, on the principle of reciprocal inhibition. The autonomic nervous system (ANS) is constructed so that the emotions of fear and anger are mediated by its sympathetic division, and relaxation is mediated by the antagonist parasympathetic division. Thus, fear and relaxation are incompatible reactions and cannot coexist. Systematic desensitization reduces a fear response to a phobic object or stimulus by conditioning an incompatible response of relaxation to the same stimulus. This incompatible learning necessarily extinguishes the fear response.

The specifics of this method can best be illustrated by considering the steps in treating a patient who is phobic for cats. The first step in the procedure is to train the patient in deep muscle relaxation. Typically training is done using Jacobson's (1962) method of relaxing specific muscle groups, progressing from the top or bottom of the body to the other end sequentially. Each muscle group is tensed to focus attention on the feelings coming from it and then relaxed. The method is tedious, quite similar to a hypnotic induction by the progressive relaxation method. Typically relaxation training extends over about six sessions, with daily home practice provided by a tape recording made during the sessions.

Even after being trained to relax, if the subject were directly presented with the phobic object, he would likely become so upset that the relaxation effect would be destroyed rather than the fear response extinguished. Hence, a hierarchy of anxiety-producing stimuli must be developed before desensitization can begin. The subject is provided with a scale of subjective units of disturbance (SUD) ranging from 100 (representing as much anxiety as he has ever experienced) to 0 (representing complete relaxation and calm). He is then asked to imagine various interactions with the phobic object and to rate the subjective feelings produced on this scale—for example, patting a cat, seeing a cat from 100 yards away, looking at a picture of a cat, and so on. From these subjective ratings, the therapist seeks to create a hierarchical arrangement of anxiety-producing situations ranging from very low levels of anxiety potential to very high ones.

When the final hierarchy is constructed, desensitization trials are commenced. Prior to each trial, the subject is instructed to attain a deep state of relaxation. He is then told to imagine the lowest item on the hierarchy and to report on his subjective state using the SUD scale. Each item on the hierarchy is paired with the relaxed state until the anxiety associated with it is completely extinguished. This extinction generalizes, with the result that the anxiety associated with the next higher item on the hierarchy is also diminished. Then it, in turn, is imagined in contiguity with a state of relaxation until its ability to produce anxiety is totally extinguished. In this systematic, steplike fashion, anxiety for the highest item on the hierarchy is finally extinguished, and, by generalization, so is the anxiety evoked by the phobic object itself.

If an individual patient is unable to generate enough anxiety for desensitization to occur by imagining hierarchical items, then an in vivo procedure, using real phobic objects, must be resorted to instead of the more convenient covert desensitization process. There are many variations of this basic procedure. For example, anger or sexual feelings may be used as responses incompatible with a fear reaction in appropriate cases. The latter may be particularly suitable for the treatment of impotency with variations of this method. The most essential element in the success of this type of treatment is the therapist's correct identification of the real nature of the phobia and the development of an appropriately graded hierarchy. For example, if a general fear of loss of control is confused with a fear of flying (a specific manifestation of the more general fear), then the results of therapy are likely to be poor.

Flooding.   Flooding is a technique used to extinguish phobic responses, not by conditioning an incompatible response, but by permitting the fear response to become extremely intense. Often this will have the effect of extinguishing the fear response to a phobic object. However, the method is not always effective and can be extremely unpleasant for the patient. Although the mechanism by which flooding is sometimes effective is not clear, it is known that in the absence of counterconditioning an incompatible response, extinction never occurs in learning situations unless the behavior to be extinguished is actually elicited and not reinforced. This method is similar to the Freudian technique of abreaction except that it is more readily producible (by simply presenting the patient with the phobic stimulus or situation). An example of flooding would be to put a patient with a flying phobia in an airplane and allow him to experience a terror-filled flight. If flooding is successful, it can produce a cure in one session; if it fails, it can exacerbate the problem.

Operant Conditioning.   Unlike systematic desensitization, which involves a classical conditioning paradigm (dealing as it does with emotional learning), operant behavior therapies use instrumental learning paradigms to shape patients' behavior. Desirable behavior (to be acquired) is reinforced, and maladaptive behavior (to be extinguished) is either not reinforced or followed by aversive stimulation. Complex new behavior patterns may be acquired or shaped by the method of successive approximations. In this method, components of the desired behavior are reinforced initially until more complex behavior can be obtained with sufficient frequency to require the complete behavior desired as a condition for a reinforcement. Modeling and imitation learning may also be used for this purpose.

Unquestionably, behavior modification was given a bad name in some circles by early attempts to employ these methods to control the behavior of institutionalized patients. Often these methods were used to train patients to eat with silverware or otherwise make them more manageable patients rather than to deal with their basic pathology. The trivial nature of these early treatment attempts caused many to lose sight of the potential of these techniques when used by an innovative and imaginative therapist. Cautela (1975) has developed a technique called covert conditioning that uses operant conditioning on imagined stimuli and responses instead of real ones. This approach seems ideally adaptable for hypnotherapy and will be described later.

Aversive Therapy.   Aversive therapy is another technique that has frequently been misused in the past. For example, it was used on convicts who were not in a position to consent meaningfully to any method of psychotherapy. Misuses such as this have contributed to the reluctance of some therapists to see much good in behaviorally oriented therapies in general (Cohn and Udolf, 1979).

Aversive therapy uses a classical conditioning paradigm in which a stimulus that produces a socially unacceptable response is rendered aversive by being paired with an aversive stimulus (Dengrove, 1973; Franks, 1966). Examples of this technique may be found in the treatment of homosexuality or alcoholism. In the former situation, male homosexuals may have pictures of nude men paired with an electric shock to extinguish the capacity of such stimuli to produce an erotic response. Typically, the termination of the shock is paired with the picture of a nude woman, which has the additional effect of associating a pleasant response with the more appropriate sexual stimulus.

Wolpe (1982) points out that aversive conditioning is never the treatment of choice in homosexuality and is contraindicated if the condition is complicated by a fear of the opposite sex, at least until this fear response is systematically deconditioned. After such deconditioning, aversive therapy may be unnecessary in many cases. Aversive therapy in alcoholism is typified by the use of drugs that produce vomiting following the ingestion of alcohol.

Eclectic Therapy.   There are very strong partisan differences between proponents of analytic and behavior therapy (Moss and Bremer, 1973). Indeed, there are strong partisan views held by proponents of specific therapeutic approaches within the analytic camp. Analytically-oriented therapists generally take the position that the behavior therapies are superficial and do not get to the root of the patient's problem. Thus, although behavior modification may be useful in specific situations like phobias, it is not thought to be useful in the wide range of other disorders seen in psychotherapy. This criticism has some truth to it, but the author believes the problem is due not to a fundamental limitation of behavior modification but rather results from its newness and the fact that behavior modification is more demanding of the therapist. He or she must be creative enough to design an individual treatment plan for each patient. Behavior modification techniques have not been around long enough for therapists to have developed adequate treatment regimens for the more complicated conditions. This is not to imply that no further progress can be made. Only a short while ago the state of the electronics art was the crystal radio set.

Concerning the issue of which of these conflicting viewpoints is correct, no method of therapy is the treatment of choice for all patients. A good therapist needs to be trained in all of these techniques to be able to choose the method most appropriate for a particular patient and his unique problems. Often the therapist will need to use techniques associated with widely different types of therapy in an eclectic and mutually supporting manner. Frequently the differences between nominally distinct modes of therapy relate more to what is going on inside the therapist's head than to differences in what he or she actually does in interacting with patients. Thus, all therapists control their patients' behavior by doling out reinforcements, whether they do it intentionally, as in behavior modification, or unwittingly, as in the case of a Freudian analyst who inadvertently trains a patient to focus on a discussion of sexual problems by reinforcing this type of material with increased interest. What most good therapists do in interacting with their patients is a great deal more similar than their theoretical views would lead one to suppose.

In summary, there are numerous theoretical approaches for effecting therapeutic change in a patient. These include but are not limited to:

1. Lowering the environmental stresses that a patient is subjected to, when possible (e.g., in a family therapy situation).
2. Breaking up or reversing feedback loops or the tendency of most psychological disturbances to feed on themselves (e.g., the tendency of some neurotics to worry about worrying too much can be reversed by any alleviation of the symptom).
3. Reducing internal conflict by strengthening the ego and making the superego more in tune with current reality.
4. Changing the patient's frame of reference or philosophic outlook on life.
5. Improving the patient's self-image.

6. Fostering the development of insight.
7. Providing emotional outlets or abreaction.
8. Removing symptoms directly.

All of these techniques and others may have therapeutic value. A good therapist is able to choose the approaches most appropriate for a particular patient based on a variety of considerations, such as the patient's diagnosis, personality, and even his cultural, ethnic, and social background (Kim, 1983; Schraa and Dirks, 1981). A poor therapist believes that there is only one way to do psychotherapy: the way he or she was originally trained.

For convenience of description, hypnotherapeutic techniques will be classified as those aimed primarily at direct symptom removal or those used in conjunction with analytic or behavior modification approaches. This is, at best, an unsatisfactory and artificial attempt to organize a large amount of clinical material. Few, if any, hypnotherapists limit their work to one or the other of these areas. Braun and Horevitz (1986) describe hypnosis as a unique constellation of perceptual alterations that permit the utilization in therapy of strengths and capacities of a patient that might otherwise not be utilized. It may do so in a variety of different ways and in conjunction with widely differing methods of psychotherapy.

Patients often come into hypnotherapy as a last resort after attempts with other types of therapy have failed. Since, if successful, hypnotherapy is often shorter than other methods, it might be more logical to make it the treatment of first resort (Van Pelt, 1975c).

Direct Hypnotic Removal of Symptoms

Treatment aimed primarily at the direct removal of maladaptive behavior, whether by direct or indirect hypnotic suggestions or by behavior modification techniques, raises the issue of symptom substitution (Rosen, 1941; Wallace and Rothstein, 1975).

Field and Kline (1974), with a strongly analytic approach, warn against the dangers of a simplistic attack on symptoms without an adequate, dynamic investigation of the value of the symptom to the patient. They cite the case of a 27-year-old man who was 130 pounds overweight and who sought hypnotic treatment for compulsive overeating. The patient was convinced that he could be cured of his problem in only one session. When asked the reason for this confidence, he revealed that two years earlier (at about the time his overeating behavior developed), he had been cured of bruxism (teeth grinding) by a dentist in only one session. The authors believed that both the bruxism and the substituted symptom were due to an underlying depression and agitation that required analytic treatment.

In the same vein, Kline (1978) reported the case of a man who had a paralyzed hand cured by direct hypnotic suggestion and who subsequently strangled his wife. It would appear that the dynamic relationship between these two events is highly speculative at best.   ·

The situation is somewhat analogous to the hypnotic control of pain. No competent psychologist or psychiatrist would undertake a procedure aimed at the hypnotic control of a pain unless the etiology of the pain had been established and required medical treatment had been initiated. In other words, pains should be treated hypnotically only when they have no value to the patient. Field and Kline argue that psychological symptoms deserve the same respect.

Montgomery and Crowder (1972) investigated the data available on the occurrence of symptom substitution. These data are not very impressive since therapists rarely do follow-ups to look for symptom substitution. Hence, if a new symptom develops, it may not be noticed. Also, if a patient develops a new symptom after the removal of an old one, it is not easy to establish that this new symptom is a substitute for the old one, particularly when the time interval between the removal of the old symptom and the establishment of the new one is long. Montgomery and Crowder found that whether a substitute symptom occurs is a function of the original condition treated. Direct symptomatic treatment of enuresis in children was not followed by substituted symptoms, whereas the removal of ulcer symptoms was.

The issue seems to be whether the maladaptive behavior to be removed is simply a useless habit, learned as the result of past contingencies of reinforcement, or whether it has some symbolic significance or other value to the patient. This question requires an answer prior to deciding on any method of psychotherapy. Even the removal of such clearly maladaptive behavior as excessive smoking can at times cause more problems than the health benefits accruing to the patient may warrant.

In a sense, any time a maladaptive behavior is removed, there is always a kind of symptom substitution. Having eliminated the old response to a stimulus, the patient must replace it with some other behavior, even if this consists of merely doing nothing. The real issue is whether this new behavior is more or less adaptive than the behavior it replaces. If it is less adaptive (or equally maladaptive), we say that symptom substitution has occurred. If it is more adaptive, we say there has been no symptom substitution. From a logical point of view, it would appear that the more clearly maladaptive the original symptom, the more likely it is that the new behavior would be an improvement, and vice-versa. One way of dealing with the problem of symptom substitution is for the therapist to specify a less disruptive replacement behavior for the symptom. The choice of the substitute behavior needs to be carefully thought out. The author recalls one patient told to chew a stick of gum every time he felt the desire to smoke a cigarette. He developed muscular aches in his jaw from constant chewing.

Another approach to the possibility of symptom substitution, and possibly a better one, is to arrange for adequate follow-up studies of the patient. If new symptoms occur, they can be treated in turn, until the patient develops a behavior in his hierarchy of responses that is more adaptive. If the patient fails to arrive at a less disruptive behavior pattern or goes on to develop a sequence of more and more severe symptoms, this might be an indication justifying a reexamination of the dynamic value of these symptoms and the consideration of a more analytic approach.

An interesting contrast to the notion of treating a psychological problem by the direct removal of a symptom was Van Pelt's (1975d) notion that a neurotic symptom could be developed inadvertently in the manner of a post-hypnotic suggestion by a parent telling a child something while the latter was in a spontaneous, self-induced, trancelike state. Thus, he thought it possible that difficulties later in life could be caused by the child's acting on such pa-rental "posthypnotic suggestions" as "You'll never amount to anything." Al-though the research on posthypnotic suggestions shows it to be unlikely that such a suggestion could have so prolonged an effect, it is still possible that it may have initiated maladaptive behavior that was subsequently reinforced by environmental factors and hence learned as a permanent feature of the per-sonality. Frankel and Orne (1976) note the high degree of hypnotic suscep-tibility displayed by phobic patients compared with patients seeking treatment for smoking behavior. Frankel (1974) suggests that spontaneous trance states precipitated as a reaction to panic or severe emotional stress may play a caus-ative role in the development of phobic behavior in a manner reminiscent of Van Pelt's theory. Consistent with this view, Kelly (1980) cites the case of dental phobia generated by a spontaneous hypnotic-like perception of dental pain while the patient was under novocaine. It should be noted that the var-ious mechanisms proposed for symptom formation by different schools of psychotherapy are not necessarily mutually exclusive. It seems probable that all of these mechanisms, and others not yet identified, can play a role in the development of symptoms. Indeed, it may be counterproductive for theorists to try to demonstrate a single mechanism for the learning of symptoms.

There are many ways of suggesting the disappearance of a symptom. One of the poorest is to suggest that it will disappear magically. Although this method may have some utility when working with children who are used to thinking in such terms in their normal fantasy life, it is not useful with adults, who typically require more reasonable explanations to develop the necessary anticipation of success. Thus, while a child may accept a suggestion that the therapist's finger is a magic wand that will cause his warts to go away, adults are more likely to respond to suggestions that the blood supply to the warts is being closed off and they are drying up and will disappear. Patients often need some face-saving rationale to account for the disappearance of symptoms to permit them to relinquish them.

Another approach to the removal of a symptom is to emphasize its negative aspects or intensify them. An example of this, in a crude form, is suggesting to a subject that in the future every cigarette he smokes will taste like burning rubber. Such a suggestion, if seen by the subject as being imposed on him, may be ineffective. Even in cases where it is accepted, it will require constant reinforcement by rehypnosis or self-hypnosis. The idea behind such a suggestion is that, if it is repeated often enough, it may be effective long enough for the patient to break his addiction and thus be able to control his future smoking behavior voluntarily. This is similar to a nonhypnotic method of smoking control in which the patient is required to smoke constantly until he becomes physically ill. Barkley, Hastings, and Jackson (1977) compared such a method with a hypnotic treatment based on suggestions of relaxation coupled with statements concerning the deleterious effects of smoking on health. They found no statistical differences in the results produced by these two methods after a 9-month follow-up and suggested that these techniques might be combined. They also made the observation that the total cessation of smoking behavior is a more appropriate measure of therapeutic success in treating smoking than a mere reduction in the rate of smoking because of the high number of subjects who return to their original rates of smoking unless they stop entirely.

Spiegel (London and Forman, 1977) has developed what he calls a single-session treatment for smoking, although it involves training the patient in self-hypnosis and having him make the same suggestions to himself several times a day. Basically it is a more sophisticated approach to emphasizing the negative aspects of smoking. The patient is given a three-part philosophy that emphasizes that smoking is a poison to his body, he needs his body to live, and his body deserves his respect and protection.

Stanton, (1978b) reports on a one-session treatment for smoking involving an adaption of the "red balloon" technique often used in pain control, (see page 244) along with specific cessation suggestions, ego-enhancing suggestions, and visualization of success. The patient is told to imagine his desire to smoke is put into a container and carried off by a red helium-filled balloon. He claims smoking cessation that was still in effect at a 6-month follow-up in 34 of 75 patients.

Barber (1978b) suggests that it is more effective to emphasize the positive aspects of life with the symptom gone than the negative side of the symptom itself. In addition to suggestions directly related to the symptom and its removal, he advocates making general positive suggestions of well-being and an enhanced capacity to enjoy the everyday experiences of life. He notes that research has shown that people are constantly thinking, whether awake or asleep, and most of the time their thoughts deal with either negative or trivial ideas. He sees one of the potentials of hypnotherapy as helping people to think more constructively and to become better able to enjoy life.

Suggestions that may make it easier for the patient to give up smoking might include a consideration of the benefits to be derived from quitting: improved general health, improved athletic ability and endurance, avoiding smoker's cough and bad breath, savings in money, improved social relationships, enhancement of the sense of taste and appreciation of food, and so on. These suggestions should be made positively rather than negatively. That is, "You will feel better and be healthier" is preferable to "Smokers run a high risk of cancer." Research in attitude changing suggests that approaches using fear to change behavior are often ineffective because they motivate subjects to develop defenses against the unpleasant consequences threatened (Janis and Feshbach, 1965).

Watkins (1976) has reported a five-session treatment for smoking. It uses a variety of strategies, including negative suggestions and imagery about smoking, and the requirement for the patient to report to the therapist by telephone daily between the second and third appointments. Sixteen of 24 patients were not smoking at a 6-month follow-up.

Perry and Mullen (1975) report that a 3-month follow-up of 54 subjects treated by Spiegel's method disclosed that success in therapy for smoking behavior was higher for subjects of greater susceptibility. They note, however, that the criterion for success was the reduction of smoking by 50%. Spiegel would regard this as a therapeutic failure because of the tendency of smokers who do not totally stop to return to their former higher rates of smoking.

Typically the initial rates of smoking reduction are quite high following therapy, but long-term follow-ups are not usually made. Barber claims the best "cure" rate obtainable after a year is about 20% and is unrelated to hypnotic depth. Pederson, Scrimgeour, and Lefcoe (1979) report a 6-month follow-up of a study of 28 male and 37 female subjects disclosed that 53% of a live hypnosis plus counseling group and 18% of a counseling alone group maintained smoking cessation. Neither exposure to antismoking material in a videotaped hypnosis session nor neutral hypnosis was effective in treatment, and the authors concluded that both the physical presence of the hypnotist and specific suggestions were necessary.

In a review of 17 studies of hypnotic treatment for smoking, Holroyd (1980) tried to evaluate the variables responsible for maintenance of smoking cessation at a 6-month follow-up. He found reported abstinence rates ranging from 4% to 88%, and he considered the effects of patient population; individual versus group treatment; standardized versus individual suggestion; the use of self-hypnosis; the number of therapy sessions; time duration of the treatment; and the use of adjunct treatments. The most important positive factor appeared to be the tailoring of suggestions to the motives and needs of the individual subjects followed by the need for some minimal number of treatment sessions (at least four), although a single 12-hour session produced good results. Also adjunctive nonhypnotic treatments were associated with good long term-results.

Jeffrey, Jeffrey, Greuling, and Gentry (1985) report that a combination of hypnotic, cognitive, and behavioral interventions in a five-session group treatment for smoking produced a 65% cessation at the conclusion of treatment and a 31% cessation at a 3-month follow-up (with dropouts and unlocatable subjects being counted as treatment failures). Even these figures, low as they are, may be unduly optimistic since the study was limited to 35 subjects who were all able to cease smoking by themselves for 48 hours as a condition of acceptance for treatment. Furthermore, as in most other studies reporting follow-up data, there was no way of checking on the accuracy of subjects' reports.

Glad, Tyre, and Adesso (1976) consider smoking behavior to have cognitive, behavioral, and affective aspects to it and discuss the need for a therapy to address each of these issues.

Sanders (1977a) reports that a mutual group hypnosis treatment provided social support for patients. Included in the treatment were brainstorming techniques, time progression, imagery, and dream induction. She reports a high success rate (13 of 19 subjects) 10 months following therapy.

Powell (1980) reports some positive results (four cessations of smoking out of seven patients) in a 6-9 month follow-up for patients who had a short-term resumption of smoking following initial therapy and were exposed to a flooding treatment followed by hypnosis.

Summarizing the clinical reports on the effectiveness of hypnosis in the treatment of smoking is difficult because many of the results may be due to specific factors or techniques used, and hence reports that appear to be in conflict may not be directly comparable. Also, adequate long-range follow-up data are rare. Nevertheless, based more on theory than on data, the author believes the most effective use of hypnosis in any problem depends on its being individualized for the specific patient and its being used as an adjunct to an appropriate method of psychotherapy rather than as a simplistic source of direct suggestions. In summary, hypnosis appears to be as good or as bad a method of eliminating smoking as any other. It certainly is not as effective a method as the newspaper ads of lay hypnotists would have the public believe.

There are verbatim accounts of specific therapeutic suggestions published in the literature, such as the collection of suggestions used by various practitioners reported in the *Handbook of Therapeutic Suggestions* (1973) of the American Society of Clinical Hypnosis or Walker, Collins, and Krass's (1982) verbatim scripts for weight control. This type of material can be useful in developing ideas to be included in one's own suggestions but should never be used verbatim with a patient. All suggestions made in hypnotherapy should be individually tailored to the needs of the individual patient (Sacerdote, 1972). The best way to frame therapeutic suggestions is by selecting, from a prearranged list of potential suggestions, those that are most appropriate to the patient, based on a preinduction interview. If the patient is made a partner in the selection and phrasing of the suggestions to be used, he will not only find the procedure less threatening but will also be helped to appreciate his own major role in the therapeutic procedure. This is a good beginning to the therapeutic relationship and will help to develop the expectations of favorable results, which are essential to their attainment (Starker, 1975). Schneck (1975) refers to the development of a set or expectation of a benefit from the treatment as "prehypnotic suggestion," and Kroger (1972) believes that it is the expectation of a cure that produces one. Stanton (1976b) explains his finding that subjects who pay for hypnotic weight reduction treatments lose more weight than patients receiving free treatment, on the basis of the former's valuing the treatment more and hence having a greater expectation of success. This finding has led to a number of experimenters requiring subjects in weight control studies to post deposits of some nominal amount, such as $20, to be refunded on the completion of the study. This, of course, is not equivalent to paying a fee, and even if it were, it would have no effect on the study's outcome being applied equally to all groups. The author believes this is a subtle way of arm twisting to prevent subjects from dropping out of the study, and hence it violates the ethical requirements of informed consent, which requires subjects to be informed that they are free to drop out at any time if they so desire.

Whether the suggestions derived should be made in an authoritative or permissive manner is a function of the needs of the patient, and this decision must be made on the basis of good clinical judgment. Hypnotic suggestions must be phrased in a manner acceptable to the patient if they are to be effective (Van Nuys, 1975). Permissive suggestions are generally better because they give the patient a feeling of mastery and control over the problem. The patient's perceived locus of control (whether he or the therapist is seen as primarily responsible for the abatement of his symptoms) is probably an important determinant of the permanence of the treatment results (Gardner, 1976a). One of the values of training a patient in self-hypnosis, beyond the resultant reduction in the number of office visits needed, is an increased sense of control over his symptoms and his life.

Another advantage of having the patient participate in the design of the suggestions to be used is the effect that this procedure has on the therapist. It aids the therapist in keeping in mind the critical role that the patient must assume in the therapy. One of the dangers of doing hypnotherapy, even among well-trained therapists, is the development of countertransference feelings of power or omnipotence. Orne (1962a), for example, has noted the interesting (and unconscious) tendency of most hypnotists to act as though the subject were literally experiencing all of their suggestions. Thus, the operator may talk to an age-regressed adult subject in a manner appropriate in addressing a young child. With his gift for an apt turn of a phrase, Orne likens this situation to a *folie a deux*. He points out that any attempt to compel a patient to behave in a manner contrary to his personality cannot succeed. The feeling on the part of a therapist that he or she and not the patient is the prime mover in the therapeutic process is not only inaccurate but counterproductive (as are all other attitudes on the part of a therapist that tend to diminish respect for the patient). It is not necessary to be a Rogerian to realize that the major part of any therapy lies in conveying to the patient feelings of respect for him and his value, since he often has little self-esteem. It is difficult for a therapist to communicate such a feeling if he does not actually have it.

Reid (1975) reports treating somnambulism hypnotically by having the patient's putting his feet on the floor become a cue to awaken him. This is a good example of using hypnosis to give a patient control over his own behavior.

If a subject presents with a symptom that is properly treatable by direct hypnotic removal but he fears the experience of hypnosis and cannot be reassured by a prehypnotic conference, several alternatives are available to the therapist. If the subject consents to hypnosis but his fears prevent a successful induction, the chaperone technique (see Chapter 3) may be employed. A better technique is to describe the procedure used as a method of inducing relaxation rather than hypnosis (Barber, 1978b). In view of Barber's work with task-motivational instructions and the lack of correlation between trance depth and therapeutic effectiveness, many suggestions may be effective even in the waking state. This was demonstrated by the remission of a large number of juvenile warts on the leg of the author's son, produced by a pediatrician painting them with water described as a magic formula that would make the warts disappear within a week.

Hypnosis can often be attained quite readily with patients who fear it or the loss of control that they erroneously think it produces by simply calling the procedure something else. This is a particularly useful technique in treating young children. Some prominent hypnotherapists such as Erickson rarely employed formal inductions. There is really no need to do so except in the case of a patient who specifically wants hypnotic treatment. Lazarus (1973) found that patients who specifically requested hypnotherapy generally did better in therapy when treated with it than with some other method. This is an additional reason for respecting the patient's wishes in therapy unless there is some cogent contraindication.

Besides smoking behavior, overeating and its resultant obesity is probably one of the most common problems for which patients seek direct hypnotic intervention.

There are some special problems in this area. The major source of concern in the treatment of overeating is not the danger that the treatment may prove ineffective but that it may prove too effective. Patients should be carefully screened for any tendency toward anorexia. This type of treatment is contraindicated in the case of young girls who are not grossly overweight or who have not been medically referred because of some physical condition whose treatment requires a weight loss that the patient is unable to attain without assistance. Any contemplated loss of weight of more than a few pounds requires a medical consultation concerning the advisability of the proposed loss and the diet by which to attain it. Also, a medical opinion is necessary to determine the rate at which this loss can safely be attained. It is possible to inflict serious physical damage by a large, precipitous weight loss. Thus, the psychotherapist needs a medical consultation and a careful follow-up of the patient to avoid this risk. The consultation is especially important in the case of young women desirous of losing weight for purely cosmetic reasons, since a medical check-up may disclose some reason why a weight loss that would be safe for the average person may be dangerous in a particular patient.

A point of clarification is in order here. What a psychologist (or for that matter a psychiatrist who, while medically trained, customarily does not perform physical examinations on his patients) requires is a medical consultation, not supervision.

The decision about how much weight can be safely lost, by what diet, and at what rate are medical issues. The decision of how to effectuate this regimen is a psychological one. A physician without special training in psychiatry is no more competent to decide this issue than a psychologist is to decide the medical ones.

Barber (1978b) maintains that behavior modification is superior to hypnosis for weight control but that the reverse is true for smoking.

Typical weight-reducing suggestions will include statements to the effect that the patient will find his diet completely satisfying, will not be hungry between meals, will find cakes and other desserts unappealing, and so on. The most effective suggestions will be those worked out in consultation with the patient that take into account his own faulty eating habits. Weight records should be kept to check the progress of the treatment. When the patient's weight approaches the target set, suggestions should be modified and directed toward maintaining the new weight rather than producing continued weight reduction.

As in the case of smoking, a great deal of eating behavior is often automatic. Any suggestions designed to make the patient more aware of his behavior and to make all eating deliberate and intentional may prove useful. Often suggestions to eat slowly and enjoy each mouthful thoroughly will prove helpful in effectuating the suggestion that the patient will find his diet completely satisfying.

Because of the typically transient nature of the effects of direct suggestions for symptom removal, it is usual to reinforce these suggestions daily either by training patients in self-hypnosis or by making an audiotape of a hypnotic session that they can listen to at home (Stanton, 1975*b*).

In the absence of an underlying symbolic meaning for overeating behavior, it is usually much easier to control hypnotically than smoking behavior, but, as in the case of the latter, a long-term follow-up is needed to evaluate the success of therapy. Typically hypnotic treatment for weight control, even when successful, is longer and more costly than treatment for smoking. Even if the suggestions are accepted and eating behavior is immediately modified, it will take time for the patient to lose any substantial degree of weight at a reasonable and safe rate. Losing weight slowly is important not just for safety considerations but to ensure that the new eating behavior becomes a permanent feature of the patient's future life patterns. Otherwise the patient will revert to his former behavior and rapidly regain any weight lost. There is medical opinion to the effect that unless the weight loss produced is permanent, the patient may be better off not losing it at all.

When overeating has a significance beyond a mere maladaptive habit, the patient may need a more dynamic approach to therapy than hypnotic suggestions aimed directly at the symptom. For example, a woman referred to the author for hypnotic treatment for obesity was found to be unconsciously using overeating as a way of making herself unattractive to men, whom she feared. It was unlikely that hypnosis would ever cause her to relinquish this defense until the reason for it was adequately worked through in therapy with the referring psychiatrist. Such a patient should have the underlying problem treated prior to any attempts at treating the symptomatic obesity. A patient in therapy with another therapist, referred specifically for hypnotherapy, should be referred back to the original therapist with a recommendation to that effect. It is not only unethical but ineffective and incompetent to do any therapy with a patient in treatment with another therapist except at his or her specific direction. A patient with a similar problem who left therapy after one session was reported by Channon (1979) who noted that the contract between patient and therapist in obesity control is symptom specific and the therapist has no license to probe into deeper problems. If a patient needs a more dynamic approach, the therapist must get the patient to understand its necessity and consent to it before proceeding.

In essence, the direct removal of symptoms by hypnotic suggestion seems to depend on several distinct mechanisms. First is the posthypnotic quality of the suggestions that originally produces the desired behavior change. By itself this probably is not sufficient to produce any lasting therapeutic change, but if the new behavior is reinforced in the patient's daily life, it can be learned and retained. Also, the general suggestions made and considered while the patient is in a receptive, suggestible state may modify his frame of reference to the point that the new behavior may be internally reinforced by increased feelings of mastery and self-control. Last, the posthypnotic suppression of some behaviors, such as smoking or overeating, may serve to break an addiction or permit a patient's appetite to diminish to a point where further control over the habit is within the capacity of a well-motivated patient.

In a review of the literature on hypnosis and weight control, Mott and Roberts (1979), note that many of the problems associated with the literature of hypnosis in smoking cessation are also present in the literature of weight control. Most of the reports are anecdotal, and few long-term follow-ups are reported.

Wadden and Flaxman (1981) compared hypnosis with covert modeling and relaxation-attention control and found all groups had weight loss at 6- and 16-week follow-ups, but there were no significant differences due to treatments. No relationship was found between susceptibility and weight loss.

Deyoub and Wilkie (1980) found that subjects given task-motivating suggestions lost more weight than subjects given the identical suggestions under hypnosis and speculated that this may have been due to hypnosis making subjects more passive, that is, expecting change without active effort. Suggestibility was unrelated to weight loss in the task-motivated groups, but highly suggestible subjects in the hypnosis group lost more weight.

Andersen (1985) also reported a positive association between susceptibility and weight loss in 38 female and seven male patients undergoing hypnotherapy for obesity.

As in the case of smoking control, it appears likely that the most effective use of hypnosis in obesity control will prove to be when it is used as a supplement to or a part of conventional methods of psychotherapy. Most of the standard therapeutic techniques reported used with hypnosis tend to be behavioral, such as covert modeling, reinforcement, and self-monitoring (Bolocofsky, Spinler, and Coulthard-Morris, 1985; Bornstein and Devine, 1980; Aja, 1977).

Analytic Hypnotherapy

Analytic hypnotherapy is the use of hypnosis as an ancillary technique in the practice of analytic psychotherapy. It uses hypnosis to investigate the dynamic meaning of symptoms and to aid in the resolution of the patient's unconscious conflicts (Deabler, 1976). The term *hypnoanalysis* subsumes a variety of specific therapies that vary in the extent to which hypnosis is employed and in the specific techniques used. In some hypnoanalyses, hypnosis may be employed in every session, while in others it may be used only on occasion for specific problems.

Hypnosis has been used in analytic psychotherapy to:

Retrieve early memories by facilitating regression and allowing greater expression of the primary process.

Generate emotional reactions and facilitate the ventilation of emotionally charged material.

Generate and analyze dreams and vivid imagery.

Intensify and exploit the transference.

Bypass resistances and defenses by increasing the patient's motivation to work through anxiety-laden material.

Build ego strength and facilitate reality testing (Baker, 1981).

Control anxiety, freeing the patient to analyze and synthesize (Astor, 1973; Sacerdote, 1972).

Hypnoanalysis, like behavior modification, is a challenging form of therapy for the analyst because the specific techniques used must be varied to meet the requirements of a particular patient. These techniques commonly include visualizations; induction of hallucinations, dreams, and fantasies; dissociative reactions; emotional abreactions; age regression and progression; relaxation; and perceptual and time distortions (Ross, 1981; Sacerdote, 1972). The capacity of hypnosis to shorten the course of analytic therapy is not only of great value in saving the patient time and money, but it may minimize the tendency of the patient to develop what Bell (1972) refers to as the "sick person self-concept."

Sacerdote (1972) notes that the essence of psychotherapy is the development of perceptual, emotional, intellectual, and behavioral change in the patient as a result of a communication with the therapist. From this viewpoint, hypnosis may be looked upon as a vehicle for the mutual communication of ideas between patient and therapist. Since it is such a potentially rich method of communication, the therapist needs an eclectic approach, selecting from among the many specific techniques available. As in any other type of psychotherapy, techniques that are most in tune with the patient's personality structure and thus most likely to be acceptable to him will usually prove the most effective.

Hypnotic Information Retrieval.   Methods of using hypnosis to acquire information about the patient's past experiences and the genesis of symptom formation include questioning under hypnosis and the fostering of regression. Sometimes regression is encouraged by special age-regression techniques, but often the circumstances of hypnoanalysis per se will produce a spontaneous regression and abreaction early in the therapy (Sacerdote, 1972). Also, questioning itself may produce a regression.

Hypnotic Questioning.   Stromberg (1975) presents what he calls a subjective questioning technique as an alternative to prolonged interviewing and directive questioning. The method consists of hypnotizing a patient, producing a relaxed state, and telling the patient to attend to nothing but what the therapist is saying. The patient is then told to remove all external thoughts from his mind and to pick out the one problem that troubles him most and concentrate on it. He is then asked what the problem is. The therapist assumes the role of a friend rather than a prying detective and encourages the patient to talk instead of cross-examining him. The advantages claimed for this method are that it permits the patient to state his problems in the order of their importance to him, not to the therapist, and it permits him to retain a feeling of being in control. Since the patient's defenses are respected, therapy is perceived as less threatening by him, and this permits the development of a better patient-therapist rapport. Stromberg believes that subjective questioning is of value with all patients who are able to achieve a reasonable depth of hypnosis and who have a desire to reveal a problem, whether or not they are able to identify it consciously.

Another type of interrogation under hypnosis is called *ideomotor questioning.* This is a dissociative phenomenon, similar to Hilgard's *hidden observer* technique, that is usually presented to the patient as a way of communicating directly with his unconscious mind. The difference is that use is made of the patient's ideomotor responses (rather than words) to communicate his answers. Typically he is told to give hand or finger signals or movements of a pendulum for a "yes" or "no" response and may also be given the option of responding with a signal for "I don't know" or "I don't want to answer" (Cheek, 1975, 1976b; Erickson and Rossi, 1975). The latter alternative would appear to be a better one because it indicates the presence of a resistance. Ideomotor questioning may be used with a "20 questions"-like format to pinpoint a time period in which the patient believes a conflict arose; for example, "Did your symptom develop before your were 10 years old?" An obvious problem with this type of technique is that if the questions require a yes or no answer, they must be of a type that lawyers call leading questions (questions that suggest an answer). Thus they may be prying and anxiety producing. This method is essentially the opposite of passive, subjective questioning. Therefore it is wise to permit the patient the alternative of responding that he does not warît to answer the question so that he can control the anxiety to which he is subjected.

Because of its focus on the patient's unconscious, which is related to his early experience, ideomotor questioning may often stimulate regressive behavior. An important value of ideomotor questioning may be that it reduces the patient's anxiety in answering questions because it gives the illusion that he is not responsible for his answers. After all, the therapist has told him that he is not questioning him but his "unconscious mind" over which he has no control.

Anderson (1977) reports an interesting demonstration involving the use of a Chevreul pendulum to permit subjects to utilize ideomotor questioning of their own unconscious. On getting answers that they did not want to get, subjects defended themselves by forgetting whether a circular motion meant "yes" or "no" or by changing the direction of motion from a "yes" response to a "no" response when it was publicly obvious that the subject could see the results. Although this demonstration used experimental subjects and not patients, it illustrates that any interpretations made (or insights developed into unconscious feelings) that a person is not ready to accept and deal with will be defended against and rejected and will not benefit a patient. The real art of doing insight therapy is gauging when a patient is ready to deal with interpretations and limiting them to such occasions. By having the patient rather than the therapist interpret the former's dreams or verbalizations, there is a built-in safeguard against premature (and anxiety-producing) interpretations, for the patient is unlikely to make discoveries he is not ready to deal with. The real value of hypnosis in therapy is not to generate new interpretations as much as it is to prepare the patient to handle this kind of material. This work must be done at the patient's own pace.

There is no reason why direct questioning of a patient under hypnosis cannot be conducted in the same manner as if the patient were undergoing therapy while awake. It may be necessary initially to tell such a patient that he is able to talk and answer questions because most hypnotized subjects are disinclined to speak or initiate any kind of spontaneous motor activity. The advantages of questioning, or for that matter of conducting analysis generally, under hypnosis is that the deeply relaxed state produced in the patient may counteract much of the anxiety associated with his verbalizations and permit him to discuss affect-laden material more readily. The author believes that the capacity of hypnosis to lower anxiety levels and to diminish the patient's feelings of responsibility for the material he produces accounts in large measure for its ability to shorten the course of psychotherapy.

In many cases, history-taking under hypnosis has proved to be productive. Spithill (1974) reports a patient who was unable to recall the events leading to the establishment of a tic when awake but was able to do so on the third session of hypnotic interviewing. The case illustrates the capacity of the hypnotic state to overcome the patient's anxiety, for in a previous session the patient had signaled, through an ideomotor response that he did not want to remember the incident. Patients should always be given the option of not remembering material that they do not want to under hypnosis or of not retaining hypnotically generated memories in the subsequent waking state. This technique will help to lower their anxiety levels to the point where they will eventually be able to deal with this material, often in the next session.

Information a therapist may get from a patient in any manner is not helpful to the patient unless and until he is ready to face up to it. Hypnosis is not effective if it is used as a means of trying to coerce information out of an unwilling patient. Its value in analysis lies in helping the patient become ready to explore unavailable material. Kaplan and Deabler (1975) report using hypnotic history taking in the investigation of the etiology of a case of violent acting-out behavior precipitated by a blow to the head in boxing. While on a conscious level the patient expressed only positive feelings toward his father, he was freely able to express much hostility toward him under hypnosis. Thus the authors viewed the patient's acting-out behavior as a form of displaced aggression derived from feelings of anger at his father.

Howland (1975) reports a special use of hypnotic questioning employed in the case of a patient suffering from a multiple personality. In this case, questioning under hypnosis was employed to permit verbal communication directly with each of the two aspects of the patient's personality. Howland addressed these two aspects of the patient as "your timid side" or "your more aggressive aspect" rather than by the names that the patient used to refer to herself to avoid subtly reinforcing her pathological dissociation. After four sessions of hypnotherapy, the patient became sufficiently communicative so that hypnosis was no longer necessary for the therapy to proceed.

Fostering Hypnotic Regression. While the ordinary dependent conditions of analytical psychotherapy or the hypnotic state are often sufficient to trigger spontaneous regression, there are also specific methods designed to induce this type of reaction. One such technique is what Kline (1975) refers to as *sensory hypnotherapy,* and another is the related technique developed by Meares (1960*b*) and modified by Raginsky (1962, 1967) called *sensory hypnoplasty.*

It is a common clinical finding that hypnosis enhances transference (and countertransference) reactions and makes their onset more rapid and their intensity greater. Sacerdote (1972) claims that a transference always develops spontaneously during a hypnotic induction, at least in a clinical context. A transference is a regressive phenomenon, dealing as it does with early emotional feelings that are reactivated and directed at the therapist. It is Kline's (1975) clinical observation that the use of sensory materials in hypnosis activates a variety of regressive mechanisms, which develop along with these rapidly emerging transference reactions. Thus, sensory hypnotherapy utilizes scene visualizations and the generation of vivid imagery as vehicles to trigger early associations and regressive behavior. Imagery may also be used not only to stimulate regression but to induce or deepen a trance, as in the cognitive induction method (see Chapter 3). That it can do so is probably related to the regressive nature of the trance state itself and the transference inherent in it. Such an induction procedure would seem particularly appropriate for use in a session employing sensory hypnotherapy.

Sensory hypnoplasty is a special type of sensory hypnotherapy in which the patient is given a piece of plastic to mold while hypnotized. The plastic serves to provide him with sensory stimuli and is a vehicle for the expression of thoughts and feelings through the products he generates. In addition to the cutaneous stimulation provided by the plastic, it is typically colored and may have odoriferous substances added to it. For example, a brown plastic scented with the odor of limburger cheese might be used to stimulate associations to the anal period. Kline claims that early memories are first expressed in the form of plastic symbols and later are verbalized.

Lindner (1973) reported recreating a psychogenic seizure by age regressing the patient to the time of a previous seizure. He was also able to demonstrate the etiology of this symptom (as a defense against the expression of the patient's feared aggressive feelings) by producing the seizure in response to suggestions that the patient act out his hostile feelings. Caldwell and Stewart (1981) and H. R. Miller (1983) also report cases of hysterical seizures treated successfully by hypnotic age regression used both to uncover the source of the seizures and to permit an abreaction and working through of the trauma.

Cheek (1975, 1976b) tentatively suggested that many symptoms that develop later in life are "imprinted" by an emotional or physiological stress that occurs with the appearance of a prototype of the symptom and, in a viewpoint reminiscent of Rank, believes that the circumstances of the patient's birth may be one such stressful event. As an example, he cites the case of a patient suffering from migraine who, on being age regressed to the event of his own birth by ideomotor questioning, recalled his mother's cries and experiencing the pain of the forceps on his head. Cheek suggests that a wide variety of psychosomatic and sexual disorders may have their origins in such birth experiences, and he advocates exploring such symptoms by regressing the patient to the time of birth.

From a theoretical point of view, the validity of the patient's birth memories and their role in the etiology of his symptom are of great interest. From a clinical point of view, they are irrelevant. The patient with the migraines developed the ability to abort them following the hypnotic regression. This benefit is just as real whether hypnosis really brought back an actual memory or the patient had simply fantasized the incident based on stories about his birth that he had heard from his mother. The method advocated is quite similar to Adler's technique of asking a patient for his earliest memory on the theory that such a memory shows the patient's basic view of the world and holds the key to his style of life. Often "memories" obtained from this type of questioning are either grossly distorted or pure fantasies, but they may still reflect much about the patient and his outlook on life. Sexton and Maddock (1979) present an unusual report utilizing age progression as well as age regression in the treatment of three cases of catatonic depression and two cases of neurotic depression. For example, catatonics were age progressed to heaven where they could talk with a deceased father or Christ. They also make the interesting point that many psychotics are in an ego state that precludes ordinary reality testing and hence may be suggestible without the need for formal trance induction.

Generation and Expression of Emotion.   Regression is not only useful for the retrieval of sensory and ideational memory; it is even more useful for the recapturing of emotional material and the context of its original occurrence. Furthermore, due to the necessary psychic connections between the present and the past, this is a two-way street. Not only can present ideational suggestions trigger regressive responses that reactivate prior emotional feelings, but present emotional states can reactivate old memories.

Barber (1978b) points out the value of hypnosis as a catalyst in producing abreactions. Sacerdote (1972) notes that because of the capacity of hypnosis to reduce the patient's fear of loss of control and the rapid development of the transference, abreactions can occur as early as the first hypnotic session, and the therapist must be prepared to cope with them.

Since all abreactions involve to some extent the linking of present emotional feelings with their origins in the past, a technique called an *affect bridge* capitalizes on this relationship (Kline, 1977; Schafer, 1981). This method starts with a present emotional state, either spontaneously developed in the course of hypnotherapy or specifically induced by hypnosis. Then the patient concentrates on it and intensifies it. He is then asked to go back in time to a situation when he felt the same way. This technique is capable of producing regressions that may identify the origins of chronic maladaptive emotional states. It may also circumvent the repression of these feelings and permit their full intensity to be developed and an abreaction to occur. The value of an abreaction to a patient is probably more than the mere ventilation and discharge of welled-up feelings that are a constant source of discomfort, for if these feelings were intense enough to have survived over the years and produce symptoms, their discharge might reasonably be expected to give only transitory relief until they build up in intensity again. The real value of the emotional reliving of traumatic experiences is that it gives the patient the opportunity to appreciate and understand the source of these feelings from his vantage point as an adult rather than as the helpless child he was at the time of the original trauma. In effect, the patient, in being able to accept and deal with his feelings, is freed from the need for the maladaptive defense of repression. Thus, these emotions are no longer forced to build up to the point that they can cause symptoms.

Age-regression techniques have been successfully used to permit ventilation of repressed emotions in Vietnam veterans suffering from delayed stress response syndrome (Brende and Benedict, 1980; D. Spiegel, 1981; Turco, 1981). MacHovec (1985) has reported similar work with four nonmilitary cases of posttraumatic stress disorder seen in brief (from five to nine sessions) hypnotherapy.

Watkins (1980) describes a technique she calls a *silent abreaction* in which a patient is asked to imagine beating a boulder that he is told represents a specific person or traumatic incident, until he is exhausted. The patient is then required to say something positive about himself before the third phase, consisting of the generation of a positive tingling feeling spreading over his body, is commenced. The latter feeling is a reinforcement for ventilating anger. Thus the treatment, while dealing with the analytical notion of abreaction, has behavioral characteristics (which shows how artificial the distinction between dynamic and behavioral therapy really is). The gist of the procedure, according to Watkins, is the complete draining of anger and the subsequent verbal interpretation and reintegration of the symbolic meanings of the situation. She introduces this method as a way of dealing with the problem of ordinary abreaction involving yelling and obscenities that might disturb people in neighboring offices. This, of course, is not the proper remedy for this common problem. The therapist should either soundproof the office or find another one more appropriate for the practice of psychotherapy.

Besides using hypnosis to build up negative emotions as grist for the analytic mill or to trigger regression, positive emotions can also be generated, and feelings of well-being, relaxation, and happiness can be used to counteract feelings of anxiety that might interfere with the progress of therapy (Bell, 1972).

Uses of Hypnotic Dreams and Imagery.   Dreams are a valuable source of material in any form of analytic psychotherapy. They have many uses beyond the translation of the manifest content into the unconscious latent content (which Freud dubbed the "royal road to the unconscious"). Dreams are often, if not always, brought to the therapist for specific reasons, such as to introduce a topic in an indirect way or to make statements without assuming responsibility for them. It is often productive to investigate why a patient brought in a particular dream for interpretation. In the author's experience, patients rarely bring a dream into therapy without having a good idea of the meaning of the dream, as well as a purpose to serve by revealing it.

The psychoanalytic position on dream interpretation is that the analyst always appears in the patient's dream, and whatever other meaning a dream may have, it always reflects the state of the transference. According to this view, a series of dreams interpreted throughout the course of therapy often reflects the progress of the therapeutic process. Many analysts feel that interpreting dreams too early in therapy can be threatening to the patient. It may give him the feeling that the therapist can get through his defenses and learn more from his verbalizations than he is ready to reveal about himself. Certainly no type of interpretation ought to be made in therapy until the relationship between the patient and therapist is strong enough to withstand the stress to which the interpretation may subject it.

Hypnosis makes it possible to expand the role of dream interpretation in therapy by the hypnotic induction of dreams, as well as by their interpretation under hypnosis. Hypnotically-induced dreams may be generated either during therapy sessions or as posthypnotic phenomena during regular sleeping periods. In the former case, interpretation may be performed by the patient while dreaming (Hodge and Wagner, 1969b; Moss and Bremer, 1973). Just as the ego may be split into a participating and an observing ego during hypnosis so, too, in dreams, whether or not hypnotically induced, an observing ego may be present that can interpret dreams while they are in progress. This phenomenon of an observing ego can be noted in naturally occurring *lucid* dreams where the dreamer is aware that he is dreaming. Under hypnosis, this observing portion of the ego can always be contacted to provide an account of an ongoing dream, as well as an interpretation of it.

One of the advantages of hypnotic dream induction, beyond its obvious value in making more dreams available for analysis (by suggestions that dreams will be remembered), is that it makes it possible to control the topics dreamed about. Patients can be told to have a dream about some significant person in their lives that reflects their real feelings toward such a person or to have a dream that will shed some light on the meaning of a symptom (Hodge and Wagner, 1969b). If a spontaneous nocturnal dream brought in for analysis is difficult to decipher, the patient can be instructed to have another dream with the same message that is less distorted. This technique assumes that at some level at least, the patient understands the meaning of the original dream. Moss and Bremer (1973) believe that hypnosis provides a special access to the patient's symbol-translating mechanism and that dream interpretation under hypnosis is therefore easier. Although they do not describe this mechanism, there are many possible factors involved in addition to the inhibition of anxiety and the apparent lowering of responsibility for hypnotic behavior. These might include freedom from the constraints of ordinary logical thinking, heightened motivation to produce material that the therapist is seeking, and the possibility of vivid sensory and affective memories of the dream experience.

As in ordinary analysis, the issue of the validity of a dream interpretation is an unanswerable question. All that the analyst can observe is whether the patient accepts or rejects a proffered interpretation. The patient's response does not demonstrate that the interpretation is correct or incorrect. Even when the patient himself produces an interpretation (the ideal procedure), its validity is not established. Fortunately, the accuracy of an interpretation is unimportant in therapy. What is important is whether the interpretation is useful. A good interpretation is one that leads to the introduction of new material into the therapy and disrupts the tendency of most patients to sound like a broken record, repeating the same material from session to session. A poor interpretation (whether correct or not) does not lead to the introduction of new material or further the progress of the analysis.

Hodge and Wagner (1969b) advocate the use of hypnotically-induced dreams to analyze the transference reaction. Dreams, whether hypnotic or natural, are often useful vehicles for analyzing this and other affect-laden relationships since they give the patient a comfortable opportunity to describe his socially unacceptable feelings indirectly. If a patient rejects the idea of dreaming or dream interpretation, the same result may be obtained by having him hallucinate. Hodge favors the use of an imaginary television set to produce hallucinated scenes, and he has the patient "switch channels" if the hallucination produces excessively upsetting results or if the therapist wishes to explore another aspect of the situation. Others have used an imaginary crystal ball for the same purpose (Bell, 1972).

If an interpretation of a dream is made or a memory is retrieved under hypnosis, Hodge (1977) advocates giving the patient the option of not remembering it when awake if he does not want to. This will limit the anxiety to which he is being exposed to what he can tolerate, and eventually the patient will be willing to remember this material.

In addition to producing dreamlike material for analysis, a hallucinated television set can be used to display much more directive material for the purpose of inducing affective states and moods (Stein, 1975).

Erickson (1977a) reports on the technique of having patients hallucinate scenes in a series of crystal balls as a method of developing historical information about affect-laden material. He also describes induced imagery involving calendar tearing as a technique for restoring memory to amnesia patients. One of the advantages he claimed for such techniques as these is that they permit patients to proceed at their own pace. He also perceived a marked dissociation between insights a patient develops unconsciously under hypnosis and consciously while awake, and he believed that whatever a patient learns in one of these states has to be learned again in the other.

Although the generation of imagery for corrective purposes rather than interpretative uses is generally associated with behavior modification, Van Rooyen (1981) reports an interesting symbolic use of concrete imagery to convey an indirect suggestion for change. A patient interested in mechanics whose reading disorder prevented him from reading his own handwriting was told to imagine himself getting smaller until he could enter the "control room of his own mind" and "repair" the mental block. This suggestion proved effective, probably because it capitalized on the patient's own interests and style of thought.

Hypnotic Overcoming of Resistances.

Hypnotic Overcoming of Resistances. Moss and Bremer (1973) conclude that insight into how maladaptive behavior is learned provides motivation for change that helps to overcome resistance. Motivation for change may also be brought about by a variety of other techniques, such as suggestions portraying the advantages of being rid of the disabling symptoms, anxiety-reducing suggestions making symptoms less necessary, and the analysis of directed experiences and fantasies. Bell (1972) takes the position that authoritative suggestions commanding a patient to get well and relinquish his symptom are not as effective as permissive ones because they do not take into account the patient's need for his ego defenses. Permissive suggestions respect both the patient and his defense structure and encourage a more effective working relationship that aids the patient in eliminating defenses by reducing his need for them.

Fogel (1976) reports using both positive and negative suggestions to increase motivation for the removal of psychogenic physical symptoms. He also reports using suggestions to counteract a patient's feelings of euphoria when such feelings had the effect of reducing motivation for improvement.

Zeig (1980a, 1980b) describes the Ericksonian technique of symptom prescription that encourages the patient to persist in the symptom. Some rationale must be given the patient for this approach—for example, "It may be instructive"— and it may be suggested indirectly. The advantage claimed is that the therapist is acting within the patient's frame of reference, and the eventual impetus for change comes from the patient when he, not the therapist, is ready.

Edelstien (1982) discusses the technique of ego stage therapy in dealing with a wide variety of resistances. He notes that these may occur at any stage of therapy: resistance to entering or terminating therapy, resistance to being hypnotized, resistance to the work of therapy, or resistance to change. The technique attempts to find the source of the resistance (e.g., repression, transference, secondary gains, or unconscious guilt) and to overcome it by communicating under hypnosis with the part of the patient responsible for the resistance and convincing it that its purpose can better be achieved by letting go of the resistant behavior. Baker (1983b) considers the meaning and management of resistance in patients with primitive ego states, (borderline, narcissistic, and psychotic patients) and concludes that in these patients, resistance is transference related. He believes that the therapist needs to support reality-based boundaries, to provide opportunity for the patient to exercise observing ego functions, and to establish positive internalized representations of the therapist. Resistance in these patients should be examined in terms of their need for increased distance and their fear of the therapeutic relationship.

The Ericksonian technique of utilization was described by Sanders (1977b) as useful in overcoming the resistance of two patients who displayed strong hostility in response to efforts to generate insight into their resistances to their prime therapy. This technique involves respecting the patient's outlook and meeting him "where he is," gaining gradual control over his behavior, and demonstrating to the patient that change is possible. This seems to be quite similar to the technique of going along with the resistance rather than attacking it head on and the technique of symptom prescription. Thus, if a patient says he cannot relax, asking him to do so will result in a battle for control with the therapist. Accepting the inability to relax and working around it will avoid this problem. Such a patient might be told to try to increase his tension as a way of demonstrating his control over his symptom. In an extreme example, that the author has mixed feelings about, Berwick and Douglas (1977) report treating paranoid schizophrenics who had the delusion that they were possessed by the devil by accepting their delusions and performing a hypnotic exorcism. The problem with this type of suggestion is that it may give the therapist the illusion that a patient has gotten better when in reality what has happened is that one delusion has been replaced with another, which results in less overt behavioral problems. In other words, the patient is a less troublesome patient with the same underlying pathology.

Miscellaneous Techniques.   Since hypnosis is a form of communication, the therapist must adapt his or her use of language and metaphor to the requirements of the patient. In working with children, it is essential to communicate with them on a level that they find meaningful. Silber (1973) used fairy tales, folklore, and symbolic metaphors to develop feelings of confidence, self-acceptance, and increased motivation in child patients. For example, he conceptualized the speech-producing mechanism of a child with a speech defect to her as a miniature version of herself. This was a metaphor that she could understand and relate to. Olness (1985) also reports the use of this type of material in child hypnotherapy.

In a similar vein, Tilton (1984) had child patients imagine interacting with comic strip characters whose communications they were more likely to accept than the therapist's, and Elkins and Carter (1981) used imagery based on science fiction to communicate ideas symbolically to children.

It is in the treatment of the more severely disturbed patients that some of the most innovative uses of hypnosis have been attempted. For example, Plapp (1976) permitted an extremely disturbed adolescent patient to hypnotize him as a means of demonstrating trust and furthering the transference. This type of role reversal also made it easier for the patient to express his fantasies indirectly through the suggestions he gave to the therapist. In view of the fact that a hypnotized subject does not actually relinquish control over the situation beyond the extent that he is willing to, this procedure may not be as risky as it might seem, and it produced good results in the case cited. On the other hand, while advocating the usefulness of this unusual type of role-reversal treatment in a proper case, Diamond (1980, 1983) regards it as contraindicated for very disturbed patients such as narcissistic, borderline, psychotic, or those with multiple personalities, poorly established ego boundaries, or low ego strength. Among the advantages claimed for this technique are the enhancement of empathy on the part of the therapist, increased rapport and a strengthening of the therapeutic alliance, increased patient motivation, the overcoming of resistances, providing the therapist with knowledge of the patient's assumptive system, and the ego strengthening produced by the role of hypnotist (as opposed to the ego-diminishing role of patient). This approach requires a particularly well-adjusted and well-trained therapist who never loses sight of his or her role as a therapist nor succumbs to countertransference feelings induced by the procedure.

Scagnelli (1976) used hypnotic dream and imagery production with eight schizophrenic and borderline patients to reduce anxiety, build ego strength, and develop insight. She reports special problems in the treatment of this kind of patient, such as fear of losing control, fear of closeness, and fear of changing a negative self-concept. These fears may appear in exaggerated form in psychotic patients, but they are by no means exclusive to this class of patient and are often seen less dramatically in neurotics and others. Scagnelli reduced the patients' fear of losing control by telling them that she was training them in self-hypnosis and letting them induce the trance themselves. Fear of closeness was dealt with by permitting the patient as much social distance as he required, and fear of changing the self-concept was controlled by using permissive techniques in ego building. The reduction of anxiety by the induction of relaxation and feelings of self-mastery was employed to enhance the patient's ability to discuss his feelings and develop insight. Hypnotic dreams were productive in generating much symbolic and primary process material. Patients were encouraged to explore their feelings, and, if negative ones developed, they were asked to express them in the form of concrete imagery. Imagery shifts were then employed, and an image of a negative or painful experience was transformed into a positive one.

Erickson and Rossi (1975) described a technique called a *double bind* that Erickson used in his indirect style of making suggestions. In essence, it involves giving a patient an illusory choice between two compatible alternatives. For example, a patient may be asked, "Will your symptom go away this week or not until next week?" or during an induction procedure, a patient might be asked if his eyes will close before or after his hand levitates. This technique is a way of making whatever a patient does become a form of compliance with the therapist's suggestion. It is somewhat similar to a therapist's getting a negativistic patient to do what the therapist wants him to by giving him an opportunity to oppose the analyst. Both techniques will succeed only if they are appropriate to the needs of the patient and are used subtly. In a similar gambit, Erickson (1966) used posthypnotic suggestion to control anxiety by telling the patient his panic states would continue but would be of shorter duration.

The use of metaphoric stories as exemplified by Erickson's teaching fables is essentially an indirect form of suggestion, and like all other indirect suggestions, it minimizes the possibility of resistance because it is difficult for a patient to resist a suggestion having little obvious relationship to an intended response. Also it is more readily acceptable to patients who resent being ordered around or who fear loss of control. By more actively involving the patient as the instigator of the desired behavior it "meets him where he is" and respects his position (Brink, 1982; Gindhart, 1981a; De Shazer, 1980; Soper and L'Abate, 1977).

Stanton (1979b), conceptualizing the major problem of most patients as demoralization produced by a low sense of self-esteem rather than any specific symptom, has demonstrated that taped hypnotic ego-enhancing suggestions and suggested images of success, relaxation, and self-confidence were effective in getting experimental subjects to develop a more internal locus of control. This carried the implication that they were not powerless victims of external events. The change in attitude remained present at a 6-month follow-up. It remains to be demonstrated how helpful this technique will be to actual patients. It probably will be useful with those whose major problems are low self-esteem and feelings of helplessness. Although these problems are common, psychopathology is often quite complex and may involve many other problems.

Kir-Stimon (1978) employed hypnosis as an aid in overcoming the anxiety of patients ready to terminate nonhypnotic therapy and become independent of the therapist.

Suicidal Patients.   Perhaps one of the most stressful situations for therapists is when they are responsible for the care of a patient with suicidal tendencies. This is a difficult situation because the therapist is required to be able to evaluate the actual risk of suicide with a degree of accuracy that the state of the art does not permit. A therapist who errs on the side of safety and either contacts the patient's relatives or seeks hospitalization of the patient unnecessarily may well destroy the therapeutic relationship (which is probably the most important safeguard against suicide that the patient has). If, on the other hand, the therapist is not cautious enough, it may cost the patient his life. Additionally, the situation may involve the therapist in a malpractice suit, particularly in California, where, in the *Tarasoff* case (1974), a court apparently unaware of the limitations of the current state of the art of psychology decided that a therapist must be able to predict the propensity of a patient for future acting-out behavior. A psychotherapist cannot rely on the erroneous notion that people who talk about suicide will not commit it. The unfortunate fact is that many patients who intend not to commit suicide but to feign an attempt to attract attention to themselves and their problems may inadvertently complete the act.

Suicidal tendencies may develop in any depressed patient, and it is not reasonable to expect patients presenting for psychotherapy to be well adjusted. Hence, sooner or later all therapists must deal with such patients.

Since suicide is often an impulsive act, if the patient can be dissuaded from it temporarily, this may be sufficient to prevent it. For this reason, many therapists who treat suicidal patients extract from them as a condition of therapy a promise that before acting on any suicidal impulse, they will first discuss it with the therapist in his or her office. (This requires the therapist to be available 24 hours a day, 7 days a week and to have a backup therapist for any period when he or she is unavailable.)

Hodge (1977) has devised a method to increase the likelihood that such an undertaking on the part of the patient will be honored. He suggests to the patient under hypnosis that he will be unable to act on such a suicidal impulse until he discusses it clearly and personally with the therapist. The reason for the requirement of a personal discussion with the therapist is that it forces the patient to delay action until a transient suicidal impulse may have time to dissipate. The reason for specifying that the patient clearly discuss the matter is to avoid the possibility that the patient may consider an unclear symbolic allusion to suicide as complying with the requirement imposed on him. Hodge says that a hypnotic suggestion to the effect that the patient would never be able to commit suicide might be seen as something being imposed on him that would invite resistance. It might even be taken as a challenge by the patient. It is not possible to say how effective this method is. Although Hodge has never had a patient treated in this manner commit suicide, the same could be said for many other therapists who simply rely on the patient's waking promise to consult with them prior to acting on self-destructive impulses. It appears that the method is not likely to be harmful to either the patient or the therapeutic relationship and that anything that may reduce the possibility of a suicide at no therapeutic cost is a worthwhile addition to a therapist's armamentarium.

In summary, the essential nature of analytic hypnotherapy is the use of hypnotic techniques to a greater or lesser degree to further the progress of an analysis. It is not the hypnosis but the analysis, with its attendant transference and the development of insight, that produces a cure. The role of hypnosis is to facilitate this process and provide an alternative means of circumventing roadblocks in therapy.

Hypnosis in Behavior Modification

Hypnosis and behavior modification are naturally compatible techniques. Although hypnosis is not essential to the practice of behavior therapy, it can facilitate it (Ascher, 1977; Astor, 1973; Dengrove, 1973; Kline, 1979a; Okhowat, 1985; Surman, 1979). Hypnosis has been used as an adjunct to all forms of behavior modification. Some of the specific purposes for which it has been employed have been to:

Enhance the depth and speed of relaxation procedures.
Shape behavior through posthypnotic suggestions so that desired responses are produced to be reinforced and learned.
Generate vivid imagery and dreams in systematic desensitization procedures, covert reinforcement paradigms, and other applications.
Facilitate communication.

Most of these uses have been within the context of a particular mode of behavior therapy, but there are some who claim that the generation of a deeply relaxed state can be therapeutic by itself as an adjunct to psychological or medical treatment (French and Tupin, 1974). Benson, Beary, and Carol (1974) write of *the relaxation response* and discuss examples of it in various religious experiences, progressive relaxation, hypnosis, yoga, Zen, and transcendental meditation. They suggest the need for research into both the benefits and possible side effects of continued use of these procedures.

On the other hand, Graham and his associates (1975) reported that in a study of 22 student volunteers suffering from insomnia, different results were obtained from nonhypnotic relaxation treatment and hypnotic relaxation treatment. Although both treatments resulted in subjective improvements, only the former produced objective benefits. These investigators attribute their results to differences in the subjects' expectations of success. However, in view of the fact that the relaxation instructions to both groups were essentially similar (both were based on the Stanford Hypnotic Susceptibility Scale, form C (SHSS:C), with suggestions to "go to sleep" or "be hypnotized" changed to "relax" for the nonhypnotic group), it seems debatable whether this study should be regarded as a test of hypnotic versus waking relaxation or simply a test of two slightly different hypnotic procedures, one an overt induction and one a covert one. This is an important issue, for often there is not much difference between what purports to be a relaxation procedure and the induction of a hypnotic state by the method of progressive relaxation, beyond the use of the term *hypnosis* in the latter procedure. Since there are no unique and universally agreed-upon indexes of a trance state, it follows that any time a study purports to investigate differences between the effects produced by a hypnotic and a waking state, a certain amount of skepticism over what the independent variable really is may be warranted (Barrios, 1973).

Hypnosis in Rational-Emotive Therapy (RET). Green (1973) notes that RET emphasizes the patient's interpretation of events in his environment and is a reeducative experience aimed at getting him to reevaluate the significance of these events. Since this is accomplished by communication with the therapist, it is essential that the patient accurately understand the therapist's messages. Psychological stress can distort the perception of these communications. Most psychological defenses, such as denial and projection, produce profound distortions in the perception of ideas and arguments, as does the transference reaction, which may develop in the relationship between any patient and therapist whether or not the latter intends it to occur. Thus, Greene advocates the use of hypnosis to increase the receptivity of the patient to the therapist's messages and to reduce distortion in communication by eliminating distracting stimuli and focusing attention on the therapeutic arguments. He reports success with this approach in getting a patient suffering from chronic alcoholism, depression, and head pains to accept ideas relating to the cause of his symptoms and a philosophic viewpoint designed to ameliorate them. The use of hypnosis to get a patient to understand and accept ideas presented in therapy was summed up by Barber (1978a) when he suggested that what is done in hypnotherapy, in essence, is to tell a patient to be quiet and listen carefully to what the therapist is saying.

Gwynne, Tosi, and Howard (1978) describe a development of RET called *rational stage-directed hypnotherapy* (RSDH), which emphasizes cognitive control over the patient's affective and behavioral responses. In the treatment of a nonassertive woman, interpersonal situations were analyzed with respect to the resulting cognitions, emotional and physiological responses, and behavior. Treatment involved cognitive restructuring under hypnosis. The patient was led through six developmental stages to develop cognitive restructuring skills. After hypnotic induction and deepening, she was told to generate an image of a previously determined self-defeating situation. She was told to experience the negative affect as much as possible and to observe herself performing in an ineffective manner. Her discomfort was intensified by pointing it out to her. Then she was instructed to discontinue visualizing the scene, and more self-enhancing behavior was suggested, which formed the basis of new imagery. Positive feelings were then enhanced by the therapist's pointing them out. This treatment seems to be a sequential combination of Cautela's covert sensitization and covert positive reinforcement (see page 231) with hypnotic enhancement of imagery and affect. (See also Boutin and Tosi, 1983; DeVoge, 1977; Tosi and Henderson, 1983).

Hypnosis in Systematic Desensitization.   Hypnosis has two distinct uses in systematic desensitization: to produce a more rapid and profound state of relaxation on cue and to assist in rendering the imagined scenes in a covert hierarchy more vivid (Astor, 1973). Thus, a hierarchical scene may be presented during desensitization trials under hypnosis and the patient told that when given a signal, such as a touch on the shoulder, he will be able to visualize the scene more vividly with ease and comfort (Dengrove, 1973). He may also be given posthypnotic suggestions of continued relaxation and a new ability to do in real life the things visualized during desensitization without experiencing anxiety.

One of the unique values of hypnotic systematic desensitization is its use with a patient who reacts with too little anxiety to imagined scenes to be deconditioned covertly but who at the same time reacts with too much anxiety to even the weakest items of a real-life hierarchy. Hypnosis may be able to make an imagined scene more realistic for such a patient and thus create enough anxiety for desensitization to occur. It may also be able to fill in gaps in a covert hierarchy (in which the difference in subjective units of disturbance [SUD] between adjacent scenes in the hierarchy is too great for the desensitization of anxiety to generalize to the next scene). Frutiger (1981) reports the use of hypnosis to counteract anxiety that prevented the patient from proceeding with an in vivo desensitization procedure for a penetration phobia that involved the insertion of glass tubes into her vagina.

Cautela (1975) cites studies that indicate that a hypnotic induction did not increase the effectiveness of procedures that involved the use of imagery, such as desensitization (Lang, Lazovik, and Reynolds, 1965; Paul, 1966, 1967). He is quick to note that these negative results of hypnotic imagery were not obtained in the covert conditioning methods that he developed and to point out the need for more research.

There are certain difficulties that must be recognized in such research. First, the value of hypnosis as an adjunct to systematic desensitization would be expected to vary greatly with individual patients. Patients who can relax deeply and visualize clearly would probably not be benefited much by the addition of hypnosis to the procedure. Neither would patients who are poor subjects. On the other hand, a potentially good subject who is having difficulty relaxing in the therapeutic situation or finding it too distracting to permit clear visualization may be markedly benefited. Such idiosyncratic results may be masked in the analysis of group data. Hence studies of this sort may have to be performed on individual subjects. More important, perhaps, is the effect of the therapist's skills as a hypnotist and his or her own conception of the value of hypnotic desensitization. This attitude may be unintentionally conveyed to the subjects and thereby affect their expectancies.

Daniels (1976c) reports completing covert desensitization of an injection phobia in only two sessions with the aid of hypnotically produced deep relaxation. He was then able to proceed with a sequence of in vivo desensitization trials.

Deiker and Pollock (1975) report a treatment technique used in phobias that integrated hypnosis and systematic desensitization. They employed systematic desensitization in a conventional manner and then followed it with Erickson's (1954) device of projecting the patient hypnotically into the future, at which time she was instructed to imagine herself cured of her phobia. Since this patient was fearful of being hypnotized and of the loss of control she believed it to entail, it was presented to her as a means of controlling her own mind. With such a patient, not only should her role in producing the hypnosis be emphasized, but also, after the initial induction, she should be trained to induce the trance herself in all subsequent sessions. Tilton (1983) reported the successful combination of this pseudo-orientation in time with other Ericksonian strategies to get a patient to prepare for the successful completion of a future situation by imagining it to be occurring during hypnosis.

Hypnotic Dream and Image Manipulation. In behavioral applications of hypnotherapy, dreams and imagery are not used primarily for interpretation and diagnosis as they are in analytic work but more directly as vehicles for the rehearsal of desirable behavior, the provision of covert corrective experiences, and the manipulation of reinforcement. Thus, imagery may be used in covert or imaginary role playing or in assertiveness training to give the patient practice in making appropriately assertive remarks in simulated situations. These situations may include a variety of social or sexual relationships where the patient is unduly inhibited and thus unable to function on an appropriate adult level (Astor, 1973). Erickson's technique of pseudo-orientation, whereby the patient is hypnotically projected into the future, is another example of the use of imagery in hypnotherapy. By this means, a patient can begin to experience himself free of his symptoms and able to do comfortably those things that his anxiety and fears prevent him from attempting (Deiker and Pollock, 1975; Dengrove, 1973).

Imagery may also be used as a means of communicating abstract ideas in a more concrete symbolic fashion, which increases their ability to evoke emotional responses. As an example of this technique, Astor (1973) asked patients to imagine themselves as a developing acorn or egg. This suggestion was intended as a supportive one designed to convey to the patient the idea that he was growing and developing. It was thus aimed at improving the patient's self-image.

Flooding is a method of therapy often done in vivo because of the intense emotions that must be developed. In view of the successful application of hypnosis in producing abreactions based on past emotion-laden events, it would appear that its potential for use in a covert flooding procedure (implosive therapy) is worthy of investigation. Hypnotic flooding would be more convenient and controllable than in vivo flooding. It would also be a safer procedure. Many responsible therapists who might be reluctant to put a patient with a severe flying phobia on an airplane might be less reluctant to expose him to a hypnotically hallucinated airplane ride where they could remain close at hand if needed. The ability of hypnosis to generate and modulate emotions may prove to be a source of substantial therapeutic leverage in such cases (Astrup, 1978). Scrignar (1981) reported successful treatment by hypnotic flooding of two patients with hand washing compulsions who resisted analytic therapy and had only limited improvement from a variety of behavioral therapies, including thought stopping, systematic desensitization, cognitive restructuring, and progressive relaxation. Hand washing rates were reduced to normal and maintained there at 2- or 7-year follow-ups.

Anderson, Basker, and Dalton (1975) used imagery as an indirect way of controlling autonomic nervous system (ANS) reactions in the treatment of migraine. In addition to general suggestions of less tension and ego enhancement, they instructed patients before and during hypnosis about the vascular mechanism underlying migraine headaches. They then asked the patients to visualize the arteries in their necks and imagine exercising control over them. All patients were then trained to use autohypnosis to abort an attack. They found that hypnosis used in this manner was superior to prophylaxis with prochlorperazine (Stemetil), with ten of 23 hypnotic patients obtaining complete remissions and only three of 24 drug patients achieving the same results. Similarly, Barabasz and McGeorge (1978) reported that hypnosis was superior to biofeedback in training peripheral vasodilation (hand warming).

Daniels (1976a) used a similar method of controlling autonomic nervous activity through suggested imagery in the treatment of migraine. After reviewing the literature with respect to the various psychological techniques found to be effective in controlling migraine headaches, he selected suggestions of hand warming and forehead cooling for use in a pilot study. These were selected because they eliminated the need for expensive biofeedback equipment and could be given by tape recorder, reducing the need for in-office treatment sessions. He then developed an integrated treatment plan combining behavioral and hypnotic techniques (Daniels, 1977). Patients were first trained to achieve deep muscle relaxation in response to a cue word. Then hypnosis was induced and suggestions of hand warming and forehead cooling given. A tape was made, and the patient was instructed to listen to it four times a day for an 18-day period. Patients were also taught to do a rational-cognitive analysis of their reactions to stressful events occurring during the day as a means of lowering their anxiety levels (Maultsby, 1971). This analysis included a specification of the event that upset the patient, his beliefs concerning this event, the feelings or emotions that these beliefs generated, and the illogical nature of his reasoning. Finally, if anxiety mounted too quickly to permit time for this kind of analysis, the patient was taught thought-stopping techniques, using the learned cue for relaxation, to reestablish a tranquil state. The patient developed the ability to produce a calm, relaxed feeling at any time and was thus able to prevent the vasoconstriction phase of a migraine attack from developing.

Cautela (1966, 1967, 1975) has developed a system of behavior modification techniques called *covert conditioning*. This therapy is based on operant conditioning, but it makes use of imagined rather than real stimuli, responses, and reinforcements. Cautela reasoned that if real aversive stimuli could be used in deconditioning homosexual responses, then imaginary ones should have the same effect, while at the same time having the advantages of requiring no special equipment and of decreasing patient attenuation rates. In addition, the use of covert aversive stimuli eliminates many ethical problems and improves patient-therapist rapport. Finally, this method is not restricted to the consulting room; the patient can be encouraged to practice imagined scenes at home, thereby developing a sense of control and mastery over his own behavior. Cautela proposes that the success of many hypnotherapies involving the use of imagery is due in part to covert conditioning and suggests that hypnotherapists might be more effective if they explicitly utilized principles of conditioning in their work. He also suggests that therapists using covert conditioning methods without hypnosis might find it worthwhile to try hypnotic imagery as a way of enhancing the treatment.

There are four basic paradigms of operant conditioning used in covert conditioning procedures: (1) covert sensitization or punishment training, (2) covert positive reinforcement (COR), (3) covert negative reinforcement (CNR), and (4) covert extinction. Covert sensitization is essentially aversive therapy performed through imagery instead of in vivo aversive stimulation. For example, a patient with a weight control problem can be instructed to imagine breaking his diet and that this imagined response is followed by feelings of nausea, social embarrassment, and the like. The patient is given practice in imagining a variety of such scenes and is required to practice them at home about ten times per day. The method has been found effective with alcoholism, sexual deviations, and smoking. Polk (1983) reports its use with hypnotic supplementation in the treatment of a case of exhibitionism. Imagined aversive stimulation followed a hypnotically imagined act of exhibitionism based on actual traumatic occurrences in the patient's past. Copemann (1977) also reports the successful use of hypnotically enhanced covert sensitization in the treatment of three cases of polydrug abuse. Two patients remained drug free at 18-month and 3-year follow-ups; one relapsed after 18 months but was successfully retreated.

Sometimes imagery is combined with in vivo procedures. For example, Dengrove (1973) describes hypnotic suggestions to a smoker that his cigarettes contained rat droppings and that he would become nauseous and ill when given one to inhale. Feamster and Brown (1963) suggested to an alcoholic in a deep trance that he would relive his worst hangover whenever he smelled, tasted, or even thought about alcohol.

Covert positive reinforcement is used as a supplement to covert sensitization. Instead of punishing inappropriate responses to diminish their frequency, more appropriate responses, which are incompatible with the undesirable behavior, are reinforced to increase their likelihood of occurring. Cautela initially has patients fill out a "reinforcement survey schedule" to determine what is highly reinforcing to them. He selects from among these items those that the patient can visualize clearly in response to the cue word *reinforcement*. Patients are instructed to imagine themselves performing some desirable behavior, and when this image is signaled to be clearly established, the therapist gives the cue word *reinforcement,* and the patient immediately shifts to imagining the reinforcing scene. Thus, immediate reinforcement follows the imagining of adaptive behavior and facilitates its acquisition. This procedure, like all other forms of covert conditioning, can also be practiced at home. It has been found effective in a variety of conditions, including cases of phobias, test anxiety, and the changing of children's self-concepts. It is easier to use with phobias than systematic desensitization since it is not necessary to employ either a hierarchial arrangement of anxiety-producing scenes or relaxation training. Lewis (1979) reports the successful use of this technique, enhanced by hypnosis, in the treatment of a schizoid personality where significant behavioral gains were maintained at a 2-year follow-up.

Covert negative reinforcement is useful for patients who are unable to state any personal source of positive reinforcement. The term *negative reinforcement* is somewhat unfortunate as it is used in the Skinnerian sense. Skinner considers the termination of an aversive stimulus to be a "negative" reinforcer instead of adopting the more straightforward terminology of saying that the termination of an aversive stimulus is positively reinforcing. Negative reinforcement in this context is not synonymous with punishment.

The technique of covert negative reinforcement is to have the patient imagine an aversive situation and then, on the verbal cue to "shift," suddenly imagine a scene depicting the behavior to be acquired. This desirable behavior is now reinforced by its association with the termination of the aversive scene. The termination of the aversive scene must be complete and rapid enough to prevent its aversive elements from becoming associated with the behavior to be learned.

Covert extinction is a method used to extinguish maladaptive behavior that is being maintained by reinforcement dispensed by people in the patient's life over whom the therapist has no effective control, such as parents or teachers. Here the patient is instructed to imagine performing the undesired behavior pattern and getting no reaction at all from these sources of reinforcement. Cautela says that it is important for the therapist to guard against the patient's developing resentment toward these people as a result of this therapy. An even greater danger of this technique may be the fact that the covert extinction procedure combined with the naturally occurring in vivo reinforcement may result in a partial reinforcement schedule being set up for the maladaptive behavior, possibly rendering it even more difficult to extinguish.

Baker and Boaz (1983) and Lamb (1985) report on a new technique reported successful in the treatment of one and three phobic patients, respectively. The method consists of age regressing the patient to the original trauma and then modifying the memory of the event with a hypnotic implant that renders the experience less traumatic. On re-regression, patients seemed to have incorporated the events of the implanted memory with the original events. Symptomatic improvement was reported maintained at follow-ups ranging from 2 to 3 years in two cases.

Aside from the relationship of this method to the observation that neurotic symptoms can be induced as well as alleviated by the implantation of false memories, the apparent ease with which pseudo-memories were incorporated into and confused with real memories has ominous implications for the dangers involved in hypnotic memory retrieval in forensic investigations.

Lamb (1982) reported essentially the same technique under a different name, calling it "the resolution of unfinished business." He cites an example of a dental phobia, caused by dental work performed at age 6 without adequate analgesia, being cured by age regressing the patient to the time of the treatment in question and having her tell the dentist she needed more novocaine.

Bourne (1975) used hypnosis in a variety of ways in the treatment of drug abuse. Hypnosis may be used to link drug usage with a variety of aversive reactions in a punishment paradigm, or it may be used to provide a substitute experience without the use of the drug. It can also be used as a relaxant in a systematic desensitization procedure to treat anxiety and other symptoms that the drug was formerly used to control. No data are yet available concerning the long-term effectiveness of these methods. It is well known that unless the psychological dependence on a drug is dealt with, merely breaking a physiological addiction will be ineffective and will be followed by readdiction. However, hypnotic treatment does address itself primarily to psychological issues and may prove to be useful.

Manganiello (1984) found hypnosis plus psychotherapy superior to psychotherapy alone in modifying the drug-taking behavior of methadone-maintained addicts. Hypnosis was used to facilitate covert conditioning and desensitization to the cues leading to drug-taking behavior, and subjects were trained in self-hypnosis. On the other hand, Wadden and Penrod (1981) found that the results of two experimental studies showed that hypnosis did not improve the effectiveness of conventional therapies in the treatment of alcoholism, and they claim that positive results reported in case studies should be viewed with skepticism because of methodological shortcomings. Perhaps the reason for this discrepancy is the fact, pointed out by Katz (1980), that a report of hypnotic treatment, with no further details given, can mean the employment of any of 20 or more specific techniques of presumably different effectiveness (e.g., direct suggestion, age regression or progression, dream induction, symptom substitution, amnesia, ego strengthening, and others). Katz views hypnosis as a "magnifying glass" that can enhance the effects of standard treatments, not as a treatment per se. Braun (1986) expresses a similar position.

Petty (1976) reports a successful attempt to enlist the aid of the patient's parents in the treatment of temper tantrums by having them refrain from reinforcing the tantrum behavior. In order for them to be able to exercise this degree of self-control, it was necessary to desensitize them to the child's behavior. The work was accomplished in one session of hypnotic relaxation and desensitization trials followed by self-administered practice at home.

Daniels (1975) reports on a patient presenting a variety of psychosomatic complaints dating from the time that she was required to speak before a class in graduate school. She was benefited by a treatment regimen combining systematic desensitization with covert positive reinforcement (COR) therapy, transcendental meditation, and hypnosis. Following the desensitization procedure, which involved a series of anxiety-producing scenes related to the patient's making oral presentations at conferences, the patient was trained in meditation as an anxiety inhibitor. In addition, she was instructed to practice COR scenes relating to successful speaking efforts at conferences. Finally, at her request, she was taught self-hypnosis procedures to produce relaxed sensations and as an aid in COR practice.

Dengrove (1973) cites the use of induced dreams as a desensitization device. The patient may be given suggested acts to perform in dreams that are paced to his progress in therapy, or he can be left to set his own pace.

O'Brien (personal communication) relates the successful use of a suggested positive dream about sycamore leaves in the treatment of a leaf phobia that was resistant to waking systematic desensitization. The desensitization hierarchy that failed had nine steps, but the patient could not be desensitized in her reaction to dead sycamore leaves (which was the original phobic object that later generalized to other types of dead leaves).

In another study, O'Brien et al. (1981) treated nine good hypnotic subjects who were snake phobic with four sessions of simple desensitization procedure involving the imagined approach to a snake at the other end of a long hall-way. This procedure was followed up in experimental subjects with five hyp-notically suggested dream scenes, all involving snakes in a very positive con-text. The dreams were designed to pair as many erotic and romantic ideas with the snake as possible. Control subjects were exposed only to the four sessions of desensitization.

There was variability among experimental subjects in the number of sug-gested dreams that individual subjects reported having. One subject reported experiencing all five dreams, and one experienced none. All subjects were pretested and posttested for how close they could approach a real snake. Following therapy, the experimental group showed a marked improvement, with all but two subjects able to touch a live snake. Control subjects with large pretest phobic reactions showed no real improvement after four desensiti-zation sessions. One of the two experimental subjects who was unable to touch the snake refused to include the snake in one of the suggested dreams and replaced it with a kitten in another. Similarly, the other unresponsive subject dreamed of a large, ugly snake instead of the cute, little one suggested and developed a nightmare that awakened her.

Attempts to treat smoking by suggesting negative dreams about the health consequences of continued smoking were unsuccessful, and five out of five subjects rejected the suggestion to have anxiety-filled dreams (O'Brien, per-sonal communication). Thus the use of hypnosis in covert sensitization may be more effective if employed for image rather than dream induction.

Taboada (1975) successfully treated night terrors in a child by exploring the child's nightmare with him under hypnosis and then modifying the dream to include positive experiences.

Fabbri (1976) reports a combination of behavioral and hypnotic techniques that were used successfully to treat a variety of sexual disorders, including frigidity, impotence, anorgasmia, premature ejaculation, and a sexual avoid-ance syndrome. Patients were first carefully evaluated and a search made for the existence of sexual anxieties (that the patient may or may not have been aware of) that inhibited their social and sexual life. Sexual counseling was given, if required. Each patient was then trained in autohypnosis and ex-posed to a series of positive suggestions and the conditioning of self-confi-dence. Relaxation training and systematic desensitization using anxiety-gen-erating scenes of sexual activity followed. Even in this behavioral setting, regressions and prior traumatic memories sometimes arose, causing abreac-tions that temporarily interrupted the desensitization process. Finally, patients were given brief sessions of assertiveness training.

An overall improvement rate of 91% is claimed for this method. Fabbri says that negative results were experienced with borderline and latent psy-chotic patients, as well as with passive-aggressive personality types driven into therapy by their spouses. The latter situation is not particularly surprising, for no method of therapy is likely to be effective unless the patient voluntarily undertakes it and is motivated to succeed in it. Therapists whose professional self-image is closely related to their success rates should not attempt treatment with patients forced into therapy by family pressures unless they initially devote their efforts to convert the nominal patient into one committed to being in therapy.

DeVoge (1975) describes a group hypnotherapy method in which each group member was asked to concentrate on a problem in her life and verbalize it to the group under hypnosis. At the initial session a discussion was held to clear up misconceptions about hypnosis, and patients were told that they would be able to talk and interact with each other under hypnosis. After each patient described a problem, the therapist, in a manner suggestive of COR, provided suggestions of contrary imagery; that is, the patient was instructed to imagine acting in a manner contrary to her normal behavior. If, for example, the patient suffered from a fear of public speaking, she was to imagine herself speaking confidently and being well accepted by the audience. The patient was required to verbalize this new fantasy to the group. This procedure was followed at all group sessions. The patients, who were four female psychologists, rotated the task of inducing hypnosis at each session. Self-hypnosis was an integral part of the treatment, which emphasized a permissive approach. Since this "therapy" was more of a personal-adjustment or growth-oriented experience than a procedure designed to deal with symptoms that drove the patients into therapy, it is difficult to evaluate its efficacy. The advantages claimed for it are that modeling aided group members with less ability to visualize scenes to improve this skill, and the rotating of the leadership role among group members prevented the development of undue dependence on the therapist.

These examples of specific therapeutic methods have been arbitrarily classified as symptomatic, analytic, or behavioral techniques, but few therapies fit naturally or exclusively into any of these categories. More commonly they contain elements of all of these approaches, either simultaneously or successively. Astor (1973), for example, points out that it is not uncommon for a person coming into hypnotherapy for symptomatic relief to stay on for further analytical work. The art of being a therapist encompasses the ability to select and combine from the vast array of therapeutic methods available those most appropriate for an individual patient and his special problems. Thus, the reason that a hypnotherapist must be well trained as a psychologist is that he or she must be able to design a program of hypnotherapy for each patient. The psychotherapist therefore needs both a large store of psychological knowledge to draw upon and creativity and imagination. Also needed is a talent for constantly evaluating the results of a procedure and a willingness to modify it as required. Unlike analytic sessions where an analyst can "play it by ear," hypnotherapy is a much more active process for the therapist, and each session requires careful preparation and planning.

Most clinical reports describe the successful use of hypnosis by the author. If one reads enough of this material, he or she is likely to get the impression that hypnosis is a panacea that has no limits on its potential. Clearly a therapeutic failure is an ego-bruising experience for most therapists, and they would be reluctant to publicize these failures. Nevertheless, the failure to help a patient is common enough for one of the author's professors to have made the comment that the prime personality attribute needed for a successful clinician is a high degree of tolerance for failure. Sanders (1982) and Lazar and Dempster (1981) refreshingly write on this subject and express the view that failures are opportunities for learning. Lazar and Dempster would classify failures according to whether they involve the induction of hypnosis, the attainment of therapeutic goals, or the development of adverse reactions. They espouse the position that most treatment failures result from failing to understand and match the patient's dynamic needs with the therapy. It is essential to realize that no canned therapy routine will be successful with all or even a majority of patients presenting with similar symptoms. Hypnosis is not a method of treatment but an adjunct to many different methods and is inappropriate unless the therapist has a specific reason to assume it may help the principal method of therapy (selected for the particular patient) achieve its goals. Last, it must be recognized that not all human problems are amenable to solution given the current state of the art in psychotherapy, and some failures will result not from mistakes of the therapist but simply from trying to treat a patient not likely to get better (Gruenewald, 1981). Such attempts are necessary because it is impossible to predict success or failure accurately with an individual patient. Statistics enable us to make good predictions about groups but have no legitimate application to individuals.

HYPNOSIS IN MEDICINE AND DENTISTRY

The medical uses of hypnosis can be divided into two major areas. The first is the treatment of the psychological aspects of and reactions to organic disease and includes such activities as the control of pain (chronic, acute, physician-induced or postoperative), hypnoanesthesia, the reduction of fear and anxiety, and the adjunctive use of hypnosis in the management of chronically or terminally ill patients. In the latter situation, hypnosis has been used to help the patient develop a philosophical acceptance of the reality of his situation, to mitigate the side effects of such treatments as chemotherapy and radiation, to motivate him to cooperate in the treatment process, and to give him a sense of control over his symptoms and pain.

The second major medical use of hypnosis, the efficacy of which still remains to be demonstrated, is to attempt to modify the process of an organic disease by the influence of the mind and the ANS over bodily functioning. In some conditions such as common and venereal warts, the effectiveness of hypnotherapy is well documented (Blum et al., 1981; Clawson and Swade, 1975; Ewin, 1974; Gravitz, 1981c; Johnson and Barber, 1978; Morris, 1985; Sheehan, 1978; Tasini and Hackett, 1977). In the following conditions, many of them psychosomatic, the results of hypnotherapy appear promising (Maher-Loughnan, 1979):

> Asthma (Kohen et al., 1984; Kroger, 1977a; Place, 1984)
> Athetoid movement in cerebral palsy (Lazar, 1977)
> Benign vocal cord nodules (Laguaite, 1976)
> Cardiac arrhythmias (Wain, Amen, and Oetgen, 1984)
> Ciliary spasm (Lupica, 1976)
> Epileptic seizures (Gravitz, 1979)
> Functional amenorrhea (Van Der Hart, 1985)
> Functional megacolon (Olness, 1976)
> Hyperreflexic bladder (Godec, 1979)
> Intention myoclonus (Stein, 1980)
> Myopia (Sheehan, Smith, and Forrest, 1982; Smith, Forrest, and Sheehan, 1983; Wagstaff, 1983a)
> Narcolepsy (Schneck, 1980)
> Neurodermatitis (Lehman, 1978)
> Psoriasis (Frankel and Misch, 1973)
> Ptyalism (Schneck, 1977a)
> Raynaud's disease (Conn and Mott, Jr., 1984)
> Reflux esophagitis (Zlotogorski and Anixter, 1983)
> Sleep paralysis (Nardi, 1981)
> Torticolliss (Avampato, 1975)
> Vaginismus (Fuchs et al., 1973)

In still other conditions, such as cancer, the potential effectiveness of hypnosis on the disease process remains speculative (August, 1975; Clawson and Swade, 1975).

In dentistry also there are many practical uses for hypnosis. Often these are analogous to medical uses, modified to meet the special requirements of dental practice, involving operative work on an outpatient basis. Probably the most important dental use of hypnosis is for the diminution of fear, anxiety, and a variety of dental phobias. It has also been used as an anesthetic and for the control of postoperative pain. In addition to its usefulness in the control of bleeding and the promoting of healing, hypnosis has special application in dentistry because of its ability to diminish salivation and the gag reflex (Colomb, 1977; Daniels, 1976a, 1976c; Dubin, 1976; Golan, 1975; Morse, 1975, 1977b, 1978; Rappaport, 1977; Stone, 1977; Weyandt, 1976).

Pulver and Pulver (1975) surveyed 102 of 280 graduates of a course in medical and dental hypnosis given by the Institute of the Pennsylvania Hospital at least 15 months after the completion of training. Their purpose was to ascertain the extent to which the graduates employed hypnosis in their practice. Respondents were divided into four classifications: family practitioners (general practitioners and internists), nonpsychiatric specialties, psychiatrists, and dentists. The percentages of respondents in each of these classifications who used formal hypnotic inductions in at least some of their cases were 70, 33, 45, and 43, respectively. If informal hypnotic procedures not involving the use of an induction routine were considered, these figures became 75, 78, 55, and 86 percent, respectively.

Pulver and Pulver believe that hypnosis warrants greater use by the medical and dental communities than it currently receives, and they investigated why it was not being used more often by the alumni sampled. Among the reasons given by practitioners for not using hypnosis were that it is too time-consuming; they felt uncomfortable using hypnosis or were insufficiently skilled in it; they were skeptical about the value of hypnosis; and both patients and colleagues had unreasonable expectations of what hypnosis could accomplish.

Fredericks (1978, 1980) describes a course of twelve 1½- to 2-hour sessions to teach hypnosis to residents in anesthesiology. Preliminary investigation, based on subjective feelings of patients, failed to establish that this training resulted in significantly superior performance in patient care as compared with residents who did not take the course. As noted by O'Brien and Weisbrot (1983), there is a dearth of research demonstrating the value of various psychological and chemical methods of pain control, and in most cases the major evidence available is based on clinical observations. On the other hand, Olness (1977) reports that in-service hypnosis training of the professional staff in a children's hospital produced positive results when evaluated by the staff rather than by patients' attitudes, and it resulted in increased use of hypnotherapy.

In this section we will consider a number of uses and objectives of hypnosis in medicine and dentistry, their advantages and disadvantages, indications and contraindications, and the specific techniques that can be used.

Pain Control and Hypnoanesthesia

Hypnoanalgesia can be used with pain having a variety of sites and causes. It is probably most valuable when employed against chronic, organic pain of known etiology. The management of chronic organic pain presents certain practical difficulties. Analgesic medications often have to be used with restraint to prevent the patient from developing a tolerance or an addiction to them. An addiction is especially undesirable in a nonterminal patient with prolonged and intractable pain. Hypnotic pain relief in a susceptible patient may provide an effective alternative with a low risk of side effects and no development of tolerance or addiction. In addition, chronic pain and its attendant restriction of activities can produce personality changes in a patient. Reactions of rage, anxiety, hostility, or depression can interact with the pain and set up a vicious cycle or feedback loop in which the emotional reaction makes the pain worse and vice-versa. Hypnosis can be used to interrupt this feedback mechanism in a manner that no drug can (Crasilneck et al., 1955; Rosen, 1941).

The first prerequisite for any program of hypnotic pain control is an adequate diagnosis of the source of the pain. It is the grossest kind of malpractice for either a physician or a psychologist to attempt to control a pain hypnotically before ascertaining that its source is not a condition requiring physical treatment or that such treatment, if required, has been instituted. The source of pain, once determined, will have a marked bearing on the prognosis for hypnotic control. Contrary to Rosen (1941), organic pain is generally easier to control hypnotically than psychogenic pain. Although secondary gains may be associated with the former, it does not have a symbolic, psychological value to the patient, as the latter always has (Kline, 1978). As Rosen himself points out, anxiety (and guilt) are less tolerable than physical pain, and, in a conversion reaction, pain often substitutes for anxiety or has a self-punishing function. Thus, psychogenic pain is not readily given up under direct hypnotic suggestion; its treatment requires a dynamic investigation into its meaning to the patient. The control of psychogenic pain is best accomplished by a psychologically trained therapist.

Even poor hypnotic subjects, when motivated enough by the pain of traumatic injuries or the need for life-saving surgery, may be able to develop effective pain control and even sufficient anesthesia for surgery to be performed under hypnosis. (See Mason, 1955, for a contrary view.) David Spiegel (1985) takes the position that hypnotic pain control is not a useful method with about one-third of patients (who are not hypnotizable), while Schafer and Hernandez (1978) argue that patients of differing susceptibilities will respond to different elements of hypnotic pain control and that any patient presenting himself for such treatment can benefit from an individually tailored treatment plan. Wain (1980b, 1986) notes that even in patients who are unable to control pain totally by hypnotic means, hypnosis may prove a valuable adjunctive treatment to reduce the need for more risky modalities, such as medications and surgery. Patients who are somnambulists may be able to achieve pain control both while under hypnosis and later as the result of posthypnotic suggestions. A patient who can obtain relief while hypnotized but is not a good enough subject to develop posthypnotic pain control may be trained in self-hypnosis (Sachs, Feuerstein, and Vitale, 1977). This training will give the patient a feeling of mastery and control over the pain and render him independent of the physical presence of the hypnotist. If the patient is unable to master self-hypnosis, the hypnotist can provide him with a ready source of relief, at a minimum expenditure of the latter's time, by preparing a tape recording of an induction procedure followed by pain-relieving suggestions (Schafer, 1975). Before the availability of inexpensive tape recorders, Butler (1954) cut phonograph records for the use of his cancer patients. He found that after a while these records became less effective because the patients began to memorize them. This problem, if it occurs, is easy to remedy because the convenience of modern tape recorders makes it possible to supply patients with as great a variety of tapes as necessary.

Olness (1981) reported that 19 of 21 pediatric cancer patients obtained substantial relief from pain and nausea by imagination exercises (a form of self-hypnosis).

Another promising approach to pain control that enables the maximum utilization of the time of the therapist is the development of group pain control therapies (Toomey and Sanders, 1983). As in all other group therapies, patients, in addition to getting the benefits of hypnosis, get social support and the knowledge that others have similar problems and are able to cope with them. Group therapy is ideally suited for inpatients in institutions having large populations of patients suffering from chronic pain.

Many factors must be considered in predicting the success of attempts at hypnotic pain control. They include:

1. The nature and origin of the pain (whether it is organic or psychogenic).
2. The expectancy and set of the patient to obtain relief.
3. Whether the patient is getting any secondary gains from his pain.
4. The motivation of the patient.
5. The rapport between patient and hypnotist.
6. The willingness of the patient to practice self-hypnosis if instructed in it (Gravitz, 1978).

The depth of trance attained is relatively unimportant. Good results can be obtained in a light to medium trance (Gravitz, 1978; Kline, 1978). (For a contrary view see Butler, 1954; Schafer, 1975).

If the patient's pain is so distracting that it interferes with a hypnotic induction, a good solution is to have him fixate his attention on the pain and use this concentration as a vehicle to induce hypnosis (Kennedy, 1977; Kline, 1977). Prior to diminishing pain, it can be useful to have the patient concentrate on the pain and intensify it because this exercise demonstrates to him the control that he has over his pain. He can then be told that any sensation that he can increase he can also decrease.

Specific Pain Control Techniques.   The following are some methods commonly used to achieve pain control under hypnosis. The methods presented are neither exhaustive nor mutually exclusive. Each is subject to many variations for adaptation to the needs of an individual patient's personality, and each may be used in combination with other techniques to provide a maximally effective treatment plan.

1. Suggestions of deep relaxation are often effective in pain control, probably because anxiety and pain are usually interrelated and each feeds upon the other. Since anxiety is incompatible with relaxation, the latter may serve to break the vicious circle and reduce both pain and suffering. In addition, the patient's expectations of relief may function as a covert suggestion that he makes to himself, which further enhances the effect. Suggestions of relaxation can be reinforced with soothing background music, subdued lighting and other appropriate environmental supplements when possible.

2. Direct suggestions of diminished pain intensity and less suffering and discomfort may be given. Some operators believe that the word "pain" is too emotionally charged and often suggests the condition that they are trying to eliminate. Hence they prefer to use the term "discomfort" or make more positive statements—for example, not "You will have less pain" but "You will be more comfortable." There may be a risk in using euphemistic expressions, however. If a person in intense pain hears a therapist describe what he would call his agony as a "discomfort," he may conclude that the therapist does not understand the severity of his problem This may interfere with the establishment of rapport.

3. Hypnotic suggestion may be used to transfer a pain from one region of the body to another, where it is less disabling. Pain may be transferred to a smaller and less sensitive region of the body. For example, the pain of bursitis in the shoulder that interferes with the patient's everyday activities may be transferred to his little finger, where it causes less suffering and disruption of the patient's life. This is a particularly useful method in dealing with psychogenic pain for which a patient has a need. It permits him to keep his pain but suffer less from it.

4. Just as hypnotic suggestion can transfer a pain from one region of the body to another, it can also be used to transform pain sensations into other sensations that are easier to tolerate, such as a tingling or feelings of warmth or cold. As in the case of transferring pain from one region of the body to another, transforming of pain may be useful when a direct attack on

psychogenic pain is contraindicated. It also shares the advantage of retaining the signaling function of organic pain while controlling the suffering experienced.

5. Pain may be controlled by suggestions of numbness in the painful area. The patient's previous experiences may be used by telling him to imagine that he has just received an injection of novocaine, and the area is beginning to become numb. A common variation of this technique is to give suggestions of numbness in one hand (*glove anesthesia*). When numbness is achieved, the patient is told he can transfer the numbness to any other part of his body by touching the part with the anesthetized hand. Thus, dental anesthesia may be obtained by touching the anesthetized hand to the face and "rubbing off the numbness." Often the testing of the anesthetized area with a sterile needle prior to any surgery will serve to demonstrate the reality of the anesthesia to the patient and increase his confidence in the procedure, thus enhancing its prospects for success. Obviously this testing is to be used only when the operator is reasonably certain it will prove successful.

A variation of this method is suitable for use with children. The child may be told that he is being given a magic finger that can prevent him from feeling pain in areas that the finger touches (or the dentist may be the one who has the magic pain-killing finger).

6. The patient can analyze the total painful experience into a series of non-painful components. For example, the patient may be trained to think of his pain as an interesting but neutral type of sensation, distinct from the suffering that it produces. This means of control may make it easier for the patient to learn to ignore the pain and live with it.

7. Dissociation may be used in a good subject to separate the patient from his pain in a variety of ways. He can be taught to think of the pain as being out in his hand and separate from himself, or a psychological amputation may be performed and an injured limb may be made to disappear. Weyandt (1976) suggested to a patient that her teeth were being taken out of her head prior to dental drilling. The patient can also be taken outside of his body during operative procedures. This is a common device used in hypnotic deliveries, where the patient is told that she will observe the procedure as though it were happening to someone else. Dissociation lends itself to combination with distractive procedures. It is even possible for patients to hallucinate minivacations and trips during surgical and dental procedures.

8. Distraction techniques are useful in hypnoanesthesia and in the control of chronic pain. They essentially use hypnotic hallucinations of pleasant experiences that are incompatible with pain or suffering. By concentrating on these pleasant experiences, the patient is able to ignore his pain. In planning this type of suggestion, it is best to ask the patient in advance about what

types of experience he enjoys most to maximize the pleasant effect sought and to avoid the possibility of suggesting something that a particular patient might find upsetting. For example, one patient found a suggestion of a family Christmas gathering upsetting because she had recently been involved in a traumatic family dispute at such an occasion (Pulver and Pulver, 1975). It is also possible to let the patient decide privately on what he wants to fantasize about by making general suggestions of having pleasant emotions and experiences but letting him fill in the details. If the therapist assures the patient that he will not inquire into the nature of these hypnotic experiences, the patient is freed to have a variety of erotic fantasies if he so desires. Patients may be told to hallucinate these experiences directly or to dream about them or, if it aids the imaginative process of a particular patient, to visualize the experience on an imagined movie screen or television set. In the latter situation, it is comparatively easy for the hypnotist to exercise control over the patient's imaginings by directing him to change channels to a different scene if for any reason the patient becomes upset.

9. Age regression to a period before the onset of the pain can control pain in a good subject.

10. Hypnotic distortion of subjective time is a useful method of making surgical and dental procedures, as well as hospitalization time and time in pain, seem to pass rapidly.

11. The final common method of pain control is to transform the pain into a visual image that can be concretely manipulated in the imagination. For example, patients have been told to imagine switches inside their bodies that can be actuated to turn off pain sensations. They have also been instructed to picture their pain being tied to a red helium-filled balloon and being carried off by it or to imagine rolling their pain into a little ball, putting it into a container, and locking it in a cabinet. Incredible as it may seem, these suggestions have been effective in controlling pain in adult patients. Most of the techniques described here, and especially this one, use ego-distorting mechanisms regularly seen in psychotics and young children. Their efficacy may be related to the capacity of hypnosis and suggestion to regress a patient into earlier, less critical, and more concrete thought processes (Barber, 1978a; Gravitz, 1978; Hodge, 1977; Kline, 1978; London and Forman, 1977).

Noting the fact that few applications of hypnosis to pain control take advantage of the remarkable alterations in perception that hypnosis is capable of producing (e.g., subjective feelings of bodily heaviness, lightness, shrinking or floating sensations, or loss of contact with the environment or time), Sacerdote (1977) describes utilizing these phenomena to produce what he calls *hypnomystical states*. While the present author finds the use of the term "mystical" in relationship to hypnosis regrettable, the paper is fascinating and describes successful pain control in cases where more conventional psychotherapy and hypnotherapy had failed.

Sacerdote classifies hypnotically generated "mystical" experiences into introvertive experiences, characterized by a withdrawal into secure isolation (induced by suggestions of the patient being securely at the center of a series of transparent spheres) and extrovertive experiences (generally induced by having the patient reach the top of a mountain peak and concentrate on the scenery). Both types of induction are essentially cognitive ones. Which experience is more appropriate is determined by a knowledge of the individual patient. Sacerdote notes that other similar approaches can be conceived. Essentially these experiences seem to provide an escape for the patient from an untenable pain-racked existence and may, like a religious experience, give him a feeling of hope and control, as well as providing a distraction. The rationale for this treatment given to the patient would appear to depend on his personality and what is most likely to be acceptable to him. Thus for a person who practices meditation or has had mystical or ESP experiences, it might be appropriate to describe the procedure in such terms. For an engineer or accountant, it might be more effective to describe it in terms of the features that it shares with the standard methods of pain control.

It is possible to consider the total effect of hypnotic intervention on pain as being the sum of a "real hypnotic effect" plus a placebo effect. Such a distinction is without practical significance, though it is of theoretical importance. As Beecher (1955) points out, a placebo effect of a drug is as much a benefit to a patient as its pharmacological effect. He found that 30% of steady postoperative incision pain was adequately relieved by placebos. This suggests that one reason hypnotic control of pain is not highly correlated with susceptibility may be that the placebo component of the total hypnotic effect is independent of the patient's trance capacity. A more interesting finding of Beecher of the diversity of adverse side reactions produced by placebos suggests not only that many apparent side reactions to real drugs may be psychogenic rather than pharmacological in origin but also that the occasional minor adverse reactions to hypnosis may be of the same nature. In any event, it is a standard procedure of many physicians to attempt to increase the effectiveness of a drug prescription by stressing the drug's effectiveness to the patient. This is an example of the use of waking suggestions and is probably employed daily by many physicians who would not ordinarily consider the use of hypnosis in their practice.

Crasilneck and his associates (1955) used hypnosis in the treatment of patients in a burn unit. Burn victims present a variety of management problems that these authors describe:

> They often have a poor psychological adjustment to their sudden disability and may be hostile, depressed, uncooperative, or negativistic (Ewin, 1984).

They need effective pain control for chronic pain and painful, recurrent dressing changes, debridements, and grafting procedures.

They need to maintain adequate food intake but suffer from loss of appetite.

They need motivation and pain control for the exercise of painfully burned parts of the body.

These problems interact and set up vicious cycles that impede the patient's recovery. For example, loss of appetite at a time when caloric and protein needs are increasing retards healing and epithelialization and may cause grafts to fail. Repeated general anesthetics for dressing changes further debilitate the patient, may produce nausea and vomiting, and require periodic withholding of food and water.

Hypnosis was found to be an effective solution to many of these problems. The starvation cycle was interrupted by motivating patients to eat and having them anticipate enjoying meals as a result of hypnotic suggestions. The improvement in nutrition produced weight gains, more successful skin grafts, spontaneous epithelialization, and healing. Patients also became more cheerful. Patients who formerly needed a general anesthetic for dressing changes were able to have them, as well as skin grafts and debridements, performed under hypnoanesthetic and to awaken feeling hungry as suggested. Also, hypnotic pain control enabled patients to perform needed exercise and become ambulatory.

Schafer (1975) studied 20 severely burned patients in a burn unit to evaluate these findings. He found that 14 patients were markedly helped in achieving pain control, especially during dressing changes, and six patients were not helped. Of the 14 patients who were benefited, half were able to achieve pain control posthypnotically, and half required the use of tape recordings to get relief between hypnotic sessions. Of the six patients who were not helped, five were under age 21, but all were suffering from so much pain and panic that they were unhypnotizable. The somewhat unusual findings that the success of hypnosis in pain control was a function of the susceptibility of the subjects may be accounted for by the fact that hypnotic susceptibility was measured on the ward rather than under normal conditions prior to or subsequent to their hospitalization. Also, it is difficult to estimate whether the failure to help the unbenefited patients may be ascribed to their lack of trance capacity or to the difficulty in establishing rapport under adverse conditions.

Schafer found that hypnosis was a valuable treatment for burn patients, but it was no longer the life-saving procedure that Crasilneck and his colleagues found it to be (because of its reversal of the starvation cycle). This was because over the years, medical management of burn patients had improved to the point where fluids and nutrition were carefully controlled and infections were nonexistent in the patient population studied.

In recent years, a number of experimental or clinical studies have been published that appear to confirm the clinical findings of Crasilneck and co-workers of the value of hypnosis to control pain and to promote healing in burn patients. Moore and Kaplan (1983) found that in patients with symmetrical burns (four on the hands and one on the thighs), when suggestions of vasodilation were directed to one side of the body only, that side had accelerated healing in four out of five patients. In the fifth patient, healing was rapid in both hands (but, of course, he was not able to serve as his own control). Hammond, Keye, and Grant, Jr. (1983) reported similar results with first-degree sunburns that they produced with ultraviolet light on a 2-inch strip on both thighs of six subjects. Ewin (1983) and Margolis and her colleagues (1983) cite evidence that early hypnotic intervention (within 10 hours of the burn) in the form of suggestions of coolness, comfort, and safety produced an increase of urinary output compared to control patients on the second day following the burn and may thus have limited the extent of local edema and inflammation. Ewin thus advocated the use of hypnosis as soon as possible in the emergency room.

Noting the evidence suggesting that anesthetized patients can react to surgeons' conversation, Ewin (1986) suggests the use of hypnosis as a method of preventing burn patients from being alarmed by the surgical team's sense of urgency or an unfortunate remark about the seriousness of the patient's condition. Such supportive use of hypnosis would appear to be of value in any major medical emergency situation. Furthermore, suggestions need not be limited to reassurance and fear reduction but could facilitate patient cooperation and expectations of rapid recovery.

Wakeman and Kaplan (1978) found that hypnosis was significantly more effective in patients from 7 to 18 years of age than in older patients with comparable burns (from 0% to 30% or 31% to 60% of body area). They speculate on the role of the higher susceptibility of younger patients or of their greater vulnerability to the severe stress occasioned by a major burn injury in accounting for the greater effect of hypnosis with them.

Van Nuys (1977) reported the successful treatment of sacroiliac pain in a physician-patient by means of waking suggestions over the telephone, demonstrating that neither a formal hypnotic induction nor face-to-face contact with the patient is necessary. Prior to the procedure, however, the therapist had developed a rapport with the patient. Since the patient's religious views led him to have reservations concerning the use of hypnosis, the procedure was presented to him as a situation involving self-directed fantasy instead of hypnosis. He was told to imagine a tenant, with whom he had experienced difficulties just prior to the development of the back pain, being "evicted from his back." This rather bizarre suggestion given to a waking, intelligent adult was followed by a substantial remission of pain within 2 hours and the patient's return to work the following day.

In addition to the treatment of cancer and burn patients, hypnotic pain control has proved successful in a variety of conditions involving severe, chronic, and disabling pain, including phantom limb pain (Siegel, 1979), pain in systemic lupus erythematosus (Smith and Balaban, 1983), intractable post-traumatic shoulder pain of 13 years' duration (Williams, 1983), and chronic low back pain (Crasilneck, 1979). It is important to note that the cases of low back pain reported by Crasilneck were primarily of organic etiology. There is some opinion (see page 311) that functional lower back pain may be a de-pressive equivalent that holds in check a severe depression with a possible suicidal threat, and its removal could be dangerous. Orne (1982) has said that hypnotic removal of psychogenic lower back pain may pose a suicide risk, and a safer method of treating it is behavior modification. (Since the present author can see no theoretical reason why a direct attack on a symp-tom by hypnosis is more likely to result in a symptom substitution than a direct removal of a symptom by behavior modification, he is inclined to believe that the generalized conclusion that functional lower pack pain is a depressive equivalent may be erroneous, based on overgeneralizing from a few reported atypical clinical examples. Nevertheless, in the face of such reports, the risk of a suicide attempt following the removal of such pain must be taken seri-ously, and it would be reckless to attempt this without a thorough investi-gation of the pain's dynamic value to the particular patient.)

Hypnoanesthesia. Hypnosis is not used as often as an anesthetic agent as it is to control nonsurgical pain. On at least two occasions, the author was unable to find a local obstetrician who employed hypnosis in deliveries for pregnant women desiring such a referral (both of whom were excellent hyp-notic subjects). Probably the principal reason for this state of affairs has been the development of reasonably safe, rapidly effective chemical agents. It has been estimated that only 25% of the population are capable of developing a sufficient degree of hypnoanesthesia for its use as the sole anesthetic in relatively minor procedures, such as fracture settings, tooth extractions, the changing of burn dressings, or the removal of sutures in frightened children. Only 10% to 15% of the population are capable of undergoing major surgery under hypnoanesthesia alone. On the other hand, chemical agents are ef-fective with all patients (Crasilneck, McCranie, and Jenkins, 1956; Crasilneck et al., 1955; Kroger and DeLee, 1957; Marmer, 1956; Raginsky, 1951).

Other reasons advanced for reluctance to use hypnoanesthesia include: the amount of time, training, and skill required for a hypnotic induction; the fact that hypnosis may be contraindicated in patients with psychological problems such as psychotics, borderlines, or depressives; and the fact that hypnosis is regarded as "quasi-scientific" in some professional circles (Crasilneck et al.,

1955; Crasilneck, McCranie, and Jenkins, 1956; Raginsky, 1951; Silberner, 1986).

Some of these objections require comment. The fact that hypnosis requires special training and skill is an objection that could be raised about any medical, dental, or psychological procedure and seems hardly necessary to comment on. However, Raginsky (1951) raises the interesting point that many anesthesiologists may have selected their specialty because it does not require the development of the close personal relationship with a patient that other branches of medicine do. If this is the case, it may be that the real objection to hypnoanesthesia on the part of some anesthesiologists is that they are uncomfortable in developing the kind of rapport with a patient required by this procedure.

With respect to the issue of time consumption, Crasilneck and his associates (1955) point out that while an initial session may take up to an hour and a half with a difficult patient, subsequent inductions usually require only a few minutes. Most patients can be given a posthypnotic cue for rapid reinduction, and rapport and control can be transferred to the attending surgeon or shared with him or her as required. An effective way of dealing with the time problem, which is used by obstetricians who employ hypnosis for deliveries, is to conduct group hypnotic training sessions for their patients. The relatively long period between the initial consultation with an obstetrician and the time of delivery makes it possible to train the patient well for her role in hypnoanesthesia, and group sessions render the process economically feasible. Dentists who are reluctant to employ hypnosis in their practice because of the time required to train patients in hypnosis might do well to conduct similar group training sessions for patients desirous of using hypnosis to make their dental visits more pleasant. Once trained, the patient can utilize hypnoanesthesia and other suggestions rapidly for all future dental work.

Kleinhauz, Eli, and Rubinstein (1985) report on the activities of a consultatory outpatient clinic for behavior dysfunctions associated with the Dental School of Tel Aviv University. A variety of dental-related behavioral dysfunctions, such as dental phobias and anxiety, extreme gagging reflex, and pain, are treated there by a multidisciplinary team using hypnosis in conjunction with a variety of psychotherapeutic methods. This may be an ideal approach for the minority of cases that are too difficult to be handled routinely by the individual dentist, but most applications of dental hypnosis will not require referral if the dentist has been adequately trained in the use of hypnosis.

With respect to the contraindication of hypnosis and hypnoanesthesia in patients with certain psychological disorders, some clarification is required. There is no absolute contraindication for hypnosis in any patient. Some patients may present a higher risk of developing adverse reactions, such as spontaneous regressions and abreactions, that are undesirable in a nonpsy-chotherapy context, and control of these requires some skill on the part of the hypnotist. Hence, with these patients, hypnoanesthesia requires a hyp-notist who is well trained in psychotherapy. It should not be attempted by a physician who lacks such training. It is unfortunate that physicians in general, and anesthesiologists in particular, do not receive more training in psycho-dynamic concepts and hypnosis, for it is not usually convenient to have a psychologist induce hypnoanesthesia except in an emergency situation. All such procedures require an anesthesiologist with chemical agents available on a standby basis should the patient require these as a supplementary mea-sure. Merely knowing that chemical agents are available can do much to re-assure a patient and increase the probability that they will not be needed. A patient should be told not to have any reluctance to ask for the aid of chemical agents if required, unless they are absolutely contraindicated for medical rea-sons. Some training and facility with hypnoanesthesia is a useful emergency tool for general practitioners or pediatricians who are often called upon to perform minor emergency procedures such as suturing a wound of a fright-ened child.

If chemical agents are generally safe, easier to administer, less time-con-suming, and effective in all patients, what then are the special indications for hypnoanesthesia? Hypnotic anesthesia may be specifically indicated in the following situations:

1. Chemical agents would be dangerous with a particular patient—for ex-ample, patients with allergies to all local anesthetics or with debilitating heart, lung, or other diseases.
2. Patients must be subjected to repeated procedures such as burn dress-ing changes or prolonged procedures where the repeated or continu-ous use of chemical agents would be debilitating.
3. Certain types of brain surgery require an anesthetic that will not inter-fere with ongoing EEG recordings.
4. The patient has an extreme fear reaction to chemical agents. Marmer (1956) notes that some patients fear the anesthetic more than the sur-gery.
5. Chemical agents are not available in emergency situations or in pris-oner-of-war camps.
6. The unique advantages of hypnoanesthesia are needed (Crasilneck, McCranie, and Jenkins, 1956; Mason, 1955; Sampimon and Wood-ruff, 1946; Scott, 1975).

Hypnoanesthesia need not be used as the sole anesthetic agent to capi-talize on its unique advantages; in fact, many consider its use in conjunction with chemical agents, in a balanced anesthesia, to be ideal (Kroger and

DeLee, 1957; Marmer, 1956; Raginsky, 1951). The use of hypnosis in conjunction with chemical agents reduces the quantitative requirements for the latter and hence reduces the deleterious aftereffects they may produce. Barber (1978b) points out that most of the internal viscera are insensitive to cutting pain. Hence, the major pain of most surgical procedures is caused by pain receptors in the area of the skin incision. The supplementing of hypnosis with the application of a local anesthetic to the site of the incision may be all that is necessary to extend the applicability of hypnoanesthesia to a larger segment of the population.

Hypnoanesthesia either alone or in combination with chemical agents has a great many unique advantages. These include:

1. Reduction in postoperative nausea and vomiting, anoxia, and other side effects of chemical anaesthetics. In childbirth, hypnoanesthesia probably serves to best advantage, for the child is born without any aftereffects of an anesthetic on vital functions.

2. Preoperative pain and anxiety can be controlled effectively, often without the use of customary medications. The patient can be helped to accept the forthcoming operation with equanimity, and it can even be made into a relatively pleasant experience. Hypnosis is an ideal way to establish a basal anesthesia with children for whom a hospital stay and surgery can be extremely traumatic, involving both separation from the parents and an exposure to frightening sights and experiences often well beyond their capacity to understand or cope with. At times surgeons and anesthesiologists are either too busy or too insensitive to the psychological needs of their patients, whether children or adults, to give these needs more than the most cursory attention. The result may be the creating of needless psychological scars that some patients may carry with them for a lifetime. Although it is not practical to require that physicians training in surgical specialties have major surgery performed on them in a manner analogous to a psychoanalyst's training analysis (so that they might be better able to appreciate how frightened most of their patients are), at least they should be given more training in the psychological sciences. This would aid them in appreciating that the machine they are repairing has a human being residing inside of it.

3. Hypnoanesthesia can be maintained for long periods of time, as in childbirth, without risk and can be terminated at will.

4. Hypnoanesthesia places no extra load on the circulatory, respiratory, hepatic, or renal systems, which contributes greatly to its safety.

5. Kroger and DeLee (1957) claim it eliminates surgical shock in childbirth and gynecological surgery. Mason (1955) claims it minimizes shock, whereas chemical agents increase it. Raginsky (1951), on the other hand,

says that in certain minor procedures, there is not much shock in any event, but in major surgery the effect of hypnosis is more to mask than to eliminate shock.

6. With hypnoanesthesia the patient may be fully conscious and can co-operate with the surgeon. A conscious state may be necessary during some spinal surgery to test for circulatory compromise or cord compression (Jones, 1977). The patient's sensitivity and protective reflexes in areas other than the surgical field are fully functional. This serves to prevent accidents, such as the burning of an unconscious patient. The inhalation of blood or vomitus is prevented by the functioning of the patient's cough reflex. The patient is also able to drink liquids during long procedures.

7. In childbirth, hypnosis gives the obstetrician additional control over the procedure. Labor can be speeded up or slowed down, and premature labor has been stopped by hypnotic suggestions (Barber, 1978b; Butler, 1954). Mason (1955) claims that many complications of childbirth are caused by a fear-induced delay in a stage of labor. Hypnosis can overcome this problem. Also, hypnosis can influence postpartum lactation (Butler, 1954). It can be used by a general practitioner or a midwife with limited training. Childbirth under hypnosis permits the mother to witness the birth of her child and hear its first cry, which some believe to be psychologically important. Werner, Schauble, and Knudson (1982), who advocate the greater use of hypnosis in childbirth, cite evidence that postpartum depression, which is common with chemical anesthesia, is rare following hypnotic anesthesia. Also, maternal fatigue is reduced.

8. In dental cases, salivation and the gag reflex can be diminished. Bleeding during surgery may be controlled. Barber (1978b) reports the successful hypnotic control of bleeding in a hemophiliac dental patient. Clawson and Swade (1975) report the control of a hemorrhage during surgery on the grandson of the senior author, who was under a chemical anesthetic at the time, by directly suggesting to the patient that he stop the bleeding. This result is supportive of Cheek's notion that chemically anaesthetized patients can hear and respond to conversations going on in the operating room (Gruen, 1972; Kroger and DeLee, 1957; Marmer, 1956; Mason, 1955; Morse, 1975, 1978; Raginsky, 1951; Sampimon and Woodruff, 1945; Scott, 1975; Stone, 1977).

9. In addition to anesthesia, hypnosis may provide the deep muscle relaxation necessary to reduce dislocations (Kubiak, 1983).

10. Perhaps the greatest advantage of hypnoanesthesia, whether used as the sole agent or in combination with chemicals, is the opportunity it presents to make therapeutic posthypnotic suggestions to facilitate the recovery proc-

ess. These have successfully included, but have not been limited to, suggestions for spontaneous postoperative voiding and bowel movements; free and easy breathing; ease in coughing; freedom from postoperative pain and reduced need for medication for its control; absence of nausea and retching; lessened discomfort when the patient must remain for prolonged periods in awkward positions (such as after flap-grafting procedures); early ambulation and comfortable exercise of parts of the body operated on; rapid healing; the toleration of intravenous needles, endotracheal tubes, and catheters; and a pleasant postoperative period with the patient enjoying good morale and time passing quickly.

Hypnoanesthesia is usually rendered more effective if the patient is trained in its use prior to the operation and, when possible, prior to hospitalization. Except in emergency situations, hypnoanesthesia should never be initiated in the operating room. If initial hypnotic inductions are performed in a leisurely, unhurried atmosphere and the patient is given the opportunity to develop an anesthesia and experience it tested successfully, his confidence in the adequacy of the procedure will be greater. Patients should be trained to enter a trance state either on a posthypnotic signal or by self-induction to save time in the operating room and render them independent of the presence of the particular hypnotist who trained them. A patient so trained may be able to have a successful hypnotic delivery under the care of another obstetrician should the one who trained her in hypnosis be unavailable at her delivery. Also, the ability to reenter hypnosis rapidly on a signal is a valuable safeguard should a patient inadvertently awaken during surgery. This contingency is quite unlikely, particularly if the hypnotist instructs the patient not to awaken until directed to and if he or she continues a steady flow of trance-maintaining chatter throughout the operation. Preliminary trials of hypnosis may be presented to patients with reservations about the procedure as exercises in relaxation to prevent their fears from producing reactions that may lead to a false impression of their abilities as subjects (Kroger and DeLee, 1957; Marmer, 1956; Mason, 1955).

Patients undergoing hypnotic deliveries should be trained with the emphasis that they are being prepared to perform a normal physiological function rather than to be subjected to a surgical procedure. When hypnosis is used in childbirth, the pain caused by uterine contractions can be used as a signal for the patient to lapse into a deep state of hypnosis as long as the contraction lasts. Patients can also be trained to dissociate the pain-generating lower halves of their bodies while the upper half remains alert (Fee and Reilley, 1982; Werner, Schauble, and Knudson, 1982).

The value of hypnosis may also extend to the prenatal period. Fuchs, Paldi, Abramovici, and Peretz (1980) report the successful treatment of 138 women suffering from severe hyperemesis gravidarum (vomiting during pregnancy) by both group and individual hypnotherapy. Results were better with the 87 patients treated in a group than for the 51 receiving individual treatment. The authors speculate on the role of common motivation in producing this unexpected result.

Fellows (1984) cites research suggesting that pregnant women may develop enhanced susceptibility as measured by form A of the SHSS or form A of the HGSHS. (Some have claimed that women are most suggestible not when they are pregnant but immediately prior to becoming pregnant!)

It is not possible to do successful hypnoanesthesia, or for that matter any other hypnotic procedure, unless the therapist takes the time necessary to establish a proper rapport with the patient and the latter develops confidence in the hypnotist's ability and concern for his welfare (Stone, 1977).

A useful procedure in the practice of hypnoanesthesia is to "walk the patient through" each step of the operating procedure to be experienced, from the time he leaves his room until the time he returns to it (Barber, 1978b; Gravitz, 1978; Kroger and DeLee, 1957). This may be done with the patient hypnotized to approximate more closely the actual procedures being simulated. The effects of this rehearsal are to reduce the patient's fear of the unknown and protect him from surprises during the surgery. If time or facility use prevents the actual walking through of these procedures, the patient should be informed in detail about what to expect, and his questions should be answered. Such a routine would probably have a reassuring and calming effect even with patients not being prepared for hypnoanesthesia.

In addition to its use as an anesthetic, hypnosis can be a valuable preoperative and postoperative adjunct to the care of surgical patients. Surman and colleagues (1974), however, report that a single psychiatric visit prior to cardiac surgery, limited to clearing up patients' misconceptions about the operative procedures and training them in a simple autohypnotic technique, was generally ineffective in lowering the incidence of postoperative delirium. Postoperative delirium is reported in from 16% to 57% of patients recovering from open heart surgery as opposed to about 0.1% of the general surgical population. It is generally self-limited and thought to be the result of anoxia produced by the heart-lung machine. Patients receiving a greater number of preoperative visits are less likely to develop this effect. Surman and his associates believe that presurgical psychotherapy can be of benefit to cardiac patients but that more than a single visit is required. On the other hand, Gruen (1972) describes a program of systematic self-relaxation and positive self-suggestions that he employed preparatory to his own cardiac bypass surgery. The operation was followed by a comfortable, rapid, and uneventful recovery. Although this is a one-subject, uncontrolled study, the results are at least suggestive.

Hart (1980) describes a taped hypnotic procedure used on 20 of 40 cardiopulmonary bypass surgical patients, preoperatively, for five sessions.

Postoperative testing disclosed that the group receiving taped hypnotic preparation required the replacement of significantly less blood and reported less anxiety than did control subjects. Blood pressure readings were not significantly different between the two groups. Hart describes these results as "thin" but promising and cites the need for additional research. In particular, the use of taped preparation needs to be compared with the effectiveness of the same treatment plan conducted by a physically present therapist.

Golan (1975) reports on a patient with aortic stenosis and an aneurysm who fainted and struck his right eye, causing a retrobulbar hemorrhage. Chemical anesthesia was ruled out by his physical condition. The hemorrhage was successfully treated with electrocauterization under hypnoanesthesia, despite the fact that the patient was normally only a grade 1 hypnotic subject. The patient was given suggestions of glove anesthesia, and, after successful testing with a needle, the anesthesia was transferred to his right eye. Prior to the surgery, the patient was given suggestions that he would heal rapidly, that the surgical procedure would seem short, that time in the hospital would pass quickly, and that he would keep his eye still and remain immobile during the operation. The hypnotic procedure took about 30 minutes, and the operation lasted for 1 hour.

J. Barber and Malin (1977) advocate the use of hypnosis during the fitting of contact lenses and emphasize the careful choice of words in the framing of suggestions. Words that denote the same thing may vary widely in their connotations and implications and thus may not be equally effective in framing suggestions.

Hypnosis in Dental Procedures. Although a dentist is in fact an oral surgeon and all of the foregoing material on the hypnotic control of organic pain and anesthesia is equally applicable to both medicine and dentistry, there are certain unique aspects of a dental practice that make hypnosis especially useful to it. Unlike the average surgeon, a dentist normally has an ongoing relationship with patients over a period of many years. This means that any efforts expended in training them in the use of hypnosis will yield dividends for both the dentist and the patient over an extended period of time and in a variety of treatment situations. In addition, most dental procedures are minor enough that a larger portion of the dentist's patient population is likely to be able to benefit from either complete or partial hypnoanesthesia. Even if a particular patient is unable to use hypnosis as an anesthetic agent, he may still receive substantial benefits from it in the control of fear, anxiety, and any number of specific dental phobias (such as fear of an injection) that are so common among dental patients. Often patients find the noise of a dental drill as upsetting as the pain, and hypnosis can aid them in ignoring this noise and similar aversive dental experiences (Golan, 1975). Merely controlling a patient's anxiety about a dental visit and relaxing him can do much to raise his threshold of pain because of the mutually enhancing relationship between pain and anxiety. Even if a patient is unable to develop enough hypnoanesthesia to be operated on without additional chemical agents, he may still be able to minimize his aversion to an injection or reduce the amount of agent needed, thus reducing the period of time that he has an uncomfortably numb face. Often hypnotic analgesia and the distracting effects of a hallucinated minivacation can turn a dental visit into a pleasant experience that a patient can look forward to instead of anticipate with dread (Morse, 1977*b*, 1978; Rappaport, 1977; Stone, 1977).

Hypnosis can also make it easier to get the patient to follow the dentist's advice on matters of prophylactic care and follow-up visits. Positive motivation for the required cooperation can be instilled by suggestions for the patient to imagine how attractive he will look with his teeth properly cared for (Golan, 1975).

Besides the obvious advantages to the patient (in experiencing less fear and tension and achieving better pain control), there are many advantages of hypnosis for the dentist. Among these are better dentist-patient relationships and improved working conditions with a relaxed, cooperative patient as well as more control over bleeding and salivation. The control of the gag reflex is relatively easy to attain, and it can be utilized both in operative work and in helping a patient to tolerate a new denture (Colomb, 1977; Eli and Kleinhauz, 1985: Morse, 1978; Stone, 1977). Morse points out that hypnosis is an interesting experience for most patients and one they are likely to tell their friends about; thus its use may enhance the dentist's reputation and practice.

The problems associated with the dental use of hypnosis are relatively minor. All practitioners need special training in this technique and need to use it enough to maintain facility with it. Dentists also have to screen patients to avoid the few likely to present psychological problems that a dentist may be unequipped to handle. Yamauchi (1981), a psychologist, reports the successful treatment of a severe dental phobia in a patient with a diagnosis of chronic paranoid schizophrenia. While this case demonstrates that hypnosis may be effective in such a severely ill patient, a dentist would be well advised to refer such a patient rather than attempt to treat him with hypnosis himself. The most common problem that a dentist may have to face is the patient who seeks nondental applications of hypnosis, such as weight control or anti-smoking suggestions (Morse, 1975, 1978; Stone, 1977). This is a problem common to all practitioners who use hypnosis in their profession. It is best dealt with by a tactful but firm refusal to perform a procedure outside the range of one's professional competence. If the reasons for refusing to perform the requested procedure are made clear to the patient and it is emphasized that this is for his own protection, the doctor-patient relationship need not be harmed and may even be improved.

Because of the ongoing relationship between a dentist and patient, it is often easy to overcome the fears that many patients may have of being hypnotized through casual general conversation. The occurrence of spontaneously developed trancelike states can be described to the patient to allay his fears of the unknown. Morse (1978) suggests the use of covert hypnotic techniques, without a formal induction procedure, for patients whose fear of hypnosis prevents its direct use.

Stone (1977) recommends a simple arm lifting and dropping demonstration for a patient who is so tense that he needs help in learning to relax enough for hypnosis to be induced. Although every operator will eventually develop a special procedure with which he or she feels most confident (often the method in which he or she was originally trained), for the beginner the most direct approach for dental anesthesia would seem to be the suggestion of a simple glove anesthesia followed by a transferring of the anesthesia to the area to be worked on (by touching or rubbing the hand against the face). In patients whose fears of hypnosis cannot be overcome, this procedure might be given as a waking suggestion, preferably following a period of relaxation instructions. Dental anesthesia may often be enhanced by suggestions that the patient enjoy pleasant hallucinatory experiences.

Hypnoanesthesia has been used successfully as the sole anesthetic in allergic patients for endodontic therapy of a vital tooth and for a dental implant (Morse and Wilcko, 1979; Gheorghiu and Orleanu, 1982). Both procedures were described by the authors as being extremely painful, normally requiring large amounts of chemical agents.

Using the measurement of the volume and chemical composition of the saliva as indexes, Morse and his associates (1981) found, as would be expected, that hypnoanesthesia was more effective than local anesthesia in reducing anxiety.

Daniels (1976c) described the treatment of a patient with a severe dental phobia who required gingival surgery. A combination of techniques was used, including covert modeling followed by covert reinforcement and pain displacement. The patient was trained to imagine another person in a variety of dental situations, each of which was followed by a positive reinforcement. Then the patient was instructed to imagine herself in similar situations, again followed by reinforcement. The patient was finally trained in self-hypnosis and taught to hallucinate cooling the gums and controlling bleeding. She was taught to displace facial pain down the right shoulder and arm into the fingertips. Following surgery the patient reported no preoperative anxiety or postoperative pain, and she required no pain control medication.

A patient who requires such a complicated treatment plan is probably rare in dental practice. If hypnosis is required for such a patient, a referral to a psychotherapist is indicated. For the majority of dental patients, simple relaxation suggestions and suggestions of glove anesthesia may be enough to produce good results.

Morse, Schoor, and Cohen (1984) report on a procedure combining hypnosis with meditation techniques that was derived from studies comparing meditation with hypnosis. Meditation-hypnosis involves induction by having the patient close his eyes and meditate on the repetition of a simple word (like a mantra in transcendental meditation). They claim the technique is nonthreatening and results in a rapid induction. This technique seems to be a particular variety of a cognitive induction and is probably less threatening to a patient because of the absence of any reference to hypnosis rather than because of anything intrinsic in concentrating on a word instead of an image or an external object.

Katcher, Segal, and Beck (1984) found that the relaxation produced in a patient by having him contemplate a poster of a tranquil scene was enhanced by hypnosis, but the relaxation produced by contemplating the changing stimulus of an aquarium was not. This result suggests that if the practitioner is considering nonhypnotic methods of relaxing patients, which will not arouse resistance in those who fear hypnosis, he can evaluate their effectiveness as compared to hypnotic relaxation by seeing if hypnosis can augment their effect.

Morse (1977a) notes the unique strains and tensions of a dental practice and observes that in addition to being the recipients of their patients' fears and anger, many dentists are perfectionists and are thus condemned to constant frustration. He therefore advocates the use of meditation and self-hypnosis by dentists as a means of coping with their practice-induced stresses. This suggestion, of course, could apply to any harassed professional who is fortunate enough to be a good hypnotic subject. Unfortunately, many good hypnotists turn out to be rather poor subjects, possibly because they are too concerned with analyzing their own hypnotic experiences and are thus unable to "let go" and participate in them. Most good subjects have very little observing ego.

On the other side of the ledger, Butler (1954), while noting that there were practically no studies on the effects of hypnosis on the hypnotist, claims that the operator may have his or her vitality drained and begin to take on the problems from which he or she seeks to free the patient. He says that this reaction may be quite severe, and the hypnotist may start identifying with patients. There is little doubt that these reactions occur and that they are quite common, but they are probably not related to hypnosis at all. They are the kind of countertransferences and patient-induced emotions that make any form of psychotherapy demanding and emotionally draining for the therapist.

Thus, hypnosis can be a double-edged sword. Self-hypnosis can help therapists cope with personal and professional problems; at the same time hypnosis may prove a demanding and exhausting tool in their work.

Adjunctive Hypnotherapy

Hypnosis has been employed in a variety of organic conditions as a supplement to standard medical treatment to control symptoms or to enhance conventional treatments by dealing with the psychological factors resulting from the disease or contributing to its etiology. These uses often go beyond the control of pain or anxiety and their feedback effects. For example, Lazar and Jedliczka (1979) report using hypnosis to control the manipulative behavior of a retarded asthmatic child by enhancing his sense of control and reducing the need to manipulate his parents. His changed behavior substantially reduced the management problem for the parents.

Hypnosis has also been used to control bleeding in hemophilia, Von Willebrand's disease, and in a case of upper gastrointestinal hemorrhage (Bishay, Stevens, and Lee, 1984; Fung and Lazar, 1983; LeBaron and Zeltzer, 1984).

Hypnosis has been used by Moldawsky (1984) as an adjunct to the treatment of Huntington's disease to allay anxiety and reduce involuntary movements not adequately controlled by drugs. It was also employed to deal with an injection phobia and low pain threshold in a kidney dialysis patient (Dimond, 1981). Dimond reports that this phobia did not appear to result from prior learning but seems to be a common reaction of dialysis patients to the sudden loss of an independent life-style produced by their dependence on a dialysis machine and the people associated with it.

Another adjunctive use of hypnotherapy is in helping patients tolerate symptoms that cannot be relieved. An example of this use of hypnosis is Brattberg's (1983) report of 22 out of 32 patients, suffering from intractable tinnitus, learning to ignore the disturbing noise after one month of therapy. Therapy consisted of an initial consultation, four weeks of home practice with an audiotape, and a final follow-up visit.

Hypnosis has proved of value in restoring or retraining motor function following an injury that produced central or peripheral neurological damage (Finkelstein, 1982; Parker, 1979; Pajntar, Jeglic, Stefancic, and Vodovnik, 1980; Vodovnik, Roskar, Pajntar, and Gros, 1979).

Murphy and Fuller (1984) report the adjunctive use of hypnosis and biofeedback in the control of blepharospasm. They found ophthalmalogic treatment had a limited effect in a particular patient, while hypnosis had a dramatic but short-lived effect. Biofeedback had a moderate but sustained effect. Since this was a one-patient case report, the results are merely suggestive and cannot be taken as an indication of the relative effectiveness of these three approaches to treatment in general. It is cited here only as an example of the range of medical problems treated with adjunctive hypnotherapy.

.

Hypnosis in the Management of Chronic and Terminal Illness

The advantages of hypnosis in the management of chronically or terminally ill patients are many. Not only can pain relief be obtained and the requirements for medication reduced, but organ dysfunction may be corrected, and the adverse effects of the patient's emotional response to the illness— his feelings of rage, depression, anxiety, and fear—may be minimized (Butler, 1954; Gardner and Lubman, 1982-1983; M. D. Hall, 1983; Kaye, 1984; Margolis, 1982-1983; Miller, 1980; Newton, 1982-1983; Oliver, 1982-1983; Shapiro, 1982-1983). J. Hilgard and LeBaron (1982) found that pain control was more effective with highly susceptible children and adolescents with cancer than with low-susceptibility patients, but the latter group still benefited from reduced anxiety. In addition to the stress produced in the patient by a chronic or terminal disease, family members are also subjected to severe stress, which may involve feelings of anger and fear as well as guilt. Family members may often require therapy (hypnotic or otherwise) for these stresses as much as or more than the patient. If the duration of life cannot be extended, its quality may be enhanced. The patient may be helped to spend his final days calmly, in good spirits, and free of dread. These days may even be productive, with the patient clearheaded rather than drugged into a zombie-like state (Butler, 1954; Clawson and Swade, 1975; LaBaw et al., 1975).

Butler describes cancer patients as people under a sentence of death who, as a result, have serious emotional disturbances. He describes what he calls a "cancer personality," which includes the failure to express feelings, the repression of anger and grudges, and stoic suffering. He believes that these patients can be helped to channel their emotional reactions from "neurotic" exaggerations of fear and self-pity to a more constructive viewpoint. Hypnosis can be used to provide the psychotherapy that all terminally ill patients need. It can be used to suppress symptoms or to facilitate the ventilation of emotion. The underlying psychotherapy rather than the hypnosis itself helps the patient come to terms with his impending demise or a future of chronic invalidism with a radical change in life-style.

In addition to helping the patient develop a philosophical acceptance of his condition, hypnotherapy may provide the patient with some feeling of control over his symptoms and pain. It may be used to motivate him to cooperate in the treatment process and to mitigate the unpleasant side effects of chemotherapy and radiation treatments (Hoffman, 1982-1983; Milne,

1982; Redd, Rosenberger, and Hendler, 1982-1983; Rosenberg, 1982-1983).

Often patients undergoing chemotherapy for cancer will develop anticipatory nausea and vomiting prior to the treatment, suggesting that much of the distress produced by such treatment may have a psychological component in addition to a physiological one. Both components may be controlled with hypnosis, as can the common feelings of rage that such patients may direct at their physicians and hospital staff. The author had occasion to treat a patient with a metastasized breast cancer who suffered severely from anticipatory emesis as the date for her chemotherapy treatments approached. In spite of having limited trance capacity, with training in self-hypnosis she was able to control both pretreatment and posttreatment nausea well enough to convert what was formerly a nightmare into merely an unpleasant experience. More important, perhaps, was the fact that in prehypnotic discussions during heterohypnosis sessions, she had the opportunity to ventilate her feelings of rage at her disease and her doctors. The increased feelings of control that the self-hypnosis gave her permitted her to retain a sense of human dignity that hospital environments (with their lack of privacy, coupled with the tendency of doctors and staff to treat hospitalized patients like objects) tend to diminish. Hypnosis may also provide a patient with some degree of hope and the feeling that something special is being done to help him (Scott, 1975).

The problem for most terminally ill patients is that the imminence of death makes ineffective the common coping mechanism of considering one's own death as occurring sometime in the future. This forces the patient to think of his death as a present reality. Many terminally ill patients experience first a social and then an intellectual death before experiencing a physical one (Price, 1972). The social death is produced by the patient's physical infirmities and the fact that friends and family avoid him because of embarrassment over what to say, feelings of guilt, and the patient's being an uncomfortable reminder of their own mortality. The intellectual or psychological death is often caused by medication designed to control anxiety and pain.

Terminal patients are often either overtreated or neglected by their physicians, usually for the same reasons. Many physicians have been unconsciously imbued with the idea that it is their function to preserve life at any cost. Hence, they view a dying patient either as a challenge that must be met with heroic surgical or medical procedures or as an ego-bruising personal failure to be avoided. Also, many dying patients may have a need to regress to the level of a clinging, dependent infant and cast the physician in the role of an omnipotent father figure (Lindner and Frank, 1973). This may place an intolerable burden on the physician and serve to magnify his irrational countertransference feelings of failure and defeat. It is interesting to note Butler's (1954) pessimistic statement that in hypnotherapy with cancer patients, the patient is being aided by the hypnotist in his struggle to survive, "but it is a losing battle and in the end cancer and death will win." This statement reflects the severe stress imposed on a physician or therapist working with dying patients, which probably is the source of Butler's belief in the debilitating effects of hypnosis on the hypnotist.

After using hypnosis in obstetrical cases, Butler (1954) went on to employ it in gynecological cancer patients with widespread metastases and pain. He did inductions in a quiet, darkened room with soft, classical background music to aid relaxation and mask distracting noise. Following induction, a series of suggestions was made to deepen the trance, and therapeutic suggestions, including posthypnotic ones, were made at the deepest level obtainable. He used hypnosis primarily to control pain and disabilities, but abreaction was used when indicated. Outpatients were seen as often as daily or as seldom as weekly, and inpatients were treated from two to four times a day. He found that if hypnotherapy was withdrawn suddenly, patients would change dramatically for the worse, but if it was gradually withdrawn, its benefits persisted for a longer period. At the time of this work, the benefits of training in self-hypnosis (to reduce the need for heterohypnotic sessions) was not fully appreciated. Also, prefrontal lobotomies were still common, and Butler regarded hypnosis as a last resort prior to surgery. In a crude way, there is an analogy between hypnotic pain control and a lobotomy, since in both cases suffering may be reduced without the elimination of ascending sensory impulses from pain receptors. On the other hand, there are many important differences between the two procedures. Hypnotic effects are completely reversible, while brain surgery is not, and hypnosis never produces the kinds of deleterious personality changes that lobotomies often did. An interesting finding Butler reported was that patients subjected to prefrontal lobotomies became poor hypnotic subjects, presumably because the operation interfered with their ability to concentrate.

Lindner and Frank (1973) report on a team approach involving a psychiatrist, a neurologist, and a psychologist in the treatment of a terminally ill patient suffering from primary familial amyloidosis. The patient was a good hypnotic subject and easily attained effective pain relief for longer and longer periods between sessions. No dynamic probing was done initially, but as the relationship with the psychologist developed, the patient was able to express his feelings of anger and fear under hypnosis and, in time, to work through his depression. Maladaptive defenses were then abandoned, and the patient was able to revive a healthy interest in life and spend his remaining time in a positive, active way rather than in a regressive, depressed fashion. The relief of pain permitted him to return to work, and the psychotherapy prepared him to face his own demise with equanimity.

Levitan (1985) reports on an interesting technique to allay the fears and anxieties of dying patients, which he calls "hypnotic death rehearsal" and describes as a method of answering the patient's question, "What is it like to die?" It, of course, does not do this; neither the patient nor the therapist knows what the subjective experience of dying is like. What the method actually does is age progress the patient to the time of his death and encourage him to verbalize his imagined experiences and feelings. Hence it provides an opportunity for the patient to verbalize his ideas and emotions about dying and gives the therapist the opportunity to correct unrealistic notions. More important is the fact that it permits the desensitization of many previously unverbalized fears. It seems to resemble the method used spontaneously by many elderly people to desensitize their fear of dying by talking about death more indirectly in the form of unnecessarily frequent estate planning sessions. Probably the major fear associated with death is the fear of the unknown, and this technique, like "walking a patient through" a surgical procedure, may serve to alleviate this fear by giving the patient the illusion that he has been there before and it was not that frightening (a conclusion that most studies of dying patients seem to support).

The use of hypnosis with hospitalized children can do much to make their stay less traumatic and more comfortable, thereby minimizing the potential for psychological damage to the child that is present in any hospitalization and rendering the child a more cooperative patient with whom it is easier for the staff to work (Moore, 1981).

Children may be very good hypnotic subjects, but there are special considerations in working with them. Sarles (1975) notes that analogies between hypnosis and going to sleep should not be made to children, and the word *sleep* should be avoided in induction procedures because children commonly resist having to go to sleep at night. Also, many young children do not produce eye closure on induction, but this need not interfere with the development of a trance (Laguaite, 1976). (Eye closure can be specifically suggested during induction to reduce distractions.) The hypnotist must take care to use language in induction procedures and in subsequent suggestions that the child can understand (LaBaw et al., 1975). Sarles further notes that children often do not give the same indications of being in a trance that adults do, probably because they do not have the same expectations. Deepening procedures are unnecessary; good results can be obtained in a light trance.

Hypnosis in children can be produced by muscular relaxation, but the methods of arm levitation or a cognitive induction utilizing an imagined television set on the child's thumb are particularly appropriate for use with children. Prior to an induction, a child, like any other patient, needs a session devoted to explaining what hypnosis is like and giving him the opportunity to have his questions answered and his fears allayed. Sarles advocates having the child produce an arm levitation prior to an induction by pressing his arm against a wall and then moving away, because the magical quality of this effect interests the child and makes him more suggestible.

Sarles was primarily concerned with the management of protracted pain or the pain of medical procedures, but LaBaw and Holton, Tewell and Eccles (1975) used hypnosis in a group setting with terminally ill children to promote better rest and sleep, ensure adequate food and fluid intake, alleviate anxiety and depression, and increase the children's tolerance for therapeutic procedures. They used hypnotically-induced tranquil scenes to provide relief from pain and anxiety.

Gardner and Lubman (1982-1983) discuss 14 different sources of resistance common in child patients, such as secondary gains, fear of death, depression, and statements to the child by parents or doctors (e.g., "The illness is God's will" or "Pain is inevitable"). These sources must be identified and dealt with in therapy.

One of the fringe benefits of hypnotherapy with terminally ill children seems to have been its effect on their physicians. It gave them the feeling that they were helping these children and their parents, and thus it reduced their own feelings of helplessness and impotence. LaBaw and associates note the use of denial by patients, parents, and physicians alike in dealing with the psychological stresses inherent in working with dying children. Thus, patients never mentioned absent group members who had expired, and parents were often upset when their child missed a day in school.

Self-hypnosis can also be taught to pediatric patients who, like adults, need a feeling of control over their symptoms and pain (Place, 1984), but Sarles believes that it should not be emphasized because the child needs an interpersonal relationship to support him.

Hypnotic Intervention in the Disease Process

In this section the effects of hypnosis on the course of organic diseases will be considered. Diseases may have a purely physical etiology such as a virus, a purely psychogenic etiology, or, more commonly, a mixture of the two in varying proportions. Because of the interrelationship between the mind and the body, mediated in one direction by the autonomic nervous system (ANS) and in the other direction by afferent pathways from receptors, the division of organic illness into psychosomatic and nonpsychosomatic conditions is a matter of degree rather than absolute. To the extent that hypnosis can have any effect on a bodily condition, there must be some such interaction present.

Although there is little doubt concerning the ability of hypnosis to affect bodily functioning, the understanding of the mechanism through which this influence is accomplished and how it may be utilized through hypnotic suggestion requires more research. This situation may be illustrated in connection with the hypnotic treatment of warts.

Warts (verruca vulgaris) are benign epidermal neoplasms caused by the papilloma virus. They regress spontaneously in normal patients, but if they are a sequel to radiation or steroid therapy or to an underlying defect in the immune system, they are unremitting and often resistant to all topical treatment (Tasini and Hackett, 1977). Tasini and Hackett successfully produced a remission of multiple warts in three children who were immunodeficient for a variety of reasons (in one case after the failure of both liquid nitrogen and chloracetic acid treatment). They suggested to the children that the warts would feel dry, turn brown, fall off, and not trouble them anymore. The treatment took an average of three sessions, and wart regressions were noticeable in from 2 weeks to a month, with total regressions obtained as early as 10 weeks. The warts did not return during follow-up periods of from 4 to 8 months.

Venereal warts (condyloma acuminatum) occur on the genitalia or perianal region. They are caused by the same virus as ordinary warts and are just as amenable to suggestion as are the former, but they may have a precancerous significance not associated with ordinary warts (Ewin, 1974). Ewin reports the successful treatment of venereal warts with direct hypnotic suggestion, hypnoanalysis (utilizing ideomotor questioning to determine the psychological value of the symptom to the patient), and waking dream interpretation or suggestion. In direct suggestions to a 22-year-old medical student suffering from penile warts, the patient was told that his body had the capacity to overcome the wart virus and heal the infection. He was told to focus his attention on the area involved and notice the sensation of warmth produced as the blood vessels dilated to bring in antibodies and white cells to fight the infection and build normal tissue. He was then told that his "inner mind" would "lock on" and maintain the warmth until the warts were healed, and he need have no further concern about them. The warts completely cleared within a month, and there was no recurrence in a 6-year follow-up.

Clawson and Swade (1975) successfully treated multiple warts in an 18-year-old girl and boys of 4 and 11 years of age by making the opposite type of suggestion. Instead of telling these patients that blood would flow into the area to fight the infection (an appropriate suggestion for a medical student), they were told that they had the ability to control the blood supply to any part of their body and that they were to cut off the supply of blood to each wart so it would dry up and die. This suggestion was successful in all cases, and the warts disappeared within 2 months. A follow-up on the girl showed no recurrence in a 3.5-year period. Since warts do spontaneously remit, the authors noted the differences observed between spontaneous remissions and the cases reported. They claim that prior to spontaneous remissions, warts often become exquisitely tender, possibly due to a hemorrhage within them, or change in size or color. No such reactions were noted in these patients. The warts, which were of long duration, simply diminished, shriveled up, and disappeared.

More important, Clawson and Swade see the hypnotic treatment of warts by suggestions of interruption of their blood supply as a prototype for the treatment of tumors, particularly those that have metastasized and whose location cannot be visualized. They speculate that it may be possible to suggest to the patient that he cut off the blood supply to the neoplasm "wherever it may be" on the somewhat tenuous theory that the subconscious mind may know the tumor's location. This approach also assumes that the effectiveness of hypnotic suggestions to cut off the blood supply to warts actually results from the alteration of this blood supply. This assumption has yet to be demonstrated. In view of the fact that suggestions of either increased or decreased blood supply produce remissions, the mechanism underlying the improvement may be quite different from what is being suggested to the patient. Suggestions have been made to cancer patients to imagine white blood cells attacking the cancer cells and the tumors shriveling up and dying or to imagine their bodies being cleansed by a waterfall passing through it washing away the cancerous cells, and these suggestions have sometimes appeared successful in producing remissions (Barber, 1978b). The mechanism behind these effects, if in fact they are real, is by no means clear.

Clawson and Swade speculate on additional ways in which hypnosis might be used as an adjunct in the physical treatment of cancer. In addition to the short-term occlusion of blood flow to the tumor during hypnotic or posthypnotic suggestion, they consider the possibility of inducing a thrombus to disrupt its blood supply permanently and the use of repeated hypnosis to prevent the development of collateral circulation. They also speculate on the possibility of hypnotically concentrating chemotherapy drugs in the region of the tumor and rendering the capillaries more permeable to the drug by suggestions of local injuries. Last, they consider the possibility of controlling oxygen distribution following radiation therapy as a way of increasing the effectiveness of the latter.

August (1975) reports preliminary positive results in an attempt to arrest further metastases in a patient with adenocarcinoma of the breast by the hypnotic lowering of the temperature of a limited area of the skin. A variety of clinical reports have been published in recent years that also suggest that hypnosis may have value not only in ameliorating the symptoms of cancer but in influencing the progress of the disease.

Several authors, noting the role of a defective immune system in the development of cancer and the vulnerability of this system to stress, suggest that hypnosis may affect the natural history of cancer indirectly by its effect on the immune system (Bowers and Kelly, 1979; M. D. Hall, 1982-1983;

H. R. Hall, 1982-1983; Newton, 1982-1983; Shapiro, 1982-1983). Some clinicians have had patients imagine their white blood cells proliferating and fighting tumor cells, and Newton (1982-1983) has published data showing longer survival time for patients "adequately" treated with adjunctive hypnosis.

There have also been reports of regression of cancers following intensive meditation (Meares, 1982-1983), and Gravitz (1985c) notes a case of tumor remission associated with hypnosis reported as early as 1846. As Gravitz pointed out, the fact that a tumor remits following hypnosis does not demonstrate that the remission was caused by the hypnosis nor does it rule out the possibility of an original misdiagnosis or a spontaneous remission.

Noting the possibility of psychogenic elements in the etiology of cancer and the role of the immune system in aborting potential cancer in young people, some authors speculate that hypnosis may prove of value in the prevention as well as the treatment of cancer (Finkelstein and Howard, 1982-1983; Weitz, 1983). Certainly the present author would agree that to the extent that hypnosis can modify behavior, such as smoking or eating habits that affect a person's exposure to known carcinogens, it can help prevent this disease. However, the author is a psychologist, not an oncologist, and hence is not qualified to evaluate how likely hypnosis is to influence the development of a potential cancer through its influence on the immune system or other physiological processes. Nevertheless, it seems bizarre to assume that having a patient visualize white blood cells proliferating and fighting cancer cells would directly influence the amount of white blood cells produced. If the cases reported in which such suggestions were effective in increasing white blood cell counts can be replicated, perhaps the effect may prove to be mediated by the positive emotional state produced by providing a patient with a sense of control and hope. If hypnosis could be demonstrated to produce an effect on the immune system, it might be tried on an experimental basis in disorders of the immune system such as AIDS.

Clearly the hypnotherapy of cancer is an area worthy of more research, for both practical and theoretical reasons. It is not possible to demonstrate the efficacy of hypnosis when it is used as an adjunct to standard medical treatment. It would be unethical and probably malpractice to use an experimental treatment exclusively in the treatment of any disease. However, improvement in cure rates with adjunctive hypnosis would be suggestive, and such treatment could easily be fitted in with palliative hypnotherapy whose value is well demonstrated. The ultimate effectiveness of hypnosis in the treatment of cancer would have to be demonstrated with the more difficult population of patients for whom all medical treatment has proved ineffective or who refuse mutilating surgical procedures and other heroic measures. Should hypnotherapy be demonstrated to have an effect on the disease process in cancer, research would then be necessary to establish the most effective use of hypnosis and the more interesting question of what the precise mechanism of intervention was.

Psoriasis is another physical condition that often is resistant to medical treatment. Noting that psoriasis often remits in the warm weather and becomes exacerbated in the winter, Frankel and Misch (1973) successfully treated a 27-year-old male patient with suggestions to imagine the feelings experienced in the skin while sunbathing. Therapy was supplemented by the use of self-hypnosis from five to six times a day. The patient also became aware under hypnosis of the secondary gains that he got from his condition, for it shielded him from social interaction, which he feared. Extensive dynamic probing was not used because the patient was involved in outside psychotherapy. As a "ripple effect," the patient also attained a needed weight loss of about 20 pounds, and his progress in psychotherapy was enhanced (Spiegel and Linn, 1969).

Herpes Simplex II is a virus-caused, sexually transmitted disease characterized by periods of remission and exacerbation of local blistering. It is known that stress (possibly by altering blood adrenaline levels) can exacerbate this condition, and, hence, hypnosis used to control stress may reduce the frequency of recurrence of lesions. Gould and Tissler (1984) cite experimental evidence that hypnotic stress manipulation has produced cold sores and clinical evidence that in two patients hypnosis coupled with self-hypnosis has reduced the frequency of exacerbation of genital herpes.

Maher-Loughnan (1975) notes that in a variety of psychosomatic disorders, spasms of smooth or striated muscles may be involved, as well as imbalance of ANS functioning associated with varying degrees of affective disturbances. Since these functions are modifiable by suggestion, he believes that any psychosomatic disorder is an indication for a trial of heterohypnotherapy and autohypnotherapy.

Bowers (1982) expressed the view that contrary to the common clinical opinion that depth of hypnosis is relatively unimportant in clinical work, it is a major factor in therapies where suggestive effects rather than the transference-enhancing ability of hypnosis is the mechanism of change. Specifically, he claims that success in treating psychosomatic conditions is highly correlated with hypnotic susceptibility even when treatment does not include the use of hypnotic rituals. Hence, he supports formal measurements of patient susceptibility rather than the more common informal estimates based on clinical experience when planning treatments or estimating prognoses. The use of autohypnosis in therapy is important for more than its ability to reduce the need for heterohypnotic sessions and to give the patient a feeling of being in control. If hypnosis is used to promote relaxation and reduce tension or to promote abreactions and facilitate an analysis, autohypnosis is not very important. When hypnosis is used for direct symptom removal, however, autohypnosis is an important safety valve. Symptom removal suggestions should always be made permissively rather than in an authoritarian manner, and the patient should be told he may keep his symptom if he wants to. In effect, autohypnosis gives the patient permission to keep a symptom for which he has a dynamic need and which would not readily be given up in any event until this need is resolved (Frankel, 1975).

Laguaite (1976) reports the use of hypnosis in the treatment of children with vocal cord nodules. These are usually bilateral growths occurring on that portion of the cord where the greatest excursion occurs during phonation. They are caused by traumata in children with excessively loud voices and will disappear if the irritation is removed. Treatment consisted of motivating the children to yell less and to speak more softly and uncovering the tensions that were the cause of their deviant vocalizations. Following a cognitive induction using an imagined television set, patients were first instructed to watch an enjoyable program and then to visualize themselves doing something related to the use of the voice. Ego-enhancing suggestions and suggestions that they would have less need to yell in the future were also given. Children were seen for an average of 11 sessions, and all but two showed improvement, with seven having complete remission of their nodules.

Cheek (1976a) reports the successful use of hypnotherapy in restoring orgasmic capacity in two young women suffering from secondary frigidity following radical gynecological cancer surgery. Therapeutic suggestions dealt with feelings of disgust produced by the aftereffects of the surgery, reactivation of memories of preoperative sexual experiences, and suggestions of "hooking up the circuits again." Fuchs and colleagues (1973) describe the use of hypnosis as a relaxant and facilitator of hallucinatory imagery in covert and in vivo systematic desensitization of vaginismus.

Cioppa and Thal (1975) used hypnosis to treat a 10-year-old girl with a case of juvenile rheumatoid arthritis who was confined to a wheelchair because of pain in her ankles. The patient was depressed and uncommunicative. In the first session, under ideomotor questioning, she said that she knew but did not want to tell why she had arthritis. The issue was not pressed, and she was simply given suggestions that she would feel better. Both the patient and her mother were disturbed by the patient's being given psychiatric treatment and thought that questioning the patient about why she had arthritis was inane. When her mother bathed her that night, she reported that her legs "felt different." Cioppa and Thal note that often patients who have little belief in hypnosis but who nevertheless are affected by it tend to use noncommittal adjectives to describe the effects experienced. Four hours after the second treatment session, the patient rode her bike for the first time in 3 months, and after the third session, she smiled for the first time and was able to jump up and down that evening without pain. She was seen for two more hypnotherapy sessions. The authors believe that the changes produced in the patient's attitude triggered a remission of her disease.

Olness (1976) described five pediatric patients with megacolon. One had an organic condition that would not have benefited from hypnotherapy, and four had functional disorders. The organic case illustrates the need for an accurate diagnosis before treating any condition with hypnosis. Olness developed a comprehensive treatment plan that comprised:

1. A preliminary effort to develop rapport with the child.
2. Informing the patient that it was possible for him to develop control over his bowels if he wanted to.
3. Giving a blackboard talk to help the child understand the functioning of his intestine and his muscles of defecation.
4. Getting the child to agree to try the treatment.
5. Hypnotic suggestions.

Hypnosis was induced in each case by having the child fixate on a smiling face drawn on his thumb while holding a coin between his thumb and forefinger. When he relaxed enough to drop the coin, he was told to close his eyes. Initial instructions for general feelings of well-being were followed up at subsequent inductions with instructions to the patient to tell himself that he had control over his anal muscles, that he would defecate only in the appropriate place, and that he was to imagine himself as a bigger boy doing something that he looked forward to and enjoying his control over himself. Parents were instructed not to remind the patient to practice these suggestions under self-hypnosis; the whole therapeutic strategy was to place active responsibility on the patient rather than have him be a passive participant in the therapy because stool retention was believed to be a manifestation of the child's desire to demonstrate control. Thus, direct efforts by parents or a physician to take away this symbolic control might strengthen the child's resolve to retain the symptom. The use of self-hypnosis and the active solicitation of the child's cooperation in the process increased rather than threatened his feeling of control. This report illustrates the need for a rational plan of hypnotherapy that takes the personality and dynamic requirements of the patient into account. Even in the treatment of medical conditions or medical aspects of psychological conditions, hypnosis must be used as an adjunct to sound psychotherapeutic principles if it is to be effective.

A number of studies have investigated the clinical use of hypnosis in the treatment of essential hypertension. Jackson (1979) reports on a longitudinal 4-year study of a single 51-year-old male patient whose systolic and diastolic pressures were lowered and stabilized by a combination of medication and hypnosis and whose medication was reduced from 20 to three tablets per day. Since hypnosis was confounded with medication, however, it is impossible to say what its effect was. It is also not possible to generalize from a one-patient study.

Friedman and Taub (1977, 1978) report a four-group study in which 12 hypertensive patients were assigned to a hypnosis-only group, 11 to a biofeedback-only group, ten to a group receiving biofeedback and hypnosis, and 11 to a control group receiving only periodic blood pressure measurements. Baseline measurements were made, and patients were followed up 1 week after the training period and monthly thereafter for 6 months.

After 1 week, the biofeedback and hypnosis groups had significant decreases in diastolic pressure from the baseline reading, but only the hypnosis group was significantly different from the other groups. Surprisingly, the combined use of hypnosis and biofeedback proved less effective than either technique alone. The authors speculate on the possibility of simultaneous hypnosis and biofeedback interfering with each other. They cite Orne's suggestion to them that a synergistic effect might be possible if there was a temporal separation between the two procedures.

At the 6-month follow-up, the hypnosis-only group was the only one having a significantly lower diastolic pressure from the baseline. Systolic pressure was significantly lower than baseline measures for the hypnosis-only group at 4, 5, and 6 months, while the biofeedback-only group maintained reductions for the first 5 months.

Case, Fogel, and Pollack (1980) report a study on the use of self-hypnosis with 15 hypnotizable patients with labile or essential hypertension. They report the unusual finding that during hypnotic induction profile testing, both hypertensive patients and 15 normotensive controls had elevations in both systolic and diastolic blood pressure. Nonhypnotizable subjects, whether hypertensive or normotensive, did not display this effect. These elevations of blood pressure during hypnosis occurred at each follow-up period and did not diminish over time.

During a 4-month period of practice of daily self-hypnosis, three subjects had a pressor effect and their blood pressure increased, seven were nonresponders, and five had decreased blood pressure. All subjects, regardless of the direction of their blood pressure change, reported subjective feelings of well-being. The authors speculate that the pressor effect during hypnosis may be similar to the pressor effect seen in subjects doing mental arithmetic tasks and may be brought about by the concentration necessary during hypnosis. They also suggest that it may be unique to Spiegel's method of hypnosis.

These issues require further investigation. The fact that the same procedure produced different long-term effects in different patients may relate to individual differences in the patients' physical state (patients with higher baseline diastolic pressures tended to have depressor effects, and those with lower baseline diastolic readings tended to have pressor effects), in how they interpreted the suggestions made, or a combination of these factors.

The authors point out that although the control of hypertension with medication has been shown to reduce the incidence of stroke, congestive heart failure, and kidney damage, it does not appear to alter heart attack or sudden death rates. Since there is evidence that there may be emotional factors in the latter conditions, they suggest that adjunctive hypnosis may be useful in the treatment of hypertension because of the emotional benefits these subjects received whether or not it reduced blood pressure. This possibility may be true in cases where blood pressure is unaffected, but it seems questionable in cases where it is actually raised and the reasons for this phenomenon require investigation.

Mount and his associates (1978) found no significant differences in blood pressure reductions in 30 normotensive, medication-free students assigned to four treatment or two control groups. Treatment groups received contingent EMG biofeedback, Jacobson's (1938) relaxation training, Mear's suggestions of well-being, hypnosis, or hypnosis plus contingent biofeedback in a counterbalanced procedure. Control groups received either noncontingent EMG feedback or a 20-minute relaxation period. Since a reduction of blood pressure in normotensive patients would necessarily involve the creation of a hypotensive state, these results would appear to have little application to the value of hypnosis as a treatment for hypertension.

Friedman and Taub (1982) present the interesting finding that difficulty in parking when visiting the laboratory had a significant effect on blood pressure studies and needs to be controlled for. This should surprise nobody who lives in a metropolitan area.

Hypnosis and Conception

Muehleman (1978) reports a case in which hypnosis was used to aid a 26-year-old woman who had difficulty conceiving a child despite the absence of a physical problem. Ideomotor questioning was used to identify a psychological problem, and an ideomotor response then indicated that she was now confident that she could conceive. On the second session, she was asked to imagine herself holding a healthy infant and project the date of this occurrence. The author estimated that her subsequent conception occurred about 3 days following her first hypnotic treatment. In view of the sensitivity of the menstrual cycle to emotional upsets, this case suggests that hypnosis (or any other type of psychotherapy) may help a couple seeking to have a child if the problem is primarily caused by emotional difficulties in the wife. Also emotional factors may affect a sperm count in the husband. Certainly emotional problems in one spouse usually affect the other, and in such a case it might prove fruitful to treat both partners. It also suggests that hypnosis might be used to disrupt the menstrual cycle and function as a contraceptive. Indeed B. J. Perry (1980) speculates on this possibility and even cites (without reference) an "unstructured observational study" of hypnotic abortions produced in 26 out of 28 women.

This notion of the potential use of hypnosis as a method of birth control requires further comment. It is one thing to say theoretically that hypnosis may interfere with the menstrual cycle and thus prevent conception; it is very different to describe the exact mechanism and to determine exactly how to suggest this effect to a particular patient. Furthermore, there is no reason why hypnosis could not be freely used on an experimental basis in an effort to aid a woman in her efforts to conceive. At the very worst, it would be of no help. On the other hand, the failure of hypnosis as a contraceptive device would be a disaster to the couple involved, and its experimental use would be reckless in the extreme.

The experimental verification of the use of hypnosis as a contraceptive would be difficult, for such research would require the participation of couples who did not care whether they had a child during the period of the research, and such couples are probably uncommon.

Hypnosis in Diagnosis

Several authors have advocated the use of hypnosis as a diagnostic aid. Boswell (1982) suggests its routine use in physical examinations to produce muscular relaxation, foster more accurate history taking, and aid in the differential diagnosis and localization of pain.

Gross (1980) claims that epileptic seizures can be distinguished from hysterical seizures in that once induced by hypnosis, hysterical seizures can be terminated by suggestion, while epileptic seizures cannot. Also, the amnesia that follows an epileptic seizure cannot be hypnotically reversed as amnesia following hysterical seizures can. Gross also says that schizophrenics are unable to control auditory hallucinations in accordance with hypnotic suggestions, while patients suffering from a dissociative reaction can. Hoffman (1985) presents a similar view.

Hypnosis has been used to communicate with the various aspects of the personality of patients suffering from multiple personality disorder, and in these cases it is of both diagnostic and therapeutic value (Ross, 1984). Abrams (1983) discusses the problems of differentially diagnosing a multiple personality from malingering by a defendant in a criminal case but offers no foolproof method of deciding this issue, which has produced marked disagreement among prominent experts in specific cases. For example, in one murder case, Orne, Dinges, and Orne (1984) concluded that the defendant was faking, while Watkins (1984) came to the opposite conclusion, and Allison (1984) believed that he displayed an atypical dissociation reaction but that it may be impossible to make a correct diagnosis in a criminal case.

Abrams (1983) advocates age regressing a suspected multiple personality patient to a period for which he is amnesic to contact another personality, but he cautions not to disclose this expectation to the patient to avoid suggesting the existence of another personality.

Bliss (1983) citing the typically high-susceptibility scores of multiple personality patients, presents arguments that the etiology of this condition may involve the occurrence of spontaneous, self-hypnotic states induced by trauma, a mechanism similar to that speculated on for phobias. Bliss believes that in view of the diversity of syndromes that may be induced by spontaneous trance states, there must be other factors involved that require investigation.

Hypnosis may be of value in distinguishing an organic condition from a hysterical reaction. For example, a patient with a hysterically paralyzed limb may be able to move it in response to a hypnotic suggestion, while a patient with an organic paralysis cannot. It is doubtful, however, that hypnosis could distinguish either of these conditions from malingering in spite of the view expressed by Spiegel and Spiegel (1984) that subjects low in susceptibility are unlikely to develop hysterical reactions, and hence if no organic pathology is present, they are likely to be faking. The problem with their viewpoint is that even if it were true on a statistical basis, it proves nothing about the etiology of an individual case. Of course, if a patient is highly susceptible, it suggests that the problem may be hysterical, and hypnosis might prove useful therapeutically.

NONTHERAPEUTIC APPLICATIONS OF HYPNOSIS

There are a variety of practical applications of hypnosis that are nontherapeutic in nature that will be discussed in this section. These include the use of hypnosis in psychological research, forensic and military applications, and the use of hypnosis in advertising and sports.

Hypnosis as a Tool in Psychological Research

Hypnosis has the potential to be useful in a variety of ways in psychological research. It may be used to manipulate or control conditions and emotional states and thus permit the latter to be used as independent variables in research (Blum and Barbour, 1979; Blum and Green, 1978; Bower, Gilligan, and Monteiro, 1981; Counts and Mensh, 1950; Hodge and Wagner, 1964; Hodge, Wagner, and Schreiner, 1966a, 1966b; Levine, Grassi, and Gerson, 1943; Maslach, 1979). Such use requires additional control groups of hypnotized subjects to avoid confounding hypnosis with the independent variable employed. Some independent method of measuring the effectiveness of the emotional manipulation is also needed. A drawback of using hypnosis in research, which may account for its infrequent use, is the fact that its employment requires the use of highly susceptible subjects, and this necessarily restricts the freedom of the experimenter to select subjects randomly. Most of the statistical analyses to which experimental data are subjected assume a random selection of subjects, and the validity of the conclusions reached depends on this assumption being met. On the other hand, the random selection of research subjects is very much like the weather—everybody talks about it, but nobody really employs it. Most experimenters compromise by randomly assigning subjects, selected on the basis of availability, to experimental groups. The practical effect of the nonrandom selection of subjects is to limit the generality of the findings to a theoretical population from which the subjects used could be deemed to be a random sample.

Hodge, Wagner, and Schreiner (1966a) report the use of hypnosis to remove the effects of previous treatments in a within-subjects, repeated-measures experimental design. They relied on the subjects' subjective reports in assessing the effectiveness of this manipulation, but this technique is open to serious question.

Kihlstrom (1979) points out the value of hypnosis as a laboratory model of the dissociative phenomena seen in psychopathology. Hypnosis has also been used to study symptom formation by means of generating internal conflicts in subjects through the implanting of paramnesias (Smyth, 1981a).

Forensic and Law Enforcement Applications of Hypnosis

Suggested forensic applications of hypnosis have included its use in lie detection, obtaining confessions, the lifting of amnesia, aiding witnesses in the recall of details, and influencing the demeanor of witnesses and defendants in court (Arons, 1977; Bryan, 1962; Gravitz, 1983b; Haward, 1984; Kroger, 1977b; Kroger and Douce, 1979, 1980; Laurence and Perry, 1983a; Reiser and Nielson, 1980; Salzberg, 1977; Stratton, 1977).

Some of these suggested uses result not only from inordinately optimistic estimates of what hypnosis can accomplish and a lack of appreciation of its limitations but also reflect serious misunderstandings of both the nature of our legal system and the constitutional rights of the accused in criminal proceedings.

Lie Detection.   The instrument most often used as a lie detector is the polygraph. A polygraph is a device that measures a variety of autonomic nervous system (ANS) responses (e.g., pulse rate, blood pressure, respiration rate, GSR) and graphs them against time. It is an excellent way of measuring these responses when they are used as dependent variables in research. When a polygraph is used as a lie detector, however, its value is questionable at best. In theory, a polygraph detects lying by measuring changes in the subject's ANS responses produced by emotional reactions accompanying a lie. Because there are wide individual differences in subjects' ANS lability, a baseline measure must be taken for each subject. Deviations from this baseline, when the subject is instructed to lie, must be calibrated in order to evaluate responses to later key questions, which are typically interspersed among neutral filler items that permit a return to the baseline. It may well be that under laboratory conditions, lying can be detected in some subjects. Whether this technique will detect lying in a psychopath or indicate the truthfulness of the responses of a frightened, innocent defendant to emotionally charged questions asked under traumatic circumstances is another question. The author knows of no study demonstrating the validity of this procedure and of no university program training students to be experts in polygraph interpretation. The state of New York (and most other jurisdictions) does not consider lie detector results reliable enough to permit such results to be admissible in evidence, in the absence of a stipulation between the parties to a lawsuit (Schathin, 1978). Nevertheless, many agencies of the federal government and some private industries seem enamored of its use. A number of marginally trained people, often former police officers, make a lucrative business of giving such tests as employment screening devices on behalf of gullible business concerns anxious to reduce their losses from employee pilfering. Evidently any device that resembles a piece of scientific equipment has the capacity to inspire confidence in its pronouncements.

Another problem with the use of lie detector tests to screen potential employees, other than the fact that such screening is both expensive and ineffective, is the fact that this procedure is likely to result in the hiring of a group of lower-class employees who are used to being treated in such an insulting manner and who may in turn treat the firm's customers in a similar manner. If the firm's clientele are mainly middle-class people, unused to such treatment, substantial loss of business may result. Furthermore, Falick (1968) argues that even if a polygraph were assumed to be reliable, its use in employment interviews should be outlawed as an unwarranted invasion of privacy.

Arons (1977) proposes the use of hypnosis as a substitute for a polygraph in lie detection. He recommends that an ideomotor response such as a finger lift or an eye blink be used as an unconscious signal that the subject be trained to give when he is lying. The usefulness of such a device in lie detection is predicated on two basic assumptions: that such a response could be imposed on an unwilling subject and that it is possible to detect when a subject is faking hypnosis in order to be in a position to make seemingly authentic, self-serving statements. Neither assumption has been demonstrated to be accurate, and both are extremely likely to prove false. There is much evidence (see Chapter 4) that experts cannot readily distinguish between real and simulating hypnotic subjects. Arons's view that hypnotic subjects fall neatly into various stages of hypnosis, with each stage having an invariant set of effects associated with it (so that faking can be detected by a subject's producing effects characteristic of the deeper stages of hypnosis while not exhibiting effects of the lighter stages), is inaccurate.

Lie detector results have been affected by feelings of guilt induced for "crimes" a subject was told under hypnosis that he committed. There is no reason to believe that a hypnotized subject cannot lie or that he will readily give up secrets under hypnosis (Barber, 1978b; Orne, 1962a).

Indeed, one of the risks of hypnotizing a potential witness is that his credibility may be rendered impeachable because it is possible to give suggestions concerning the facts in issue to such a subject that he may later be unable to distinguish from reality. For this reason the decision to employ hypnosis to improve the memory of a potential witness is primarily a legal rather than a psychological decision. This decision must be made by the attorney in charge of the case. All such hypnotic sessions should be made in the presence of this attorney and should be preserved on tape, preferably videotape, with a continuously running clock shown in the picture to avoid claims of tape editing (Hibler, 1979). Questions must be carefully planned in advance with the attorney to avoid the adversary party's successfully claiming that ideas concerning the facts of the case were implanted in the witness. Unless there is a compelling reason for a contrary course of action (such as a need to probe for information concerning the whereabouts of a kidnapping victim whose life may be in danger), it is a good rule never to hypnotize a witness whose testimony is the sole proof available of a fact in issue at a trial.

Hypnotic Confessions. Hypnotically obtained confessions have been defended by some writers on the grounds that hypnosis could be used merely to remove a defendant's amnesia for the event and the decision to confess could still be made voluntarily. This decision could even be deferred until the subsequent waking state (Arons, 1977). There is a great danger that hypnosis may be used, sometimes inadvertently and sometimes by overzealous law enforcement agencies, to instill false beliefs in a suspect concerning the facts of a crime and his involvement in it or the advantages to himself of making a confession or other statement. The fact that a subject has been returned to the waking state does not ensure that the hypnotist's influence over him is no longer effective. Many subjects are extremely suggestible following hypnosis. The problem in law enforcement of false confessions made by mentally disturbed people who are not under the influence of hypnotic suggestions has made it necessary for the state of New York.to require the corroboration of any confession before a conviction can be based on it. The risk of obtaining a false confession or of violating the defendant's constitutional right against self-incrimination, even if a confession is true, is too great to permit the introduction of hypnotically obtained confessions into evidence. All confessions and statements obtained, in whole or part, by the use of hypnosis ought to be regarded as the product of psychological coercion and be deemed involuntary and inadmissible as a matter of law. The courts have uniformly adopted this position, and convictions have been set aside when confessions or other statements have resulted from indirect or even inadvertent hypnosis (Udolf, 1983). Prosecutors would be well advised to prohibit anyone on their staffs from hypnotizing a suspect who is likely to make a statement or confession, lest it be rendered inadmissible.

The use of procedures to induce hypnosis surreptitiously by describing the procedure as an exercise in relaxation or by some other subterfuge (Arons, 1977), although justifiable in some clinical situations, is clearly an outrageous violation of an accused person's constitutional right against self-incrimination.

As a practical matter, the Miranda warnings (required to be given to persons charged with a crime as soon as they are in police custody) inform the defendant of his right to remain silent and to consult a lawyer before making any statement. This warning may reduce the opportunity the police have for hypnotic interrogations. These warnings, however, apply only to people who are arrested. They need not be given to persons "invited" to come to the police station and be interviewed "voluntarily."

Use of Hypnosis to Affect Witness Demeanor.   Bryan (1962) suggests the use of hypnosis to affect the courtroom demeanor of witnesses or the defendant in order to render them calm, more self-possessed, and confident. Such demeanor is designed to help them make a more favorable impression on the jury and, hence, make their testimony more likely to be believed. This is not subornation of perjury since the witness is not being told what to testify but only how to testify. Such instructions given to a witness in the waking state are not only proper but commonplace, and indeed it is an attorney's duty to prepare a witness or a client for all facets of his or her courtroom appearance. If, however, this preparation is done by hypnotic suggestion and the fact of the hypnosis is brought out under cross-examination, the jury may believe that an attempt was made to deceive them. In addition, such hypnosis may render the witness's testimony incompetent in some jurisdictions. Thus, the decision to employ hypnotic preparation is a matter of trial strategy that must be made by the attorney. It is the author's opinion that any use of hypnosis on a witness, even if it has no relationship to the facts about which he is to testify, renders the witness' credibility impeachable and is ill advised in the absence of a clear and cogent reason for its employment. Such a reason might be the need to call a witness who is too emotionally distraught to testify coherently without help. In such a case, the induction might best be performed in the presence of the court and opposing counsel, with the jury absent.

Investigative Use of Hypnosis.   The use of hypnosis to recover forgotten details of an event or to resolve an emotionally caused amnesia in witnesses is one of the forensic applications of hypnosis that has most potential value to law enforcement agencies and attorneys. This use is particularly valuable for police agencies looking for leads, clues, or a description of the perpetrators of a crime from a witness whom they do not have to rely on exclusively to prove any major element of the People's case. The real value of the method is its ability to develop leads that may ultimately help uncover independent evidence. For example, Kroger was able to have a witness "relive" the scene of the kidnapping of 26 school children in California and recall all but one digit of the license number of the van driven by the kidnappers (*Time*, 1976; Kroger, 1977b).

There is a large literature pointing out serious problems with hypnotically refreshed memories in forensic application (AMA Council on Scientific Affairs, 1985; Loftus and Loftus, 1980; Orne, 1979; Perry and Laurence, 1983; M. C. Smith, 1983; Timm, 1983; Udolf, 1983; Worthington, 1979; Zelig and Beidleman, 1981). These problems include, but are not limited to, subjects' developing confabulations to fill in the gaps between memories and then confusing these confabulations with reality, thereby rendering their detection under cross-examination more difficult. Also, real memories may be permanently destroyed or altered by suggestions made in the form of leading questions, whether this is done inadvertently, by poor technique, or deliberately to suborn perjury. Research has shown that hypnotized witnesses are more prone to error produced by leading questions but no more accurate than waking subjects in response to nonleading questions (although they typically verbalize more material). The more directive the questioning, the greater is this effect (Dywan and Bowers, 1983; Hilgard and Loftus, 1979; Laurence and Perry, 1983b; Putnam, 1979; Rafky and Bernstein, 1984; Udolf, 1983; Zelig and Beidleman, 1981).

One study found that hypnotic subjects were more accurate than waking subjects in lineup identifications, but neither hypnotic nor waking control subjects demonstrated any relationship between confidence in their identifications and accuracy (Sanders and Simmons, 1983). On the other hand, Wagstaff (1982a) found that 13 hypnotized subjects were not better than 12 control subjects in identifying a face shown 7 days earlier, and he says that there was some evidence that hypnosis may have increased the number of false positive identifications.

In clinical work, the accuracy of hypnotically retrieved memories is unimportant; there the interest is in the subjective reality of the patient, not objective truth. In forensic work, the accuracy of this material is vital; human life and liberty may hinge on it.

Common memory retrieval techniques include age regressing a witness back to the time of the crime or having him visualize it on a television screen. The latter method is often used in cases where reexperiencing the original event would prove unduly upsetting to the witness. The accuracy of information obtained in this manner is, of course, open to serious question. It would be unsuitable for use as evidence, for it is likely to be a mixture of fact and fantasy. The witnesses did not observe the events of the crime safely on a television screen but in real life under traumatic circumstances, and what is being obtained here is a fantasy, not a memory.

Because hypnotically refreshed memories are typically mixtures of real memories, confabulations, and other fantasies in indeterminant proportions and neither the witness nor the hypnotist can say which is which, the value of this material is primarily in investigations where it might provide leads to independent evidence. Such material, if used as evidence in a trial, may result in the presentation of false testimony by honest witnesses. Hence, investigative use of hypnosis ought to be limited to witnesses whose testimony is unlikely to be necessary at a trial. It is not always easy to predict early in an investigation how likely a witness is to be needed at a trial, and thus investigative hypnosis should not be rushed into. The common police practice of using hypnosis on victims of crimes is shortsighted, for a victim is likely to be needed to testify, and in some jurisdictions the pretrial hypnosis may render much of his testimony inadmissible and destroy the People's case. In all jurisdictions it will at least render his testimony impeachable.

Schafer and Rubio (1978) cite examples of some 14 cases employing hypnotic crime investigation and the results obtained.

The Los Angeles and Israeli national police have hypnosis squads that specialize in this type of investigation (*U.S. News and World Report,* 1978). The FBI has gained helpful information from dozens of crime victims in its hypnotic investigation program, which employs only professionals as hypnotists (*New York Times,* 1979).

Both the FBI and the U.S. Air Force have established rigid guidelines controlling the circumstances under and the purposes for which hypnosis may be used in criminal investigations to guard against the foregoing problems and sources of error (Ault, Jr., 1979; Hibler, 1979, 1984, 1984a; Stratton, 1977; Teten, 1979). The Civil Aeronautics Board uses hypnosis in air-crash investigations (Teten, 1979). Hiland and Dzieszkowski (1984) describe how important information concerning six accidents involving naval aircraft was obtained by hypnotic interviewing of eight witnesses.

Use of Hypnosis in Court.   The two major uses of hypnosis in court are to show the basis of an expert's opinion concerning the mental condition of a defendant and to enhance the memory of a witness or break an amnesia. In general, hypnotically-produced evidence is admissible for the first purpose, since hypnosis is generally recognized by the appropriate scientific community as being a reliable (in the legal sense of the term. i.e., valid) procedure for purposes of diagnosis. The trial judge, however, has discretion to refuse to admit such evidence if he or she believes it is likely to be unduly prejudicial or if there is a danger that the jury may regard it as substantive proof of the facts stated under hypnosis.

With respect to the enhancement of a witness   memory by hypnosis, different jurisdictions take different positions. The general rule is that all witnesses (with the exception of a witness qualified as an expert) must testify to matters of fact, not opinion, and must testify from memory. If a witness cannot remember the events in question, the courts will permit him to "refresh his recollection" with a variety of memory-jogging devices, such as notes, newspaper clippings, and even leading questions, but before being permitted to testify to the facts in issue, he must state that he is now able to testify from memory.

No U.S. court, to the author's knowledge, has ever permitted a witness to testify while under hypnosis, probably because of the prejudicial effect of such a dramatic event on the jury, who might be misled into thinking that hypnosis ensures the accuracy of the testimony or at least prevents lying. (Neither conclusion is correct.) Another legal problem in permitting a witness to testify under hypnosis is the fact that, in general, witnesses are required to testify under oath, and there is a question concerning the capacity of a hypnotic subject to take an oath (Scott, 1977). There is also the question of whether a hypnotized witness has the legal capacity to commit perjury. Furthermore, no court has ever admitted a recording or testimony concerning what a witness previously said under hypnosis as evidence of the facts stated, for this evidence would be hearsay and effectively deprive the opposing party of the right to cross-examine the witness.

Thus, the major use of hypnosis on witnesses is as a memory-jogging device prior to testifying. Different jurisdictions where the issue has arisen have taken one of two positions. Some jurisdictions treat hypnosis like any other memory-enhancing device and permit the witness to testify from the hypnotically refreshed memory in the subsequent waking state. These jurisdictions leave the issue of the credibility of such testimony to the jury. They generally require that the opposing party be given notice of the use of hypnosis and be provided with a videotape of the proceedings to aid in cross-examination. Even these jurisdictions give the trial judge discretion not to admit this evidence if its proponent fails to establish it was competently done by an expert or if the hypnotic questioning was unduly suggestive.

Other jurisdictions, noting the potential for confabulation and memory distortion inherent in the hypnotic situation, regard any evidence not reported by a hypnotized witness prior to the hypnosis as suspect and inadmissible. In such a jurisdiction, the investigative use of hypnosis on a key witness may destroy a party's case.

No jurisdiction that the author is aware of holds that a previously hypnotized witness is totally incompetent and cannot testify to matters he related prior to the hypnosis, nor does any object to solely investigative hypnosis on non-court witnesses or to the use of evidence derived from such investigation. (For a sampling of the controversy over the use of hypnotically refreshed testimony, see Appelbaum, 1984; Bateman, 1980; Brown, 1985; Gibson, 1982; Karlin, 1983; Reiser, 1984; Roberts, 1982; Scholder, 1982; Udolf, 1983.)

A more adequate treatment of the subspecialty of forensic hypnosis would require a book of its own. Interested readers are referred to *Forensic Hypnosis* (Udolf, 1983) for a more detailed description of the psychological and legal issues involved and a comprehensive review of legal cases. (For a less legalistic viewpoint and a very different perspective on the psychological issues, see Reiser, 1980.)

Military Uses of Hypnosis

Since military and espionage applications of hypnosis are necessarily kept secret, it is difficult to estimate the extent to which hypnosis is used in these areas.

Estabrooks (1957) in a James Bond vein, suggests that hypnosis could provide a secure method for sending secret messages. He proposes that good hypnotic subjects be used as couriers. They could be hypnotized, given a secret message, and then instructed to forget that they have been given the message until hypnosis is reinduced at a prearranged signal by a designated person. The courier would be instructed that he would not be hypnotizable by anyone else. Thus, the message would be secure not only from careless disclosure on the part of the messenger but even under torture, for the courier could not disclose a message that he was unaware of.

Certain problems are inherent in this procedure, however. First, hypnotic amnesia does not last indefinitely. Often it will dissolve spontaneously, particularly after an event that triggers a partial memory retrieval. Second, hypnotic memory improvement is not so impressive as to preclude the possibility of error in the repetition of the message. Couriers with good rote memories would have to be employed and given short, clear messages. With respect to enabling couriers to withstand physical torture, the use of self-hypnosis techniques would appear to have more promise (Kline, 1978). Balson, Dempster, and Brooks (1984) discuss styles of coercive persuasion (commonly called brainwashing) and victims' responses to them. They found that persons subjected to such tactics who detached themselves by the spontaneous use of self-hypnosis and imagery were best able to resist ideological conversions and suffered least from posttraumatic effects when liberated. The selection of couriers with the proper personality attributes would be of even more importance. If an enemy knew that a person was carrying a hypnotic message, instructions designed to make him insusceptible to future attempts at hypnosis could be overcome, particularly by induction attempts disguised as relaxation procedures, exercises in imagination, or concentration. After all, the subject would have no conscious reason to avoid these innocuous-sounding activities.

The possible use of a hypnotic subject as an unwitting agent in espionage or assassination activities is a special case related to whether a hypnotic subject can be induced to commit a crime and will be dealt with in Chapter 7. However, whether an agent is an unwitting one or a voluntary one, Estabrooks suggests that hypnosis may be used to enhance his performance. A person convinced of his innocence may act less suspiciously and be more convincing to others. In this regard, Shaw (1978) has reported the use of self-hypnosis in an acting school to render student performances more realistic. Based on blind audience ratings, hypnotically aided scenes appear to have been portrayed more convincingly. As Shaw notes, the extent to which self-hypnosis is informally used by actors in general is difficult to estimate. It seems to the author that any method of acting, where the actor imagines himself to be the character portrayed, is really a variety of informal self-hypnosis.

Hypnosis in Advertising

The goal of advertising is to influence the target person's motivation to buy a product, support a political cause, or contribute to a fund-raising campaign. Because of the commercial importance of this effort, much of the creative talent available in the television industry is employed in this activity. The problems of the advertiser are many. He must, first of all, get the target's attention to his message. In a magazine or similar medium, there are a host of other ads and materials competing for this attention. On television, an ad must capture the viewer's attention in a matter of seconds for he is likely to be awaiting a commercial break to prepare a snack or go to the bathroom. This is why advertisers try to capitalize on the attention-getting qualities of sex and humor. On the other hand, if these devices are too effective, they can detract from the perception and memory of the product. There was a commercial for a vacation island featuring a statuesque girl walking out of the water in a bikini, which had an excellent attention-getting quality. However, only a very small percentage of the author's students (male or female) were able to recall the name of the sponsor when asked. (As a matter of fact, in the first edition of this book the author referred to this ad as being for an airline!) This is the reason that some ads employ characters associated with the product name.

Having captured the attention of the target, the ad must then motivate him to buy the product, often one for which he either has no need or which he could just as well obtain from a competitor. It is in this effort that the principles of the psychology of motivation and persuasion come into play. Prior to the application of psychodynamic investigation and motivational research in advertising, there were techniques used to sell products that were based on the application of general psychological principles. They involved no specific research with a particular product.

With the advent of motivational research techniques in advertising, psychologists began to investigate the real reasons why people buy particular products and found that these reasons were often unconscious and quite different from the rationalizations given when people were asked why they used a certain brand. Motivational research involves the use of various projective techniques to investigate a consumer's associations to products and the images that these products connote. It permits advertisers to aim sales appeals directly (and indirectly) to the actual consumer motives that affect buying behavior. Often these motives are strong because they are kept at a high level by frustration in daily life, for example, sexual needs or needs for power and dominance. Sometimes these motives involve common and powerful emotions such as fear or guilt.

There is little need to illustrate sexual motivation in ads because it is so common. The ad with a sexy model describing the product as a "man's beer" and challenging the viewer's virility with the question, "You are a man, aren't you?" is an example of subtly equating the drinking of the product with having an affair. Ads for automobiles often appeal to the need for dominance and power by their emphasis on the number of "horses" at the owner's command or with statements such as, "A man must be in control." The toothpaste ad that gives absolution to the negligent mother who fails to see to it that her children brush their teeth regularly, obviously appeals to her feeling of guilt. Most deodorant ads appeal to both sexual motives and fear of social ostracism. Having utilized powerful, and often unconscious, motives to create a desire to buy the product, effective advertising still requires providing the consumer with a good reason for buying. He needs an excuse for doing what he already unconsciously wants to do because all people like to believe that they behave rationally.

An example of psychological research in marketing involved an instant cake mix that could simply be mixed with water and baked to produce a delicious cake with little effort. Housewives, however, refused to buy this product and researchers were employed to investigate the reasons the product did not sell. They prepared two identical shopping lists, except for the inclusion of the instant cake mix on one, and asked a sample of housewives to rate the hypothetical woman who prepared the lists on a variety of attributes related to how good a wife and mother she was. They found that the housewife who prepared the list containing the instant cake mix was rated significantly poorer on most counts and they concluded that the cake mix was so easy to prepare that housewives felt guilty about using it. They therefore recommended packaging the product in a new container and changing the directions to include a fresh egg. Sales improved radically, for now the housewife was given an opportunity to contribute her efforts to the end product and protect her family by seeing to it that "the ingredients that should be fresh, are."

The use of hypnosis as an advertising technique to generate purchasing motivation rarely involves a direct trance induction. It usually involves the application of indirect waking suggestions in a manner similar to Erickson's style. Occasionally, however, examples of more direct methods can be observed. For example, one headache remedy was advertised in a metronome-like ad describing how "pain mounts up." This ad was invariably successful in triggering a migraine attack in an associate of the author who had to avoid watching the commercial.

Indirect suggestions are often made in the name of a product. Calling a perfume Tabu gives it a sexual connotation, for sex is also "tabu." Often indirect suggestions are made nonverbally in the form of body language, facial expression, and tone of voice. Since most human communication normally uses these modalities, the viewer is familiar with this language. Thus, he accepts uncritically messages that if expressed verbally would be instantly recognized as misleading, ridiculous, or even in violation of FCC standards for broadcasting. Often these nonverbal messages have no relationship to the spoken messages or may directly contradict them. A pair of gyrating hips in an advertised pair of jeans, or a protruding posterior in a seamless brief, convey a very different message than the associated verbal pronouncements concerning comfort and style.

The use of the hypnotic technique of having concrete images serve as symbols to represent abstract ideas can also be seen in many advertisements in the form of dramatizations. For example, pain may be depicted physically, or a calorie in food represented by a caricature of a demon.

The repetition of suggestions used in hypnosis is also used in advertising.

It has been found that repetition of a message with a slight change in motif (such as the omission of the final portion of a familiar ad) is particularly effective, possibly because of a Zeigarnik effect produced by the failure to provide the closure anticipated by the viewer.

Packard (1958) described the efforts made by marketing psychologists to capitalize on color and package design to create an attention-commanding hypnotic effect designed to make the product stand out from its competitors and encourage impulse buying. He described a study of eye-blinking rates of housewives in a supermarket that suggested that the effect of the supermarket environment is to induce a relaxed hypnoidal state in the shoppers, which may render them less critical in their purchasing behavior.

Perhaps the most valuable use of hypnosis in marketing is as an information-gathering device as opposed to influencing consumer behavior directly. Packard describes the use of hypnotic in-depth interviews to discover the unconscious attitudes of consumers toward products and what factors cause them to buy or avoid buying specific products.

There was concern for a while among both legislators and psychologists about the possible effectiveness of subliminal advertising. This is a technique whereby a target person is subjected to a subthreshold advertisement of which he is supposedly not consciously aware but which may affect his behavior. Research in this area typically utilizes a time limen and consists of flashing messages to the subject for a shorter period of time than is normally required for perception. The fear was that these messages would be able to motivate a person to buy a product or to take some action without his being consciously aware of the source of this motivation. Thus, he would be unable to use his higher mental processes in evaluating the desirability of his behavior. This is exactly what most psychologically oriented advertising attempts to do. The evidence, however, seems unimpressive that subliminal advertising has any effect at all. Its very name is a contradiction in terms. Those effects that have been produced in a small percentage of subjects might more parsimoniously be attributed to these people having a lower than average threshold, or to other factors relating to the failure of experimental controls. The fact that subjects in "perceptual defense" studies fail to repeat four-letter Anglo-Saxon words that are not normally used in polite society, when they are flashed on a screen for an interval long enough to produce measurable physiological responses, may indicate that the subjects are defending themselves by raising their time limens. It seems more likely to indicate that they are simply embarrassed to repeat these words or they doubt the accuracy of their own perceptions.

While subliminal advertising is probably not much of a danger, the reduction of the viewer's critical faculties is often accomplished by working advertising into the plot of a TV drama, either by having the actors use a brand name product or by means of background signs.

There is a pseudo-ethical issue in the use of hypnotic and other psychological techniques for such socially questionable purposes as motivating people to buy products that they may neither need nor want and often cannot afford. The reason that this is referred to as a pseudo-ethical question is that all science, by its nature, is basically amoral. It is a scientist's task to discover natural laws and learn what antecedents produce what consequences. The application of these principles, whether for socially acceptable or unacceptable ends, while of concern to a scientist as a citizen or as a practitioner of a profession, is irrelevant to his role as a scientist. Physicists have given us the potential for tapping almost limitless amounts of energy. They have also given us the capacity to terminate all life on earth either in a nuclear holocaust or more gradually through the poisoning of the environment. One thing seems certain; any scientific discovery that can be applied for practical ends will be, even when these ends are not universally thought to be good ones. This is a risk inherent in all research.

Hypnosis in Sports

A major part of an athlete's performance is a function of his mental state, which can be profoundly influenced by suggestions, both hypnotic and waking. One of the major functions of the sympathetic division of the autonomic nervous system (ANS) is the mobilization of bodily resources for emergency situations, enabling the organism to fight or flee more efficiently when angry or frightened. Increases of up to 33% in strength or endurance can be produced by the emotions of anger or fear. Hence, hypnotic or self-hypnotic suggestions are often used to "psych up" athletes prior to a performance. In addition to its use in mobilizing appropriate emotional responses, hypnosis is valuable in providing relaxation and increased self-confidence (Krenz, 1984). This is particularly important in athletic activities that require highly developed skills and concentration such as golf or archery. Kroger (1977b) improves the confidence of golfers in their putting ability by suggesting to them that the hole is the size of a sewer. Training in self-hypnosis is a valuable adjunct to the use of hypnosis in sports, and it renders hypnotic aid available to the athlete whenever needed. Heavyweight boxer Ken Norton habitually used self-hypnosis to prepare himself psychologically for a fight (Stevenson, 1978). Callen (1983) had 423 long-distance runners complete a questionnaire concerning their mental state and activities during running and found similarities between their thoughts and events commonly occurring during hypnosis. Fifty-four percent of respondents reported subjective feelings of being in an altered state of consciousness, which they produced by such methods as rhythmical breathing, repeating a phrase, counting, imagining music, or imagery. Fifty-nine percent claimed to be more creative while running, and 58%

engaged in imagery, often to improve their time or distance. Callen suggests the large population of runners is a valuable resource for the study of spontaneous self-hypnotic phenomena.

Simek and O'Brien (1981) used hypnosis to develop the mental state required for optimal performance in members of a collegiate fencing team and in a professional boxer. One fencer was given the effective suggestion that every opponent with whom she fenced would remind her of a rival for her boyfriend. Relaxation instructions were given to the boxer to deal with his anxiety, which was causing him to "freeze up" in the first round. These instructions were followed with suggestions that his opponent was responsible for all of his problems, to marshal anger.

Professional sports are major industries with large amounts of money dependent on successful team performances. Hence, organizations like major league baseball teams have not been hesitant to employ staff psychologists to deal with players' personal problems that may interfere with their job performance or to use hypnosis in the securing of peak performance from players. Rod Carew used hypnotism to improve his concentration at the plate. Eric Solderholm also used hypnosis to improve his hitting. Paul Blair, after being hit with a pitched ball, used hypnosis to deal with his fear of being hit again.

Although hypnosis may be an aid in optimizing an athlete's performance, it cannot create an ability that he does not have. A fighter may be made more aggressive by hypnotic suggestion but, if he cannot box well, hypnosis may result in his being hurt more than if he retained his more cautious boxing style. One major league pitcher who had problems with wild pitches and loss of control was aided by hypnosis in getting the ball over the plate more regularly, only to have the number of hits against him dramatically increase.

The use of hypnosis in sports, both professional and amateur, gives rise to ethical questions as to whether this is equivalent to psychologically drugging an athlete and whether the practice should be prohibited. It is theoretically possible to use pain-reducing suggestions to improve the performance of a runner or even to permit an athlete with an unhealed injury to play, in a manner analogous to drugging a racehorse that has an injured leg. There is a distinction, of course, between a racehorse and a human professional athlete who is able to understand the risks involved and provide an informed consent to the procedure. On the other hand, a high school or even a college athlete is often not mature enough to resist the pressure produced by feelings of "duty" to his teammates or school. He may thus be subjected to undue influence to consent to such an ill-advised procedure. The author regards the employment of hypnosis by a psychologist in such a case as both a violation of professional ethics and malpractice.

Proponents of the use of hypnosis with athletes argue that it is really nothing more than a more effective variation of a pep talk. They note that, as in all other hypnotic effects, it is the subject himself, not the hypnotist, who produces whatever results occur. The only effect of hypnotic suggestion is to produce the optimal performance of which the athlete is already capable. No new or artificial ability is created. They argue that the fans are entitled to see the best performance possible in a professional contest.

Hypnosis and ESP

There are a number of articles discussing a purported relationship between hypnosis and ESP phenomena that are cited here because they raise issues that require comment (Eisenberg, 1978; Fourie, 1981; Nash, 1982; Sargent, 1978; Shaposhnikov, 1982).

The author is not unprejudiced concerning the ESP literature. He tends to have a mechanistic view of the world and psychological phenomena. Thus, when someone talks about clairvoyance (communication from inanimate objects to people), telepathy (communication between people via non-sensory means) or psychokinetics (the influence of thoughts on inanimate objects), he would ask what is the medium of communication and upon what receptor it acts. This is not to say that research in ESP cannot be well designed and scientifically valid. Such research is respectable and it should be conducted, but it seems that if there were any basis for the belief that ESP phenomena are real, then the amount of such research conducted since the 1920s ought to have produced more convincing evidence than is currently available as well as some reasonable theory of the mechanisms involved.

Tests of statistical significance can never establish that a difference between an experimental and control group is not due to chance, only that the probability of it being so is at some given level. Thus, if there is only one chance in 100 that this difference occurred by chance, and the null hypothesis is rejected at the 0.01 level, this particular result may still be due to chance. If enough research is done, such spuriously significant results will occur.

Most journals are reluctant to publish nonsignificant findings unless they contradict previously published results (although it is just as much an increment of knowledge to learn that an independent variable does not produce an effect as it is to learn that it does). Thus, most research is tested at the 0.05 level of significance to make it easier to get it published. It therefore follows that fully 5% of the psychological and other scientific literature is spurious, reporting as real results that are actually due to chance.

Such spurious results are usually not replicable, but many journals will not publish replication studies, thereby preventing the necessary verification of results. To evaluate whether a particular experimental result found to be significant is in fact real, it would be helpful to know how many times this experiment was run without finding significance. This information is not generally available.

If a researcher proposes a view that is intrinsically reasonable, it is generally accepted in scientific circles that he or she has the burden of establishing this view by a certain amount of evidence. If the view advocated is contrary to all prior human experience and intrinsically unreasonable, then its proponents ought to have an even greater burden of proof imposed on them.

There may be a certain amount of heuristic value in much ESP research. For example, the author would be inclined to attribute Sargent's (1978) finding that a hypnosis group performed better than a waking control group in a clairvoyance task with ESP cards either to a greater sensitivity on the part of hypnotic subjects to subtle, unintended cues (which are not apparent in the report of the study) or to hypnotic relaxation and concentration facilitating the subjects "playing bridge" or counting the cards correctly guessed.

The problem with ESP research involving hypnosis is basically a public relations one. Most people regard ESP phenomena as having a supernatural basis, with the ordinary laws of the universe not applying. Hypnosis has suffered much in the past from its association with magic, mysticism, and the like, and even today many professional people have misgivings about its scientific validity because of these past associations. Hence, claims that hypnosis can enhance ESP abilities, like some extravagant claims for its clinical effectiveness, are likely to make many professionals leery of its use in situations where it may be quite appropriate and helpful.

Miscellaneous Applications of Hypnosis

Hypnosis has been used in education as a learning aid, and as a method of dealing with examination anxiety, and for self-improvement suggestions (e.g., of greater self-confidence) in social and business situations (Boutin, 1978; Cohen, 1979; Hebert, 1984; Porter, 1978; Spies, 1979; Wollman, 1978).

Cole (1979) found that hypnosis was no more effective in improving the academic performance of 31 students in a college preparation course (who were exposed to a 40-minute induction and deepening tape plus four subsequent 15-minute hypnotic tapes making suggestions of enhanced academic performance) than exposing students to control tapes making the same suggestions without hypnosis or lectures. These results are not particularly surprising. Hypnosis would not be expected to improve academic performance unless poor performance was caused by psychological factors (other than a low level of ability) and these factors were identified and addressed by the hypnotic technique used. Van Pelt (1975a, 1975b) suggested the use of hypnosis in business as a method of coping with interpersonal problems and in space travel to deal with boredom, nervous strain, and problems produced by weightlessness, interruption of sleep cycles, and space sickness. Christie (1982) discusses a variety of industrial uses of hypnosis, such as attitude change, performance facilitation, vocational counseling, advertising, and consumer research, both with and without formal trance induction.

Hypnotic phenomena play an indirect role in entertainment. Most members of a movie audience resemble people in a hypnotic trance. The movie itself probably functions similarly to the word picture painted by a hypnotist in a cognitive induction and detaches the audience members from their immediate surroundings. Good subjects trained in self-hypnosis can probably use this skill to enhance the vividness of the private fantasies in which all people engage. It is likely that creative people like authors or playwrights can use hypnotic fantasy productively to generate new ideas for their work. Robert Louis Stevenson got the idea for Dr. Jekyll and Mr. Hyde from a nocturnal dream (Dement, 1974). Hypnotic suggestions have not only been used to help actors assume a character but also to generate appropriate facial expressions in photographers' models (Kondreck, 1963).

Hypnosis even comes into play in modern religious life. Many people have had the experience of being so entranced by the charismatic style of a television evangelist that they listened captivated for an entire sermon without having had prior interest in the message being conveyed. Indeed, the ability to attract and hold the attention of an audience is much like a hypnotist's getting a subject to concentrate on a fixation object or instructing him to "attend only to the sound of my voice."

Matheson (1979b) points out the similarities between religious experiences and healing and hypnotic phenomena. Tappeiner (1977), a theologian who notes the operation of hypnotic factors in several varieties of religious experience, argues that the fact that religious phenomena can be explained in terms of hypnotic principles does not negate their spiritual validity, that is, God works through natural mechanisms.

The present author would agree that noticing the hypnotic qualities and techniques of an evangelist commits the observer to nothing regarding the spiritual validity of his message.

Walker (1984) notes the common factor of what he calls "inadequate religious attitudes," which can complicate psychotherapy, and suggests a role both for hypnosis and ministers of religion in an effort to correct these and facilitate therapy. This thought-provoking article suggests that perhaps psychotherapists, as part of their training, should be exposed to the major tenets of the various religious denominations, for guilt is commonly seen in patients with overly strict religious beliefs, and psychotherapists are often reluctant to address such issues. Perhaps if they were more knowledgeable concerning the beliefs of the major religious denominations, they might recognize when their patient's beliefs were idiosyncratic or "inappropriate" and when a consultation with a clergyman might prove helpful in correcting them (just as therapists are trained to recognize when a medical consultation is necessary).

Shepperson and Henslin (1984) and Andrich (1978) consider some of the historical objections to hypnosis raised by theologians and caused by the kinds of misconceptions discussed in Chapter 1.

The diverse applications of hypnosis discussed in this chapter tend to obscure the fact that hypnosis is basically a phenomenon rather than a technique. It would be strange indeed if a natural phenomenon like hypnosis did not occur often in daily life, but when it does occur naturally in such prosaic settings as the movies or while watching television, we usually fail to recognize a spontaneous trance for what it is. Sometimes naturally occurring trances can have unfortunate consequences, as in the case of highway hypnosis. Recognizing that effects of this nature can occur makes it possible for engineers to design cars and highways to minimize or eliminate such risks.

Training in self-hypnosis opens the door for the employment of hypnosis in many minor applications, such as the control of normal levels of anxiety before giving a speech or prior to an important business interview, where it would normally not be practical to incur the expense of a professional consultation.

While this chapter has considered some of the major applications of hypnosis, it is not possible to consider all of its potential uses, for these extend to any situation that requires relaxation; the stimulation of imagery, emotion or motivation; or the enhancement of the ability to concentrate on something and become detached from the environment.

CHAPTER 6

Self-Hypnosis

Self-hypnosis or autohypnosis is a procedure in which the subject both induces the hypnotic state and makes suggestions to himself. When self-hypnosis is to be employed as part of a therapeutic regimen, it is necessary for the therapist to train the patient in its use. Often training is done under heterohypnosis, and the initial self-inductions are aided by a posthypnotic signal to go into the hypnotic state. There is some experimental evidence that inexperienced subjects can hypnotize themselves about as well as they can be hypnotized by another person (Johnson and Weight, 1976; Ruch, 1975; Shor and Easton, 1973).

There is ambiguity, however, concerning the nature of the self-hypnosis procedures typically employed in such studies, involving, as they do, an experimenter giving a subject either initial verbal instructions or a booklet of directions on hypnotizing one's self, as well as a set of suggestions. There may be elements of both self-hypnosis and heterohypnosis present in such a procedure. The main value of heterohypnosis in training a subject to induce autohypnosis is not providing him with a posthypnotic signal for induction but in letting him experience the subjective feelings of the hypnotic state that he must seek to attain self-induction.

Shor (1970) developed a scale called an Inventory of Self-Hypnosis (ISH), patterned after form A of the Harvard Group Scale (HGSHS), which measures heterohypnotic susceptibility. Shor and Easton found that scores on the

ISH and the HGSHS correlated only 0.39; but Johnson and Weight (1976) point out that the reliabilities of these two instruments are 0.55 and 0.74, respectively, and, hence, the maximum possible correlation after correcting for attenuation would be only 0.64. Thus, Shor and Easton's results indicate some consistency in subject susceptibility to these two hypnotic modes. Generally, it appears that the same factors that are related to heterohypnotic susceptibility are involved in self-hypnotic susceptibility, and good subjects for heterohypnosis usually (not always) are good subjects for self-hypnosis. For example, Singer and Pope (1981) found that people involved in fantasy and imaginative activities are usually good subjects for self-hypnosis. J. Hilgard (1979) reported a similar conclusion for heterohypnosis and found that good subjects were involved in imagery, daydreaming, and absorption in reading or movies from early childhood.

The view is often expressed that all hypnosis is self-hypnosis because it is the subject's imagination that produces all of the effects in heterohypnosis. On the other hand, it could be argued that all hypnosis is basically heterohypnosis, and self-hypnotic effects result from posthypnotic suggestions given while training subjects in self-hypnosis. As early as 1928, Young researched this issue. He had hypnotic subjects instruct themselves prior to hypnosis to modify specific aspects of rapport behavior and posthypnotic amnesia. He found that subjects could do this successfully and concluded that there was no sine qua non of hypnosis. Posthypnotic amnesia was dependent on the subject's set or expectancy, and hypnotic behavior could be modified in many ways without affecting its depth. He concluded that the essential element in heterohypnosis was the autosuggestion of the subject.

Ruch (1975) also supports the notion that active self-hypnosis is the primary phenomenon and that heterohypnosis is, in effect, a case of guided self-hypnosis. He found that initial self-hypnosis facilitated subsequent heterohypnosis but that conventional heterohypnosis (of a passive subject by an active hypnotist) inhibited later attempts at self-hypnosis. This inhibitory effect was eliminated when "first-person instructions" were used in heterohypnosis. That is, instead of saying to the subject, "I am going to give you suggestions to help you to relax," the experimenter would say, "I am going to give myself instructions to help me relax." Thus the subject was able to regard the hypnotist's voice as his own, making suggestions to himself.

Ruch's view of the primacy of self-hypnosis is contrary to the conventional idea that heterohypnosis is an aid in training a person in self-hypnosis. It is premature to say whether the foregoing results are generalizable or are limited to the particular induction procedures tested. However, it seems questionable to label the procedure used as self-hypnosis, since, in the initial instructions, the experimenter made suggestions concerning the sequence of events that were to occur and then left the subject to count to himself and experience them. This is similar to the Flower method of heterohypnosis in which all instructions to the subject are massed at the beginning of the induction. For an induction to qualify as an example of true autohypnosis, the subject should be responsible for all elements of the induction, and the hypnotist should make no suggestions of any kind beyond requesting the subject to commence the procedure.

Johnson (1981) notes that any study of self-hypnosis must be contaminated to some degree by heterohypnotic influence unless the study is limited to spontaneously developed trance states.

Gardner (1981) proposed making a distinction between self-hypnosis (which she used to indicate self-hypnosis preceded or aided by heterohypnosis) and autohypnosis (which referred to spontaneous autohypnosis with no prior heterohypnosis). However, since these two terms are generally used interchangeably, such a distinction will probably prove as futile as the distinction between susceptibility and hypnotizability made in this book. If such distinctions are to be made (and they probably should be), then perhaps it will be necessary to coin new terms.

Most researchers have found few, if any, differences in success in inducing self-hypnosis as a function of previous heterohypnotic experience (Johnson, 1979; Kroger, 1977a; LeCron, 1964; Sacerdote, 1981; Shor and Easton, 1973). Sacerdote (1981) points out that with the modern trend toward more permissive inductions, the distinction between heterohypnosis and self-hypnosis is becoming vaguer.

Fromm (1975) notes that until recently, most of the serious research in hypnosis was in heterohypnosis; the literature of self-hypnosis was often the product of "quacks and laymen." She questioned on theoretical grounds the common assumption that heterohypnosis and self-hypnosis are basically the same and undertook to investigate the similarities and differences between the two. She conceptualizes hypnosis as an ego-splitting process. In heterohypnosis, the ego splits into two parts: the experimenter (participating ego) and the observer (observing ego). In autohypnosis, the ego splits into three parts: the experimenter and observer plus a director who gives the hypnotic instructions and suggestions. She found that in some subjects, a third or fourth aspect of the ego, a skeptic, was also present.

In a preliminary study, Fromm gave 18 males and 18 females one session each of heterohypnotic and autohypnotic experiences using a counterbalanced order of presentation. The 12 least-susceptible subjects described both experiences as essentially the same, but the 24 most-susceptible subjects described subjective differences between the experiences. Idiosyncratic fantasy and visual imagery arose spontaneously with a much higher frequency in autohypnosis. There was also more rational, cognitive activity going on in this condition, and subjects were unanimous in reporting the greater number of ego splits predicted. Autohypnosis was found, as predicted, to require more effort on the part of the subjects.

Some subjects were able to reach a deeper state under heterohypnosis, while others went deeper under autohypnosis. Fromm accounts for this difference in terms of differences between subjects with respect to their need for surrender versus their need for autonomy and control. In a second study, three males and three females were instructed to practice self-hypnosis once a day for a month. Subjects were required to keep a daily diary of their experiences and were interviewed by telephone every few days. They were also subjected to two interviews plus a follow-up group discussion one month after the study.

Fromm found that with practice, self-inductions were easier to achieve. Eventually subjects began to employ methods of induction exclusively of their own design. Some used dissociative methods, such as producing an arm levitation by forgetting about the arm or commanding it to rise. Others simply "let go" and developed a passive-receptive ego state. After 2 or 3 weeks, most subjects who did not incorporate self-hypnosis into their life-style became bored with the procedure and had to be coaxed to continue the experiment. One of the causes of this problem was thought to be the tendency of prolonged self-hypnosis to reduce the transference with the experimenter. It was found that imagery was stimulated to a much greater extent in self-hypnosis but that some effects, such as positive hallucinations, profound ego regression, and role playing, were easier to produce in heterohypnosis.

The major advantage claimed for self-hypnosis in this study was that the subject was always attuned to his own responses during induction, and hence suggestions could be optimally timed. An outside hypnotist can at best make an educated guess as to the subject's subjective state. Johnson and Weight (1976), using factor analysis, found that behavioral and subjective experiences of subjects under heterohypnosis and self-hypnosis were generally similar. However, heterohypnosis invoked more feelings of unawareness of the environment, passivity, and loss of control, while autohypnosis was associated with more feelings of time distortion, disorientation, active control, and variations of trance depth.

In a later longitudinal study, Fromm and her associates (1981) essentially confirmed her earlier results. They concluded that "expansive free-floating attention" and ego receptivity to internal stimuli were state-specific for self-hypnosis, while concentrated attention and receptivity to a single external source of stimuli were state-specific for heterohypnosis. Again imagery was found to be much richer in self-hypnosis, while suggestions of age regression or positive and negative hallucinations were markedly more effective in heterohypnosis.

As noted by Johnson (1981) and Orne and McConkey (1981), there are both important similarities and differences between self-hypnosis and heterohypnosis, and to a large extent the design of the research tends to emphasize one or the other of these two factors. Thus, research measuring behavior tends to emphasize the overall similarities, while studies assessing experiential factors tend to highlight differences. Johnson (1979) found that while self-hypnosis produced more feeling of time distortion, active direction, and variation of trance depth, subjective experiences and behavioral scores were comparable for the two forms of hypnosis, and, hence, they are similar enough to be "conceptualized under the same label." Since subjects in this study were not selected on the basis of susceptibility, it is not possible to compare these results with Fromm's (1975) work in which self-hypnotic or heterohypnotic states were compared in high-susceptibility subjects.

Johnson, Dawson, Clark and Sikorsky (1983) found that if two sessions of hypnosis were used, there was a general decrement effect in the second hypnotic session regardless of whether the second session involved self-hypnosis or heterohypnosis, but the initial use of self-hypnosis mitigated this decrement, as did switching from one mode to the other. As in previously reported studies, there was no main effect of the sex of the hypnotist, nor did this factor interact with either the order of presentation of the two modes of hypnosis or the sex of the subject.

Frankel (1975) compared a variety of techniques that have been used to induce a relaxation response: hypnosis, transcendental meditation, autogenic training, Zen, and yoga. Most of these, like autohypnosis, are self-induced states. Although Frankel believes that it is premature to conclude that these are all different names for the same phenomenon, he points out four elements that these techniques share: (1) a fixation of attention on either an external object or a mental image; (2) the development of a passive attitude, ignoring distracting thoughts and environmental stimuli; (3) decreased muscle tone; and (4) a quiet, nondistracting atmosphere gives optimal results.

Several good hypnotic subjects who practiced transcendental meditation have told the author, subsequent to an initial hypnotic session, that the subjective effects of hypnosis were identical to those experienced in meditation. Although, it is only an unverified impression, the fact that many people who practice meditation seem to make excellent hypnotic subjects suggests a very close relationship, if not an identity, between meditation and self-hypnosis. It seems probable that a mantra (the secret phrase that a meditator is taught to concentrate on) is a conditioned stimulus for rapid trance induction.

Milton Erickson's original experience with hypnosis appears to date back to early in his life and to have involved spontaneous self-hypnosis. The probable influence of these early experiences on the subsequent development of his unique therapeutic approach can be seen in his interview with Rossi (Erickson and Rossi, 1977).

ADVANTAGES AND DISADVANTAGES
OF SELF-HYPNOSIS

Many of the practical advantages of autohypnosis have been alluded to in the previous chapter. These advantages include the following:

1. Reducing demands on the therapist's time by diminishing the number and frequency of required heterohypnotic sessions.
2. Providing the patient with the benefits of hypnotic suggestions whenever required and without regard to the availability of the hypnotist.
3. Lessening the intensity of the transference relationship when this is desirable. (This can be a double-edged sword, for often psychotherapy will require the intensification rather than the weakening of this reaction).
4. Developing the patient's sense of self-mastery and control and an ego-building feeling of independence.
5. Employing autohypnosis as a safety valve against the danger of premature attack on a defense still needed by the patient. This permits him to decide whether he is ready to relinquish his symptom.
6. Using self-hypnosis as a way of focusing on the patient's role and his prime responsibility for the progress of his own therapy. This may be its most important function for many patients.

The disadvantages of self-hypnosis are few and relate mainly to its weakening of a desirable transference relationship. Also, the therapist has necessarily given up direct control over the therapeutic suggestions to be made. This may be a positive or a negative factor, depending on the particular case. Some therapists have expressed concern about how the patient will use self-hypnosis once he is instructed in it (Maher-Loughnan, 1975), but it seems that these fears are based more on groundless (and often vaguely perceived) beliefs in the magical potency of hypnotic suggestions than in the realities of the situation. Training subjects in self-hypnosis is a common and accepted procedure in hypnotherapy and one that appears extremely unlikely to produce any adverse effects. The use of self-hypnosis in psychotherapy is by no means a method of self-treatment in the conventional sense of this term. The therapist will carefully instruct the patient as to the type of suggestions to be employed. A patient trained in self-hypnosis is given no ability or propensity to make harmful suggestions to himself that he did not always possess. Self-hypnotic training has been used with children and severely disturbed adult patients without any report of untoward incidents that the author is aware of.

Some therapists attempt to prevent problems, particularly with young patients, by imposing posthypnotic conditions on the occasions when, or the purposes for which, self-hypnosis is to be employed. For example, Maher-Loughnan (1975) suggested to children that they would use self-hypnosis only at home when a parent was present. Although the necessity for such suggestions may be questionable, it is difficult to criticize a therapist for being cautious. However, just as the dangers may be more imagined than real, so too may be the effect of such attempted safeguards. Trance-limiting suggestions would be expected to have varying degrees of effectiveness with different patients, although their effectiveness with a particular patient would diminish with the passage of time and the development of proficiency in self-hypnosis.

Suggestions made to an adult without his prior consent that are designed to limit his future susceptibility to hypnosis, except for "therapeutic or research purposes" by a specified subgroup of hypnotists, are an unethical and outrageous interference with his right to freedom of choice.

Another limitation of autohypnosis is that it requires motivation on the part of the patient to practice daily in order to develop skill in the technique. As suggested by Fromm, this can become tedious. Many patients in psychotherapy will not make the effort required to be successful at it. On the other hand, medical patients taught self-hypnosis to control intractable pain are much more likely to be motivated to do the required homework by their need for relief.

Gardner (1981) says that the indications and contraindications for teaching self-hypnosis to children are the same as for adult patients. Self-hypnosis with children is appropriate in cases where daily practice is needed to reinforce appropriate new behaviors, control pain, extend insights, or if the child is likely to encounter emergencies (e.g., an asthmatic attack). It is also appropriate to enhance feelings of control and self-esteem. Gardner believes that self-hypnosis may be contraindicated for acting-out children or children with poor judgment or impulse control. The contraindications for self-hypnosis training are, in general, the same as those for heterohypnosis. Some of these will be discussed in the next chapter under the rubric of problems in hypnosis.

TECHNIQUES OF AUTOHYPNOSIS

Just as there are a great number of ways of inducing heterohypnosis, there is also almost no limit to the varieties of autohypnotic techniques. Some of the works listed in the References and Bibliography of this book that were addressed to lay audiences provide an idea of this variety. It is improbable, however, that even a good subject would be successful in inducing self-hypnosis as a result of reading a book. What is generally required is personal training by a hypnotist, and this always includes some degree of heterohypnosis, whether in the form of a formal trance induction or in the form of helpful suggestions and supervision. An example of a self-hypnosis training procedure that the author has found effective (and which the reader may modify as he desires, to meet the requirements of his own personality and the needs of his patients) will now be described.

If a subject is to be trained in self-hypnosis by means of heterohypnosis, this should be taken into account in the selection of the heterohypnotic in-duction procedure. Specifically, hypnosis should be attempted in the most permissive manner possible and the subject's own role in producing all of the hypnotic phenomena emphasized. Following the induction phase, time should be spent in deepening the trance as much as possible so that the subject can experience the subjective feelings accompanying hypnosis. These feelings should be suggested to be pleasant and positive ones. The fact that the subject is always in control of what he thinks, feels, and does and is in no way under the control of the hypnotist should also be made clear. After the subject has had a chance to experience and enjoy the deep relaxation of the hypnotic state and his fears of the new experience have been allayed, he should be told that he can reproduce this pleasant, secure, relaxed state whenever he desires, without the aid of the hypnotist, by going through an induction ritual that he is then taught.

The particular ritual described is not important. Few subjects will be able to go into a self-hypnotic state instantly on a posthypnotic signal, and it is preferable to give the subject an induction ritual that permits him to enter the state gradually. For example, he may be told to say to himself: "When I reach the count of 10, I will be in a very deep, relaxed, hypnotic state," and then to start counting. Whatever posthypnotic quality may result from giving these instructions under hypnosis will aid the subject in his early efforts, but the method does not depend on posthypnotic suggestion and could be taught to a waking subject as well. Even in the latter case, however, a previous hyp-notic induction is desirable to permit the subject to experience the state he is trying to produce.

The subject should also be instructed, while still under hypnosis, to per-form all self-hypnosis in a quiet, private place and to sit or lie comfortably in a position appropriate for heterohypnosis before commencing. The subject should be told that following the self-induction, he can make the same kind of deepening suggestions to himself that the hypnotist has used. One or two of these techniques should be described to him. He should be told that each time he induces hypnosis, it will be easier, and he will go deeper than the last time. A good practice is to train a subject in a self-induction technique related to the one by which he has been successfully hypnotized since he will have experience and confidence in such a method. Thus, if heterohypnosis was induced by an arm levitation, the subject can be trained to levitate his arm to induce hypnosis. In the initial induction, the hypnotist will elect the method he or she believes will be easiest for the subject, and, if it is successful, will use it as the basis of the self-induction method to be taught. If the hypnotist had difficulty with the method originally attempted and had to switch to another technique to induce a trance, then he or she will also have to modify the self-induction procedure taught.

The subject should be told that following self-induction and deepening, he will be able to make any desired suggestions to himself, just as an external hypnotist could. He is then told that when he is finished making the suggestions, he is to awaken himself by the use of a simple formula, such as counting to 3, to ensure a comfortable and gradual return to the waking state. It should be suggested that he will never experience any unpleasant after effects of hypnosis, such as headache, muscle cramp, or a feeling of numbness, and that if any emergency occurs while he is under hypnosis, he will instantly awaken and be able to deal with the situation. Just how effective this latter suggestion is, or whether the same result would not occur without it, is uncertain, but it is never a mistake to err on the side of caution. Just making such a suggestion may have the effect of putting some of a subject's unspoken fears to rest.

After explaining the procedure to the subject under hypnosis and ensuring that he understands what is required of him, the subject should be returned to the waking state. Any additional questions he may have should be answered, and then he should immediately be given the opportunity to try out the procedure with the hypnotist present. The subject should be told to go ahead and induce the hypnotic state by himself, enjoy the pleasant, relaxed feeling for a few minutes, and then awaken himself. It is useful to tell him to raise his hand when he has attained a state as deep as or deeper than that induced by the hypnotist so that the instructor-hypnotist can gauge the subject's progress.

The immediate practice of the self-hypnotic procedure makes it most likely to succeed because it capitalizes on the subject's heightened expectancy produced by the successful heterohypnosis. It also permits any misunderstandings or problems to be corrected while the hypnotist is present to supervise the procedure. If the patient reports he is unable to produce hypnosis by himself it may be helpful to point out to him that he has already proved that he can do it (under heterohypnosis), for he and not the hypnotist was responsible for whatever effects were obtained.

Following the successful completion of this exercise, the subject should be told that he must practice the procedure one or more times daily to attain proficiency in it and to reinforce the therapeutic suggestions that he has been instructed to make to himself. These will be specific to the patient's treatment plan but may additionally include general positive suggestions of well-being. These final instructions give the hypnotist the opportunity to repeat his suggestion, this time while the subject is in the waking state, that with each subsequent induction, the subject will go deeper. (For examples of other variations in the teaching of patients to induce or utilize self-hypnosis, see Garver, 1984, and Sacerdote, 1984).

If self-hypnotic suggestions are part of a patient's treatment plan, the patient should always be the one to induce the trance state, even in hetero-hypnotic sessions in the therapist's office. The therapist can thus monitor the patient's technique, and it motivates the latter to do his homework, for in effect,he is being tested on his performance.

Once a patient masters the generation of an autohypnotic state, he is free to modify it in a variety of useful ways. For example, he can learn to induce this state with his eyes open and without any external indications of being hypnotized. He can then induce a brief trance in a public place without attracting attention to himself, a useful skill should he have a need for an immediate, supportive self-suggestion, such as one to diminish a desire he may be experiencing to smoke a cigarette while trying to stop smoking (Spiegel, 1974a).

If a patient is unable to learn self-hypnosis because he is unwilling to devote the time necessary for practice (or for any other reason) but is a good enough subject for heterohypnosis, some of the advantages of self-hypnosis (such as the daily repetition of therapeutic suggestions) may be attainable by making a tape recording for the patient to listen to at home. These tapes should be tailor-made for the requirements of a particular patient, and ideally they should be made during an actual hypnotic session with the patient so that suggestions may be timed in response to the patient's reactions. If the issue of control is important to a patient, it may be worthwhile to have him prepare the tape himself from a script. This sort of tape may lack the professional quality of one made by the therapist and may not be optimally timed, but it has the advantage of requiring a patient who resents being controlled by others to follow no one else's suggestions but his own.

Much of the potential of self-hypnosis or heterohypnosis to benefit a patient may reside in the opportunity it affords him to detach himself from the external world and devote his full attention to a consideration of the positive ideas and suggestions presented. Not only are these ideas focused on intensely, but, because of their careful selection in consultation with the therapist, they are less likely to be the trivial or negative type of ideation that Barber claims is typical of most people's routine thought processes.

In addition to teaching a patient how to induce self-hypnosis, the therapist must train him or her in the preparation of the suggestions to be employed in this state. In general, these should be carefully thought out and planned by the patient prior to the induction (just as heterosuggestions should) to avoid disruption of the trance state. They should emphasize the benefits being sought rather than the negative aspects of the symptom and should be made with an attitude of belief and expectancy. Self-hypnosis provides more than the opportunity to reinforce suggestions made during heterohypnotic sessions; it permits the patient to expand and enlarge on these, drawing from his own resources, and to internalize these new outlooks and attitudes (Eisen and Fromm, 1983).

Although the use of hypnoanesthesia is not unusual, Rausch (1980), a dentist who uses hypnosis in his work, published a report on his own cholecystectomy using self-hypnosis as the sole anesthetic with a surgical team inexperienced in hypoanesthesia. The principal reason for this mode of anesthesia was Rausch's desire to experience hypnoanesthesia. It was completely successful and was followed by a rapid recovery.

There are styles in psychological research just as there are styles in clothing, and in recent years much has been published concerning death and dying. It was inevitable that attention would begin to be focused on the survivors and the mourning process. Studies in both areas have much broader implications than the issue of death and many of the findings may be applicable to reactions to any other major loss, such as divorce or chronic disease.

Fromm and Eisen (1982) describe three stages of the mourning process: (1) denial of the reality of the loss, (2) a period of turmoil and hypercathexes of memory, and (3) detachment of libido from the lost love object and the formation of new relationships. They contend that self-hypnosis may aid the adjustment of the bereaved by its capacity to stimulate primary process imaging and evoke affective rather than intellectual responses.

Handelsman (1984), on the other hand, takes the position that the value of self-hypnosis in facilitating the mourning process resides in its ability to increase feelings of self-efficacy rather than its ability to enhance imagery. Probably both factors and others are involved, and the predominant ones may prove to be a function of the individual patient and the therapeutic approach employed. The important point is that there is a consensus of opinion that mourning is essential to working through feelings of grief, anger, and abandonment attending a death or other major loss. Hypnosis or self-hypnosis should be used to facilitate such a process and speed the transition to a new life without the lost love object rather than simply to suppress the initial painful feelings.

A noteworthy technique in the use of self-hypnosis to control chronic pain proposed by Fogel (1984) seems appropriate for patients who may equate self-hypnosis with abandonment by the therapist. This technique consists of instructing the patient to imagine himself talking to a sympathetic listener (a "sympathetic ear") who is eager to hear all of his symptoms, feelings, and complaints. This technique of internal ventilation produced substantial pain relief in the two patients presented.

In recent years, a variety of reports have appeared that question the common clinical opinion that susceptibility is not a major factor in hypnotic or self-hypnotic pain relief (Sacerdote, 1978; D. Spiegel, 1980). The present author suspects that the conflicting clinical results on this issue may be due to the subtle communication by the clinician to the patient of his or her expectations for success or failure. This factor requires investigation prior to forming any conclusion as to which side of this controversy is correct.

A listing of the types of conditions for which self-hypnosis was employed in treatment would include every problem for which heterohypnosis was used. Gardner (1981) has published such a list of problems of children from 3 to 20 years of age who were treated with self-hypnosis. This sampling may reassure some therapists reluctant to use self-hypnosis on child patients, even when it would be appropriate, for fear the child may misuse the technique.

Kohen, Olness, Colwell and Heimel (1984) report on the use of self-hypnosis, based on relaxation-mental imagery exercises (RMI), which capitalize on children's skill in imagery, to treat 505 children and adolescents ranging in age from 3 to 20. These patients presented with such problems as enuresis, asthma, headache, habit disorders, encopresis, anxiety, pain, and obesity. Some needed self-hypnosis as an aid to pelvic examinations. Overall 51% of these patients achieved complete resolution of the presenting problem, and another 32% attained significant improvement. Considering the short attention span and limited verbal ability of a typical 3-year-old, the successful use of self-hypnosis in this age group probably requires an unusually skilled and experienced therapist as well as a bright child.

PROBLEMS WITH SELF-HYPNOSIS

Baker (1983c), noting the increased use of hypnosis with patients with preoedipal pathology (narcissistic, borderline, or psychotic), suggests that permissive techniques and self-hypnosis are most appropriate because they decrease the patient's feeling of vulnerability and foster a sense of self-control. However, he finds that such patients sometimes become resistant to self-hypnosis because they associate it with object loss or a sense of abandonment. He advocates the use of dream induction with such patients and likens dreams to a transitional object in linking inner and outer reality and the past with the present. Thus, the constant availability of the therapist through a dream mitigates the patient's fear of loss.

Citing arguments that multiple personality disorders are created and maintained by spontaneous self-hypnosis, Miller (1984) argues that in such cases, the self-hypnosis may also function as a resistance against fusion to protect the patient from feelings of guilt. He cites a clinical example in support of this position. Unfortunately, the case involved a criminal prosecution, and thus the issue of self-hypnosis as a resistance was complicated by the possibility of both secondary gains and deception even after conviction.

A more interesting problem with self-hypnosis was reported by Smith and Kamitsuka (1984). A 13-year-old girl with leukemia had been taught self-hypnosis to control headaches, anxiety, and the effects of medical procedures. On admission to a hospital, her unannounced use of self-hypnosis for symptom control produced neurological symptoms that were misdiagnosed by the staff (who were unaware of the self-hypnosis) as a possible sign of central nervous system deterioration. This case suggests that patients trained to use self-hypnosis ought to be instructed to inform the staffs of hospitals when they are using it in such settings.

Once trained in self-hypnosis for therapeutic purposes, the patient is free to use the method for a variety of other purposes, including the making of suggestions for self-improvement, greater self-confidence, and, if he desires, the enrichment of his own private fantasy life. Holloway and Donald (1982) describe a self-hypnosis group organized by a college counseling center to provide this type of benefit to a non-patient population of students. This use is reminiscent of Perle's view that there may be benefits of psychotherapy for essentially normal people in providing them with better self-understanding, new experiences, and increased richness of living.

To therapists who believe that extensions of the application of autohypnosis beyond the uses contemplated in therapy are undesirable and thus a risk inherent in this method of treatment, it can only be said that it is hard to conceive of anything more demeaning to a patient than the notion that he cannot be trusted with control over his own thought processes.

CHAPTER 7

Psychological, Legal, and Legislative Problems and Alleged Dangers of Hypnosis

This chapter will discuss some of the problems that occur with reasonable frequency in the employment of hypnosis or about which some writers have expressed concern. The opinions of experts concerning the degree of risk in the practice of hypnosis vary widely. They range from those maintaining there is little or no risk of any kind (Conn, 1972; Erickson, 1939a) to those claiming that hypnosis, particularly in incompetent hands, may present many substantial dangers (Kleinhauz and Beran, 1981, 1984; Rosen, 1960a; West and Deckert, 1965). Some of the statements concerning the dangers of hypnosis found in the literature seem unduly alarmist in view of the data presented to support them. Actually there is very little conflict in the data. It is in the interpretation of the data that conflict exists. If an untoward event follows the application of hypnosis in therapy, there are several questions that must be answered in evaluating its significance. First, is there a causal connection between the hypnotherapy and the adverse reaction? If this question can be answered in the affirmative (and often it cannot be answered one way or the other), the next issue raised is how much of this effect has been caused by the hypnosis per se and how much has resulted from either the specific suggestions made or from the interpersonal relationship present in any therapeutic situation. These questions are not easy to answer and must be taken into account in the design of research examining this issue.

Fortunately, those untoward reactions that most commonly follow hypnosis tend to be minor, self-limited sequelae that are easy to deal with. The more serious reactions referred to in the literature are much rarer, and it is questionable that they are primarily due to hypnosis.

The undesirable effects and problems of hypnosis to be considered in this chapter will be of a psychological or a legal nature, or both. Usually with psychological problems, the "danger," if any, of a procedure is primarily to the subject; in legal problems, it is principally to the hypnotist. This separation is, of course, not complete; an adverse reaction that resulted from the failure of the therapist to exhibit the degree of skill common to competent members of his or her profession would meet the legal definition of malpractice. Thus it would be a problem for the hypnotist, as well as the subject. Also, the question of whether a hypnotic subject can be induced to engage in self-destructive or antisocial behavior against his will necessarily involves both psychological and legal issues.

PSYCHOLOGICAL PROBLEMS IN HYPNOSIS

Some of the minor problems of hypnosis have already been discussed. They sometimes result from carelessness on the part of the hypnotist and can usually be prevented by the use of proper technique. They include delayed effects of posthypnotic or uncancelled hypnotic suggestions, misunderstanding by the subject of the suggestions made, and the rare difficulties encountered in the termination of hypnosis.

All hypnotic suggestions given during a session that are not intended to affect posthypnotic behavior should be cancelled prior to terminating hypnosis, even if the subject did not appear to accept them. Subjects should be tested in the waking state prior to being dismissed to ensure that these suggestions have in fact been cancelled. The evidence is that in most cases the subject himself will cancel these suggestions, but it is better not to rely on his implicit understanding that the suggestions were not meant to outlast the session.

Because of the literalness with which most hypnotic subjects react to suggestions, hypnotists should always avoid the use of idiomatic expressions that, if taken literally, would produce results different from those sought. (For example, a patient told to "Let her hair down" and describe how she really feels about something may actually undo her hair arrangement.) Particular care is required when making suggestions to subjects with limited ability in English who are foreign born, uneducated, or of low intelligence. Precautions must also be taken to ensure that a child patient understands the suggestions clearly. Often very bright children give the hypnotist the illusion that he or she is dealing with a small adult; but even bright children may not understand some words in a suggestion.

Orne (1965*a*) notes that amateurs are the hypnotists most likely to have difficulty with subjects refusing to terminate a hypnotic state, probably because such a reaction is an ideal passive-aggressive response on the part of a subject who has become angry at the hypnotist. The reason that professionals using hypnosis rarely get such reactions is that they fail to reinforce them by getting upset, as does a suddenly frightened and terrified amateur hypnotist.

The possibility of problems with symptom substitution has also been previously discussed. It should be noted that this is not properly considered a problem of hypnosis but is a problem of any type of psychotherapy that seeks to directly remove a symptom having a dynamic value to the patient. Some symptoms may have such value; many do not. There is no general agreement as to what percentage of symptoms fall into either category. The significance of a particular symptom in an individual patient is always a matter of clinical judgment on the part of the therapist.

The remaining psychological problems to be considered here are those reactions that occur either during or immediately after hypnosis and are usually discussed under the rubric of sequelae.

Orne (1965*a*) finds both qualitative and quantitative differences in the types of hypnotic sequelae seen in the laboratory and in therapeutic settings. If the hypnosis is perceived by the subject as episodic and he has no expectation of permanent change, there are very few sequelae, and any that do occur are of a minor nature. This is the case in laboratory research, where the emphasis is impersonal and on the phenomena studied, not the subject, or in dental treatment where effects are also perceived by the subject as temporary.

In experimental work with thousands of "normal college students," in a setting specifically defined as experimental and with subjects told that no treatment, however minor, would be given, Orne reports virtually no serious reactions to hypnosis. Anxiety reactions, symptom formations, depressions, or decompensations, which have occasionally been reported in clinical contexts did not occur. The complications that did appear were such minor disturbances as an occasional mild and transient headache, drowsiness, nausea, or dizziness. If these complications occur, they typically do so on the first induction and are easily suggested away. The incidence of such reactions was reported by Orne to be from 2% to 3%, which is in close agreement with J. Hilgard's (1965) findings. Orne points out that due to the superficial screening of his subjects and the large numbers of them, it is quite likely that some of them may have had serious psychopathology. Since these results were in an experimental context, they are more likely to reflect the effects of hypnosis per se than the effects of either a therapeutic relationship or therapeutic suggestion, and these results suggest that hypnosis itself is a safe procedure. Orne further notes that although minor problems experienced by amateur hypnotists might be concealed, it would be hard for them to hide major problems. Although major problems can occur, they are quite rare, in spite of the incompetence and irresponsibility of the hypnotist. This scarcity of untoward reactions is probably due to the episodic and nontherapeutic nature of the hypnotic session.

The low incidence of serious aversive reactions in experimental work is in contrast to their relatively high incidence in the reports of experienced clinicians. Levitt and Hershman (1961, 1963) surveyed 866 hypnotherapists and found that about 27% of the 301 respondents reported observing major or minor untoward reactions to hypnosis, including anxiety, panic, depression, headache, crying, vomiting, fainting, dizziness, excessive dependency, and eight cases of sexual difficulties and psychotic behavior. Forty-three percent of the psychologists (as compared to 27% of the other respondents) reported these difficulties. J. Hilgard (1974) notes that often the more experienced hypnotists reported the most problems.

Orne (1965a) and Conn(1972) interpret this finding quite differently. Conn believes the prevalence of sequelae reflects an incompetence on the part of the hypnotist, who failed either to dehypnotize subjects properly or to screen them adequately prior to hypnosis. Orne, on the other hand, suggests that only the better-trained therapists adequately observed and recorded sequelae.

Wineburg and Straker (1973) report an acute, self-limiting depersonalization reaction in a 26-year-old female paraprofessional hospital worker. This woman was used as a demonstration subject in a hospital training course in hypnosis and was given weight reduction suggestions. They believe that the adverse reaction was due to the subject's misconceptions about hypnosis and the fear that it could weaken superego controls over her sexual fantasies. The authors recommend that to prevent reactions such as this, all patients should be observed after hypnotic treatment. Moreover, the patients' beliefs and expectations concerning hypnosis should be investigated beforehand, at which time they should be given an explanation of the true nature of hypnosis. This type of reaction, although certainly a risk in hypnotherapy, seems clearly to be the result not of hypnosis but of the patient's fears and intrapersonal dynamics. It should be preventable by an adequate consideration of these factors prior to and during hypnosis. Straker (1973) presents two other cases in which patients developed emotional upsets during a therapeutic induction because of intrapersonal dynamic reasons. In one instance, the induction resulted in a rapid regression and enhanced transference that flooded the patient with childhood memories of early fears and recurrent nightmares. In the other instance, a hypnotic induction took on the significance of a sexual attack to a 36-year-old female patient because of her previous beliefs about hypnosis. This resonated with earlier rape fantasies, greatly upsetting her. These types of reactions are not different from those obtained in ordinary psychotherapy, but the fostering of regression and transference by hypnosis can make them occur more rapidly and dramatically and give the illusion that they are caused primarily by hypnosis.

Sometimes the unusual nature of the hypnotic state causes even an experienced therapist to forget that a hypnotic induction does not cause all of the usual principles of human behavior and interaction to cease to operate. As an illustration, Orne (1965a) cites the case of a dentist whose wife was constantly asking him to hypnotize her for weight reduction suggestions, which he steadfastly refused to do. Instead, he insisted that she see a physician to get diet recommendations. The dentist finally relented and hypnotized his wife, but, instead of making weight loss suggestions, he made the suggestion that she would see her doctor. This suggestion was unsuccessful and resulted in the formation of a minor symptom. The idea of consulting a doctor was unacceptable to this woman in the waking state, and it was equally unacceptable under hypnosis.

Rosen (1960a) cited clinical examples of what he considered to be very serious dangers of hypnosis. These included the development of psychoses and a suicide following the hypnotic removal of phantom limb or low back pain and pruritus. He believes that pain that persists for emotional reasons may be a depressive equivalent and hold a severe depression in check. He is quite critical of weekend hypnotic courses touting hypnosis as an uncovering device and believes that neither uncovering techniques nor regressions are safe in the hands of persons ignorant of psychodynamics. Although it is hard to disagree with his contention that no one should treat a patient under hypnosis beyond his competence to treat him while awake, it is equally hard to agree with his view concerning the dangers of hypnosis. The cases he cited are clinical examples and as such cannot establish the causal agency of either the hypnosis or the symptom removal in producing the sequelae claimed. The fact that a psychosis follows hypnosis does not logically demonstrate that it was caused by the hypnosis. Conn (1972), after 30 years of practicing hypnotherapy on over 3,000 patients, denies ever seeing a psychosis precipitated by hypnosis. Also, even if such causality could be established, it seems clear that the cause of adverse reactions reported is less likely to be the hypnosis than the method of psychotherapy. These cases really relate to the issue of symptom substitution, not hypnosis, and the weight of the literature does not support the view that symptom substitution involving new, psychotic, or life-threatening symptoms is a high-risk phenomenon (Wolpe, 1982).

Kleinhauz and Beran (1981, 1984) present six cases of severe and/or chronic reactions to hypnosis, five involving either inadequate dehypnotizing of the subject by a lay or stage hypnotist and one involving a dentist exceeding his area of competence by treating a patient for smoking without consideration of the dynamic value of the symptom to the patient. One of the patients was reported to be a member of the audience at a stage demonstration, and another claimed to have stolen a pistol as a result of the misinterpretation of a remark by a stage hypnotist that he should act like a cowboy and crack shot. The present author is skeptical of this latter case since the claim was raised as a defense in a criminal prosecution. The authors conclude that all therapists should inquire about prior hypnotic experiences to discover such influence in the genesis of the patient's condition so that they can provide adequate treatment. They also advocate the outlawing of stage hypnosis and criticize the "contamination" of the relationship with the subject by the hypnotist by using it not for the benefit of the patient but to make him an instrument for the purpose of entertaining an audience.

On the other hand, they do not object to experimental hypnosis because, while the researcher seeks to accomplish research goals rather than help the subject, the latter is aware of this, and the procedures are carefully designed and monitored. This position seems to present a problem in logical consistency. The subject in stage hypnosis is also aware of the purposes of the hypnotist (often to a greater extent than in experimental hypnosis), and there is usually little concern with the subject in most experimental work but rather a focus on some hypnotic phenomenon. Often researchers are not clinically experienced, and little follow-up work on possible sequelae is undertaken. It is possible that the unstated reason for the belief of the authors that experimental hypnosis is acceptable while stage hypnosis is not is that the value of the former justifies whatever risks may be involved.

Other reactions to hypnosis reported to have occurred in the course of psychotherapy include a spontaneous 72-hour atypical paranoid reaction, a spontaneous cataleptic reaction, and a spontaneous age regression (Hall, 1984; Kornfeld, 1985a; J. Miller, 1983; D.Spiegel and Rosenfeld, 1984). Although such reactions would be a disaster to a lay hypnotist, when they occur in the course of therapy and are properly managed, they may contribute to a dynamic understanding of the patient. Certainly anyone undertaking to do hypnotherapy needs to be prepared for such atypical reactions.

Orne (1965a) suggests that some of the severe anxiety reactions that may occur in therapeutic inductions result from the fact that the patient expects permanent changes in his personality and that he is ambivalent about these changes. This ambivalence is demonstrated by the fact that the anxiety reactions can often be controlled by assuring the patient that the induction is intended simply to test his ability as a subject and that no therapeutic suggestions will be made during the session. Also, transference and countertransference issues may contribute to this anxiety. Orne believes that these issues should be dealt with under hypnosis, for if the therapist awakens the patient, the latter may interpret this as meaning that the therapist is unable to deal with the anxiety reaction.

J. Hilgard also reported on the incidence of sequelae in laboratory hypnosis and agrees with Orne's conclusion that most reported cases of serious difficulties with hypnosis arise in clinical rather than laboratory settings (Hilgard, Hilgard, and Newman, 1961; J. Hilgard, 1974). Hilgard concludes that most of the fears expressed concerning reactions to hypnosis are groundless and are based on inaccurate preconceptions of the hypnotist having undue influence over a subject. Untoward reactions obtained from subjects experiencing experimental hypnosis, although theoretically interesting, are not severe. The 1974 study was undertaken because of a change in the characteristics of the student body available for research since the study of 1961. It was found that of the 120 university students studied, 15% had some kind of reaction to the hypnotic experience (SHSS, form C) that lasted an hour or longer. This figure rose to 31% if short-term reactions (lasting from 5 minutes to an hour) were included. Thus, she warns against the premature dismissal of hypnotic subjects.

Some of the reactions (e.g., headache, confusion, or anxiety) began during hypnosis and either terminated with it or persisted for a while after the session. The chief short-term aftereffects reported were drowsiness and confusion (16 of 19 sequelae). Hilgard suggests that these may be regarded as a continuation of the hypnotic state rather than a reaction to it. It is similar to the experience of many people who require a period of readjustment after awakening in the morning.

Longer sequelae were experienced by 18 of 120 subjects in the 1974 study as opposed to only 7 of 220 subjects in the 1961 study. The much higher percentage in the later study may be due to the fact that form A of the SHSS was used in the earlier study, and form C, which includes age regression and dream induction, was used in the later one. Half of the long-term reactions (9 of 18) were a continuation of drowsiness and confusion, but more complex ones were also reported. One delayed response reported involved nocturnal dreaming about hypnosis, but it is not clear whether this response should be considered a sequelae or the hypnosis simply regarded as a day residue that appeared in the dream. Headaches were also reported that lasted from 1.5 to 2 hours but disappeared following sleep. Headaches were interpreted as representing a conflict between the desire to be hypnotized and anxiety concerning the experience or a desire to avoid it. Little, if any, relationship was found between hypnotic susceptibility and sequelae. There was, however, a positive relationship between pleasant aftereffects (which were not considered sequelae, such as feelings of relaxation, calm, and well-being) and susceptibility. Although these reactions were always suggested at the termination of hypnosis, only about 60% of the subjects reported experiencing them. It was found that there were wide individual differences in how subjects react following a hypnotic experience, but, in an experimental setting at least, there were no alarming sequelae. In the 1961 study, a significant relationship was found between sequelae and adverse childhood experience with anesthesia.

This result was partially confirmed by Orne (1965a) with some subjects; it was not replicated in the 1974 study, however.

Faw, Sellers, and Wilcox (1968) criticized the 1961 study for not employing an unhypnotized control group. They hypnotized half of 207 subjects on three occasions and did not hypnotize the others. They found that hypnosis produced fewer sequelae than the control condition as measured by MMPI score changes, self-referrals to the campus counseling center, and the need for medical attention. These measures, of course, involve more serious reactions than those reported by J. Hilgard.

In a 1982 study, Crawford, Hilgard, and MacDonald found that 72% of 107 college student subjects reported feelings of relaxation after hypnosis on form C of the SHSS, and 29% reported minor transitory sequelae, while only 5% developed adverse reactions following the administration of form A of the SHSS.

Ryken and Coe (1977) compared sequelae reported by two groups of hypnotized subjects with those of four groups of nonhypnotized subjects in a verbal learning study, attending class, taking an exam, or just participating generally in college life. Although the details of the results are complicated, they indicate that sequelae are not unique to hypnosis and that there are no more adverse effects of experimental hypnosis than there are of attending class, taking an exam, or college life in general. In addition, the hypnotic treatment resulted in more positive effects than these other experiences.

Readers may wonder how well-trained, experienced professional observers can differ so radically on the issue of how safe hypnosis is in a particular context, with both extremes of the spectrum having advocates. It is the present author's view that adherents of a position emphasizing the dangers of hypnosis recognize that severe reactions can occur (especially in a therapeutic context) but fail to consider their low probability of occurrence. As an analogy, most physicians regard penicillin as an extremely safe drug, but rarely, it can produce a fatal anaphylactic shock in a sensitized individual. Also severe adverse reactions can occur in nonhypnotic therapy. For example, a suicide attempt may follow a temporary improvement in a depressed patient or result from a premature removal of a symptom, particularly one involving self-destructive behavior.

Although the evidence appears overwhelming that hypnosis is a safe procedure with little risk to a subject, no such claim is made here with regard to the effect of ill-advised suggestions that have been made to subjects. Usually such suggestions are made by either lay hypnotists or persons with no psychological training, practicing outside the limits of their professional competence. Van Pelt (1952) cites examples of neurotic problems caused by "foolish" suggestions made by stage hypnotists, and Kline (1978) cites what can only be characterized as an idiotic suggestion made to a religious woman by a lay hypnotist that if she failed to stick to her diet and lose weight, God would punish her. This suggestion resulted in considerable problems for her when she failed to lose weight as required. Kline (1972b) also cites the case of an obstetrician, angered by a patient's not complying with his suggestions for weight reduction, who told her that if she did not stick to her diet, she would kill her pet dog. Although this suggestion may have been given by the physician with the intent of motivating the patient, it probably resulted from his own unrecognized countertransference feelings in response to his ego-bruising therapeutic failure. The patient killed the dog and subsequently was hospitalized with a diagnosis of paranoid schizophrenia. Kline, having had an opportunity to see the patient later, believes that she experienced a psychotic episode superimposed on a neurotic personality as a result of the incident.

This last case also illustrates some of the potential psychological dangers of hypnotherapy to the therapist. Perhaps the most serious potential danger of hypnosis to the therapist is that its magical qualities and associations may cause him or her to lose sight of its limitations. The therapist still needs to understand the reasons behind the patient's maladaptive behavior and to employ sound psychological principles in their correction. Even a well-trained psychotherapist may be seduced by the illusory power he or she seems to have over a hypnotized patient and may begin to develop feelings of grandiosity and an unwarranted confidence in his or her ability to change a patient by direct commands (West and Deckert, 1965).

The apparent power that a hypnotist has over a subject is called illusory because it results from the hypnotist's being sensitive enough to the personality and motivation of the subject to be able to predict what suggestions the subject is willing to accept and what suggestions he is likely to reject. By limiting suggestions to the former group, the hypnotist appears to have far more control over the subject than is actually the case (Orne, 1972). This limitation may seem to conflict with previous statements made to the effect that inappropriate suggestions can be damaging to a subject. The point is that although a subject may not accept such a suggestion in most instances (unless it is able to upset a delicate balance of opposing tendencies within him), it can generate a conflict within the subject. Indeed, the generation of internal conflict is a valuable use of hypnosis in the study of psychopathology and symptom formation. Smyth (1981a, 1982) used hypnotically-implanted paramnesias to generate and study psychopathology in the laboratory and to provide material for the training of graduate students in psychoanalytic theory. However, it is one thing for an experimenter deliberately to produce a conflict under controlled conditions and with full understanding of what he or she is doing, and another for such a conflict to be inadvertently created and possibly go unnoticed.

The effect of hypnosis in producing feelings of power and grandiosity in the hypnotist may be enhanced by contrast with nonhypnotic therapy, where the difficulties, slow progress, and high failure rates are often very self-depreciating experiences for a therapist. On the other hand, Conn (1972) points out that there are a lot of grandiose people in politics, public life, and professional societies who are not practicing hypnotherapy.

Orne (1965a) makes the point that hypnosis can intensify a therapist's own counter transference reactions and make handling them as well as maintaining the proper distance from the patient more difficult. He, like Lindner (1977), concludes that therapists often use hypnosis in the service of their own neurotic needs rather than the needs of the patient. Some may even derive symbolic sexual gratification from its induction, presumably because of the illusion of dominance and control involved.

Rosen (1959) reports that a number of physicians employing hypnosis have developed serious psychopathology, usually of a paranoid nature. Pulver and Smith (1965) fail to report such findings, and Orne (1965a) reports having seen only one such case. It is important to realize that physicians can develop mental disorders just as anyone else can (perhaps more readily due to the frequently stressful nature of their work). If the incidence of serious psychopathology among hypnotherapists were sufficiently high to indicate a relationship between the two (and to the author's knowledge it is not), an important question that would have to be answered would be, Did the psychopathology result from the work with hypnosis, or did interest in hypnotherapy result from premorbid personality factors in the therapist? Neither possibility could be dismissed out of hand.

Orne (1972) suggests that hypnotherapists must recognize their own power fantasies, neurotic needs, and countertransferences to avoid using hypnosis in a manner to support patients' destructive instead of positive tendencies. He thinks that the following attitudes and behaviors are signs that a therapist may have problems:

1. The use of hypnosis indiscriminately with all patients.
2. The therapist's finding the process of induction enjoyable.
3. Undue concern with the depth attained by the patient.
4. Concern about the patient's faking hypnosis.
5. The therapist's viewing an induction as a battle of wills.
6. The therapist's looking forward to hypnotizing attractive patients.

Effective therapists need to be able to distinguish their own needs from those of the patient and to be guided in their work exclusively by the latter.

If a patient sees hypnosis as a situation involving power or dominance on the part of the hypnotist and submission on the part of the subject or as a symbolic type of seduction, hypnotherapy is contraindicated unless and until such misconceptions are corrected. Rosen (1960a) reports one such patient who talked a dentist into giving her hypnotic treatments for smoking as an excuse to see the dentist, to whom she was attracted. A therapist with similar attitudes about the nature of hypnosis ought to avoid using hypnosis in therapeutic work unless his or her own feelings are fully understood and worked through in personal therapy.

If these misconceptions about the nature of hypnotherapy are shared by both patient and therapist, then all of the ingredients for a full-blown therapeutic disaster are present.

SELF-DESTRUCTIVE, ANTISOCIAL, IMMORAL, OR CRIMINAL BEHAVIOR AS POSSIBLE RESULTS OF HYPNOTIC SUGGESTION

The issue of whether a hypnotized person can be compelled to engage in self-destructive, antisocial, immoral, or criminal behavior is one about which there is very little conflict in the experimental data. The issue does not revolve as much around the experimental facts as it does around the meaning and significance of these facts. It is one thing to ask if antisocial, immoral, self-destructive, or criminal behavior can be elicited from hypnotized subjects. The answer to this question is clearly, yes. It is another thing to ask if the hypnosis was necessary or sufficient to produce this behavior or if it played a part in facilitating it. An important auxiliary question is how much of the behavior in question resulted not from the hypnosis but from the interpersonal relationship or transference between the hypnotist and subject. There is also the issue of how the subject perceives the behavior. Should the behavior be called criminal or antisocial if the subject is misled into believing that circumstances exist that would justify it? Is behavior self-destructive or antisocial if, because of the experimental setting and the subject's confidence in the integrity of the experimenter, he does not believe that the experimenter would expose him to any real danger or permit him to do anything harmful to others in spite of appearances? It is in the answers to these important auxiliary questions that conflict exists among authorities. A review of the experimental findings in this area will serve to clarify the current state of the controversy.

In 1939 Rowland reported a classic study in which a newly developed sheet of nonreflecting (and hence invisible) glass was placed over a box containing a diamondback rattlesnake. Two hypnotized subjects were told to reach into the box and pick up the snake, which was described to them as a "coiled rubber rope." One subject reached for the snake and was surprised when her hand struck the glass. The other awakened immediately when he saw the snake. The subject who complied, when questioned later, said that although she had no memory of the incident, she must have been confident that the experimenter would not expose her to any danger.

Two other subjects were asked if they knew how dangerous a rattlesnake was and replied in the affirmative. They were then directed to reach in and pick up the snake with no attempt made to deceive them into believing that the snake was something else. Both subjects complied, although one needed additional urging.

Finally, two additional subjects were shown a glass full of sulfuric acid, which reacted violently when a piece of zinc was added to it. The experimenter instructed them to throw this acid into Rowland's face, which, unknown to them, was protected behind another sheet of the invisible glass. One subject complied without hesitation. The other required some urging but complied. She then covered her face with her hands and was very disturbed.

Forty-two control subjects were asked to pick up the snake. With one exception, all refused to come close to the box. The exception was a woman who was convinced that the snake was artificial.

From these findings, Rowland concluded that persons in deep hypnosis will allow themselves to be exposed to unreasonable dangers or perform acts unreasonably dangerous to others because their confidence in the hypnotist causes them to forgo their better judgment. Therefore, he argued, only psychologists or other trained people should be permitted to use deep hypnosis. He felt that the common belief that subjects would not accept self-injurious or antisocial suggestions was badly in need of a reexamination. Young (1952) replicated these results with respect to both the deception and the direct coercion treatment. Only one of eight subjects refused to touch the snake or throw the acid.

In 1942, Brenman selected six female subjects ranging in age from 17 to 20, all of whom were capable of attaining a deep somnambulistic state and showed complete amnesia for the first hypnotic session. She sought to test these subjects for the production of antisocial or self-injurious actions that were minor enough to permit their complete expression without any deception of the sort Rowland employed to avoid any problem with the subjects' not believing in the reality of the situation. She was able to get several subjects to "steal" a dollar from a jacket by having the subject believe that the dollar and the jacket were her own. She also got a subject to steal a pencil from a professor's desk with a similar deception and had one subject verbally attack a classmate in response to suggestions that the victim had criticized her. One subject was induced to invade the privacy of another by looking through her purse after being told it was her own. In addition, a subject was induced to violate her own privacy by being told she was in bed alone, in the dark, and to verbalize her bedtime fantasies. In response to this suggestion, the subject verbalized a sexual fantasy concerning a young man and her feelings of guilt about it. The experimenter provided the subject with complete amnesia for this episode, presumably to save her embarrassment; but such an intrusion into the privacy of a research subject suggests that Rowland was unrealistically optimistic when he implied that the dangers of the misuse of hypnotism could be prevented by limiting its use to psychologists or other professionals.

This study indicates not that subjects can be compelled to commit antisocial or self-injurious acts but that they can be deluded into thinking that the suggested acts are innocuous.

In 1947 Watkins reported a series of studies on the use of hypnosis to get military personnel to reveal secrets or to attack superior officers or friends. Like Rowland's studies, these demonstrations used either deception or coercion. In one case, seven soldiers in the waking state were given a message by a captain and told not to disclose it, either because it was a military order or to earn a ten dollar reward. Hypnosis was induced by a posthypnotic signal, and subjects were then told that Watkins was the captain who gave them the message and they were asked to repeat it to be sure that they had it right. All subjects complied and had a posthypnotic amnesia for the disclosure. In addition, all were unable to resist the reinduction of hypnosis by means of the signal even though they had been instructed to try to resist it.

An enlisted WAC (Women's Army Corps) was compelled to repeat a message in a light hypnotic state while fully aware that she was not supposed to, by being told that she could not prevent the words from coming out of her throat and would endure "intense suffering" until they came out.

A 20-year-old private with a good military record was induced to attack a lieutenant colonel and try to strangle him by being told that the colonel was a "dirty Jap soldier" trying to kill him. It took three others to break the soldier's grip. This demonstration was repeated with a young lieutenant who attacked a friend; but in this case the subject pulled a pocket knife that the experimenter was unaware of, and a serious accident was narrowly averted.

In another case, a WAC volunteer was induced to disclose confidential information about the office in which she worked before a professional audience of 200 people. The demonstration was stopped for security reasons by a senior military officer present. This disclosure was obtained by Watkins' simply telling the subject that he was her first sergeant and questioning her as such.

Finally, Watkins reported hypnotizing a corporal "against his will" by having him fixate on a ten dollar bill and telling him he could keep it if he successfully resisted hypnosis but that he would not be able to, and he would be sound asleep by the time the author counted to 25. It is, of course, an illusion that this subject appeared to have hypnosis imposed upon him. He was just as responsible for bringing about the hypnotic state as any other subject; the only difference was that he was tricked into concentrating on the ten dollar bill and the suggested ideation that produced the trance response. Had he known how not to cooperate with the author by simply ignoring him, no effect could have been produced. The situation is quite similar to what Hodge (1977) has called the "rhinoceros principle." If you tell a person that no matter what else he does he must be sure not to think of a low-probability concept, like a rhinoceros, his effort to avoid the idea will cause it to be constantly brought to mind.

Watkins, like all other researchers in this area, worked with only highly susceptible subjects and does not claim generality for these results except in such subjects. He estimates that his population is limited to about 10% of volunteers. It will be remembered that volunteers as a group tend to be much better than average subjects.

In a study using 50 deeply hypnotized subjects, Erickson (1939a) failed to get them to commit such actions as stealing small sums of money or important papers or reading the mail of others. Unlike Brenman, who successfully elicited this type of behavior by deception, Erickson did not try to get the subjects to believe that their actions were proper. He believed that an act cannot be regarded as antisocial unless the subject believes it to be. Hence, he neither disguised the nature of the proposed act nor assumed responsibility for it. Under these circumstances, he found that hypnotic subjects will not perform antisocial acts when commanded to do so by the hypnotist (Conn, 1972).

Barber (1961a) critically reviewed the literature concerning the hypnotic production of antisocial behavior and concluded that the essential condition to elicit such behavior was not hypnosis but:

1. The careful preselection of subjects.
2. Previous practice sessions conditioning the subject to obey the experimenter.
3. The subject's belief that he is supposed to obey all instructions.
4. The understanding that the experimenter will take responsibility for the results of the acts requested.

It is not particularly surprising that the enlisted personnel in Watkins's study followed the directions of an officer. All had considerable training and experience in following orders, and knowing that they were in an experiment was ample reason for them to believe that it was proper for them to behave as the experimenter obviously expected them to. Merely hypnotizing a subject carries with it the strong implication that the subject is expected to carry out all suggestions.

Orne (1972) points out that it is all but meaningless to investigate whether a subject will attempt to carry out antisocial behavior in what he perceives to be an experimental situation, for his confidence in the experimenter to protect him and others from apparent harm and to assume responsibility for the results precludes a real test. Milgram's (1963, 1969) work on the obedience of subjects to the demands of experimenters to administer painful or apparently dangerous electric shocks to other subjects illustrates aggressive behavior legitimized by being perceived as part of a research project. Orne and Evans (1965) note the wide range of bizarre and apparently senseless or dangerous behaviors that subjects in experiments willingly perform without question. These behaviors are produced not by hypnosis but because of the experimental context in which they are requested. Indeed, Coe, Kobayashi, and Howard (1972b) suggest that the best way to get subjects to commit a criminal act is not to hypnotize them but to convince them that the act requested is part of a research project.

On the other hand, when Erickson (1939a) refused to assume responsibility for the immoral acts he asked subjects to perform or to protect them from the consequences of these acts, they did not comply.

Levitt and Baker (1983) note that the more outrageous the experimental behavior requested, the more likely the subject is to comply, for the more convinced he is that a responsible investigator would not expose him or others to such dangers. They, therefore, investigated the ability of hypnotized subjects to resist innocuous hypnotic suggestions. They believe that testing the coercive power of such suggestions is of practical value because the use of hypnotic suggestions to treat maladaptic ego syntonic symptoms, like smoking, involves the hypnotic coercion of patients to cease such behavior. (This is a conclusion that the present author finds untenable. He believes that hypnotic suggestions are effective only if they reflect the patient's own desires. Efforts to compel an unwilling patient to give up a symptom will fail.) Levitt and Baker found that the propensity of subjects to resist innocuous hypnotic suggestions was a function of their attitude toward the hypnotist and the experimenter requesting the resistance.

In a study designed to investigate the role of hypnosis in eliciting antisocial or self-injurious behavior, Orne and Evans (1965) replicated the studies of Rowland and Young. However, they used a variety of control groups, which included hypnotic subjects in a subsequent waking state as their own controls, simulating subjects with the experimenter unaware of their actual status, and ordinary waking controls. They found that simulators and waking controls, as well as hypnotized subjects, complied with suggestions to pick up a venomous snake, to pick up a coin in a container of acid, or to throw acid at an assistant. This study demonstrates that it is not possible to draw any conclusions about the role of hypnosis in the elicitation of antisocial or self-injurious behavior from studies such as Rowland's or Young's because the behaviors performed were found to be perceived by waking subjects as within the range of "experimentally legitimized behavior."

Coe, Kobayashi, and Howard (1972a, 1972b) tried to separate the effects of the relationship between the experimenter and the subject, the knowledge on the part of the subject that he is in an experimental situation, and the hypnotic state per se. They found that the relationship alone was as likely as hypnosis to get a subject to aid the experimenter, a graduate student, in stealing an examination. The combination of a relationship and hypnosis was no more effective than either of these conditions by themselves. However, since they were not totally successful in deluding hypnotic subjects about the experimental nature of the behavior requested, hypnosis was confounded with knowledge of being part of an experiment, which has been shown to be enough to produce compliance by itself.

Parrish (1974) found 12 subjects who were morally opposed to calling someone a "dirty son of a bitch" and 12 subjects without such scruples. They were divided into three groups, all of which were instructed to call a confederate who interrupted them by this appellation, as a result of hypnotic suggestion (with or without amnesia for the suggestion) or a waking suggestion. This mild "antisocial" act was selected because it appeared to the experimenter that subjects who were opposed to performing it would find it equally reprehensible in or out of an experimental context. The results appear to indicate that moral principles were stronger than hypnosis; only one of the subjects who found the language morally objectionable complied, as compared to six who had no such compunction. The suggestion generated conflict in some morally opposed subjects who, while failing to make the response, found themselves upset by experiencing a desire to do so.

Levitt and his associates (1975) report on a group of studies where hypnotized and simulating subjects were requested to cut up an American flag or mutilate a Bible. These tasks were selected because the experimenters believed them to be more objectionable than the use of bad language. At the same time, the tasks were sufficiently innocuous that the experimenter could permit the subjects to carry them to completion without the need for subterfuge to protect the subject or others. The experimenters believed that it would be obvious to the subjects that what they were doing was real, and there was no way that the researchers could protect them from the consequences of their actions. In contrast to previous studies such as Rowland's or Young's, which produced high compliance rates, these studies found that 19.7% to 25% of the subjects refused to perform one or both of the tasks requested. There were no significant differences between hypnotic subjects and simulators, but more of both groups refused to mutilate the Bible than to cut the flag, presumably because they perceived the former as an act of blasphemy and hence more reprehensible than an unpatriotic action. In post experimental interviews, subjects who complied with the requests gave as their reasons that the act was not really objectionable or that it was rendered acceptable because of the experimental context or the influence of hypnosis. The point is made that, contrary to "the lore of hypnosis," no subject spontaneously awakened from the hypnotic state when an unacceptable suggestion was made, as evidenced by subsequent testing for hypnotic depth.

Watkins, in a 1972 article concerning the possibility of hypnosis producing antisocial behavior, lists impressive collections of authorities on both sides of the issue and acknowledges that each side supports its position with anecdotal reports and uncontrolled studies. While maintaining that experimental, legal, and ethical difficulties prevent answering the question with hard data, he argues on theoretical grounds that since hypnosis has elements of being both a state and a relationship and since other states (e.g., drunkenness or epilepsy) and other relationships can produce criminal behavior, hypnosis probably also can. Conn (1972), while reaching the opposite conclusion with respect to the ability of hypnosis to produce atypical criminal behavior, also cites a series of conflicting personal opinions communicated to him by well-known authorities on hypnosis.

Most of the conflict among the authorities cited by Watkins and Conn is more apparent than real and results from their addressing different questions. The issue is not whether antisocial or self-destructive behavior can be obtained from hypnotized subjects. The data clearly show that it can and has been. It can also be elicited from nonhypnotized experimental subjects and from subjects having a close relationship with the person seeking to produce the behavior. The real issue is whether antisocial or self-injurious behavior can be obtained from a subject in the absence of a relationship between himself and the hypnotist in a situation that the subject does not perceive as experimental.

Since the author knows of no reported instance in the laboratory or in occasional real-life reports in which such behavior has clearly been produced in the absence of these other factors (which are themselves adequate to account for the behavior), and since, in studies where these factors seem minimized, compliance rates tend to be low, he would vote with those who doubt that hypnosis per se is likely either to deceive or compel a subject into committing behavior that he considers wrong. Pointing out the common observation that subjects responding to negative hallucinations do not walk into negatively hallucinated objects in their pathway, Orne (1972) makes the point that attempts to produce perceptual distortions to deceive subjects are never completely successful. In situations where hypnosis is commonly employed, such as in therapy, research, or on the stage, the hypnotist has a great deal of influence over a subject prior to the hypnosis. He doubts that hypnosis is likely to be more successful than other methods of persuasion in getting people to do things that they do not want to, but he concedes that, like alcohol or group pressure, it may facilitate persuasion attempts even before it is actually induced. It certainly has not been demonstrated to deprive a subject of his will or freedom of choice, nor does it turn him into a mere robot.

To support this position, Orne cites an instructive report of Janet describing a demonstration given to a group of magistrates in 1889 at the Salpêtrière. The subject was a woman who readily carried out a broad range of "criminal" behaviors in response to hypnotic suggestions. These included stabbing victims with a pseudo-dagger and "poisoning" them with sugar. The subject was then left with a group of unscrupulous medical students who were told to awaken her. Instead, one made the suggestion that she was alone and she should start to undress. In response to this suggestion, which obviously had to be performed in reality if it was accepted, the subject, who recently appeared willing to commit murder on command, simply awakened.

Hypnosis can be used to give a subject an excuse to do something that he wants to do but is inhibited from doing. This is exactly how it is used in therapy: to get a patient to produce verbal material that he wants to talk about but is prevented from expressing by anxiety, shame, or guilt.

Perhaps the most important reason for the persistence of conflict over whether hypnosis can produce antisocial behavior relates not so much to the difficulty of experimental designs to tease apart the influence of hypnosis from confounding factors but to what Orne calls the logical unassailability of either position to experimental evidence. This is related to the impossibility of demonstrating a negative proposition. If, for example, a subject fails to perform an injurious act requested, it can be argued that he was not a good enough subject or that the hypnotist was inept. On the other hand, if he does perform the act (and all causative factors other than hypnosis were eliminated), it could be argued that he did not really find his action morally objectionable.

Neither Barber (1961a) nor Orne (1972) was able to find any adequately reported cases of the alleged use of hypnosis to produce actual criminal behavior where there was not a long-standing and close relationship between the hypnotist and the subject, sufficient in itself to account for the influence of the former over the latter.

In addition, all such cases involve legal proceedings, and, hence, the facts of the case are in dispute. It is thus impossible to know if hypnosis was actually employed in such a case, or if it was merely offered as an excuse by the defendant. Many cases of alleged seduction or rape by means of hypnosis are equally questionable, and in some instances plaintiffs have admitted that their allegations of hypnotic influence were fabricated. It is for this reason that two cases reported by Kline (1972b) involving hypnosis used to effectuate a heterosexual and a pedophilic homosexual seduction are of interest, for they were reported by the hypnotists involved, who sought therapy as a result of their behavior. These reports are more likely to be accurate than most other accounts by alleged victims, for here there was little motivation to lie.

In the first case, an obstetrician had developed an elaborate technique of using repeated hypnotic sessions as a means of developing erotic feelings in his patients. Over a period of several months he gradually included himself in these fantasies and eventually got the patient to want to act out these fantasies with him.

In the second case, a graduate psychology student was in the habit of seeking out babysitting jobs with boys of 10 or under. He would introduce hypnosis in a context of magical performances, usually by having the child imagine enjoyable television programs. He proceeded with his sexual molestation only when he felt confident of his ability to produce an amnesia in his victim.

In both cases, the hypnotists seem to have had marked psychopathic tendencies. They came to therapy not because of guilt feelings over their unethical or criminal behavior but because of fear of exposure if they continued.

Whether these cases demonstrate that hypnosis, when employed by an amoral hypnotist, poses a serious danger of being used as a vehicle for seduction is another matter. It must be pointed out that the obstetrician was by no means always successful in his attempts. Second, the prolonged period of interaction with the offender's patient was ample for the development of transference reactions, which by themselves would be adequate to account for the doctor's ability to seduce the patient. Orne (1972) notes the unique quality of a doctor-patient relationship and how readily it may become sexualized to the point that many patients would be willing to have sex with their therapist. That a disturbed physician or therapist is able to take advantage of the patient's vulnerable position and subvert the doctor-patient relationship for his own advantage seems to be a risk inherent in all therapeutic relationships, not of hypnosis in particular.

It could be argued that the use of hypnosis in therapy may provide a patient with some protection from being exploited sexually by an unethical practitioner. If, as suggested here, the seduction was successful because of the transference and the relationship between the parties rather than the hypnosis, then such a seduction in the absence of hypnotic suggestions would make the therapist guilty of only an aggravated form of unprofessional conduct in most states. On the other hand, if hypnosis was employed and a court was convinced that it overcame the will of the patient, it would be the equivalent of the use of force in many states, and the therapist would be guilty of rape. Although the author does not believe that hypnosis would be successful as a method of seduction with a person not predisposed to having sex with the hypnotist, it is obviously not possible to test this proposition in ethically acceptable research. Given the state of controversy in this area, the People in a rape prosecution based on hypnotic influence would be likely to find reputable expert witnesses willing to testify that such a seduction is possible. Hence, the use of hypnosis in seduction would be needless and risky for the hypnotist.

In this connection, it is interesting to note that Conn (1972) quotes Erickson as advising him of a number of unsuccessful attempts on the part of skilled hypnotists to have sex with their wives or lovers while the latter were hypnotized. In all cases, the women, who were willing in the subsequent waking state, refused under hypnosis because they felt the hypnosis "deprived" them. Conn also cites a number of cases of apparent hypnotic seduction where therapy disclosed that the reason for having sex with the hypnotist was based on other factors in the patients' dynamics, such as underlying feelings of inadequacy with males of their own social class or masochistic tendencies. The hypnosis merely provided the excuse needed.

Although the case of the psychology student who sexually abused children is more disconcerting than cases involving the seduction of adult victims, there, too, relational factors beyond mere hypnosis were probably involved. Lest such unfortunate occurrences cause a clamor for ill-advised legislation seeking to restrict the use of hypnosis, it should be recognized that the reliably reported incidence of such cases is quite small (even allowing for the possibility of many such attempts being successfully concealed) and the action of the student is presently a serious crime. Furthermore, the obstetrician, as a physician, would probably have been included in the class of people authorized to practice hypnosis under any restrictive legislation likely to be proposed.

While concerned with the misuse of hypnosis by either incompetent or immoral hypnotists, Kline (1958a, 1972b) discusses other factors involved in the influence of a hypnotist over a subject. One such factor is the former's rating on the Machiavellianism scale. He notes that in his 1958 study, which attempted to get a reputable subject to commit an act of indecent exposure in what appeared to be a public setting, some experimenters were able to get the subject to comply, and some were not. Kline asserts that the hypnotist's attitude toward the experiment and his or her emotional involvement in it are the important factors. The results seem to support equally well the alternative explanation: that the relationship between the subject and hypnotist is the key factor.

Coe, Kobayashi, and Howard (1972a, 1972b) in a 2 × 2 factorial study testing the efficacy of the variables of hypnosis and subject-hypnotist relationship in inducing a subject to attempt to buy what he believed was heroin, found that the relationship was the only variable that affected task performance.

In an effort to devise a task that was aversive in itself and not as the result of future consequences, O'Brien and Rabuck (1976) suggested to seven female subjects, either under hypnosis, posthypnotically, or in the waking state, that each would make a homosexual pass at a female confederate by trying to arrange a date with her. Only the waking subjects complied with this suggestion.

Coe (1977) discusses the design and ethical standards required in studies to investigate the ability of hypnosis to produce antisocial behaviors. He says that there are four crucial variables that the design must take into account:

1. Highly susceptible subjects are needed.
2. The antisocial act requested must be seen by the subject and society as serious and antisocial.
3. The coercive effect of the subject-hypnotist relationship must be separable from the coercive effect of hypnosis.
4. Subjects must be unaware that they are taking part in an experiment.

Since the last requirement demands the deception of subjects, it is in conflict with the American Psychological Association's general ethical standard for research that requires the informed consent of all research subjects. Although these standards do not absolutely forbid deviations in a proper case, they are, unfortunately, not very helpful in setting forth guidelines as to when such deviations are acceptable. They say only that such departures impose even greater responsibility on the experimenter for the protection of subjects. Certainly the opinion of an advisory ethics committee will be influenced by both the importance of the research and the steps taken to protect subjects from harm.

Coe discusses these issues and describes a variety of precautionary steps to protect both subjects and experimenters. Since his research has involved simulated illegal drug purchases, he not only enlists the cooperation of law enforcement agencies in his research but recommends that experimenters unknown to the subject carry with them official letters describing what they are doing and telephone numbers where these facts can be verified. In addition, an experimenter known to the subject should be available in case the subject or a bystander reacts by attacking or trying to arrest an experimenter. The one precaution that Coe seems to have omitted is the obtaining of legal advice prior to any research involving apparent criminal behavior on the part of the subject. In many states, an attempt to commit a criminal act that is prevented from being consummated only by the deception of the experimenter or even by the legal impossibility of its completion is an indictable attempt to commit the crime in question. In New York, for example, if a subject with the mental capacity to commit a crime (and many subjects in this type of research clearly have this) tries to buy a packet of sugar thinking it is heroin, he is guilty of a crime. Unless a legally sufficient agreement not to prosecute such subjects is worked out with the local prosecutor's office in advance of the research, the subject is not adequately protected.

Levitt (1977) also discusses factors in the design of studies to evaluate the coercive power of hypnosis and recommends that the crucial portion of such studies take place away from the laboratory and involve people other than research personnel as an aid in deceiving the subject about the experimental nature of the situation. Also, he advocates using objectionable but not dangerous or antisocial acts (e.g., cleaning up vomitus) so that the subject can be permitted to perform the coerced behavior in actuality.

LEGAL AND LEGISLATIVE PROBLEMS
IN HYPNOSIS

Criminal Responsibility

For a variety of reasons, the present author does not believe that hypnosis is a likely vehicle for inducing a subject not ordinarily so inclined to commit a crime. There is no evidence that a hypnotist has any real power to compel a subject to commit an act that is repugnant to him in a situation that the subject does not perceive as experimental. Conn (1981) refers to the belief that subjects can be coerced into any behavior through hypnosis as a myth and says that myths, like rumors, are difficult to stop once they gain a foothold.

Second, all subjects retain a certain amount of observing ego, and it is difficult, if not impossible, to deceive a subject totally as to the existence of circumstances that would render the proposed criminal actions justifiable or appropriate. In addition, the principal reason for using hypnosis to induce a person to commit a crime would appear to be to insulate the hypnotist from criminal prosecution by creating an amnesia in the subject for the source of his motive to commit the act. However, posthypnotic amnesia is neither permanent nor resistant to attempts to break it down, either by subsequent hypnosis or ordinary probing methods of interrogation. In reality, it would afford the criminal hypnotist little protection.

On the other hand, whether or not hypnosis can be said to cause the act, a subject can commit a criminal act while under hypnosis or subsequent to it, and the question arises as to the criminal liability of the subject or the hypnotist under such circumstances. There is little question concerning the criminal liability of a hypnotist who suggests the commission of a crime to a subject. Under common law, he or she would have been guilty as an accessory before the fact. Today, in many jurisdictions, common-law distinctions between accessories before and after the fact have been abolished, and all co-conspirators are equally guilty of any crime committed, whether or not they were present at the scene of the crime. In addition to the crime suggested, they may be guilty of the additional crime of conspiracy, which is an agreement between two or more persons to commit a crime. Whether a hypnotist would be guilty of the separate crime of conspiracy would depend on whether the facts in a particular case would permit a court to draw the conclusion that the hypnotist and the subject entered into an agreement to commit the crime in question. If the hypnotist attempted to get the subject to commit a crime by means of suggestion, this probably would not amount to a conspiracy, but in New York, the hypnotist would be guilty of the additional crime of criminal solicitation. This offense consists of attempting to induce, persuade, or cajole a person to commit a crime. It does not amount to a conspiracy because the other person does not agree to do so. If, however, hypnosis is used not to induce a subject to commit a crime but to facilitate the criminal performance (e.g., to make a bank robber less nervous and more self-assured during the crime), then there is a clear criminal conspiracy between the hypnotist and the subject, and both are equally guilty of the crime planned and the crime of conspiracy. Since the conspiracy is perfected, the underlying criminal solicitation is merged into it and is, in fact, a lesser included offense. Hence, the hypnotist could not be convicted of both the conspiracy and the criminal solicitation.

The criminal liability of a hypnotic subject is not so clear-cut. If the subject submits to hypnosis with the intent of improving his criminal performance, he is criminally liable for his actions. If the hypnotist tries to impose the criminal behavior on the subject, the issue becomes one of fact. Has the hypnotic suggestion overcome the will of the subject by rendering him powerless to resist or deceiving him into believing that the act was proper under the circumstances, or did it merely give him an excuse to do what he was already willing to do? What is the legal effect on his criminal responsibility of these various possibilities? These questions are difficult to answer for a variety of reasons. There is very little case law on the subject, since this type of situation is quite rare, and the answers may be different in different jurisdictions.

The first basic question to be answered is whether hypnosis would be treated by the courts as a special type of insanity. The author is inclined to believe that it would be. The reason that there are special rules for determining the criminal responsibility of mentally ill defendants is not, as many psychologists and psychiatrists may believe, to give special consideration to a defendant who cannot conform his behavior to social requirements because he is ill. The real reason for excusing what would otherwise be criminal behavior in such people is that they have not committed a crime under the law. In order to be guilty of a crime, a defendant must perform each element of the crime as defined in the statute creating it. These elements are collectively referred to by lawyers as the corpus delicti of the crime, literally the "body of the wrong." The corpus delicti of most crimes includes both the criminal acts and a coexisting criminal state of mind (mens rea). All elements of the corpus delicti of a crime must be proved beyond a reasonable doubt, including the defendant's required mental state at the time. Normally since it is not possible to look inside the mind of another to determine his mental state, this requirement is met by relying on the presumption that a person is deemed to have intended the natural consequences of his or her actions. However, this presumption is not reasonable in the case of severely disturbed or psychotic people. Hence, special rules are needed to determine whether they had the capacity to form the mental state required to be guilty of a crime.

The most common test of mental capacity to commit a crime is the so-called M'Naghten rule: a person is excused from criminal liability for an otherwise criminal act if, at the time of the commission of the offense, he suffered from a "defect of reason" such that he *either* did not know the nature and quality of his actions or, if he did know this, he did not know that they were wrong. Under this rule, if the court treated hypnosis as a defect in reason and if it were persuaded that the subject was compelled to commit the act by hypnosis, he would still be criminally liable if he understood what he was doing and that it was wrong. In most states that have adopted the M'Naghten rule, an "irresistible impulse" is no defense in a criminal action. Thus, a kleptomaniac who knows that shoplifting is wrong but cannot restrain this behavior is criminally liable, though he suffers from a "mental illness." Similarly, even if an irresistible hypnotic suggestion to commit a crime were possible (or if the court were persuaded that it was), it would be no defense. On the other hand, some jurisdictions, such as the federal courts in Washington, D.C., have adopted the proposed American Law Institute insanity test as enunciated in the *Brawner* case. This test holds that a person is not criminally responsible for his actions if he lacks substantial capacity to appreciate their wrongfulness *or* to conform his conduct to the requirements of the law (Cohn and Udolf, 1979). Under this rule, behavior proved to be compelled by hypnotic suggestion would be excused.

If a subject were deluded into believing that circumstances rendered the criminal behavior justifiable, he would be excused under either rule because he did not know that the behavior was wrong. Sometimes lawyers deal with this situation by referring to the legal fiction of "a sane man with an insane delusion." Here the delusion is treated as a mistake of fact. In other words, if it would have been a defense had the facts been as the defendant believed them to be, he would be excused; if not, he would be criminally liable. Thus, a paranoid who kills a person he believes is following him would not be excused because it is not justifiable to kill a person for following you. On the other hand, if the same paranoid killed a person he believed was trying to kill him, he would be excused because he had a right to use deadly physical force to defend his own life. These results are exactly the same as would be obtained by a straightforward application of the M'Naghten rule.

Sometimes it is alleged that hypnosis has produced criminal behavior not as a result of the intent of the hypnotist but through a misunderstanding on the part of the subject. Deyoub (1984) reports the case of a 30-year-old man who claimed he robbed a bank as a result of the misinterpretation of what was intended as an ego-enhancing suggestion, made by a lay hypnotist, to the effect that he could do anything he wanted to, even rob a bank. A similar defense was raised by a prisoner tried for escape from a California prison. In this case, the defendant claimed that an age-regression suggestion made by a fellow prisoner and amateur hypnotist that the defendant should go back to where "he was having a good time" was instrumental in causing him to escape and return to his home (where he was arrested) (*People v. Marsch*, 17 Cal. App 2d 248; 338 P2d 495). In both cases, these claims were made as a defense in a criminal trial and should be viewed with skepticism (1959). The author knows of no American criminal case where the defense of hypnotic influence was successful.

Orne (1972) expressed concern over what he considered would be the grave social consequences of the courts' believing that it is possible for hypnosis to be used to cause antisocial behavior. In view of the effect of the M'Naghten rule, claiming hypnotic influence as a means of escaping criminal liability by a guilty defendant would probably not be as effective as he fears. Also, there have been few instances where such a defense has been asserted. Nevertheless, in view of the conflicting literature on this issue, it is probably possible for both defense and prosecuting attorneys to find reputable and honest expert witnesses willing to support either side of this issue. The fact that a spurious issue of hypnotic influence may be raised as a defense in a criminal action seems to be of no greater concern than the fact than an unfounded defense of insanity is often raised. In one case, a defense attorney contended that his client was not criminally responsible for his actions because he was unduly influenced by violent television programs. Clearly the legal system must depend on the good judgment and common sense of the courts and jurors; in most cases, confidence in the soundness of their decisions appears justified to the author.

Another situation that may involve the hypnotist in criminal or civil liability, or both, is the claim that he or she used hypnosis not to induce a subject to commit a crime but to victimize the subject—perhaps for purposes of sexual molestation or to influence a subject for the financial or other advantage of the hypnotist. This type of situation can best be illustrated by considering charges of sexual molestation or seduction. As in the case of induced criminal behavior, the present author does not believe that such victimization is possible in the absence of the kind of interpersonal relationship between the subject and hypnotist that could accomplish the same purpose without the hypnosis. Nevertheless, it is clearly possible for a hypnotist to have sexual relations with a subject under hypnosis, and there have been reliably reported cases of this. Hence, the legal effect of such conduct must be considered.

If such behavior occurs within a psychotherapeutic context, it seems clear that in spite of an occasional advocate of the "therapeutic" effects of sex between therapist and patient, such conduct violates the professional ethics of the "therapist" in question, whether a physician or a psychologist. It is also an act of malpractice, and the therapist is civilly liable for it because it is clearly not an acceptable therapeutic procedure. At best, it is employed for the "therapist's," not the patient's needs; at worst, it may inflict substantial psychological damage on the patient. It is also a type of malpractice that is often specifically excluded from coverage in standard professional malpractice insurance policies under the rubric of "immoral behavior." Sexual relations between a therapist and patient amount to malpractice and unprofessional conduct, whether or not hypnosis is employed, and without regard to the question of whether hypnosis was used to compel the patient to comply with the therapist's wishes or merely gave her an excuse to do what she was willing to do. In a criminal prosecution based on this behavior, the latter issue would become vital. If a court were convinced that the hypnotic suggestion had the effect of compelling the patient to submit to sex relations with the therapist, this would be regarded in most states as the equivalent of force, and the hypnotist could be convicted of rape. In the unlikely event that the patient was charged with the crime of adultery because one or both of the parties were married to another person at the time of the sex act in question, the same rules described in the case of criminal behavior would apply.

Although it is difficult to have much, if any, sympathy for a therapist who misuses his therapeutic relationship with a patient for the purpose of having sexual relations with her, the possibility of an ethical practitioner being falsely accused of misusing a therapeutic relationship with a patient for the purpose of having sexual relations with her is a matter of concern. This type of accusation is rare, however, possibly because of the greater sophistication of the public who are no longer willing to believe stories of hypnotists having Svengali-like power over helpless, robot-like subjects.

It is possible that an honest patient may accuse a therapist of an impropriety on rare occasions because of a misinterpretation, particularly of some physical action on his part, or the confusion of an erotic fantasy or hallucination with reality. This is especially likely in view of the fact that many patients seen in therapy may be severely maladjusted to begin with and have difficulty in reality relationships. There are several ways to minimize this admittedly improbable risk. First, hypnotherapy should not be used on a patient without a careful initial evaluation. Second, in a therapeutic context, the hypnotist would do well to avoid procedures requiring any physical contact with the patient whenever possible. Some earlier writers have made it a point to have a third party present during hypnotic sessions with members of the opposite sex, but this is generally not feasible. The presence of a third party during psychotherapy will have an inhibitory effect on the patient. It is difficult enough for many patients to discuss the intimate details of their lives with a therapist with whom they have a strong interpersonal relationship. They can hardly be expected to do so in the presence of a stranger. Even the use of a tape recorder may inhibit a patient, for he will wonder who may eventually listen to the tape. Furthermore, unless the tape is a videotape, it may not be of much value in protecting the therapist against unfounded claims.

There are some elementary things that therapists can and should do to protect themselves from such claims. They should never see a member of the opposite sex, except in emergency situations, unless either a secretary or some other reputable person is present in the office. This rule is often difficult to follow, and it can be relaxed with patients whom the therapist knows well and whose integrity is unquestionable. It ought to be observed with new patients or unstable ones given to erotic fantasies. Although the secretary will not be in the consulting room, she will be able to support the therapist's denial of subsequent charges of misconduct by testifying as to the demeanor of the patient on leaving the office and the fact that no claims of impropriety were made at the time. Perhaps the best protection any therapist has from claims of unethical conduct is his own professional reputation. People who violate the standards of conduct of their profession usually do so repeatedly and not as isolated incidents. It is extremely unlikely that a previously ethical therapist will suddenly depart from customary professional conduct and engage in sexual activities with a patient.

All therapists owe at least two duties to their profession beyond conducting themselves in accordance with its ethical standards. The first is to do everything possible to ensure that practitioners clearly guilty of this type of offense are removed from the profession and have their license to practice or certification permanently revoked. It is misplaced compassion to permit such a person to resume professional status after a course of psychotherapy on the theory that even therapists become ill and he or she has now been restored to fitness to practice. This type of behavior is too damaging to the good name of the entire profession and everyone in it to permit ourselves the luxury of acting on our charitable impulses. The second duty is to encourage practitioners unjustly accused by dishonest patients to prosecute such patients fully, both civilly for damages sustained to a professional reputation and criminally for extortion or perjury, as the facts may establish. Too often, the therapist may be reluctant to prosecute because of the embarrassment that such a charge may engender. This is analogous to a rape victim's refusing to prosecute for the same kinds of reasons, and it produces the same result: the criminal is free to commit the same crime again on another victim.

Malpractice Liability

One of the regrettable tendencies of most psychotherapists (including the present author) is that they often describe their theories, opinions, and personal prejudices, which are based on clinical experience and anecdotal reports, as though they were demonstrated facts. This tendency is particularly unfortunate because of the effect of such writings on establishing what is and is not regarded as malpractice by the courts.

Until recently, relatively few malpractice cases were brought against psychiatrists or psychologists. Thus, the courts have done little to set guidelines for acceptable professional behavior. Recently insurance carriers have claimed large increases in malpractice claims paid, and malpractice insurance premiums are increasing at a geometric rate. Malpractice insurance costs are rapidly approaching the point where it may no longer make economic sense for many therapists to continue in private practice.

Ultimately the cost of malpractice insurance must be passed on to the patient, and there are limits to how much professional fees can be increased. Quality psychotherapy, like quality medical care, is already out of the reach of many, and an undesirable side effect of this situation is the flourishing of incompetent lay hypnotherapists.

Malpractice is a tort or civil wrong, which is closely related to the tort of negligence. The tort of negligence is based on the legal principle that everyone has a duty to act like a "reasonable man" and thereby protect others from harm. When a person breaches this duty and as a result another person suffers a financial loss proximately caused by this breach, he is liable for the tort of negligence. The legal theory behind this liability is that the loss should be taken off the shoulders of the person suffering it and placed on the shoulders of the person whose breach of a duty caused it. Malpractice is a special type of negligence, committed by a professional person. All professional people have a duty to behave in a manner similar to reasonable and competent people in their profession under similar circumstances. A failure to meet this standard of professional performance will render the practitioner liable for damages in malpractice.

The standard of professional conduct against which a practitioner's performance is judged is not the highest standard of the profession but the average standard. Thus, a theoretically brilliant new method of treatment that proves unsuccessful may expose the practitioner to malpractice liability because it does not represent the usual method of treatment and standard of care of the profession. When new or experimental methods of treatment are employed, the therapist should seek prior legal consultation as to what measures need to be taken for protection from future claims. At the very least, patients should be clearly informed as to the experimental nature of the procedures and of any possible adverse effects. This information and the patient's informed assent to the procedure should be reduced to writing and signed by the patient. A therapist should not attempt to be a lawyer or believe that a consent form that he or she draws up will be adequate protection. Legal advice concerning the peculiarities of one's own jurisdiction should always be sought.

One of the unfortunate consequences of clinicians writing as if their opinions concerning unproved theories were fact is that such writings may be used to establish the acceptable standards of professional performance, even if they prove to be erroneous. For example, if there is an extensive literature citing the dangers of hypnosis based on atypical and poorly controlled clinical examples, it may convince a court that hypnosis is an intrinsically dangerous procedure requiring special precautions. The result will be increased risk of malpractice suits against its practitioners, in spite of the fact that the larger body of carefully controlled research indicates that it is a very safe procedure, involving less risk to subjects than ordinary daily activities.

Indeed, the former Department of Health, Education and Welfare (now the Department of Health and Human Services) declared hypnosis to be an at-risk experimental procedure in spite of all of the evidence cited that hypnosis (in an experimental context) is an extremely safe procedure (Coe and Ryken, 1979). Coe and Ryken note that this ruling will be a great impediment to future research, for it will make it more difficult to get institutional ethical review boards to approve research projects in hypnosis. They express concern that the reasons for the department's ruling were not given, particularly in view of all of the evidence that there is minimal risk, if any, to subjects in hypnotic research.

The real reason for declaring hypnosis an "at risk" experimental procedure appears to be a failure on the part of this Department and its personnel to investigate the matter adequately before making the ruling.

Legislative Problems

Many people, including professionals who are not lawyers, are of the opinion that all human problems could be solved if only the proper law were enacted. Actually few human problems are so readily soluble, and often poorly thought-out legislation creates greater problems than those it was designed to rectify (Cohn and Udolf, 1979). Each instance of proposed legislation related to hypnosis needs to be carefully considered before advocating that it be enacted.

A case in point is the use of stage hypnosis as an entertainment vehicle. Many, if not the majority of, professional workers advocate that this be outlawed. Kline (1976) reports on the efficacy of such attempted legislation in the United States and Europe. The arguments for the outlawing of stage hypnosis range from its being dangerous to its being in poor taste or that it is a medical device whose use should therefore be restricted.

The arguments that stage hypnosis is dangerous are for the most part based on atypical and anecdotal reports, such as the case Kline cited of a woman who sustained a serious burn to her hand because of the incomplete removal of suggestions of anesthesia made by a stage hypnotist. The bulk of the evidence appears to indicate that stage hypnosis, even in incompetent hands, is no more dangerous than experimental hypnosis because of the episodic character of the session and the fact that neither the subject nor the hypnotist expects to produce permanent changes in the subject's behavior. The argument that stage hypnosis can be humiliating to the subject or in bad taste is a more interesting one but would be difficult to resolve. The problem is in deciding whose standards of good taste to adopt.

The argument that hypnosis is a medical device is neither true nor relevant. First, if hypnosis were to be looked upon as a device, it would clearly be a psychological and not a medical one. Second, it is neither a device nor the exclusive property of any professional group but is, in fact, a naturally occurring phenomenon. If it were a medical device, it would make no sense to restrict its nonmedical uses to physicians anymore than it would to prevent an auto mechanic from listening to a noisy engine with a stethoscope to localize the noise. Stage hypnosis is neither a medical nor a psychological use of hypnosis.

There are three major reasons why legislation restricting the practice of stage hypnosis should not be enacted. First, there is no need for such legislation to protect subjects. If a stage hypnotist did something either to harm or embarrass a subject, he or she would presently be fully liable in tort for these actions. Merely consenting to be a subject in such a performance in no way waives the participant's rights against the hypnotist for any injury sustained, and if a demonstration subject (or an experimental subject for that matter) were induced to sign a release of all claims prior to the procedure, such a document would be without legal effect in most jurisdictions.

A more important reason for opposing this type of legislation is that hypnosis involves nothing more than a hypnotist talking to a subject. Legislation restricting the freedom of one person to talk to another seems to be a dangerous violation of the freedom of speech assurances of the Constitution. If the government can restrict the freedom of one citizen to talk to another, to protect the latter from some undefined "danger" of hypnosis, it is a simple step to take similar action to protect him from the "dangers" intrinsic in unpopular political ideas. For this reason alone, legislation to limit stage hypnosis should be opposed, even if it could be shown to have substantial capacity to harm a subject. No psychotherapist questions that verbalizations of parents and peers have the ability to cause psychological damage to children. Indeed, the major part of a psychotherapist's practice is attempting to rectify this damage. On the other hand, few would advocate placing restrictions on what parents or others can say to children.

A third reason for reluctance to support antistage hypnosis legislation is of particular concern to psychologists. Kline (1976) believes that hypnosis can be defined clearly enough to enable legislation concerning it to be drafted and that the medical and psychological professions can and should join in efforts to make stage hypnosis illegal. It is hard to agree with the first conclusion, for in the light of the theoretical views already presented, it is often difficult, if not impossible, to say whether a particular procedure, such as relaxation or meditation, differs from hypnosis merely in name or in substance. In clinical practice, this distinction is unimportant, but in the case of a prosecution based on a hypnosis statute, it would be vital. Furthermore, some theorists, like Barber, deny that there is any such thing as a hypnotic state over and above the effects produced by the antecedent procedures used.

As to the second conclusion, it is not only inaccurate but dangerous to psychology as a profession. A long legislative history attests to the fact that many in organized medicine are dedicated to the goal of convincing the public and the state legislatures that psychology is not an independent profession but merely a highly specialized branch of medical technology whose practitioners are less competent than physicians and need to work under medical supervision. This fiction probably originated because psychology as a science is only 100 years old. Since in the past there were always patients needing psychological help and there was no science of psychology on which to base scientific methods of therapy, it was natural for physicians to fill this vacuum and create the specialty of psychiatry. When psychologists began to apply the findings of their new science to practical problems and the treatment of patients, it was natural for them to come into conflict with the physicians who had preempted the field. Similar conflicts occurred in the past when physicians began to recognize that mental disturbances were not due to pacts with the devil and began treating psychotic patients, formerly treated by the church with exorcism.

Psychologists need to be particularly cautious in supporting legislation restricting the practice of hypnosis. Often such legislation has been used by medical lobbyists as a means of downgrading psychologists. For example, although some states, such as California, have statutes defining the practice of psychology and specifically listing hypnosis as included within it, other states, such as Florida, have a hypnosis law that reduces a psychologist to the level of a hypnotechnician and authorizes only physicians, dentists, and a variety of other unqualified practitioners, to practice hypnosis without medical supervision. In effect, such a law requires a psychologist with over six years of graduate training to be supervised in the practice of his or her profession by a layperson who may have no training at all in either psychiatry or hypnosis.

This unfortunate (and basically economic) conflict between some in organized medicine and psychology, coupled with the concern of other professional groups, such as social workers, over threats to their right to practice psychotherapy and the lobbying efforts of a variety of totally untrained practitioners have made it impossible in many states to pass an adequate psychology licensing law. This has permitted a large variety of quacks and incompetents to enter the field. Recently an advertisement appeared in a New York paper touting a training program that claimed that in two weeks, a high school graduate could be "fully certified" as a hypnotherapist, and went on to describe the large income he or she could then command. The remedy to this situation must ultimately involve cooperation rather than conflict between the professional workers in the field. Perhaps modification of the training programs of mental health workers to produce a single program combining the best features of the programs of the different disciplines is required.

Although the author does not believe that the alleged dangers of stage hypnosis are comparable to the dangers involved in attempting to outlaw it, there is a danger associated with it that is both real and serious: the propensity of many stage hypnotists to engage in private practice as "professional hypnotists" or "hypnotechnicians." This danger is really one of laypersons practicing psychotherapy rather than a danger of stage hypnosis with which it is not necessarily connected.

Byers (1975) found that hypnotechnicians carefully supervised in a program of treatment for alcoholics were as successful as the professional staff in their therapeutic work. The arguments made by stage hypnotists and other laypersons who have been trained to induce hypnosis and seek to go into practice as hypnotechnicians are that they will not practice psychotherapy but merely limit themselves to making nontherapeutic suggestions for self-improvement, such as antismoking or weight control suggestions, and they will limit therapeutic suggestions to those made by prescription in cases referred to them by physicians or psychologists under whose supervision they will work.

With respect to the first argument, any suggestion made with the intent to produce a permanent change in behavior is a therapeutic one. No patient should be given weight control, confidence-building, or even antismoking suggestions without a careful psychological assessment. In addition, the proper method for using hypnosis with a particular patient must take into account the underlying dynamics of his personality. There is no doubt that many lay hypnotists are extremely skillful in inducing hypnosis, and some have taught this technique to professional people. There is no reason why they should not do so; but it is a very different thing to be able to induce a hypnotic state, which can be learned in a few minutes, and to use it to help a patient, which takes many years of training.

The second argument is worthy of more consideration. First, if a hypnotechnician were to obtain medical supervision in this work, it would, in most cases, be a matter of the blind leading the blind, for the average nonpsychiatrist physician may receive about two weeks of training in psychiatry in medical school, and the training may include nothing at all about hypnosis. Second, even if the technician were to be supervised by a well-trained psychiatrist or psychologist, this would still not solve the problem, for the notion that a layperson can be supervised by a professional while working in hypnotherapy results from a fundamental misunderstanding of the nature of supervision in psychotherapy. A therapeutic supervisor does not treat a patient indirectly through the supervisee. This is impossible to do. What a clinical supervisor actually does is discuss progress, problems, and techniques used by the therapist and make suggestions that the supervisee considers and adopts or rejects for his work with his patient. The practice of any psychotherapy requires the therapist to react immediately to the patient's verbalizations with the appropriate response. It cannot be conducted effectively by anyone except a well-trained person with a clear idea of both therapeutic goals and methods of attaining them. A supervisor's role is to act as a consultant and to sharpen the therapeutic skills of the prime therapist, not to replace them. For this reason, it is a fiction when a layperson practicing hypnosis claims to do so under medical supervision or by prescription. Thus, although the author believes that stage hypnosis is a proper activity, he does not believe that the practice of hypnosis by hypnotechnicians is. Professionals should decline to refer patients to such individuals for treatment. This view may seem to contradict the view that stage hypnosis should not be outlawed because it involves the issue of freedom of speech. Hence, this matter needs clarification. After all, the practice of psychotherapy also is nothing more than two people talking to each other. It is the author's belief that freedom must necessarily include the right to do something that others may consider ill advised or even stupid. If a person wants to be treated psychologically (or medically for that matter) by an untrained layperson, he should have the right to do so, and this treatment should not be made illegal. What should be illegal is not the conducting of therapy by a layperson but his or her charging a fee. If it were unlawful for a layperson to charge a fee for practicing psychotherapy, this restraint would effectively prevent him or her from making a living by practicing psychology and at the same time preserve the rights of the patient.

It is an interesting tribute to the effectiveness of the political lobbying of the medical societies that even a biochemist with diabetes cannot self prescribe insulin, although he or she is as knowledgeable about the drug as the physician and will require it for the rest of his or her life. This is an example of a paternalistic government concerned about protecting citizens from themselves. People are so used to accepting this situation they no longer question it, but perhaps it should be questioned. For example, the legal profession has always recognized the right of the individual to represent himself in court however disastrous this could prove, and there is no requirement that a person's will be drawn by an attorney. It is extremely doubtful that the average layperson could execute a will that would be both admitted to probate and have the legal effect intended. Yet affording citizens the dignity of being in charge of their own personal affairs has not resulted in any widespread legal disasters, nor has it prevented the vast majority of people from seeking legal assistance when they require it.

CHAPTER 8

Hypnosis in Perspective

Until now this book has dealt primarily with the empirical facts of hypnosis and their practical application, both demonstrated and potential. Theoretical issues and experimental designs were discussed when necessary in connection with empirical findings rather than in a separate section for a variety of reasons. In the first place, theoretical differences arise from differences in the interpretation of research data and are quite meaningless without a broad familiarity with these data. Second, the author believes that in a book designed for professional readers empirical and practical issues are more important than theoretical ones. However, in this concluding chapter a few words appear in order relating to the role of theory in hypnosis and the place of hypnosis in psychology. No attempt will be made here to describe the details of the major theoretical positions and issues with respect to hypnosis. Such an undertaking would result in a chapter many times the size of the rest of this book and would be unduly redundant. Hence, material is provided in the References and Bibliography section of this book for readers who are interested in more of the details of the theoretical positions which have been mentioned.

The term *theory* according to Hall and Lindzey (1957) may be applied to a wide variety of devices ranging from a set of formal postulates and their logical derivatives, having a precise syntax and terminology, to an informal hypothesis or hunch about the nature of reality. Theories may vary in the scope and range of the phenomena that they attempt to account for and in the precision with which they seek to predict. All theories are generated by inductive reasoning. In other words, they seek to tie a number of specific observations together into a general principle. Having done this, the theory can then be used deductively to predict future specific results that lend themselves to experimental verification. To the extent that these predictions are verified, the theory is supported, and, if supported enough, it is ultimately called a law. To the extent that a theory's predictions are disconfirmed, the theory needs to be modified to account for the new as well as the old data. At present, psychology is a science with many theories and few laws.

Theories have many functions, some of which are more important than others. One function of a theory is to serve as a mnemonic device to tie together and organize a large number of isolated facts. Another function is to satisfy the human need for explanation and organization. Some theories are reductionistic in that they explain the phenomena they deal with in terms of simpler or better-understood phenomena or relate one universe of events to another universe. For example, Dollard and Miller's theory explains the vaguer principles of psychoanalysis in terms of scientifically validated principles of learning, and the DNA theory explains the mechanics of heredity in terms of biochemical principles. Some theories are more descriptive than explanatory and only give the illusion of explaining the phenomena with which they deal. For example, calling all of a person's innate drives an id and other sets of psychological processes an ego or a superego really explains nothing. It simply names what is observed and gives the satisfying illusion that by naming or classifying a phenomenon, we understand it.

These functions of a theory are not the more important ones, and the characteristics of a given theory are largely matters of the personal taste of the theorist. Because of his own personality and professional background, the present author has a preference for mechanistic, reductionist theories but they cannot be demonstrated to be better or worse than any other kind. Indeed, the so-called law of parsimony, which states that the simplest explanation for any phenomenon (the one that makes the fewest assumptions) is the best, is also nothing more than a matter of personal preference.

The most important value of a theory is to generate research by producing testable predictions. If a theory does this effectively, it is a good theory, no matter how erroneous it may be and no matter how frequently it may be disconfirmed. The function of a theory is to be productive of new knowledge, not to be right or wrong. If a theory were 100% correct but did not generate research, it would be sterile and useless except as a mnemonic device. Some theories, like Freud's, are incapable of generating testable propositions, since they can account for all possible behaviors after they occur and hence can predict little, if anything. Nevertheless, they may stimulate much research because of their heuristic value or because of the opposition they generate (Hall and Lindzey, 1957).

Judged by this standard, all current theories of hypnosis are good ones, for all have resulted in substantial amounts of research, which have contributed significantly to the empirical data available concerning hypnotic phenomena.

In a real sense, a theory is a set of guidelines for the systematic throwing away of data. Since it is impossible for an experimenter to observe and record all aspects of even the simplest behavior of a research subject, his or her theoretical position defines those aspects of the behavior that are important and should be noted and those aspects that are irrelevant and may be ignored. Since it is never possible to observe everything occurring within an experiment, all researchers must be guided by some theory in their experimental design. People like Skinner who disavow theory and claim to work on a purely empirical level simply substitute implicit and unstated theoretical assumptions for explicit and clearly stated ones (Hall and Lindzey, 1957).

An ideal theory of hypnosis would have to accomplish all of the following:

1. Describe the essential nature of hypnotic phenomena and provide either some invariant criteria for the existence or absence of a hypnotic state or account for why such criteria do not exist.
2. Account for all of the empirical facts of hypnosis within its scope. These empirical facts include not just the types of phenomena described in Chapter 4 but also individual variations in these effects and individual differences in susceptibility.
3. Relate hypnotic phenomena to other psychological phenomena and/ or to physiological principles and place them within a context in psychology.
4. Be precise enough in terminology and syntax to generate testable predictions for future research.

No present theory of hypnosis meets all of these standards, but most attempt to deal with at least some of these issues. Salter's (1973) notion that hypnosis is an example of conditioning and Graham's (1978) view that it results from the functioning of the nondominant cerebral hemisphere are both attempts to put the phenomenon in context and relate it to a body of existing knowledge. Some theorists try to relate all hypnotic phenomena within a common conceptual scheme, while others tend to deal with only a limited group of phenomena, presumably with the goal of later extending the principles derived to other areas. Some theorists, like Barber, tend to develop several minitheories for different phenomena within the context of a broader overall theory. Thus, while Barber believes that what should be studied in hypnotic research are the antecedent events that produce subsequent results, he generally finds different specific antecedent events for different hypnotic phenomena.

There is a confusing array of seemingly contradictory theoretical views of hypnosis among researchers, but there appear to be certain major points of agreement among all of these positions. Often the differences among theories relate more to semantic issues, terminology, or matters of emphasis than to substantive differences. It would be strange indeed if this were not so, for most theorists are intelligent, well-trained observers and they are all observing the same phenomenon.

There are few, if any, differences among theorists concerning the empirical facts of hypnosis. Also, there are no theorists whom the author is aware of who deny the reality of hypnotic phenomena. Although investigators like Barber and his associates do not believe that a trance state is necessary to account for these effects, they do not regard the phenomenon as any less real because they believe it may be accounted for in terms of task motivation rather than a trance state. Indeed, Barber regards the types of behavior typically elicited under hypnosis as evidence of the enormous potential of the mind to influence the human condition.

Both nonstate theorists like Barber and state theorists like Orne have addressed the issue of the lack of external and objective criteria for the presence of a trance state, but they have done so from different perspectives. Barber would deny the existence of a special state of consciousness called a trance that is capable of producing the phenomena commonly labeled hypnotic. Orne would be inclined to believe that, theoretically, the essential criteria of this condition could be specified, though at present he admits the presence or absence of hypnosis is merely a clinical diagnosis (Orne, 1959).

The state versus nonstate issue of hypnosis, while appearing to be a major one, seems to be largely a semantic one produced by different theorists' interpreting the word *state* differently. Barber seems to be using the term *trance state* to mean a special condition of consciousness that is capable of rendering a subject hypersuggestible by itself and thus producing all of the effects commonly attributed to hypnosis. State theorists, on the other hand, seem to regard a trance as a set of subjective feelings experienced by people under hypnosis that makes it more likely that they will accept and act on suggestions that have a low probability of being accepted under ordinary waking conditions. Who is right in this controversy? Probably both sides are. The situation is analogous to the story of the blind men who examined different aspects of an elephant and came up with different ideas of what the total entity called an elephant is like.

In view of the wide variations in the nature of trance states attainable (ranging from the seizure-like states produced by Mesmer through the hyperempiric trance of Gibbons to the more common deeply relaxed states conventionally produced), it is reasonable to assume that a trance state should be viewed as a response to induction procedures and suggestions and is much the same as any other response to hypnotic suggestions. This viewpoint is also supported by the fact that subjects generally develop the kind of trance reactions that they either expect to develop or that they have been instructed to produce. This is the real reason why there are no universal criteria of hypnosis. On the other hand, the fact that a hypnotic trance is a response to suggestions does not preclude it from facilitating the acceptance of subsequent suggestions. It probably does so as the result of the formation of a set to respond and also because the subjective experiences of the subject increase his belief in the reality of the state and his expectations of future compliance. Every salesperson knows that a prospect can be eased into buying a product if he or she can be induced to agree with statements in the early phase of a sales pitch. The fact that results similar to those produced under hypnosis are obtainable without previous trance-inducing suggestions does not establish that a trance state cannot also produce these results or, for that matter, that a different specific type of trance state may not have developed as a result of task-motivating instructions.

Orne's notion that the behavior of a hypnotic subject is influenced by the "demand characteristics" of the situation is quite similar to Coe's idea that hypnosis is a "social role." These views have been incorrectly taken by some to indicate that the behavior of a hypnotized subject may be accounted for by assuming that he is faking in order to please the hypnotist by producing the effects that he knows the latter wants. This is the rationale behind the postexperimental questioning of subjects with exhortations to them to be honest in their reports. If this interpretation were correct, it would seem equally likely for the subject to report he did not experience an effect that he really did because now he can only please the experimenter by denying the effect previously claimed.

Barber's (1978d) explanation of stage hypnosis seems to equate responding to the demand characteristics of a situation with faking. He notes how difficult it would be for a subject in front of a large audience to reject the suggestion that a broom presented to him was an attractive woman whom he should dance with. Although in such a situation it may be easier for a subject to go along with the suggestion, this does not establish that in all instances, a subject responding to the demand characteristics of a situation or enacting the social role of a hypnotic subject is faking in the usual meaning of this term.

A social role is a set of behaviors that society imposes in certain common situations. We all have many social roles such as husband, father, professor, and scientist, and we normally behave appropriately to each role. As Coe (1977) points out, no one would regard a person conforming to the requirements of his social role of a father as "faking."

Orne (1971) advocates the use of unhypnotized subjects simulating hypnosis as a control group in hypnotic research. It is essential when such subjects are used that the experimenter working with them be blind as to their status to avoid his or her unconsciously treating them differently from hypnotic subjects and thus introducing experimenter bias. Orne does not advocate the use of simulators for the purpose of testing the reality of hypnotic phenomena, for even if their behavior were identical to that of hypnotized subjects, it would not logically establish that hypnosis could be accounted for by faking or that the identical behaviors of hypnotized and simulating subjects were not caused by different factors. Although simulators are often successful in deceiving experimenters in short studies, their behavior is rarely identical to that of real subjects. The function of simulators in research, according to Orne, is to establish a baseline of behavior when the ability of hypnosis to transcend the limits of volitional abilities is in issue or to evaluate a subject's willingness to perform suggestions. Simulators are also useful when the effectiveness of an experimental deception needs to be evaluated.

The reason that some people confuse simulation studies with faking studies is again a semantic difficulty caused by the imprecision of the English language. All effects produced by a subject under hypnosis must result from his imaginative efforts unless one is prepared to accept a theory of hypnosis that equates it with magic or experimenter control over the subject. Few, if any, modern psychologists would subscribe to such a theory. The difficulty is in establishing a precise line between a subject striving to experience what he has been asked to and one simply pretending to do so. For example, the fact that a subject age regressed to an earlier period in life typically acts less maturely than his actual age but more maturely than the age suggested does not demonstrate that he is acting in the sense of trying to deceive the hypnotist. It does establish that he is acting in the sense of attempting to experience the effects suggested. Although these attempts typically do not amount to an actual revivification of the earlier experiences, they are no less real or experiential in nature.

To avoid questions of whether simulating subjects have been inadvertently hypnotized by the experimental procedures used, Orne (1971, 1977) advocates the use of low-susceptibility subjects for simulation groups. Unfortunately, this results in confounding the variable of hypnosis with the variable of susceptibility in all such studies. If a second control group of simulators having high-susceptibility were used, this confounding could be eliminated (provided that they behaved similarly to the low-susceptibility simulators). If they behaved differently from low-susceptibility simulators but the same as hypnotized subjects, then there would be ambiguity as to whether susceptibility rather than hypnosis was the operant variable or whether the group was inadvertently hypnotized. If the high-susceptibility simulation group behaved differently from both other groups, more complex issues would arise, including the possibility of group artifacts in which some of the subjects were inadvertently hypnotized and some were not.

The problem of confounding hypnosis with susceptibility is a serious one in much hypnotic research. Since subjects in hypnotic groups must frequently be selected not only on the basis of high susceptibility but often on the basis of the ability to develop a particular phenomenon, such as age regression or hallucinations, such subjects cannot be randomly selected but must be chosen on the basis of an organismic variable. This violates the basic assumption of most of the statistical procedures used to evaluate research results. Normally the way this situation is resolved is to consider the subjects used as comprising a random sample taken from a hypothetical population and limiting the generality of the findings to such population. For example, findings from a study on age regression could be limited to a population comprised of high-susceptibility people capable of developing age-regression phenomena. However, if control group subjects must be selected from low-susceptibility subjects in an effort to prevent unintentional hypnosis, there is no longer any one population from which all research subjects can be regarded as being sampled. This situation casts serious doubt on the generality of the results of the research, and the use of additional groups of high-susceptibility control subjects may be required in future studies.

In a perceptive article, Frankel (1978) points out the need for experimental procedures to be developed to deal with issues arising in clinical practice. He describes the case of a young man hospitalized following a cholecystectomy who developed chronic debilitating hiccups that abated following hypnotic treatment. Frankel notes that although it is convenient to say that the hypnotic intervention produced the remission of the symptom, actually the hypnotic treatment was confounded with a variety of other conditions, including a relationship with a supportive therapist, relaxation, a placebo effect, and distraction. It is thus not possible to say which of these factors, alone or in combination, may have produced the effect observed. Nor is it possible to do an experimental study with a large number of identical patients, each being randomly assigned to treatment groups with only one of these factors in operation per group.

Frankel believes that the answer to clinical questions like this can be obtained only through the cooperation of clinical and experimental workers. Clinicians will be needed to identify problems requiring investigation, and creative researchers will be needed to devise new experimental procedures to deal with problems that current methodology cannot address.

Nugent (1985) discusses the requirements of case study reports with respect to their ability to support inferences concerning the effect of an intervention on a problem (internal validity) and the generality of the findings (external validity or replicability). He classifies case reports into five categories:

1. Purely anecdotal reports having no basis, beyond the author's opinion, for making a claim of change or of a causal relationship between a change and intervention.
2. Reports involving before and after objective measures.
3. Reports involving repeated objective measures during treatment.
4. Reports involving repeated measures and stability projections to the past and future.
5. Reports having repeated measures, stability projections, and multiple patients.

An analysis of 74 case study reports published in the *American Journal of Clinical Hypnosis* from January 1978 to January 1983 showed that 67 of these were in the first category, 2 were in the second category, 2 were in the third category, and none was in categories four or five. Although this study argues for the need to upgrade the quality of case reports to enable sounder inferences to be drawn from them concerning the causal relationship between a therapeutic intervention and change in a patient, it fails to concern itself with other uses of case reports and their requirements.

Perhaps the greatest value of a case report to a clinician is not to make inferences about causation (it can no more establish this than a correlation study can) but to suggest new approaches to clinical problems and impasses. For this purpose, case reports need to give more details concerning etiological and diagnostic factors and a more precise description of the intervention than is usual. The experimental standard of giving enough detail so that the procedure could be replicated should be employed. What case reports do not need (and should not contain) is information about the patient that could be characterized as gossip rather than operative factors in the case, such as statements like, "The patient was an attractive woman who liked baseball." The elimination of this type of irrelevant information may make it easier to disguise the identity of patients with a minimum of demographic and factual distortions (which if not limited to nonessential features of the case can lead to erroneous conclusions). Although it is legitimate for journals to inquire into compliance with ethical standards prior to accepting research or case study reports for publication, statements in a report to the effect that the research was approved by an institutional ethical review board or that the identity of patients was disguised are a waste of time and space. Readers have a right to assume that members of their profession conduct themselves in an ethical manner, unless there is evidence to the contrary.

Another important, and often unappreciated, value of case reports is the legal protection they may afford a practitioner. Since malpractice is generally defined as the failure to exhibit that degree of care and skill common to the average member of a profession, the fact that a method of treatment is reported in the literature as efficacious provides some legal safety for a clinician using it.

A survey of 500 members of the American Society of Clinical Hypnosis conducted by Rodolfa, Kraft, and Reilley (1985) suggests that many experienced practitioners in psychology, medicine, and dentistry rely more on a few books (by authors they regard as highly ranked authorities) than on journal articles to keep their knowledge of hypnosis current. Thus journal articles may need to be more attuned to the needs of busy clinicians. Ninety percent of the respondents reported the *American Journal of Clinical Hypnosis* as their primary source of articles about hypnosis, and 40% said that the *International Journal of Clinical and Experimental Hypnosis* was their second source.

Although theoretical issues are the lifeblood of research, the applied worker or the clinician is often troubled by the widely divergent viewpoints presented in the literature. Often these positions are advocated in a manner evincing a great deal of ego involvement on the part of their proponents, and acrimonious personal controversy between adherents of differing sectarian views is unfortunately not rare.

Perhaps the best way to deal with this situation is to remember that it is not the function of theories to be correct but to be useful. A theory can aid a clinician in the preparation of a treatment program and give some realistic view of what he or she can and cannot hope to accomplish with a particular patient. Often the empirical data of hypnosis will be more valuable in this regard than any theory, but theories can be valuable to a clinician in developing new or modified methods of treatment and in giving direction to his or her work. Some theories may be more useful than others for a particular kind of problem, and there is no reason why a clinician cannot use different theories for different problems in an eclectic manner, just as a good therapist uses different methods of treatment for different patients.

When Einstein's theory of relativity was demonstrated to be a more accurate description of the universe than Newtonian physics, engineers did not suddenly stop using Newtonian physics. They simply used the approach most applicable to the problem at hand and often mixed the two. For example, an electronic engineer may use conventional physics in designing a cathode ray tube, while at the same time make a relativistic correction in the mass of the electrons in a beam accelerated to a high velocity, as required by relativity theory.

Since the major value of a theory to clinicians is to give them a feeling of knowing where they are with a patient and where they are trying to go, perhaps the most useful theoretical outlook is one that the individual practitioner has developed based on familiarity with the literature and personal experience. Such a theoretical outlook will probably not be very different from the prevailing theories but will have the advantage of being expressed in the clinician's own idiom. This will ultimately eliminate a lot of pseudo-issues caused by ambiguity of language. In any event, the increase in the clinician's self-confidence produced by such a theoretical orientation to hypnosis will be subtly conveyed to patients, and it will increase their confidence in the treatment. The expectation of success is a major factor in any kind of psychotherapy. In hypnotherapy it often spells the difference between success and failure.

It would be difficult to conclude this book without indulging a little in the dangerous practice of prognosticating the future of hypnosis in psychology and related fields. Since the best predictor of future behavior is past behavior, it is likely that hypnosis will continue to experience cycles of enthusiasm and neglect in psychology and medicine. At the time of this writing, it is experiencing a continuing crest of renewed interest and seminars and writings about it are proliferating. Rodolfa, Kraft, Reilley and Blackmore (1982, 1983) found that 30% of APA-approved clinical and/or counseling doctoral programs and 39% of non-APA-approved programs offered formal course work in hypnosis, while 55% of 123 APA-approved clinical-counseling internships offered training in hypnosis. Descriptions of medical school or professional courses in hypnosis are beginning to appear in the literature (Burrows and Dennerstein, 1979; Taub-Bynun and House, 1983).

There are certain differences between the present revival of interest in hypnosis and past periods of popularity that may serve to reduce the extreme variations between the high and low phases of this cycle. In the past 25 years, there has been a rapid development of research activity in hypnosis, and this research has been improving in quality. Hypnosis has become a popular topic for doctoral dissertations (Clark, Hungerford, and Reilley, 1984). The Reference and Bibliography section of this book cites about 100 such dissertations conducted in the last ten years. Hypnosis will probably continue to be regarded as respectable area for research in most universities if the unreasonable application by nonscientists of governmental regulations, designed to protect research subjects from unethical practices, can be prevented from making research in hypnosis too onerous to undertake.

Current research has done much to increase our knowledge of what hypnosis can and cannot accomplish and to disprove many common misconceptions in this regard. This work should serve to ameliorate the severity of periods of professional rejection of hypnosis. In the past, these periods often resulted from rejection by marginally trained hypnotherapists who were led to expect miraculous results from hypnosis, and when these miracles were not forthcoming, they became disenchanted with hypnosis and discarded it.

The future of hypnosis in therapy will depend on many factors. The most important of these are the quantity and quality of future research and the training and ability of the clinicians who practice hypnosis. It may also be affected by such extraneous factors as the development of alternative and better methods of treatment. Whatever its status in applied psychology, hypnosis will always remain a fascinating phenomenon for study in its own right.

Glossary

ABREACTION. An intense emotional discharge. In psychoanalysis, an emotional reliving of an earlier traumatic incident.

ACQUISITION. The part of a learning curve that describes the increase of habit strength or the development of stimulus control over a response.

ADDICTION. A physiological dependence on an addictive drug (as opposed to a psychological dependence or habituation). Characterized by: (1) the presence of withdrawal symptoms when the drug is withheld, and (2) tolerance, a phenomenon that results in larger doses of the drug being required to produce the former effect.

AFFECT BRIDGE. A technique by which significant memories are recovered by inducing an intense emotional state in a subject and asking him to remember a past instance when he felt the same way.

AGE PROGRESSION. A technique in which it is suggested to a subject that he is going forward in time and becoming older.

AGE REGRESSION. A technique in which it is suggested to a subject that he is going back in time and becoming younger.

AGNOSIA. Loss of the ability to recognize persons, things, or other integrated sensory patterns.

ALEXITHYMIA. The inability to express feelings through the use of language, and thought content bound to external stimuli with a paucity of fantasy.

AMNESIA. Loss of memory; inability to recall.

ANALGESIA. The loss or reduction of pain sensation.

ANESTHESIA. The loss of all sensory modalities.

ANIMAL HYPNOSIS. A misnomer. A state of immobility in animals resembling hypnotic catalepsy in people. Produced in many animals by holding them immobile for a short period. In some species (e.g., a possum) this may be an adaptive mechanism, probably not related to hypnosis at all. (See Carli, 1982; Crawford, 1977; Gibson, 1977).

ANIMAL MAGNETISM. The magnetism that Mesmer believed resided in his own body and was responsible for producing cures in his patients.

ANOREXIA NERVOSA. A life-threatening neurosis in which the patient, usually a young woman, diets to the point of emaciation.

ANOSMIA. Loss of sense of smell.

ANXIETY, Neurotic. Free-floating fear. The patient is afraid but is unaware of the source of the fear. In psychoanalytic terms, it is the fear that the ego feels concerning the threatened expression of id impulses, as repression begins to fail to hold them in check.

ARM LEVITATION. The lifting of an arm by an ideomotor reaction without the subject's voluntary intent to perform the action suggested.

AUTHORITARIAN SUGGESTION. A suggestion made to the subject in a manner to convey the impression that it is being imposed by the hypnotist.

AUTOHYPNOSIS. *See* Autosuggestion.

AUTOMATIC WRITING. A dissociative phenomenon in which a subject is instructed that his unconscious will write a message without any conscious intent or even knowledge that the writing is occurring.

AUTOSUGGESTION. Self-hypnosis; hypnosis induced by the subject. Also refers to suggestions made by the subject to himself.

BABINSKI SIGN. An abnormal reflex in response to a scratching of the plantar surface of the foot. Instead of the toes curling down, they spread apart and the big toe flares out. In adults a sign of pyramidal tract damage. There is conflict over the significance, if any, of this sign in children.

BEAT NOTE. A waxing and waning in intensity of a tone that is heard when two tones, close together in frequency, are sounded simultaneously. This effect is due to the wave crests alternately reinforcing or opposing each other as they slip in and out of phase. The two tones must be within a JND (just noticeable difference) of each other, so that they cannot be discriminated as different tones and sum and difference frequencies cannot be detected.

BIOFEEDBACK. A technique by which a subject is given information about the status of some autonomic nervous system response to enable him to learn to exercise control over this response by instrumental conditioning.

BLIND STUDY. A research design in which a subject does not know what experimental group he is in or what experimental manipulation he is to receive. This design is used to eliminate placebo and expectation effects.

BRAIDISM. A method of hypnotic induction devised by James Braid, which involves having the subject stare at a target above his line of vision to produce fatigue of the extrinsic eye muscles.

BRUXISM. Involuntary teeth grinding during sleep.

CATALEPSY. A rigidity of the skeletal muscles. May be accompanied by "waxy flexibility" (the subject keeps his limbs in any position in which they are placed).

CHALLENGES. A suggestion to a subject that he try to break a previous suggestion but will be unable to do so—for example, a challenge to open the eyes after closure of the eyes and catalepsy of the eye muscles have been suggested.

CHAPERONE TECHNIQUE. A technique of inducing hypnosis in a reluctant subject by having him ostensibly witness the induction of another (pseudo) subject.

CHARACTER DISORDER. A condition marked by a faulty development of a personality (as opposed to a neurosis which is characterized by symptom formation). Symptoms are ego alien; character disorders are ego syntonic and more in the nature of maladaptive habits. In psychoanalytic terms, a character disorder results from a fixation at a preoedipal level of psychosexual development.

CHEVREUL PENDULUM. A weight on the end of a chain or string used to demonstrate ideomotor responses.

CLASSICAL CONDITIONING. Also known as Pavlovian conditioning or stimulus substitution learning. The method by which autonomic nervous system responses are learned in accordance with the following paradigm:

$$
\text{Continguous Pairing} \begin{cases} \text{Unconditioned} \longrightarrow \text{Unconditioned} \\ \text{Stimulus} \qquad\qquad \text{Response} \\ \text{(e. g., meat} \qquad \text{(e.g., salivation)} \\ \text{powder)} \\ \\ \text{Conditioned} \longrightarrow \text{Conditioned} \\ \text{Stimulus} \qquad\qquad \text{Response} \\ \text{(e.g., bell)} \qquad \text{(e.g., salivation)} \end{cases}
$$

CLINICAL HYPNOSIS. The use of hypnosis in psychotherapy or in the treatment of psychological aspects of medical conditions.

COGNITIVE INDUCTION. An induction procedure in which the subject's attention is captured by his being directed to imagine a certain scene (as opposed to being told to fixate on a visual target).

COLD PRESSOR PAIN. Pain produced in a body appendage by subjecting it to intense cold. Usually produced by the immersing of a hand or limb in ice water.

COMMAND. An instruction directing a subject to do something (as opposed to a suggestion that he *should* do or experience something).

CONFOUNDING VARIABLES. If there is a difference between an experimental and a control group in some variable other than the independent variable, the latter. is said to be confounded with the former. It is then impossible to say which of the two variables (or combination of their effects) produced any differences obtained in the criterion, or dependent, variable.

CONSCIOUS. Referring to the state of being subjectively aware.

CONTENT AMNESIA. An amnesia in which what is unavailable to recall is the content of the person's memory.

CONTROL GROUP. A group of subjects treated identically to an experimental group except for the independent variable. Designed to provide a baseline for the dependent variable and to establish logically that any difference between the two groups in the dependent variable must be due to the action of the independent variable.

CONTROL VARIABLE. A variable that is either eliminated or held constant between an experimental and control group to avoid confounding. Any variable that could reasonably be expected to affect the results of a study must be treated as an independent variable or a control variable.

COUNTERBALANCED DESIGN. A research design technique to eliminate differential effects of practice and fatigue, used in studies whose subjects are successively exposed to different levels of the independent variable. For example, in a Latin Square design, an equal number of subjects get each experimental condition at every successive level of practice. For example:

Trial Number:	1	2	3	4
Group 1	A	B	C	D
Group 2	B	C	D	A
Group 3	C	D	A	B
Group 4	D	A	B	C

(A, B, C, and D are different levels of the independent variable.)

COUNTERTRANSFERENCE. A transference reaction formed by the therapist and directed at the patient.

CRISIS. The convulsive-type reaction characteristically produced by Mesmer's hypnotic inductions.

DAY RESIDUE. The events of the day that are represented, usually with minimal distortion, in the manifest content of the dreams of the same night. They are differentiated from the latent or unconscious meanings of the manifest content that Freudians believe date back to early childhood. Freud believed that day residues were vehicles to which latent thoughts attached themselves to be carried into the manifest dream.

DECOMPENSATION. The breaking down of a patient's defense structure and the appearance of overtly psychotic behavior.

DEFENSE (Mechanism). An unconscious behavior developed in order to cope with anxiety. Usually a compromise reaction to an unconscious conflict. Differs from a symptom in that the defense is neither maladaptive per se nor a problem to the patient.

DELUSION. An irrational belief tenaciously held in spite of all evidence to the contrary.

DEMAND CHARACTERISTICS. The cues in an experimental situation that suggest to the subject that the experimenter's expectations and the social pressures on him to conform to these.

DENIAL. A defense mechanism by which a person refuses to recognize an unpleasant external reality.

DEPENDENT VARIABLE. The variable measured in an experiment. The criterion variable. The variable that is affected by the action of the independent variable.

DEPRESSION. A feeling of hopelessness, despondency, and, often, apathy and guilt. A way of dealing with stress by giving up. Like anxiety, it is a form of psychic pain.

DICHOTIC. Referring to different stimuli simultaneously applied to each ear.

DISSOCIATION. The dividing up of the psyche into two or more parts functioning independently at the same time (for example, automatic writing or talking).

DOUBLE BIND. A technique of getting a patient to comply with a request by giving him an illusory choice between doing what is requested or not doing the contrary.

DOUBLE BLIND STUDY. A research design in which neither the subject nor the experimenter collecting data knows which experimental group the subject is in. In addition to seeking to eliminate placebo or subject expectation effects, this design seeks to eliminate experimenter bias and inadvertent differential treatment of research subjects that would confound the effect of the independent variable.

DYNAMICS. In psychoanalytic theory this refers to the interaction among the components of the psyche (id, ego, and superego). Used to refer to the unconscious mechanisms underlying symptoms and the symbolic significance of a symptom.

ECTOMORPHY. A component of a somatotype (body type) according to Sheldon (1954) characterized by the predominance of skin and the central nervous system over other tissue, (i.e., predominance of components derived from the ectoderm).

EGO BUILDING. The therapeutic repair of an ego structure made defective by a fixation. In the psychoanalytic treatment of character disorders, this is thought necessary before a patient can be treated by psychoanalysis, which requires the ego to be at least at the oedipal or neurotic level of development.

EGO SPLITTING. A dissociation of the ego into functional components (for example, an observing and participating ego in a dream or hypnotic state).

EIDETIC IMAGERY. A photographic memory; the production of a visual memory with perceptual vividness.

ELECTROCARDIOGRAM (EKG). A graph of the electrical activity of the heart muscle as a function of time.

ELECTROENCEPHALOGRAM (EEG). A recording of the electrical activity of various major regions of the cerebral cortex taken from the scalp of a subject.

ELECTROMYOGRAM (EMG). A record of the electrical activity of a muscle in response to various forms of stimulation.

EMOTION. A series of autonomic nervous system responses plus the subjective feelings they produce and the accompanying ideation (for example, anger, fear, or joy).

ENDOMORPHY. A component of a somatotype according to Sheldon (1954) characterized by a predominance of the viscera and fat (i.e., derived from the endoderm).

ENURESIS. Involuntary urination. Usually nocturnal but may be diurnal. Often but not always psychogenic in origin.

ESP. Extrasensory perception.

EXPERIMENTAL HYPNOSIS. Hypnosis used in an experimental as opposed to an applied context.

EXPERIMENTALLY LEGITIMIZED BEHAVIOR. A wide range of apparently dangerous, antisocial, self-injurious, or pointless behaviors that research subjects are willing to engage in on request in what they perceive as an experimental situation.

EXPERIMENTER BIAS. An effect produced by an experimenter who unintentionally treats experimental and control subjects differently.

EXTINCTION. The portion of a total learning curve where habit strength is weakened by the withholding of reinforcement; an active unlearning process. Not the same as passive forgetting, which occurs with the passage of time.

FACTORIAL DESIGN (A × B). A study involving the simultaneous manipulation of two or more independent variables in the same experiment. Typically different experimental groups are given all permutations of the variables used. The purpose of this design is not primarily to measure the main effects of the variables but the interactions between them.

FANTASY. In the generic sense of the term, synonomous with primary process thinking; includes nocturnal dreaming and hallucinations. In the specific sense of the term, it refers to daydreaming. All fantasy involves the formation and manipulation of images.

FEAR. A reaction of the automatic nervous system to a stimulus believed to be threatening or dangerous. Synonymous with reality anxiety.

FEEDBACK LOOP. A mechanism by which psychological conditions tend to feed on themselves. For example, a paranoid who perceives others as enemies and treats them as such will find that they in turn will become hostile toward him, thus confirming his original belief.

FIXATION. A Freudian term to indicate arrested development, or the leaving behind of an undue amount of psychic energy at an earlier stage of psychosexual development.

FLEES BOX. A box with two viewing holes that presents the left-handed image on a card to the right eye and vice-versa, without the subject's being aware of it. Used to detect malingering.

FLOODING. A technique to extinguish phobic reactions by causing a patient to develop an intense and prolonged phobic response.

FOLIE a DEUX. An unusually close interpersonal relationship in which two people have a similar pathology.

FORENSIC HYPNOSIS. Legal applications of hypnosis.

FRACTIONATION. A process for deepening a trance by repeatedly hypnotizing and dehypnotizing a subject.

FREE ASSOCIATION. What Freud called "the patient's work." The obligation on the part of a psychoanalytic patient to verbalize his train of thought without censorship. The term is a misnomer, for the value of the method lies in the psychically determined connections between the associations. If the association were truly free, it would be valueless.

FRIGIDITY. The lack of desire or ability of a woman to achieve sexual satisfaction.

g. Usually regarded as a general intellectual ability common to all subtests of specific abilities on an intelligence test. The degree of commonality or correlation between tests of different specific abilities. Really the result of the impossibility of designing a test of a single ability. For example, tests of rote memory correlate to some degree with tests of arithmetic ability because the former is necessarily involved in the latter.

GALVANIC SKIN RESPONSE (GSR). The indirect measurement of the activity of the sweat glands as a function of time by measuring the electrical resistance of the skin.

GENERALITY OF FINDINGS. Refers to the utility of findings based on a sample for making inferences about the population from which the sample was drawn.

GENERALIZATION, Stimulus. The learning phenomenon in which stimuli other than the stimuli used during acquisition acquire evocation control over conditioned responses.

GLOVE ANESTHESIA. A hypnotically suggested or a hysterical anesthesia in the area of a hand normally covered by a glove. A condition that is neuroanatomically impossible.

GOAL-DIRECTED FANTASY. A fantasy designed to facilitate the production of a suggested response. (for example, having a patient imagine a helium-filled balloon attached to his hand to facilitate an arm levitation).

GUILT. Feelings of self-blame and self-condemnation for what the patient considers a reprehensible action or thought. Called moral anxiety by Freud.

HERING REFLEX. A reflex mediated by receptors in the carotid sinus, which lowers the heart rate in response to an increase in blood pressure.

HIDDEN OBSERVER. A form of automatic talking developed by Hilgard to elicit reports of pain sensations of which a subject given suggestions of pain relief is not consciously aware. Similar to automatic writing.

HIGHWAY HYPNOSIS. A spontaneous hypnotic trance induced by the monotony of a straight highway, which offers little to distract the motorist from staring at the roadway.

HYPEREMPIRIC TRANCE. A hypnotic trance state in which the subject is given suggestions of increased rather than decreased motor activity.

HYPERMNESIA. Enhancement of memory produced by hypnosis or other means.

HYPNOANALYSIS. Psychoanalysis conducted with the patient under hypnosis.

HYPNOIDAL STATE. A very light or prehypnotic condition; the lightest of Charcot's three stages of hypnosis.

HYPNOSIS. The trance state produced by an induction procedure.

HYPNOTECHNICIAN. *See* Lay Hypnotist.

HYPNOTHERAPY. The use of hypnosis as a method of psychotherapy or as an adjunct to a method of psychotherapy.

HYPNOTIC SUSCEPTIBILITY. A personality characteristic that determines a subject's ability to be hypnotized and to attain a given depth of trance.

HYPNOTISM. The study and science of hypnotic phenomena as opposed to the trance state.

HYPNOTIZABILITY. The ability of a subject to be hypnotized; takes into account both basic hypnotic susceptibility and transient motivational factors.

IDEOMOTOR QUESTIONING. A questioning technique in which a hypnotized subject is asked questions requiring answers like "yes" and "no" and responds with an ideomotor signal such as a raised finger.

IDEOMOTOR RESPONSE. A motor response produced without conscious intent by concentrating and imagining that the response is occurring spontaneously.

ILLUSION. A common misperception of some sensory stimulus. All sensory modalities are subject to illusions.

IMAGERY SHIFT. A sudden change of images developed by a subject. Changes are made on cue.

IMPOTENCE. Male sexual dysfunction. The term includes erectile difficulties, premature ejaculation, and delayed ejaculation.

INDEPENDENT VARIABLE. The variable that an experimenter manipulates in an experiment.

INDIRECT SUGGESTION. A suggestion that is implied rather than directly stated.

INDUCED DREAM. A dream that is a response to a hypnotic suggestion to dream. It may be induced either during hypnosis or posthypnotically.

INDUCED EMOTION. 1. An emotion suggested under hypnosis. 2. The emotional state generated in the therapist or patient by the actions of the other.

INSIGHT. Self-understanding; awareness of the real reasons for one's feelings, behavior, and symptoms.

INSTRUMENTAL CONDITIONING. Also known as Operant Conditioning; Trial and Error Learning. The mechanism for learning responses of the voluntary nervous system in accordance with the following paradigm:

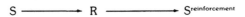

$$S \longrightarrow R \longrightarrow S^{reinforcement}$$

INTERPRETATION. An attempt to develop insight in a patient by the therapist's presenting his or her opinions concerning the unconscious meanings of the patient's behavior and symptoms.

ISCHEMIC PAIN. Pain produced by depriving part of the body of its blood supply.

LAY HYPNOTIST. A layperson who has learned to induce hypnosis but is untrained in psychology and psychotherapy.

LETHARGY. The middle state of trance depth according to Charcot.

LIMEN, Absolute. The minimum stimulus duration or intensity on some dimension that can just be perceived on 50% of the trials.

LIMEN, Difference. The minimum difference between two stimuli that can just be perceived on 50% of the trials. Also known as a just noticeable difference (JND).

LUCID DREAM. A nocturnal dream in which the dreamer (observing ego) knows that he is dreaming. Also called a dream of knowledge.

MACHIAVELLIANISM. The tendency to view others as objects to be manipulated and used without regard for their interests. The name derives from Machiavelli's essay *The Prince* in which he advocates a course of conduct for rulers based on expediency and duplicity.

MAGNETIZER. The term used for hypnotist prior to Braid's introduction of the term *hypnosis*.

MANTRA. The secret word that a meditator is supposed to concentrate on during transcendental meditation; likely to function as a conditioned stimulus for the relaxation response.

MEDICAL MODEL. A concept of psychopathology describing a mental illness as analogous to a physical illness: symptoms are said to reflect an inner disorder of the personality that requires correction (in contrast to the behavior modification approach that the symptom *is* the behavior disorder, and if it is removed, it no longer makes sense to regard the patient as ill).

MESOMORPHY. A component of a somatotype according to Sheldon (1954) characterized by a predominance of bone and muscle (i.e., derived from mesoderm).

MINITRANCE. A spontaneous trance that some investigators believe is reinstated automatically when a subject is given a posthypnotic cue for the performance of a posthypnotic suggestion.

MIRANDA WARNINGS. A statement of an arrestee's rights that the police are required to give him as soon as he is taken into custody and before he may be questioned. These include advising him that he has the right to remain silent, that anything he says can and will be used against him, and that he has a right to consult a lawyer prior to making any statement. He must then be asked if he understands these rights and if he desires to consult a lawyer. He may not be questioned unless he affirms that he understands the warning and, if he requests a lawyer, until he has consulted with the lawyer. In addition, he must affirmatively state that he desires to make a statement.

MONOIDEISM. Literally, "concentration on a single idea," which Braid ultimately believed was the essence of hypnosis. He unsuccessfully tried to change its name to this.

MORAL ANXIETY. *See* Guilt.

MULTIPLE PERSONALITY. An uncommon dissociative disorder characterized by the patient's behaving at different times as though he had a variety of different personalities. Often there is selective amnesia of one personality for the others.

NANCY SCHOOL. A school of hypnosis founded by Bernheim that subscribed to the view that hypnosis was basically a heightened state of suggestibility and was a normal phenomenon elicitable in most people.

NEGATIVE AFTERIMAGE. Seeing a visual stimulus as a negative after the stimulus is turned off. In the case of a color image, the afterimage is seen in terms of the complementary colors of the original.

NEGATIVE HALLUCINATION. A hallucination in which the subject fails to perceive a stimulus that is physically present.

NEGATIVE REINFORCEMENT. 1. In the Skinnerian sense, a reinforcement produced by the turning off of an aversive stimulus. 2. An alternative (and opposite) usage is as a synonym for punishment.

NEGATIVISM. The tendency of a patient to resist doing what he is asked. Passive negativism involves ignoring instructions. Active negativism involves doing the opposite of what is asked.

NEODISSOCIATION THEORY. The position, developed by Hilgard, that when two tasks are performed simultaneously, one on a conscious and one on an unconscious level, each is performed less efficiently because of (1) the effort required for the other task and (2) the effort required to keep the unconscious task out of awareness.

NEUROSIS. A condition characterized by symptom formation where the symptoms, while painful, are not so disabling as to prevent the patient from functioning in daily life or to require institutionalization. In Freudian terms, neurotic symptoms are not merely maladaptive behavior but are a symbolic way of dealing with an intrapsychic conflict.

NEUTRAL HYPNOSIS. Hypnosis per se. The condition produced by a hypnotic induction procedure alone without the use of any specific, additional suggestions.

NREM. Non-REM stages of sleep. *See also* REM.

NONSENSE SYLLABLE. A meaningless arrangement of letters designed to provide stimuli or responses that have minimal amounts of preexperimental associations to them. Used in learning studies so that the learning process may be studied from the beginning.

OBSERVING EGO. That part of the ego that does not participate in a dream or hypnotic situation but stands back and observes the procedure as if a third party.

OPERANT CONDITIONING. *See* Instrumental Conditioning.

ORGANIC DISEASE. A disease with either a physiological or psychological etiology characterized by structural changes in the body.

ORGANISMIC VARIABLE. Something that is used like an independent variable in an experiment but that the experimenter cannot manipulate because it is a characteristic of the organism (e.g., intelligence). Since this variable cannot be manipulated, it must be varied by the selection of subjects, and, hence, random experimental samples cannot be used.

PAIN. In hypnotic studies, pain usually refers to the afferent sensory impulses associated with pain receptors. The term may be used to refer to either the sensory or perceptual aspects of these impulses.

PAIRED-ASSOCIATES LIST. A list of words or nonsense syllables to be learned, where the stimuli and responses are organized into fixed pairs presented in a different random order on each learning trial. Items on such a list have either a stimulus or a response function. Hence, this type of list is useful in studies designed to separate the effects of stimulus and response variables in rote learning.

PARAMNESIA. A false memory.

PARIS SCHOOL. The school of hypnosis founded by Charcot in Paris that had the view that hypnotic phenomena were manifestations of hysteria and only hysterics could be hypnotized. It also held that hypnosis was a physiological phenomenon that had definite stages and could be induced by physiological manipulations.

PARTIAL REINFORCEMENT SCHEDULE. A reinforcement schedule in which not every response made to a training stimulus is reinforced. Generally results in slower acquisition but also more resistance to extinction.

PARTICIPATING EGO. The part of the ego subjectively experiencing the hypnotic responses suggested.

PASSIVE-AGGRESSIVE PERSONALITY. A personality type that expresses hostility by passivity and ineptness.

PERCEIVED LOCUS OF CONTROL. Refers to whether a subject perceives that his fate is determined by forces outside himself (fate or powerful others) or by factors from within himself (talent or intelligence).

PERCEIVED SELF. *See* Self-Image.

PERCEPTION. Sensation plus organization; the subjective awareness of external stimuli organized into enduring figures and grounds. Perception combines sensory information and notions of the significance of this information.

PERMISSIVE SUGGESTION. A suggestion made in such a manner as to give the subject the option of responding. The subject, not the hypnotist, is made the perceived source of the response.

PERSONALITY. All of the factors within a person that play a role in determining his unique responses to his environment.

PHOBIA. A neurosis involving an unrealistic fear of an innocuous object or a fear out of all proportion to the actual danger.

PLACEBO EFFECT. An effect of a drug or treatment based on the patient's expectations of benefit rather than the pharmacological or physical effects of the drug or treatment.

PLANARY TRANCE. A stuporous trance, described by Erickson, that is even deeper than a somnambulistic state.

POSITIVE AFTERIMAGE. The continuing perception of a visual stimulus in its original form and color, after it has been terminated.

POSITIVE HALLUCINATION. A perception in the absence of a real external stimulus.

POSITIVE REINFORCEMENT. Anything that makes a response more likely to occur in the presence of a training stimulus. A reward.

POSTHYPNOTIC AMNESIA. Amnesia for the events of a hypnotic trance that occurs in the subsequent waking state.

POSTHYPNOTIC CUE/ SIGNAL. A signal given in the posthypnotic period for the performance of previously suggested posthypnotic behavior.

POSTHYPNOTIC SUGGESTION. A suggestion given during a trance designed to be carried out in the subsequent waking state.

PRECONSCIOUS. The repository within the nervous system of those memories that are freely accessible to consciousness but are not currently in conscious awareness. A Freudian construct.

PREHYPNOTIC SUGGESTION. Suggestions given prior to a hypnotic induction designed to produce a set or expectancy of success.

PRIMARY PROCESS. A primitive modality of thinking characterized by imagery. The earliest mode of thought according to Freudians. The term includes fantasy or daydreaming, nocturnal dreaming, and hallucinations.

PROJECTION. A defense mechanism in which an anxiety-producing thought is dealt with by projecting it onto another person (for example, "I do not hate him; he hates me")

PSEUDO-AMNESIA. The initial failure to learn material, which gives the illusion of its being forgotten in the posthypnotic state.

PSYCHOGENIC. Conditions stemming from a psychological etiology as opposed to organic causes.

PSYCHOPATH. A character disorder defined by a marked underdevelopment of the superego or sense of morality. Not a synonym for a mentally ill person but a specific type of psychopathology.

PSYCHOSIS. A disorder characterized by symbolic symptom formation where the symptoms are so disabling that the person cannot function in daily life. Often characterized by the presence of hallucinations and/or delusions.

PSYCHOSOMATIC ILLNESS. An organic condition produced in part or whole by psychogenic causes.

RANDOM SAMPLE. A sample selected in such a manner that each element in the population sampled has an equal chance of being selected and the selection of one element has no effect on the selection of any other element.

RAPPORT. 1. A reality-oriented relationship between two people. A mutual understanding and acceptance of the duties and expectations of the parties to a relationship. 2. The hypnotic phenomenon in which the subject responds only to suggestions from the hypnotist and from no one else unless the hypnotist so directs.

REAL TIME. Objective time as measured by a clock.

RECALL. A method of demonstrating memory in which the subject has to produce the material without cueing.

RECIPROCAL INHIBITION. A method of eliminating an undesired behavior by training the patient to produce an incompatible substitute behavior. For example, since relaxation and anxiety are incompatible responses, phobic anxiety can be reciprocally inhibited or counterconditioned by making the phobic object elicit a relaxation response.

RECOGNITION. A method of testing memory requiring a subject to recognize material previously learned from among incorrect items.

REGRESSION. The replacing of more mature behavior with behavior appropriate to an earlier period of life. In psychoanalysis, it means going back to an earlier period of psychosexual development.

RELEARNING. A method of demonstrating learning that involves relearning the material and comparing the number of trials needed for relearning with the original number of learning trials. The savings in relearning trials is an index of the amount of retention of the original learning. Sometimes this retention cannot be demonstrated in any other way.

RELEASE SIGNAL. A signal given during the posthypnotic period to terminate ongoing posthypnotic behavior.

RELIABILITY. The consistency of a psychological test. The ability of a test to yield consistent results when given to the same subjects repeatedly.

REM. Rapid eye movements occurring during stage 1 sleep and correlated with visual dreaming.

RESISTANCE. A reaction of a patient during psychotherapy that is unconsciously designed to defeat the therapy.

RESPONSE. A reaction to an internal or external stimulus. Overt responses change the relationship between the organism and its environment. Modern behaviorists also regard covert reactions, such as a thought, to be responses.

RETROACTIVE INHIBITION. The effect of subsequent learning in weakening the retention of previous learning; an active interference model of forgetting.

REVIVIFICATION. A reliving of a prior period of life.

SAVINGS METHOD. *See* Relearning.

SECONDARY GAINS. The primary function of a symptom in psychoanalytic theory is to control anxiety. Any additional benefits that a patient gets from his symptom, such as avoiding responsibility or controlling others, are called secondary gains.

SECONDARY PROCESS. A more advanced logical mode of thinking, reality-oriented, logical, analytical, or integrative and more involved with language than images. In psychoanalytic terms, it is a function of a more developed ego system than the primary processes.

SELF-HYPNOSIS. *See* Autosuggestion.

SELF-IMAGE. The sum of all the beliefs, attitudes, perceptions, and opinions that a person has about himself.

SENSATION. The physiological processes that occur as a result of the stimulation of sense organs and receptors.

SENSORY HYPNOPLASTY. A technique of developing regression under hypnosis by having the patient mold a piece of plastic.

SENSORY HYPNOTHERAPY. A form of hypnotherapy in which sensory imagery plays a major role.

SEQUELAE. In hypnotic literature refers to deleterious consequences of hypnosis.

SERIAL LIST. A list of words or nonsense syllables used in learning studies where the subject is required to learn both the items and their order. Each item on the list functions as a stimulus, a response, and a reinforcement.

SET. *See* Prehypnotic Suggestion.

SIMULATION GROUP. A group of nonhypnotized subjects instructed to act as though they were hypnotized and to attempt to deceive the experimenter concerning their true status.

SOCIAL ROLE THEORY. As applied to hypnosis, the notion that being a hypnotic subject imposes a role or a set of social expectations on the subject that affects his behavior.

SOMNAMBULISM. 1. Sleepwalking; 2. a deep hypnotic stage; 3. the deepest stage of hypnosis according to Charcot.

SOURCE AMNESIA. A posthypnotic amnesia where the subject remembers an unusual fact told to him under hypnosis but is unaware of the source of this information. Often occurs spontaneously.

SPECIFIC POSTHYPNOTIC AMNESIA. A suggested posthypnotic amnesia for a specific area of recall or memory.

SPONTANEOUS ABREACTION. An abreaction under hypnosis that was not deliberately produced by the hypnotist.

SPONTANEOUS POSTHYPNOTIC AMNESIA. A posthypnotic amnesia that occurs without specific suggestions to the subject to produce it.

SPONTANEOUS RECOVERY. The recovery of a portion of habit strength previously extinguished, following a period of rest and without any intervening relearning trials or practice.

SPONTANEOUS REGRESSION. A hypnotic regression obtained without the hypnotist's making any direct or indirect suggestions designed to produce it.

SPONTANEOUS TRANCE. A naturally occurring trance state that is not produced by either heterohypnosis or autohypnosis.

STIMULUS. Any form of physical or chemical energy to which an organism has a receptor capable of reacting. Anything capable of eliciting a response. May be overt (external) or covert (internal).

SUBCONSCIOUS. A commonly used corruption of the term *unconscious.*

SUBJECTIVE QUESTIONING. A passive technique of hypnotic questioning.

SUBJECTIVE TIME. Time as perceived by a subject (as opposed to real time).

SUBLIMINAL. A stimulus below the limen and thus not perceivable. (The term *subliminal perception* is therefore a self-contradictory expression).

SUD. Subjective unit of disturbance. A scale running from 0 to 100 on which a subject is instructed to rate the amount of anxiety he is experiencing.

SUFFERING. The psychological aspect of the total pain experience; the unpleasant component of the pain experience that includes both perceptual and cognitive aspects.

SUGGESTIBILITY. The propensity of a subject to accept and act on suggestions.

SUGGESTION. An attempt to get a subject to produce a behavior without commanding or directing him to do so.

SYMBOL. 1. Something that stands for something else or a referent. 2. In psychoanalysis, a concrete image representing a repressed infantile wish. 3. The expression of an abstract idea in a more primitive, concrete manner.

SYMPTOM. 1. Any maladaptive behavior. 2. In psychoanalysis, a compromise reaction between the two elements of an internal conflict. Symptoms are learned to control the anxiety associated with the inner conflict.

SYMPTOM SUBSTITUTION. The notion that since symptoms have a symbolic meaning and the patient needs them to hold anxiety in check, their direct removal, without first resolving the inner conflict, will result in a substitute and possibly worse symptom being acquired in their place.

TASK MOTIVATION. Barber's notion that the main determinant of "hypnotic-like" behavior is the subject's motivation to produce the responses that the experimenter wants him to rather than a trance state.

TIME DISTORTION. The ability of hypnotic suggestion to make subjective time seem to pass more rapidly or more slowly than real time.

TORT. A civil wrong rendering the tort-feasor liable for damages in a lawsuit. A breach by the defendant of a primary right (i.e., a right not arising out of a contract) of the plaintiff.

TRANCE. An altered state of consciousness rendering a subject hypersuggestible (Nonstate theorists question the existence of such a special state.)

TRANCE CAPACITY. *See* Hypnotic Susceptibility.

TRANCE DEPTH. Generally defined in terms of the number of low-probability responses a subject makes in response to suggestions.

TRANCE LOGIC. The suspension of critical judgement on the part of a hypnotized subject and his ability to tolerate the coexistence of logically incompatible phenomena. Similar to the reaction of dreamers who are not upset by bizarre effects occurring during nocturnal dreams.

TRANSFERENCE. An intense and inappropriate emotional reaction of a patient directed at the therapist. In psychoanalysis this emotion is thought to be transferred to the therapist from more significant people in the patient's earlier life.

TRICHOTILLOMANIA. Pulling one's own hair out.

TRUE EFFECT. The pharmacological or physiological effect of a drug or treatment with the placebo effect removed.

UNCONSCIOUS. A part of the psyche that contains memories not freely accessible to conscious awareness. The material in the unconscious, in psychoanalytic theory, was forced there and is held there by the process of repression.

VAGINISMUS. A spasm of muscles surrounding the vagina that makes penetration and intercourse impossible.

VALIDITY. The degree to which a psychological test measures what it purports to measure.

VARIABLE INTERVAL SCHEDULE (VI). A reinforcement schedule in which only the first response in a time interval is reinforced.

VICARIOUS REINFORCEMENT. The learning of a behavior by observing a model displaying the behavior and being reinforced for it.

VICIOUS CIRCLE. *See* Feedback Loop.

WAKING SUGGESTION. Suggestions given to a waking, as opposed to a hypnotized, subject.

WITHIN-SUBJECTS, REPEATED-MEASURES DESIGN. An experimental design in which each subject sequentially receives every level of the independent variable and hence functions as his own control.

ZEIGARNIK EFFECT. The tendency to remember an uncompleted task. A motivational concept related to the need to complete a task and develop a feeling of closure.

ZEITGEIST. The spirit of the times.

References and
Bibliography

Abrams, S. (1983). The multiple personality: A legal defense. *American J. of Clinical Hypnosis* **25**(4):225-231.

Abramson, M., and Heron, W. T. (1950). An objective evaluation of hypnosis in obstetrics: Preliminary report. *American J. of Obstetrics and Gynecology* **59**:1069-1074.

Acosta, E., Jr., and Crawford, H. J. (1985). Iconic memory and hypnotizability: Processing speed, skill, or strategy differences? *International J. of Clinical and Experimental Hypnosis* **33**(3):224-235.

Adams, P. (1977). *The New Self-Hypnosis*. Hollywood: Wilshire Book Co.

Aja, J. H. (1977). Brief group treatment of obesity through ancillary self-hypnosis. *American J. of Clinical Hypnosis* **19**(4):231-234.

Akstein, D. (1977). Socio-cultural basis of terpsichoretrancetherapy. *American J. of Clinical Hypnosis* **19**(4):221-225.

Albert, I. B., and Boone, D. (1975). Dream deprivation and facilitation with hypnosis. *J. of Abnormal Psychology* **84**(3):267-271.

Albert, I., and Williams, M. H. (1975). Effects of post-hypnotic suggestions on muscular endurance. *Perceptual and Motor Skills* **40**(1):131-139.

Allen, B. P. (1978). *Social Behavior: Fact and Falsehoods about Common Sense, Hypnotism, Obedience, Altruism, Beauty, Racism, and Sexism*. Chicago: Nelson-Hall.

Allison, R. B. (1984). Difficulties diagnosing the multiple personality syndrome in a death penalty case. *International J. of Clinical and Experimental Hypnosis* **32**(2):102-117.

Alman, B. M. (1980). Consequences of direct and indirect suggestions on success of post-hypnotic behavior. *Dissertation Abstracts International* **40**(10-A):5369.

Alman, B. M., and Carney, R. E. (1980). Consequences of direct and indirect suggestions on success of posthypnotic behavior. *American J. of Clinical Hypnosis* **23**(2):112-118.

AMA Council on Scientific Affairs. (1985). Scientific status of refreshing recollection by the use of hypnosis. *J. of American Medical Association* **253**(13):1918-1923.

American Society of Clinical Hypnosis: Education and Research Foundation. (1973). *A Syllabus on Hypnosis and a Handbook of Therapeutic Suggestions.*

Andersen, M. S. (1985). Hypnotizability as a factor in the hypnotic treatment of obesity. *International J. of Clinical and Experimental Hypnosis* **33**(2):150-159.

Anderson, J. A. D.; Basker, M. A.; and Dalton, R. (1975). Migraine and hypnotherapy. *International J. of Clinical and Experimental Hypnosis* **23**(1):48-58.

Anderson, J.W. (1977). Defensive maneuvers in two incidents involving the Chevreul pendulum: A clinical note. *International J. of Clinical and Experimental Hypnosis* **25**(1):4-6.

Anderson, O. (1979). A supplement to Freud's case history of "Frau Emmy v. N." in Studies on Hysteria 1895. *Scandinavian Psychoanalytic Review* **2**(1):5-16.

Andrick, J. M. (1978). Hypnosis and the Emmanuel movement: A medical and religious repudiation. *American J. of Clinical Hypnosis* **20**(4):224-234.

Angelos, J. S. (1978). A comparison of the effects of direct and indirect methods of hypnotic induction on the perception of pain. *Dissertation Abstracts International* **39**(6-B):2972-2973.

Ansel, E. L. (1977). A simple exercise to enhance response to hypnotherapy for migraine headache. *International J. of Clinical and Experimental Hypnosis* **25**(2):68-71.

Appelbaum, P. S. (1984). Hypnosis in the courtroom. *Hospital and Community Psychiatry* **35**(7):657-658.

Araoz, D. L. (1978). Clinical hypnosis in couple therapy. *J. of the American Society of Psychosomatic Dentistry and Medicine* **25**(2):58-67.

Araoz, D. L. (1979). Hypnosis in group therapy. *International J. of Clinical and Experimental Hypnosis* **27**(1):1-13.

Araoz, D. L. (1983). Hypnosex therapy. *American J. of Clinical Hypnosis* **26**(1):37-41.

Araoz, D. L. (1986). Uses of hypnosis in the treatment of psychogenic sexual dysfunctions. *Psychiatric Annals* **16**(2):102-105.

Arnold, M. B. (1946). On the mechanism of suggestion and hypnosis. *J. of Abnormal and Social Psychology* **41**:107-128.

Arons, H. (1961). *Master Course in Hypnotism.* South Orange, NJ: Power Publishers.

Arons, H. (1975). *Handbook of Self-hypnosis.* South Orange, NJ: Power Publishers.

Arons, H. (1977). *Hypnosis in Criminal Investigation.* South Orange, NJ: Power Publishers.

Arons, H., and Bubeck, M. F. H. (1971). *Handbook of Professional Hypnosis.* South Orange, NJ: Power Publishers.

As, A. (1962). The recovery of forgotten language knowledge through hypnotic age regression: A case report. *American J. of Clinical Hypnosis* **5**:19-21.

As, A.; Hilgard, E. R.; and Weitzenhoffer, A. M. (1963). An attempt at experimental modification of hypnotizability through repeated individualized hypnotic experience. *Scandinavian J. of Psychology* **4**:81-89.

Ascher, L. M. (1977). The role of hypnosis in behavior therapy. *Annals of New York Academy of Sciences* **296**:250-263.

Asher, R. (1956). Respectable hypnosis. *British Medical J.* **1**:309-313.

Ashford, B., and Hammer, A. G. (1978). The role of expectancies in the occurrence of posthypnotic amnesia. *International J. of Clinical and Experimental Hypnosis* **26**(4):281-291.

Ashton, M. A., and McDonald, R. D. (1985). Effects of hypnosis on verbal and non-verbal creativity. *International J. of Clinical and Experimental Hypnosis* **33**(1):15-26.

Astor, M. H. (1973). Hypnosis and behavior modification combined with psychoanalytic psychotherapy. *International J. of Clinical and Experimental Hypnosis* **21**(1):18-24.

Astrup, C. (1978). Physiological mechanisms of flooding (implosion) therapy. *Pavlovian J. of Biological Science* **13**(4):195-198.

August, R. V. (1975). Hypnotic induction of hypothermia: An additional approach to postoperative control of cancer recurrence. *American J. of Clinical Hypnosis* **18**(1):52-55.

Augustynek, A. (1978). Remembering under hypnosis. *Studia Psychologica* **20**(4):256-266.

Ault, R. L. (1979). FBI guidelines for use of hypnosis. *International J. of Clinical and Experimental Hypnosis* **27**(4):449-451.

Austrin, H. R., and Pereira, M. J. (1978). Locus of control as a predictor of hypnotic susceptibility. *American J. of Clinical Hypnosis* **20**(3):199-202.

Avampato, J. J. (1975). Hypnosis: A cure for torticollis. *American J. of Clinical Hypnosis* **18**(1):60-62.

Baer, L. (1979). Effect of a time-slowing suggestions on rate of emission of an operant response. *Psychological Record* **29**(3):389-400.

Baer, L. (1980). Effect of a time-slowing suggestion on performance accuracy on a perceptual motor task. *Perceptual and Motor Skills* **51**(1):167-176.

Baer, L. (1981). Effects of a time-slowing suggestion versus rate-changing directions on operant response rate. *Dissertation Abstracts International* **42**(2-B):739.

Bakal, P. A. (1981). Hypnotherapy for flight phobia. *American J. of Clinical Hypnosis* **23**(4):248-251.

Baker, E. L. (1981). An hypnotherapeutic approach to enhance object relatedness in psychotic patients. *International J. of Clinical and Experimental Hypnosis* **29**(2):136-147.

Baker, E. L. (1983a). The use of hypnotic techniques with psychotics. *American J. of Clinical Hypnosis* **25**(4):283-288.

Baker, E. L. (1983b). Resistance in hypnotherapy of primitive states: Its meaning and management. *International J. of Clinical and Experimental Hypnosis* **31**(2):82-89.

Baker, E. L. (1983c). The use of hypnotic dreaming in the treatment of the borderline patient: Some thoughts on resistance and transitional phenomena. *International J. of Clinical and Experimental Hypnosis* **31**(1):19-27.

Baker, R. A. (1982). The effect of suggestion on past-lives regression. *American J. of Clinical Hypnosis* **25**(1):71-76.

Baker, R. A.; Haynes, B.; and Patrick, B. S. (1983). Hypnosis, memory and incidental memory. *American J. of Clinical Hypnosis* **25**(4):253-262.

Baker, S. R., and Boaz, D. (1983). The partial reformulation of a traumatic memory of a dental phobia during trance: A case study. *International J. of Clinical and Experimental Hypnosis* **31**(1):14-18.

Balaam, M. (1984). Further comment on Benson's "Short-term hypnotherapy with delinquent and acting out adolescents." *British J. of Experimental and Clinical Hypnosis* **2**(1):47-49.

Balaschak, B.; Blocker, K.; Rossiter, T.; and Perin, C. T. (1972). The influence of race and expressed experience of the hypnotist on hypnotic susceptibility. *International J. of Clinical and Experimental Hypnosis* **20**(1):38-45.

Baldwin, B. A. (1978). Crisis intervention and enhancement of adaptive coping using hypnosis. *American J. of Clinical Hypnosis* **21**(1):38-44.

Ballinger, S. E. (1983). "I'm not hypnotized": A patient's perception of hypnosis. *Australian J. of Clinical and Experimental Hypnosis* **11**(2):111-113.

Balson, P. M.; Dempster, C. R.; and Brooks, F. R. (1984). Auto-hypnosis is a defense against coercive persuasion. *American J. of Clinical Hypnosis* **26**(4):252-260.

Bandler, R., and Grinder, J. (1975). *Patterns of the Hypnotic Techniques of Milton H. Erickson, M.D. Volume 1.* Cupertino, CA: Meta Publications.

Banyai, E. I., and Hilgard, E. R. (1976). A comparison of active-alert hypnotic induction with traditional relaxation induction. *J. of Abnormal Psychology* **85**(2):218-224.

Barabasz, A. F. (1976). Treatment of insomnia in depressed patients by hypnosis and cerebral electrotherapy. *American J. of Clinical Hypnosis* **19**(2):120-122.

Barabasz, A. F. (1980a). Effects of hypnosis and perceptual deprivation on vigilance in a simulated radar target-detection test. *Perceptual and Motor Skills* **50**(1):19-24.

Barabasz, A. F. (1980b). EEG alpha, skin conductance and hypnotizability in Antarctica. *International J. of Clinical and Experimental Hypnosis* **28**(1):63-74.

Barabasz, A. F. (1982). Restricted environmental stimulation and the enhancement of hypnotizability: Pain, EEG alpha, skin conductance and temperature responses. *International J. of Clinical and Experimental Hypnosis* **30**(2):147-166.

Barabasz, A. F. (1984). Antarctic isolation and imaginative involvement— Preliminary findings: A brief communication. *International J. of Clinical and Experimental Hypnosis* **32**(3):296-300.

Barabasz, M.; Barabasz, A. F.; and Mullin, C. S. (1983). Effects of brief Antarctic isolation on absorption and hypnotic susceptibility—Preliminary results and recommendations: A brief communication. *International J. of Clinical and Experimental Hypnosis* **31**(4):235-238.

Barabasz, A. F., and Lonsdale, C. (1983). Effects of hypnosis on P300 olfactory-evoked potential amplitudes. *J. of Abnormal Psychology* **92**(4):520-523.

Barabasz, A. F., and McGeorge, C. M. (1978). Biofeedback, mediated biofeedback and hypnosis in peripheral vasodilation training. *American J. of Clinical Hypnosis* **21**(1):28-37.

Barber, J. (1977). Rapid induction analgesia: A clinical report. *American J. of Clinical Hypnosis* **19**(3):138-147.

Barber, J. (1980). Hypnosis and the unhypnotizable. *American J. of Clinical Hypnosis* **23**(1):4-9.

Barber, J., and Adrian, C. (Eds.). (1982). *Psychological Approaches to the Management of Pain.* New York: Brunner-Mazel.

Barber, J., and Gitelson, J. (1980). Cancer pain: Psychological management using hypnosis. *Ca—A Cancer Journal for Clinicians* **30**(3):130-136.

Barber, J., and Malin, A. H. (1977). Hypnosis and suggestion for fitting contact lenses. *J. of the American Optometric Association* **48**(3):379-382.

Barber, T. X. (1956a). Comparison of suggestibility during "light sleep" and hypnosis. *Science* **124**:405.

Barber, T. X. (1956b). "Sleep" and "hypnosis": A reappraisal. *J. of Clinical and Experimental Hypnosis* **4**:141-159.   ·

Barber, T. X. (1956c). A note on "hypnotizability" and personality traits. *J. of Clinical and Experimental Hypnosis* **4**:109-114.

Barber, T. X. (1957a). Experiments in hypnosis. *Scientific American* **196** (4):54-61.

Barber, T. X. (1957b). Hypnosis as perceptual-cognitive restructuring. I. Analysis of concepts. *J. of Clinical and Experimental Hypnosis* **5**:147-166.

Barber, T. X. (1957c). Hypnosis as perceptual-cognitive restructuring. III. From somnambulism to autohypnosis. *J. of Psychology* **44**:299-304.

Barber, T. X. (1958a). The concept of "hypnosis." *J. of Psychology* **45**:115-131.

Barber, T. X. (1958b). The "good" hypnotic subject. *Science Digest* **43**(1):36-41.

Barber, T. X. (1958c). Hypnosis as perceptual-cognitive restructuring. II. "Post" hypnotic behavior. *J. of Clinical and Experimental Hypnosis* **6**:10-20.

Barber, T. X. (1958d). Hypnosis as perceptual-cognitive restructuring. IV. "Negative hallucinations." *J. of Psychology* **46**:187-201.

Barber, T. X. (1959a). Toward a theory of pain. Relief of chronic pain by prefrontal leucotomy, opiates, placebos and hypnosis. *Psychological Bulletin* **56**(6):430-460.

Barber, T. X. (1959b). The "eidetic image" and "hallucinatory" behavior: A suggestion for further research. *Psychological Bulletin* **56**(3):236-239.

Barber, T. X. (1959c). The afterimages of "hallucinated" and "imagined" colors. *J. of Abnormal and Social Psychology* **59**(1):136-139.

Barber, T. X. (1960a). "Hypnosis," analgesia and the placebo effect. *J. American Medical Association* **172**(7):680-683.

Barber, T. X. (1960b). The necessary and sufficient conditions for hypnotic behavior. *American J. of Clinical Hypnosis* **3**(1):31-42.

Barber, T. X. (1961a). Antisocial and criminal acts induced by "hypnosis": A review of experimental and clinical findings. *Archives of General Psychiatry* **5**:301-312.

Barber, T. X. (1961b). Physiological effects of "hypnosis." *Psychological Bulletin* **58**:390-419.

Barber, T.X. (1961c). Experimental evidence for a theory of hypnotic behavior. II. Experimental controls in hypnotic age-regression. *International J. of Clinical and Experimental Hypnosis* **9**(4):181-193.

Barber, T. X. (1962a). Experimental controls and the phenomena of "hypnosis": A critique of hypnotic research methodology. *J. of Nervous and Mental Disease* **134**(6):493-505.

Barber, T. X. (1962*b*). Toward a theory of "hypnotic" behavior: The "hypnotically induced dream." *J. of Nervous and Mental Disease* **135**:206-221.

Barber, T. X. (1962*c*). Toward a theory of hypnosis: Posthypnotic behavior. *Archives of General Psychiatry* **7**:321-342.

Barber, T. X. (1962*d*). Hypnotic age regression: A critical review. *Psychosomatic Medicine* **24**(3):286-299.

Barber, T. X. (1963). The effects of "hypnosis" on pain—a critical review of experimental and clinical findings. *Psychosomatic Medicine* **25**:303-333.

Barber, T. X. (1964*a*). Hypnotizability, suggestibility and personality: A critical review of research findings. *Psychological Reports.* Monograph Supp. **14**(3):299-320.

Barber, T. X. (1964*b*). "Hypnosis" as a causal variable in present day psychology: A critical analysis. *Psychological Reports* **14**:839-842.

Barber, T. X. (1964*c*). Hypnotic "colorblindness," "blindness" and "deafness": A review of research findings. *Diseases of the Nervous System* **25**:529-537.

Barber, T. X. (1964*d*). Hypnotically hallucinated colors and their negative after images. *American J. of Psychology* **77**(2):313-318.

Barber, T. X. (1964*e*). Toward a theory of "hypnotic" behavior: Positive visual and auditory hallucinations. *Psychological Record* **14**:197-210.

Barber, T. X. (1965*a*). Hypnosis throughout the world. *Archives of General Psychiatry* **12**:109-110.

Barber, T.X. (1965*b*). Measuring "hypnotic-like" suggestibility with and without "hypnotic induction"; Psychometric properties, norms, and variables influencing response to the Barber Suggestibility Scale (BSS). *Psychological Reports.* Monograph Supp. **16**(3):809-844.

Barber, T.. X. (1965*c*). The effects of "hypnosis" on learning and recall: A methodological critique. *J. of Clinical Psychology* **21**:19-25.

Barber, T. X. (1965*d*). Physiological effects of "hypnotic suggestions": A critical review of recent research (1960-64). *Psychological Bulletin* **63**(4):201-222.

Barber, T. X. (1965*e*). Experimental analysis of "hypnotic" behavior: A review of recent empirical findings. *J. of Abnormal Psychology.* **70**:132-154.

Barber, T. X. (1966). The effects of hypnosis and suggestions on strength and endurance: A critical review of research studies. *British J. of Social and Clinical Psychology* **5**:42-50.

Barber, T. X. (1967*a*). "Hypnotic" phenomena: A critique of experimental methods. In J. E. Gordon (Ed.), *Handbook of Clinical and Experimental Hypnosis* (pp. 444-480). New York: Macmillan.

Barber, T. X. (1967b). Reply to Conn and Conn's "discussion of Barber's 'hypnosis as causal variable.' " *International J. of Clinical and Experimental Hypnosis* **15**(3):111-117.

Barber, T. X. (1969a). An empirically based formulation of hypnotism. *American J. of Clinical Hypnosis* **12**(2):100-130.

Barber, T. X. (1969b). Controls in hypnotic research: Comment on Schneck's (1969) critique of Barber. *Perceptual and Motor Skills* **28**:630.

Barber, T. X. (1969c) Invalid arguments, postmortem analysis, and the experimenter bias effect. *J. of Counseling and Clinical Psychology* **33**(1):11-14.

Barber, T. X. (1970a). *LSD, Marijuana, Yoga and Hypnosis.* Chicago: Aldine.

Barber, T. X. (1970b). *Suggested ('Hypnotic') Behavior: The Trance Paradigm versus an Alternative Paradigm.* Harding, MA: Medfield Foundation.

Barber, T. X. (1974). Implications for human capabilities and potentialities. In T. X. Barber, N. P. Spanos, and J. F. Chaves, *Hypnosis, Imagination and Human Potentialities* (pp. 109-126). New York: Pergamon Press.

Barber, T. X. (1975). Responding to "hypnotic" suggestions: an introspective report. *American J. of Clinical Hypnosis* **18**(1):6-22.

Barber, T. X. (Ed.). (1976a). Self-control: Temperature biofeedback, hypnosis, yoga, and relaxation. Introduction to *Biofeedback and Self-control: 1975/76.* (pp. xiii-xxix). Chicago: Aldine.

Barber, T. X. (1976b). *Hypnosis: A Scientific Approach.* New York: Psychological Dimensions.

Barber, T. X. (1978a). Hypnosis, suggestions, and psychosomatic phenomena: A new look from the standpoint of recent experimental studies. *American J. of Clinical Hypnosis* **21**(1):13-27.

Barber, T. X. (1978b). Proseminar on hypnosis and psychosomatics in New York City. September.

Barber, T. X. (1978c). "Hypnosis," suggestions and psychosomatic phenomena: A new look from the standpoint of recent experimental studies. In J. L. Fosshage and P. T. Olsen (Eds.), *Healing: Implications for Psychotherapy.* New York: Human Sciences Press.

Barber, T. X. (1978d). Seminar at Molloy College, Rockville Centre, New York, May.

Barber, T. X. (1980). Effects of a traditional trance induction on a response to "hypnotist-centered" versus "subject-centered" test suggestions. *International J. of Clinical and Experimental Hypnosis* **28**(2):114-125.

Barber, T. X., and Calverley, D. S. (1962). "Hypnotic behavior" as a function of task motivation. *J. of Psychology* **54**:363-389.

Barber, T. X., and Calverley, D. S. (1963a). Toward a theory of hypnotic behavior: Effects on suggestibility of task motivating instructions and attitudes toward hypnosis. *J. of Abnormal and Social Psychology* **67**:557-565.

Barber, T. X., and Calverley, D. S. (1963b). The relative effectiveness of task-motivating instructions and trance-induction procedure in the production of "hypnotic-like" behaviors. *J. of Nervous and Mental Disease* **137**(2):107-116.

Barber, T. X., and Calverley, D. S. (1963c). "Hypnotic-like" suggestibility in children and adults. *J. of Abnormal and Social Psychology* **66**:589-597.

Barber, T. X., and Calverley, D. S. (1964a). Effect of E's tone of voice on "hypnotic-like" suggestibility. *Psychological Reports* **15**:139-144.

Barber, T. X., and Calverley, D. S. (1964b). Hypnotizability, suggestibility and personality: I. Two studies with the Edwards Personal Preference Schedule, the Jourard Self-Disclosure Scale, and the Marlowe-Crowne Social Desirability Scale. *J. of Psychology* **58**:215-222.

Barber, T. X., and Calverley, D. S. (1964c). Hypnotizability, suggestibility and personality: III. A study using teachers' ratings of children's characteristics. *J. of Psychology* **57**:275-280.

Barber, T. X., and Calverley, D. S. (1964d). Hypnotizability, suggestibility and personality: IV. A study with the Leary Interpersonal Check List. *British J. of Social and Clinical Psychology* **3**:149-150.

Barber, T. X., and Calverley, D. S. (1964e). Toward a theory of "hypnotic" behavior: Enhancement of strength and endurance. *Canadian J. of Psychology/Rev. Canad. Psychol.* **18**(2):156-167.

Barber, T. X., and Calverley, D. S. (1964f). Toward a theory of hypnotic behavior: Effects on suggestibility of defining the situation as hypnosis and defining response to suggestions as easy. *J. of Abnormal and Social Psychology* **68**:585-592.

Barber, T. X., and Calverley, D. S. (1964g). Comparative effects on "hypnotic-like" suggestibility of recorded and spoken suggestions. *J. Consulting Psychology* **28**(4):384.

Barber, T. X., and Calverley, D. S. (1964h). Empirical evidence for a theory of "hypnotic" behavior: Effects of pretest instructions on response to primary suggestions. *Psychological Record* **14**:457-467.

Barber, T. X., and Calverley, D. S. (1964i). Toward a theory of "hypnotic" behavior: An experimental study of "hypnotic time distortion." *Archives of General Psychiatry* **10**:209-216.

Barber, T. X., and Calverley, D. S. (1964j). Experimental studies in "hypnotic" behavior: Suggested deafness evaluated by delayed auditory feedback. *British J. of Psychology* **55**(4):439-446.

Barber, T. X., and Calverley, D. S. (1964k). An experimental study of "hypnotic" (auditory and visual) hallucinations. *J. of Abnormal and Social Psychology* **68**(1):13-20.

Barber, T. X., and Calverley, D. S. (1964l). The definition of the situation as a variable affecting "hypnotic-like" suggestibility. *J. of Clinical Psychology* **20**:438–440.

Barber, T. X., and Calverley, D. S. (1965*a*). Empirical evidence for a theory of hypnotic behavior: Effects on suggestibility of five variables typically included in hypnotic induction procedures. *J. of Consulting Psychology* **29**(2):98–107.

Barber, T. X., and Calverley, D. S. (1965*b*). Empirical evidence for a theory of "hypnotic" behavior: The suggestibility-enhancing effects of motivational suggestions, relaxation-sleep suggestions and suggestions that the S will be effectively "hypnotized." *J. of Personality* **33**(2):256–270.

Barber, T. X., and Calverley, D. S. (1965*c*). Hypnotizability, suggestibility and personality: II. Assessment of previous imaginative-fantasy experiences by the As, Barber-Glass, and Shor questionnaires. *J. of Clinical Psychology* **21**(1):57–58.

Barber, T. X., and Calverley, D. S. (1966*a*). Toward a theory of hypnotic behavior: Experimental evaluation of Hull's postulate that hypnotic susceptibility is a habit phenomenon. *J. of Personality* **34**(3):416–433.

Barber, T. X., and Calverley, D. S. (1966*b*). Effects on recall of hypnotic induction, motivational suggestions, and suggested regressions: A methodological and experimental analysis. *J. of Abnormal Psychology* **71**(3):169–180.

Barber, T. X., and Calverley, D. S. (1966*c*). Toward a theory of "hypnotic" behavior: Experimental analysis of suggested amnesia. *J. of Abnormal Psychology* **71**(2):95–107.

Barber, T. X., and Calverley, D. S. (1968). Toward a theory of "hypnotic" behavior: Replication and extension of experiments by Barber and coworkers (1962–65) and Hilgard and Tart (1966). *International J. of Clinical and Experimental Hypnosis* **16**(3):179–195.

Barber, T. X., and Calverley, D. S. (1969). Multidimensional analysis of "hypnotic" behavior. *J. of Abnormal Psychology* **74**(2):209–222.

Barber, T. X.; Calverley, D. S.; Forgione, A.; McPeake, J. D.; Chaves, J. F.; and Bowen, B. (1969). Five attempts to replicate the experimenter bias effect. *J. of Consulting and Clinical Psychology* **33**(1):1–6.

Barber, T. X., and Coules, J. (1959). Electrical skin conductance and galvanic skin response during "hypnosis." *International J. of Clinical and Experimental Hypnosis* **7**(2):79–92.

Barber, T. X.; Dalal, A. S.; and Calverley, D. S. (1968). The subjective reports of hypnotic subjects. *American J. of Clinical Hypnosis* **11**(2):74–88.

Barber, T. X., and Deeley, D. C. (1961). Experimental evidence for a theory of hypnotic behavior. I. "Hypnotic colorblindness" without "hypnosis." *International J. of Clinical and Experimental Hypnosis* **9**:79–86.

Barber, T. X., and De Moor, W. (1972). A theory of hypnotic induction procedures. *American J. of Clinical Hypnosis* **15**(2):112–135.

Barber, T. X., and Glass, L. B. (1962). Significant factors in hypnotic behavior. *J. of Abnormal and Social Psychology* **64**(3):222-228.

Barber, T. X., and Hahn, K. W., Jr., (1963). Hypnotic induction and "relaxation." *Archives of General Psychiatry* **8**:295-300.

Barber, T. X., and Hahn, K. W., Jr. (1964). Experimental studies in "hypnotic" behavior: Physiologic and subjective effects of imagined pain. *J. of Nervous and Mental Disease* **139**(5):416-425.

Barber, T. X.; Hilgard, E. R.; Morgan, A. H.; Hilgard, J. R.; Stern, D. B.; Spiegel, H.; and Nee, J. C. (1978-1979). Glossary. *American J. of Clinical Hypnosis* **21**(2-3):238-246.

Barber, T. X., and Silver, M. J. (1968a). Fact, fiction and the experimenter bias effect. *Psychological Bulletin Monographs* **70**(6 part 2):1-29.

Barber, T. X., and Silver, M. J. (1968b). Pitfalls in data analysis and interpretation: A reply to Rosenthal. *Psychological Bulletin Monographs* **70**(6 part 2):48-62.

Barber, T. X., and Wilson, S. C. (1977). Hypnosis, suggestions, and altered states of consciousness: Experimental evaluation of the new cognitive-behavioral theory and the traditional trance-state theory of "hypnosis." *Annals of New York Academy of Sciences* **296**:34-47.

Barber, T. X., and Wilson, S. C. (1978-1979). The Barber Suggestibility Scale and the Creative Imagination Scale: Experimental and clinical applications. *American J. of Clinical Hypnosis* **21**(2 and 3):84-108.

Barber, T. X.; Wilson, S. C.; and Scott, D. S. (1980). Effects of a traditional trance induction on response to "hypnotist-centered" versus "subject-centered" test suggestions. *International J. of Clinical and Experimental Hypnosis* **28**(2):114-126.

Barkley, R. A.; Hastings, J. E.; and Jackson, T. L., Jr. (1977). The effects of rapid smoking and hypnosis in the treatment of smoking behavior. *International J. of Clinical and Experimental Hypnosis* **25**(1):7-17.

Barmark, S. M., and Gaunitz, S. C. B. (1979). Transcendental meditation and heterohypnosis as altered states of consciousness. *International J. of Clinical and Experimental Hypnosis* **27**(3):227-239.

Barnett, E. A. (1981). *Analytical Hypnotherapy: Principles and Practice.* Kingston, Canada: Junica.

Barrett, D. (1979). The hypnotic dream: Its relation to nocturnal dreams and waking fantasies. *J. of Abnormal Psychology* **88**(5):584-591.

Barrett, D. L. (1980). The hypnotic dream: Its relation to nocturnal dreams and waking fantasies. *Dissertation Abstracts International* **40**(9-B):4470.

Barrios, A. A. (1973). Posthypnotic suggestions as higher order conditioning: A methodological and experimental analysis. *International J. of Clinical and Experimental Hypnosis* **21**(1):32-50.

Bateman, W. (1980). The use of hypnosis in the interrogation of witnesses. *Australian J. of Clinical Hypnotherapy* **1**(2):87-90.

Bauer, H.; Berner, P.; Steinringer, H.; and Stacher, G. (1980). Effects of hypnotic suggestions of sensory change on event-related cortical slow-potential shifts. *Archiv fur Psychologie* **133**(3):161-169.

Bauer, K. E. (1981). Temporal sequencing and goal directed fantasy in suggested amnesia. *Dissertation Abstracts International* **41**(7-B):2745.

Bauer, K. E., and McCanne, T. R. (1980a). An hypnotic technique for treating insomnia. *International J. of Clinical and Experimental Hypnosis* **28**(1):1-5.

Bauer, K. E., and McCanne, T. R. (1980b). Autonomic and central nervous system responding: During hypnosis and simulation of hypnosis. *International J. of Clinical and Experimental Hypnosis* **28**(2):148-163.

Baum, D., and Lynn, S. J. (1981). Hypnotic susceptibility level and reading involvement. *International J. of Clinical and Experimental Hypnosis* **29**(4):366-374.

Beahrs, J. O. (1977). Integrating Erickson's approach. *American J. of Clinical Hypnosis* **20**(1):55-68.

Beahrs, J.O. (1983) Co-consciousness: A common denominator in hypnosis, multiple personality and normalcy. *American J. of Clinical Hypnosis* **26**(2):100-113.

Bean, B. W., and Duff, J. L. (1975). The effects of video tape, and of situational and generalized locus of control, upon hypnotic susceptibility. *American J. of Clinical Hypnosis* **18**(1):28-33.

Beecher, H. K. (1946). Pain in men wounded in battle. *Annals of Surgery* **123**(1):96-105.

Beecher, H. K. (1955). The powerful placebo. *J. American Medical Association* **159**(17):1602-1606.

Beigel, H. G., and Johnson, W. R. (1980). *Application of Hypnosis in Sex Therapy.* Springfield, IL: Charles C. Thomas.

Bell, G. K. (1972). Clinical hypnosis: Warp and woof of psychotherapies. *Psychotherapy: Theory, Research and Practice* **9**(3):276-280.

Bender, V. L.; Navarrete, F. J.; and Nuttman, D. (1975). Effects of "neutral hypnosis" on a conditioned physiological response. *Psychological Reports* **37**(3):1155-1160.

Bennett, L., and Scott, N. (1949). The production of electrocardiographic abnormalities by suggestion under hypnosis: A case report. *American Practit.* **4**:189-190.

Benson,G. (1984a). Short-term hypnotherapy with delinquent and acting out adolescents. *British J. of Experimental and Clinical Hypnosis* **1**:19-27.

Benson, G. (1984b). Comments on M. Gibson's review of the literature on hypnosis with children. *British J. of Experimental and Clinical Hypnosis* **2**(1):43-45.

Benson, H. (1983). The relaxation response: Its subjective and objective historical precedents and physiology. *Trends in Neurosciences* **6**(7):281-284.

Benson, H.; Arns, P.A.; and Hoffman, J. W. (1981). The relaxation response and hypnosis. *International J. of Clinical and Experimental Hypnosis* **29**(3):259-270.

Benson, H.; Beary, J. F.; and Carol, M. P. (1974) The relaxation response. *Psychiatry* **37**(1):37-46.

Bergerone, C.; Cei, A.; and Ruggieri, V. (1981). Suggestibility and cognitive style: A brief communication. *International J. of Clinical and Experimental Hypnosis* **29**(4):355-357.

Bergman, A. R. (1981). A signal detection analysis of the effect of hypnosis on pain. *Dissertation Abstracts International* **42**(3-B):1159-1160.

Bergmann, M.S.; Graham, H.; and Leavitt, H. D. (1947). Rorschach exploration of consecutive hypnotic age level regression. *Psychosomatic Medicine* **9**:20-28.

Berman, R.; Simonson, E.; and Heron, W. (1954). Electrocardiographic effects associated with hypnotic suggestions in normal coronary sclerotic individuals. *J. of Applied Physiology* **7**:89-92.

Bernhardt, R., and Martin, D. (1977). *Self Mastery through Self-Hypnosis*. New York: Bobbs-Merrill.

Bernheim, H. (1973). *Hypnosis and Suggestion in Psychotherapy.* 1886. Reprint. New York: Jason Aronson.

Bernstien, A. E. (1977). *Hypnosis: A Handbook*(2d ed.). Perth, Australia: Pilpel.

Berry, G. C. (1982). Discriminating groups of hypnotized and meditating subjects from normal subjects with the Altered States of Consciousness Inventory (ASCI). *Dissertation Abstracts International* **43**(5-B):1594.

Bertrand, L. D.; Spanos, N. P.; and Parkinson, B. (1983). Test of the dissipation hypothesis of hypnotic amnesia. *Psychological Reports* **52**(2):667-671.

Berwick, P. R., and Douglas, R. R. (1977). Hypnosis, exorcism and healing: A case report. *American J. of Clinical Hypnosis* **20**(2):146-148.

Best, H. L., and Michaels, R. M. (1954). Living out "future" experiences under hypnosis. *Science* **120**:1077.

Biasiotto, J. L. (1978). Effects of hypnosis and/or task-motivating suggestions upon muscular endurance. *Dissertation Abstracts International* **38**(7-A):4034-4035.

Bishay, E. G., and Lee, C. (1984). Studies of the effects of hypnoanesthesia on regional blood flow by transcutaneous oxygen monitoring. *American J. of Clinical Hypnosis* **27**(1):64-69.

Bishay, E. G.; Stevens, G.; and Lee, C. (1984). Hypnotic control of upper gastrointestinal hemorrhage: A case report. *American J. of Clinical Hypnosis* **27**(1):22-25.

Bliss, E. L. (1980). Multiple personalities: A report of 14 cases with implications for schizophrenia and hysteria. *Archives of General Psychiatry*
37(12):1388-1397.

Bliss, E. L. (1983). Multiple personalities, related disorders and hypnosis.
American J. of Clinical Hypnosis **26**(2):114-123.

Blum, G. S. (1978-1979). A conceptual model for hypnotic alterations of
consciousness. *J. of Altered States of Consciousness* **4**(2):189-201.

Blum, G. S., and Barbour, J. S. (1979). Selective inattention to anxiety-
linked stimuli. *J. of Experimental Psychology: General* **108**(2):182-224.

Blum, G. S., and Green, M. (1978). The effects of mood upon imaginal
thought. *J. of Personality Assessment* **42**(3):227-232.

Blum, G. S., and Nash, J. K. (1982). EEG correlates of posthypnotically
controlled degrees of cognitive arousal. *Memory and Cognition*
10(5):475-478.

Blum, G. S.; Nash, J. K.; Jansen, R. D.; and Barbour, J. S. (1981). Posthypnotic attenuation of a visual illusion as reflected in perceptual reports
and cortical event-related potentials. *Academic Psychology Bulletin*
3(2):251-271.

Blum, G. S., and Porter, M. L. (1974). Effects in the restriction of conscious
awareness in a reaction time task. *International J. of Clinical and Experimental Hypnosis* **22**(4):335-345.

Blum, G. S.; Porter, M. L.; and Geiwitz, P. J. (1978). Temporal parameters
of negative visual hallucination. *International J. of Clinical and Experimental Hypnosis* **26**(1):30-44.

Bolocofsky, D. N.; Spinler, D.; and Coulthard-Morris, L. (1985). Effectiveness of hypnosis as an adjunct to behavioral weight management. *J. of
Clinical Psychology* **41**(1):35-41.

Bongartz, W. (1985). German norms for the Harvard Group Scale of Hypnotic Susceptibility, Form A. *International J. of Clinical and Experimental
Hypnosis* **33**(2):131-139.

Boring, E. G. (1954). *A History of Experimental Psychology*. New York:
Appleton-Century-Crofts.

Bornstein, P. H., and Devine, D. A. (1980). Covert modeling-hypnosis in
the treatment of obesity. *Psychotherapy: Theory, Research and Practice*
17(3):272-276.

Bornstein, P. H.; Rychtarik, R. C.; McFall, M. E.; Winegardner, J.; Winnett,
R. L.; and Paris, D. A. (1980). Hypnobehavioral treatment of chronic
nailbiting: A multiple baseline analysis. *International J. of Clinical and Experimental Hypnosis* **28**(3):208-217.

Boswell, L. K., Jr. (1982). Introduction of hypnosis during the initial physical
examination. *Medical Hypnoanalysis* **3**(2):67-72.

Botto, R. W. (1977). Cognitive mediation of pain: Behavioral, physiological, and personality correlates. *Dissertation Abstracts International* **37**(7-B):3640-3641.

Botto, R. W.; Fisher, S.; and Soucy, G. P. (1977). The effect of a good and a poor model on hypnotic susceptibility in a low demand situation. *International J. of Clinical and Experimental hypnosis* **25**(3):175-183.

Bourne, P. G. (1975). Non-pharmacological approaches to the treatment of drug abuse. *American J. of Chinese Medicine* **3**(3):235-244.

Boutin, G. E. (1978). Treatment of test anxiety by rational stage directed hypnotherapy: A case study. *American J. of Clinical Hypnosis* **21**(1):52-57.

Boutin, G. E., and Tosi, D. J. (1983). Modification of irrational ideas and test anxiety through rational stage directed hypnotherapy (RSDH). *J. of Clinical Psychology* **39**(3):382-391.

Bower, G. H.; Gilligan, S. G.; and Monteiro, K. P. (1981). Selectivity of learning caused by affective states. *J. of Experimental Psychology: General* **110**(4):451-473.

Bowers, K. S. (1966). Hypnotic behavior: The differentiation of trance and demand characteristic variables. *J. of Abnormal Psychology* **71**(1):42-51.

Bowers, K. S. (1973). Hypnosis, attribution and demand characteristics. *International J. of Clinical and Experimental Hypnosis* **21**(3):226-238.

Bowers, K. S. (1975). *Responding to unattended information: Is it affected by hypnotizability or by posthypnotic suggestions?* Paper presented at the 27th annual meeting at the Society for Clinical Hypnosis, Chicago.

Bowers, K. S. (1976). *Hypnosis for the Seriously Curious* (2d ed.). New York: Norton.

Bowers, K. S. (1977). Hypnosis: An informational approach. *Annals of New York Academy of Sciences* **296:**222-237.

Bowers, K. S. (1979a). Hypnosis and healing. *Australian J. of Clinical and Experimental Hypnosis* **7**(3):261-277.

Bowers, K. S. (1979b). Time distortion and hypnotic ability: Underestimating the duration of hypnosis. *J. of Abnormal Psychology* **88**(4):435-439.

Bowers, K. S. (1981a). Has the sun set on the Stanford Scales? *American J. of Clinical Hypnosis* **24**(2):79-88.

Bowers, K. S. (1981b). Do the Stanford Scales tap the "classic suggestion effect"? *International J. of Clinical and Experimental Hypnosis* **29**(1):42-53.

Bowers, K. S. (1982). The relevance of hypnosis for cognitive-behavioral therapy. *Clinical Psychology Review* **2**(1):67-78.

Bowers, K. S., and Brenneman, H. A. (1979). Hypnosis and the perception of time. *International J. of Clinical and Experimental Hypnosis* **27**(1):29-41.

Bowers, K. S., and Brenneman, H. A. (1981). Hypnotic dissociation, dichotic listening, and active versus passive modes of attention. *J. of Abnormal Psychology* **90**(1):55-67.

Bowers, K. S., and Kelly, P. (1979). Stress, disease, psychotherapy, and hypnosis. *J. of Abnormal Psychology* **88**(5):490-505.

Bowers, P. (1978). Hypnotizability, creativity and the role of effortless experiencing. *International J. of Clinical and Experimental Hypnosis* **26**(3):184-202.

Bowers, P. (1982). The classic suggestion effect: Relationships with scales of hypnotizability, effortless experiencing and imagery vividness. *International J. of Clinical and Experimental Hypnosis* **30**(3):270-279.

Bozick, B. J. (1976). An investigation into the effects of posthypnotic suggestion on the performance of selected motor skills by males under stress conditions which produce anxiety. *Dissertation Abstracts International* **38**(2-A):692.

Brabender, V., and Dickhaus, R. C. (1978). Effect of hypnosis on comprehension of complex verbal material. *Perceptual and Motor Skills* 47(3 part 2):1322.

Braid, J. (1960). *Braid on Hypnotism — The Beginnings of Modern Hypnosis*. New York: Julian Press.

Bramwell, J. M. (1956). *Hypnotism: Its History, Practice and Theory*. London: Grant Richards, 1903. Reissued, New York: Julian Press.

Brassfield, P. A. (1983). Unfolding patterns of the multiple personality through hypnosis. *American J. of Clinical Hypnosis* **26**(2):146-152.

Brattberg, G. (1983). An alternative method of treating tinnitus: Relaxation-hypnotherapy primarily through the home use of a recorded audio cassette. *International J. of Clinical and Experimental Hypnosis* **31**(2):90-97.

Braun, B. G. (1983a). Neurophysiologic changes in multiple personality due to integration: A preliminary report. *American J. of Clinical Hypnosis* **26**(2):84-92.

Braun, B. G. (1983b). Psychophysiologic phenomena in multiple personality and hypnosis. *American J. of Clinical Hypnosis.* **26**(2):124-137.

Braun, B. G. (1984a). Hypnosis and family therapy. *American J. of Clinical Hypnosis* **26**(3):182-186.

Braun, B. G. (1984b) Hypnosis creates multiple personality: Myth or reality? *International J. of Clinical and Experimental Hypnosis* **32**(2):191-197.

Braun, B. G. (1986). Introduction: The uses of hypnosis in psychiatry. *Psychiatric Annals* **16**(2):75-77.

Braun, B. G., and Horevitz, R. P. (1986). Hypnosis and psychotherapy. *Psychiatric Annals* **16**(2):81-86.

Brende, J. O., and Benedict, B. A. (1980). The Vietnam combat delayed stress response syndrome: Hypnotherapy of "dissociative symptoms." *American J. of Clinical Hypnosis* **23**(1):34-40.

Brenman, M. (1942). Experiments in the hypnotic production of anti-social and self-injurious behavior. *Psychiatry* **5**:49-61.

Brink, N. E. (1981). Hypnosis and control. *American J. of Clinical Hypnosis* **24**(2):109-116.

Brink, N. E. (1982). Metaphor creation for use within family therapy. *American J. of Clinical Hypnosis* **24**(4):258-265.

Brodsky, A. M., and McNeil, D. W. (1984). Hypnotizability and volunteering for hypnosis experiments. *American J. of Clinical Hypnosis* **26**(3):206-211.

Brown, D. P. (1977). A model for the levels of concentrative meditation. *International J. of Clinical and Experimental Hypnosis* **25**(4):236-273.

Brown, D. P. (1985). Hypnosis as an adjunct to the psychotherapy of the severely disturbed patient: An affective development approach. *International J. of Clinical and Experimental Hypnosis* **33**(4):281-301.

Brown, D. P., and Fromm, E. (1977). Selected bibliography of readings in altered states of consciousness (ASC) in normal individuals. *International J. of Clinical and Experimental Hypnosis* **25**(4):388-391.

Brown, J. M., and Chaves, J. F. (1980). Hypnosis in the treatment of sexual dysfunction. *J. of Sex and Marital Therapy* **6**(1):63-74.

Brown, R. J. (1985). Hypnosis in Canadian criminal law. *American J. of Clinical Hypnosis* **27**(3):153-158.

Browning, C. H., and Friesen, D. D. (1974). The relationship between hypnotic induction modality and locus of control expectancy. *American J. of Clinical Hypnosis* **17**(2):108-114.

Bruhn, R. A. (1983). Effects of hypnosis on counselor trainee skill acquisition and self-perceived confidence. *Dissertation Abstracts International* **43**(11-A): 3509.

Brumley, W. (1979). When is therapy indicated for female sexual concerns? A clinician's views. *Australian J. of Clinical and Experimental Hypnosis* **7**(3):231-234.

Bryan, W. J., Jr. (1962). *Legal Aspects of Hypnosis*. Springfield, IL: Charles C. Thomas.

Bryan, W. J., Jr. (1976). Anxiety and depression and emotional instability. *J. of American Institute of Hypnosis* **17**(1):16-27.

Buckner, L. G., and Coe, W. C. (1977). Imaginative skill, wording of suggestions and hypnotic susceptibility. *International J. of Clinical and Experimental Hypnosis* **25**(1):27-36.

Burns, A. (1977). The distribution and factor structure of hypnosis scores following intervention. *International J. of Clinical and Experimental Hypnosis* **25**(3):192-201.

Burns, B., and Reyher, J. (1976). Activating posthypnotic conflict: Emergent uncovering, psychotherapy, repression and psychopathology. *J. of Personality Assessment* **40**(5):492-501.

Burrows, G. D., and Dennerstein, L. (1979). Teaching hypnosis in Victoria. *Australian J. of Clinical and Experimental Hypnosis* **7**(3):207-213.

Burrows, G. D., and Dennerstein, L. (Eds.). (1980). *Handbook of Hypnosis and Psychosomatic Medicine.* New York: Elsevier/North Holland Biomedical Press.

Burrows, G. D.; Dennerstein, L.; and Frenader, G. (1982). A note on hypnosis and the law. *Australian J. of Clinical and Experimental Hypnosis* **11**(2):83-88.

Bushnell, J. A. (1984). Hypnosis and single case experimental design: Some ruminations on a theme. *Australian J. of Clinical and Experimental Hypnosis* **12**(1):1-8.

Butler, B. (1954). The use of hypnosis in the care of the cancer patient. *Cancer* **7**:1-14.

Byers, A. P. (1975). Training and use of technicians in the treatment of alcoholism with hypnosis. *American J. of Clinical Hypnosis* **18**(2):90-93.

Bynum, E. B. (1977). Hypnotic age regression: An experimental investigation. *Dissertation Abstracts International* **28**(5-B):2394-2395.

Caldwell, T. A., and Stewart, R. S. (1981). Hysterical seizures and hypnotherapy. *American J. of Clinical Hypnosis* **23**(4):294-298.

Call, J. D. (1976). Children, parents and hypnosis: A discussion. *International J. of Clinical and Experimental Hypnosis* **24**(2):149-155.

Callen, K. E. (1983). Auto-hypnosis in long distance runners. *American J. of Clinical Hypnosis* **26**(1):30-36.

Carasso, R. L.; Peded, O.; Kleinhauz, M.; and Yehuda, S. (1985). Treatment of cervical headache with hypnosis, suggestive therapy, and relaxation techniques. *American J. of Clinical Hypnosis* **27**:(4):216-218.

Carli, G. (1982). Animal hypnosis: An attempt to reach a definition. *Archives italiennes de biologie* **120**(1-3):138-159.

Carona, A. J. (1981). The effects of hypnotic induction procedures, relaxation instructions, and normal wakefulness on the recall of violent and nonviolent stimuli. *Dissertation Abstracts International* **41**(10-B):3881.

Carter, B. D.; Elkins, G. R.; and Kraft, S. P. (1982). Hemispheric asymmetry as a model for hypnotic phenomena: A review and analysis. *American J. of Clinical Hypnosis* **24**(3):204-210.

Case, D. B.; Fogel, D. H.; and Pollack, A. A. (1980). Intrahypnotic and long-term effects of self-hypnosis on blood pressure in mild hypertension. *International J. of Clinical and Experimental Hypnosis* **28**(1):27-38.

Cautela, J. R. (1966). Treatment of compulsive behavior by covert sensitization. *Psychological Record* **16**:33-41.

Cautela, J. R. (1967). Covert sensitization. *Psychological Reports* **20**:459-468.

Cautela, J. R. (1970). Covert reinforcement. *Behavior Therapy* **1**:33-50.

Cautela, J. R. (1975). The use of covert conditioning in hypnotherapy. *International J. of Clinical and Experimental Hypnosis* **23**(1):15-27.

Cerio, J. E. (1983). The use of hypnotic elements and audio recordings with the fantasy relaxation technique. *Personnel and Guidance J.* **61**(7):436-437.

Cescato, M. (1981). Barber's view of hypnosis: A review of the evidence for. *Australian J. of Clinical Hypnotherapy* **2**(1):37-45.

Channon, L. D. (1979). Resistance by "not hearing" in weight control therapy. *Australian J. of Clinical and Experimental Hypnosis* **7**(3):282-283.

Channon, L. D. (1982). A case of nailparing. *Australian J. of Clinical and Experimental Hypnosis* **10**(2):120-122.

Channon, L. D. (1984a). Some preconceptions about hypnosis among pre-clinical medical students: A brief communication. *International J. of Clinical and Experimental Hypnosis* **32**(4):356-361.

Channon, L.D. (1984b). A script for reluctant runners. *Australian J. of Clinical and Experimental Hypnosis* **12**(2):139-141.

Channon, L. D. (1984c). Some areas where care may be needed in instruction about self-hypnosis. *Australian J. of Clinical and Experimental Hypnosis* **12**(1):61-62.

Channon, L. D. (1984d). Extrasensory communication in hypnosis: Some uncomfortable speculations. *Australian J. of Clinical and Experimental Hypnosis* **12**(1):23-29.

Channon, L. D., and Diment, A. D. (1979). Spontaneous use of a "screen" technique. *Australian J. of Clinical and Experimental Hypnosis* **7**(3):288-289.

Chapman, C. R., and Feather, B. W. (1973). Effects of diazapam on human pain tolerance and pain sensitivity. *Psychosomatic Medicine* **35**:330-340.

Charlesworth, E. A., and Doughtie, E. B. (1982). Modification of baseline by differential task presentation as either hypnosis or "learned" relaxation. *Perceptual and Motor Skills* **55**(3, part 2):1131-1137.

Chaves, J. F. (1968). Hypnosis reconceptualized: An overview of Barber's theoretical and empirical work. *Psychological Reports* **22**:587-608.

Chaves, J. F., and Barber, T. X. (1976). Hypnotic procedures and surgery: A critical analysis with applications to "acupuncture analgesia". *American J. of Clinical Hypnosis* **18**(4):217-236.

Cheek, D. B. (1959). Unconscious perception of meaningful sounds during surgical anesthesia as revealed under hypnosis. *American J. of Clinical Hypnosis* **1**:101-113.

Cheek, D. B. (1964). Surgical memory and reaction to careless conversation. *American J. of Clinical Hypnosis* **6**:237-240.

Cheek, D. B. (1965). Further evidence of hearing under chemo-anesthesia: Detailed case report. *American J. of Clinical Hypnosis* **7**:55-59.

Cheek, D. B. (1966). The meaning of continued hearing sense under general chemo-anesthesia: A progress report and report of a case. *American J. of Clinical Hypnosis* **8**:275-280.

Cheek, D. B. (1975). Maladjustment patterns apparently related to imprinting at birth. *American J. of Clinical Hypnosis* **18**(2):75-82.

Cheek, D. B. (1976a). Hypnotherapy for secondary frigidity after radical surgery for gynecological cancer: Two case reports. *American J. of Clinical Hypnosis* **19**(1):13-19.

Cheek, D. B. (1976b). Short-term hypnotherapy for frigidity using exploration of early life attitudes. *American J. of Clinical Hypnosis* **19**(1):20-27.

Cheek, D. B., and LeCron, L. M. (1968). *Clinical Hypnotherapy.* New York: Grune & Stratton.

Chertok, L. (1975). Hysteria, hypnosis, psychopathology. *J. of Nervous and Mental Disease* **161**(6):367-378.

Chertok, L. (1977). Freud and hypnosis: An epistemological appraisal. *J. of Nervous and Mental Disease* **165**(2):99-109.

Chertok, L. (1978). Hypnosis: The psychobiological crossroads: A 200-year query. *J. of Nervous and Mental Disease* **166**(4):231-233.

Chertok, L. (1981). *Sense and Nonsense in Psychotherapy: The Challenge of Hypnosis.* New York: Pergamon.

Chertok, L. (1982). The unconscious and hypnosis. *International J. of Clinical and Experimental Hypnosis* **30**(2):95-107.

Chertok, L. (1983). Psychoanalysis and hypnosis theory: Comments on five case histories. *American J. of Clinical Hypnosis* **25**(4):209-224.

Chertok, L. (1984a). On the centenary of Charcot: Hysteria, suggestibility and hypnosis. *British J. of Medical Psychology* **57**(2):111-120.

Chertok, L. (1984b). Hypnosis and suggestion in a century of psychotherapy: An epistemological assessment. *J. of the American Academy of Psychoanalysis* **12**(2):211-232.

Chertok, L.; Michaux, D.; and Droin, M. C. (1977). Dynamics of hypnotic analgesia: Some new data. *J. of Nervous and Mental Disease* **164**(2):88-96.

Chiofalo, L. C., and Coe, W. C. (1982). A failure to support the relationships of selected traits and hypnotic responsiveness in drama students. *American J. of Clinical Hypnosis* **24**(3):200-203.

Christenson, J. A. (1949). Dynamics in hypnotic induction. *Psychiatry* **12**:37-54.

Christie, B. (1982). Hypnosis in occupational psychology. *Bulletin of the British Society of Experimental and Clinical Hypnosis* **1982**(5):21-26.

Chubb, H. (1978). Organismic involvement, hypnotic involvement, imaginative involvement: A physiological investigation. *Dissertation Abstracts International* **39**(4-B):1945.

Cioppa, F. J., and Thal, A. D. (1975). Hypnotherapy in a case of juvenile rheumatoid arthritis. *American J. of Clinical Hypnosis* **18**(2):105-110.

Citrenbaum, C. M.; King, M. E.; and Cohen, W. I. (1985). *Modern Clinical Hypnosis for Habit Control.* New York: W. W. Norton.

Clark, B. D.; Hungerford, L. E.; and Reilley, R. R. (1984). Doctoral dissertations on hypnosis: 1923-1980. *Psychological Reports* **54**(1):203-209.

Clarke, J. C., and Jackson, J. A. (1983). *Hypnosis and Behavior Therapy: The Treatment of Anxiety and Phobias.* New York: Springer.

Clawson, T. A., and Swade, R. H. (1975). The hypnotic control of blood flow and pain: The cure of warts and the potential for the use of hypnosis in the treatment of cancer. *American J. of Clinical Hypnosis* **17**(3):160-169.

Cleveland, C. T. (1982). A comparison of hypnosis, frontalis EMG biofeedback, and the two combined for training relaxation. *Dissertation Abstracts International* **42**(7-B):2981.

Coe, W. C. (1965). The heuristic value of role theory and hypnosis. *Dissertation Abstracts* **25**(a):5371-5372.

Coe, W. C. (1966). Hypnosis as role enactment: The role demand variable. *American J. of Clinical Hypnosis* **8**(3):189-191.

Coe, W. C. (1973a). A further evaluation of responses to an uncompleted posthypnotic suggestion. *American J. of Clinical Hypnosis* **15**(4):223-228.

Coe, W. C. (1973b). Experimental designs and the state-nonstate issue in hypnosis. *American J. of Clinical Hypnosis* **16**:118-128.

Coe, W. C. (1973c). The concept of role skills: Hypnotic behavior. Paper presented at the Annual Meeting of the American Psychological Association, Montreal, August.

Coe, W. C. (1974). A reply to Lieberman's "The state-nonstate issue in hypnosis: A closer look." *American J. of Clinical Hypnosis* **16**(3):199-201.

Coe, W. C. (1976a). Effects of hypnotic susceptibility and sex on the administration of standard hypnotic susceptibility scales. *International J. of Clinical and Experimental Hypnosis* **24**(3):281-286.

Coe, W. C. (1976b). The elusive nature of completing an uncompleted posthypnotic suggestion. *American J. of Clinical Hypnosis* **18**(4):263-271.

Coe, W. C. (1977). The problem of relevance versus ethics in researching hypnosis and antisocial conduct. *Annals of New York Academy of Sciences* **296**:90-104.

Coe, W. C. (1978). The credibility of posthypnotic amnesia: A contextualist's view. *International J. of Clinical and Experimental Hypnosis* **26**(4):218-245.

Coe, W. C.; Allen, J. L.; Krug, W. M.; and Wurzmann, A. G. (1974). Goal-directed fantasy in hypnotic responsiveness: Skill, item wording, or both? *International J. of Clinical and Experimental Hypnosis* **22**(2):157-166.

Coe, W. C.; Basden, B.; Basden, D.; and Graham, C. (1976). Posthypnotic amnesia: Suggestions of an active process in dissociative phenomena. *J. of Abnormal Psychology* **85**(5):455-458.

Coe, W. C.; Baugher, R. J.; Krimm, W. R.; and Smith, J. A. (1976). A further examination of selective recall following hypnosis. *International J. of Clinical and Experimental Hypnosis* **24**(1):13-21.

Coe, W. C.; Buckner, L. G.; Howard, M. L.; and Kobayashi, K. (1972). Hypnosis as role enactment: Focus on a role specific skill. *American J. of Clinical Hypnosis* **15**(1):41-45.

Coe, W. C.; Kobayashi, K.; and Howard, M. L. (1972a). An approach toward isolating factors that influence antisocial conduct in hypnosis. *International J. of Clinical and Experimental Hypnosis* **20**(2):118-131.

Coe, W. C.; Kobayashi, K.; and Howard, M. L. (1972b). More on experimental design in evaluating the influence of hypnosis in antisocial conduct. In *Proceedings, 80th Annual Convention of the American Psychological Association* (pp. 861-862).

Coe, W. C., and Ryken, K. (1979). Hypnosis and risks to human subjects. *American Psychologist* **34**(8):673-681.

Coe, W. C., and Sarbin, T. R. (1966). An experimental demonstration of hypnosis as role enactment. *J. of Abnormal Psychology* **71**:400-406.

Coe, W. C., and Sarbin, T. R. (1971). An alternative interpretation to the multiple composition of hypnotic scales. *J. of Personality and Social Psychology* **18**(1):1-8.

Coe, W. C., and Sarbin, T. R. (1977). Hypnosis from the standpoint of a contextualist. *Annals of New York Academy of Sciences* **296**:2-13.

Coe, W. C., and Scharcoff, J. A. (1985). An empirical evaluation of the neurolinguistic programming model. *International J. of Clinical and Experimental Hypnosis* **33**(4):310-318.

Coe, W. C., and Steen, P. (1981). Examining the relationship between believing one will respond to hypnotic suggestions and hypnotic responsiveness. *American J. of Clinical Hypnosis* **24**(1):22-32.

Coe, W. C.; St. Jean, R. L.; and Burger, J. M. (1980). Hypnosis and the enhancement of visual imagery. *International J. of Clinical and Experimental Hypnosis* **28**(3):225-243.

Coe, W. C.; Taul, J. H.; Basden, D.; and Basden, B. (1973). An investigation of the dissociation hypothesis and disorganized retrieval in posthypnotic amnesia with retroactive inhibition in free-recall learning. *Proceedings of the 81st Annual Convention of the American Psychological Association* **8**:1085-1086.

Cohen, S. B. (1981). Phobia of bovine sounds. *American J. of Clinical Hypnosis* **23**(4):266-268.

Cohen, W. (1979). Hypnosis helps a driver obtain a license. *Australian J. of Clinical and Experimental Hypnosis* **7**(3):285-287.

Cohn, A., and Udolf, R. (1979). *The Criminal Justice System and Its Psychology.* New York: Van Nostrand Reinhold Co.

Cole, R. D. (1977). Increasing reading and test taking skills with hypnosis and suggestion. *Dissertation Abstracts International* **37**(8-A):4859.

Cole, R. D. (1979). The use of hypnosis in a course to increase academic and test-taking skills. *International J. of Clinical and Experimental Hypnosis* **27**(1):21-28.

Coleman, J. C., and Broen, W. E., Jr. (1972). *Abnormal Psychology and Modern Life* (4th ed.). Glenview, IL: Scott, Foresman.

Collison, D. (1979). Hypnotherapy and clinical ecology. *Australian J. of Clinical and Experimental Hypnosis* **7**(3):215-218.

Colomb, C. (1977). Why sophology in dental anesthesiology? In A. R. Guerra, *Modern Anesthesia in Dentistry* (p. 11-18). Philadelphia: Franklin Institute Press.

Comins, J. R.; Fullam, F.; and Barber, T. X. (1975). Effects of experimenter modeling, demands for honesty, and initial level of suggestibility on response to "hypnotic" suggestions. *J. of Consulting and Clinical Psychology* **43**(5):668-675.

Conn, J. H. (1972). Is hypnosis really dangerous? *International J. of Clinical and Experimental Hypnosis* **20**(2):61-79.

Conn, J. H. (1981). The myth of coercion through hypnosis. *International J. of Clinical and Experimental Hypnosis* **29**(2):95-100.

Conn, J. H., and Conn, R. H. (1967). Discussion of T. X. Barber's " 'Hypnosis' as a causal variable in present day psychology: A critical analysis." *International J. of Clinical and Experimental Hypnosis* **15**(3):106-110.

Conn, L., and Mott, T., Jr. (1984). Plethysmographic demonstration of rapid vasodilation by direct suggestion: A case of Raynaud's disease treated by hypnosis. *American J. of Clinical Hypnosis* **26**(3):166-170.

Connors, J. R., and Sheehan, P. W. (1978). The influence of control comparison tasks and between- versus within-subjects effects in hypnotic responsivity. *International J. of Clinical and Experimental Hypnosis* **26** (2):104-122.

Cooper, L. M., and Erickson, M. H. (1954). *Time Distortion in Hypnosis.* Baltimore: Williams and Wilkins.

Cooper, L. M., and London, P. (1973). Reactivation of memory by hypnosis and suggestion. *International J. of Clinical and Experimental Hypnosis* **21**(4):312-323.

Cooper, L. M., and London, P. (1978-1979). The Children's Hypnotic Susceptibility Scale. *American J. of Clinical Hypnosis* **21**(2, 3):170-185

Cooperman, S. B. (1983). Hypnotically induced changes in visual perception. *Dissertation Abstracts International* **43**(9-B):3070.

Cooperman, S., and Schafer, D. W. (1983). Hypnotherapy over the telephone. *American J. of Clinical Hypnosis* **25**(4):277-279.

Copemann, C. D. (1977). Treatment of polydrug abuse and addiction by covert sensitization: Some contraindications. *International J. of the Addictions* **12**(1):17-23.

Council, J. R.; Kirsch, I.; Vickery, A. R.; and Carlson, D. (1983). "Trance" versus "skill" hypnotic inductions: The effects of credibility, expectancy, and experimenter modeling. *J. of Consulting and Clinical Psychology* **51**(3):432-440.

Counts, R. M., and Mensh, I. N. (1950). Personality characteristics in hypnotically induced hostility. *J. of Clinical Psychology* **6**:325-330.

Cowell, D. (1984). Hypnosis with children: Research and some professional issues. *British J. of Experimental and Clinical Hypnosis* **2**(1):35-40.

Cox, T. H. (1978). Post-hypnotic suggestion in behavior modification. *J. of the American Society of Psychosomatic Dentistry and Medicine* **25**(2):68-73.

Crasilneck, H. B. (1979). Hypnosis in the control of chronic low back pain. *American J. of Clinical Hypnosis* **22**(2):71-78.

Crasilneck, H. B. (1980). The case of Dora. *American J. of Clinical Hypnosis* **23**(2):95-97.

Crasilneck, H. B. (1982). A follow-up study in the use of hypnotherapy in the treatment of psychogenic impotency. *American J. of Clinical Hypnosis* **25**(1):52-61.

Crasilneck, H. B., and Hall, J. A. (1959). Physiological changes associated with hypnosis: A review of the literature since 1948. *International J. of Clinical and Experimental Hypnosis* **7**:9-50.

Crasilneck, H. B., and Hall, J. A. (1975). *Clinical Hypnosis: Principles and Applications.* New York: Grune and Stratton.

Crasilneck, H. B.; McCranie, E. J.; and Jenkins, M. T. (1956). Special indications for hypnosis as a method of anesthesia. *J. of American Medical Association* **162**(18):1606-1608.

Crasilneck, H. B., and Michael, C. M. (1957). Performance on the Bender under hypnotic age regression. *J. of Abnormal and Social Psychology* **54**:319.

Crasilneck, H. B., Stirman, J. A.; Wilson, B. J.; McCranie, E. J.; and Fogelman, M. J. (1955). Use of hypnosis in the management of patients with burns. *J. of the American Medical Association* **158**(2):103-106.

Crawford, F. T. (1977). Induction and duration of tonic immobility. *Psychological Record* **27**(special issue):89-107.

Crawford, H. J. (1982). Cognitive processing during hypnosis: Much unfinished business. *Research Communications in Psychology, Psychiatry and Behavior* **7**(2):169-179.

Crawford, H. J., and Allen, S. N. (1983). Enhanced visual memory during hypnosis as mediated by hypnotic responsiveness and cognitive strategies. *J. of Experimental Psychology: General* **112**(4):662-685.

Crawford, H. J.; Crawford, K.; and Koperski, B. J. (1983). Hypnosis and lateral cerebral function as assessed by dichotic listening. *Biological Psychiatry* **18**(4):415-427.

Crawford, H. J.; Hilgard, J. R.; and MacDonald, H. (1982). Transient experiences following hypnotic testing and special termination procedures. *International J. of Clinical and Experimental Hypnosis* **30**(2):117-126.

Crawford, H. J.; MacDonald, H.; and Hilgard, E. R. (1979). Hypnotic deafness: A psychophysical study of responses to tone intensity as modified by hypnosis. *American J. of Psychology* **92**(2):193-214.

Crosson, B. A. (1979). Control of skin temperature through the use of suggestion and biofeedback during hypnosis. *Dissertation Abstracts International* **39**(9-B):4639.

Crosson, B. (1980). Control of skin temperature through biofeedback and suggestion with hypnotized college women. *International J. of Clinical and Experimental Hypnosis* **28**(1):75-87.

Crosson, B.; Meinz, R.; Laur, E.; Williams, D.; and Andreychuk, T. (1977). EEG alpha training, hypnotic susceptibility, and baseline techniques. *International J. of Clinical and Experimental Hypnosis* **25**(4):348-360.

Crosswell, G. L., and Smith, E. W. L. (1974). Evaluation of a hypnotist by subjects in hypnotic, hypnotic simulator and control conditions. *American J. of Clinical Hypnosis* **17**(2):102-107.

Crouse, E., and Kurtz, R. (1984). Enhancing hypnotic susceptibility: The efficacy of four training procedures. *American J. of Clinical Hypnosis* **27**(2):122-136.

Crowley, R. J. (1980). Effects of indirect hypnosis (rapid induction analgesia) for the relief of acute pain associated with minor podiatric surgical procedures. *Dissertation Abstracts International* **40**(9-B):4549.

Cummings, C. P. (1978). The effects of hypnotic ego-strengthening and assertion training on levels of assertiveness and psychological growth. *Dissertation Abstracts International* **39**(1-B):372-373.

Cunningham, P. V., and Blum, G. S. (1982). Further evidence that hypnotically induced color blindness does not mimic congenital defects. *J. of Abnormal Psychology* **91**(2):139-143.

Cupples, D. E. (1984). The effects of cognitive arousal upon visual persistence. *Dissertation Abstracts International* **44**(11-B):3506-3507.

Cutcomb, S. D. (1982). Studies in the brain correlates of human cognitive function. *Dissertation Abstracts International* **42**(11-B):4609-4610.

Dalal, A. S. (1966). An empirical approach to hypnosis: An overview of Barber's work. *Archives of General Psychiatry* **15**:151-157.

Dalal, A. S., and Barber, T. X. (1969). Yoga, "Yogic feats" and hypnosis in the light of empirical research. *American J. of Clinical Hypnosis* **11**(3):155-166.

Dampier, Sir William C. (1949). *A History of Science* (4th ed.). Cambridge: Cambridge University Press.

Daniels, L. K. (1974). Rapid extinction of nail biting by covert sensitization: A case study. *J. of Behavior Therapy and Experimental Psychiatry* **5**:91-92.

Daniels, L. K. (1975). The treatment of psychophysiological disorders and severe anxiety by behavioral therapy, hypnosis and transcendental meditation. *American J. of Clinical Hypnosis* **17**(4):267-270.

Daniels, L. K. (1976a). The effects of automated hypnosis and hand warming on migraine: A pilot study. *American J. of Clinical Hypnosis* **19**(2):91-94.

Daniels, L. K. (1976b). The treatment of acute anxiety and postoperative gingival pain by hypnosis and covert conditioning: A case report. *American J. of Clinical Hypnosis* **19**(2):116-119.

Daniels, L. K. (1976c). Rapid in-office and in-vivo desensitization of an injection phobia utilizing hypnosis. *American J. of Clinical Hypnosis* **18**(3):200-203.

Daniels, L. K. (1976d) Covert reinforcement and hypnosis in modification of attitudes toward physically disabled persons and generalization to the emotionally disturbed. *Psychological Reports* **38**(2):554.

Daniels, L. K. (1977). Treatment of migraine headache by hypnosis and behavior therapy: A case study. *American J. of Clinical Hypnosis* **19**(4):241-244.

Das, J. P. (1961). Learning and recall under hypnosis and in the waking state: A comparison. *Archives of General Psychiatry* **4**:517-521.

Dash, J. (1981). Rapid hypno-behavioral treatment of a needle phobia in a five-year-old cardiac patient. *J. of Pediatric Psychology* **6**(1):37-42.

Dauven, J. (1969). *The Powers of Hypnosis*. New York: Stein & Day.

Dave, R. (1979). Effects of hypnotically induced dreams on creative problem solving. *J. of Abnormal Psychology* **88**(3):293-302.

Dave, R. P. (1980). An exploratory investigation into the efficacy of post-hypnotically suggested sleep talking as a paradigm for eliciting verbal descriptions of nocturnal dreams in process. *Dissertation Abstracts International* **40**(9-B):4532.

Davidson, R. J., and Goleman, D. J. (1977). The role of attention in meditation and hypnosis: A psychobiological perspective on transformations of consciousness. *International J. of Clinical and Experimental Hypnosis* **25**(4):291-308.

Davis, S.; Dawson, J. G.; and Seay, B. (1978). Prediction of hypnotic susceptibility from imaginative involvement. *American J. of Clinical Hypnosis* **20**(3):194-198.

Deabler, H. L. (1976). Hypnotherapy of impotence. *American J. of Clinical Hypnosis* **19**(1):9-12.

Debetz, B., and Stern, D. B. (1979). Factor analysis and score distributions of the HIP—Replication by a second examiner. *American J. of Clinical Hypnosis* **22**(2):95-102.

Deforest, F. D. (1979). Modification of stimulation seeking behavior in psychopaths using hypnotic sensory imagery conditioning. *Dissertation Abstracts International* **40**(1-A):161.

Deforest, F. D., and Johnson, L. S. (1981). Modification of stimulation seeking behavior in psychopaths using hypnotic sensory imagery conditioning. *American J. of Clinical Hypnosis* **23**(3):184-194.

Degun, M. D., and Degun, G. (1982). The use of hypnosis in the treatment of psychosexual disorders: With case illustrations of vaginismus. *Bulletin of the British Society of Experimental and Clinical Hypnosis* **1982**(5):31-36.

Deiker, T., and Counts, D. K. (1980). Hypnotic paradigm-substitution therapy in a case of hypochondriasis. *American J. of Clinical Hypnosis* **23**(2):122-127.

Deiker, T. E., and Pollock, D. H. (1975). Integration of hypnotic and systematic desensitization techniques in the treatment of phobias: A case report. *American J. of Clinical Hypnosis* **17**(3):170-174.

Delmonte, M. M. (1984). Meditation: Similarities with hypnoidal states and hypnosis. *International J. of Psychosomatics* **31**(3):24-34.

Delprato, D. J. (1977). Pavlovian conditioning of Chevreul's movement. *American J. of Clinical Hypnosis* **20**(2):124-130.

Delprato, D. J., and Holmes, P. A. (1978). Facilitation of arm levitation by responses to previous suggestions of a different type. *International J. of Clinical and Experimental Hypnosis* **26**(3):167-177.

Dement, W. C. (1974). *Some Must Watch While Some Must Sleep.* San Francisco: W. H. Freeman.

DeMers, G. E. (1980). Effects of post-hypnotic suggestion on the performance of a fine motor skill under stress. *Dissertation Abstracts International* **40**(9-A):4955-4956.

Dempsey, G. L., and Granich, M. (1978). Hypno-behavioral therapy in the case of a traumatic stutterer: A case study. *International J. of Clinical and Experimental Hypnosis* **26**(3):125-133.

Dengrove, E. (1973). The uses of hypnosis in behavior therapy. *International J. of Clinical and Experimental Hypnosis* **21**(1):13-17.

Dengrove, E. (Ed.). (1976). *Hypnosis and Behavior Therapy.* Springfield, IL.: Charles C. Thomas.

Dennerstein, L., and Burrows, G. D. (1979a). The role of hypnosis in the management of psychosexual dysfunction. *Australian J. of Clinical and Experimental Hypnosis* **7**(3):247-252.

Dennerstein, L., and Burrows, G. D. (1979b). Psychosexual dysfunction: Therapy approaches. *Australian J. of Clinical and Experimental Hypnosis* **7**(3):235-245.

Denver, D. R.; Grove, R. N.; De Varennes, S.; and Gagnon, F. (1979). Effects of two language modalities on hypnotic induction by groups. *American J. of Clinical Hypnosis* **21**(4):252-257.

DePiano, F. A., and Salzberg, H. C. (1979). Clinical applications of hypnosis to three psychosomatic disorders. *Psychological Bulletin* **86**(6):1223-1235.

DePiano, F. A., and Salzberg, H. C. (1981). Hypnosis as an aid to recall of meaningful information presented under three types of arousal. *International J. of Clinical and Experimental Hypnosis* **29**(4):383-400.

De Shazer, S. (1978). Brief hypnotherapy of two sexual dysfunctions: The crystal ball technique. *American J. of Clinical Hypnosis* **20**(3):203-208.

De Shazer, S. (1979). On transforming symptoms: An approach to an Erickson procedure. *American J. of Clinical Hypnosis* **22**(1):17-28.

De Shazer, S. (1980). Investigation of indirect symbolic suggestions. *American J. of Clinical Hypnosis* **23**(1):10-15.

DeStefano, R. F. (1977). The "inoculation" effect in think-with instructions for "hypnotic-like" experiences. *Dissertation Abstracts International* **38**(4-B):1875.

DeVoge, S. (1975). A behavioral analysis of a group hypnosis treatment method. *American J. of Clinical Hypnosis* **18**(2):127-131.

DeVoge, S. (1977). Use of hypnosis for assertive training and self-concept change in women: A case study. *American J. of Clinical Hypnosis* **19**(4):226-230.

DeVoge, J. T., and Sachs, L. B. (1973). The modification of hypnotic susceptibility through imitative behavior. *International J. of Clinical and Experimental Hypnosis* **21**(2):70-77.

DeWitt, G. W., and Averill, J. R. (1976). Lateral eye movements, hypnotic susceptibility and field independence-dependence. *Perceptual and Motor Skills* **43**(3):1179-1184.

Deyoub, P. L. (1984). Hypnotic stimulation of antisocial behavior: A case report. *International J. of Clinical and Experimental Hypnosis* **32**(3):301-306.

Deyoub, P. L., and Epstein, S. J. (1977). Short-term hypnotherapy for the treatment of flight phobia: A case report. *American J. of Clinical Hypnosis* **19**(4):251-254.

Deyoub, P. L., and Wilkie, R. (1980). Suggestion with and without hypnotic induction in a weight reduction program. *International J. of Clinical and Experimental Hypnosis* **28**(4):333-340.

De Zulueta, F. I. S. (1984). The implications of bilingualism in the study and treatment of psychiatric disorders: A review. *Psychological Medicine* **14**:541-557.

Dhanens, T. P., and Lundy, R. M. (1975). Hypnotic and waking suggestions and recall. *International J. of Clinical and Experimental Hypnosis* **23** (1):68-79.

Diamond, M. J. (1977*a*). Issues and methods for modifying responsivity to hypnosis. *Annals of New York Academy of Sciences* **296**:119-128.

Diamond, M. J. (1977*b*). Hypnotizability is modifiable: An alternative approach. *International J. of Clinical and Experimental Hypnosis* **25**(3):147-166.

Diamond, M. J. (1980). The client-as-hypnotist: Furthering hypnotherapeutic change. *International J. of Clinical and Experimental Hypnosis* **28**(3):197-207.

Diamond, M. J. (1982). Modifying hypnotic experience by means of indirect hypnosis and hypnotic skill training: An update (1981). *Research Communications in Psychology, Psychiatry and Behavior* **7**(2):233-239.

Diamond, M. J. (1983). Therapeutic indications in applying an innovative hypnotherapeutic technique: The client-as-hypnotist. *American J. of Clinical Hypnosis* **25**(4):242-247.

Diamond, M. J. (1984). It takes two to tango: Some thoughts on the neglected importance of the hypnotist in an interactive hypnotherapeutic relationship. *American J. of Clinical Hypnosis* **27**(1):3-13.

Diamond, M. J.; Gregory, J.; Lenny, E.; Steadman, C.; and Talone, J. M. (1974). An alternative approach to personality correlates of hypnotizability: Hypnosis-specific mediational attitudes. *International J. of Clinical and Experimental Hypnosis* **22**(4):346-353.

Dillon, R. F., and Spanos, N. P. (1983). Proactive interference and the functional ablation hypothesis: More disconfirmatory data. *International J. of Clinical and Experimental Hypnosis* **31**(1):47-56.

Diment, A. D.; Walker, W. L.; and Hammer, A. G. (1981). Response to poetry in hypnosis and the waking state: A study of non-suggested aspects of the hypnotic state. *Australian J. of Clinical and Experimental Hypnosis* **9**(1):19-40.

Dimond, R. E. (1981). Hypnotic treatment of a kidney dialysis patient. *American J. of Clinical Hypnosis* **23**(4):284-288.

Dolby, R. M., and Sheehan, P. W. (1977). Cognitive processing and expectancy behavior in hypnosis. *J. of Abnormal Psychology* **86**(4):334-345.

Dollard, J., and Miller, N. E. (1950). *Personality and Psychotherapy.* New York: McGraw-Hill.

Dorcus, R. M. (1937). Modification by suggestion of some vestibular and visual responses. *American J. of Psychology* **49**:82-87.

Dorcus, R. M. (1960). Recall under hypnosis of amnestic events. *International J. of Clinical and Experimental Hypnosis* **8**:57-60.

Dorcus, R. M. (1963). Fallacies in predictions of susceptibility to hypnosis based upon personality characteristics. *American J. of Clinical Hypnosis* **5**:163-170.

Dougherty, R. E. (1983). Cerebral hemispheric dominance, hypnotic trance depth, and hypnotizability. *Dissertation Abstracts International* **43**(7-B): 2332.

Douglass, V. L. (1978). Relationship of spontaneous amnesia, ego states, and hidden observers to post-hypnotically dissociated task interference. *Dissertation Abstracts International* **39**(4-B):1951.

Dubin, L. L. (1976). Subjective apperception and use of color during dental procedures under hypnosis: Report of a case. *American J. of Clinical Hypnosis* **18**(4):282-284.

Dubreuil, D. L.; Spanos, N. P.; and Bertrand, L. D. (1982-1983). Does hypnotic amnesia dissipate with time? *Imagination, Cognition and Personality* **2**(2):103-113.

Duff, J. L. (1978). A comparison of procedures for enhancing hypnotic susceptibility. *Dissertation Abstracts International* **38**(7-B):3390.

Dull, R. A. (1980). The effects of hypnotic techniques on linguistic productivity. *Dissertation Abstracts International* **41**(4-B):1499.

Dumas, L. (1964). A subjective report of inadvertent hypnosis. *International J. of Clinical and Experimental Hypnosis* **12**(2):78-80.

Dumas, R. A. (1980). Cognitive control in hypnosis and biofeedback. *International J. of Clinical and Experimental Hypnosis* **28**(1):53-62.

Duncan, B., and Perry, C. (1977). Uncancelled hypnotic suggestions: Initial studies. *American J. of Clinical Hypnosis* **19**(3):166-176.

Dynes, J. B. (1947). Objective method for distinguishing sleep from hypnotic trance. *Archives Neur. Psychiat.* **57**:84.

Dywan, J., and Bowers, K. (1983). The use of hypnosis to enhance recall. *Science* **222**(4620):184-185.

Edelstien, M. G. (1982). Ego state therapy in the management of resistance. *American J. of Clinical Hypnosis* **25**(1):15-20.

Edmonds, G. M. (1979). Hypnotic facilitation of temperature biofeedback training. *Dissertation Abstracts International* **39**(9-B):4611.

Edmonston, W. E., Jr. (1960). An experimental investigation of hypnotic age regression. *American J. of Clinical Hypnosis* **3**:127.

Edmonston, W. E., Jr. (1977a). Conceptual and investigative approaches to hypnosis and hypnotic phenomena. *Annals of the New York Academy of Sciences* **296**:314.

Edmonston, W. E., Jr. (1977b). Neutral hypnosis as relaxation. *American J. of Clinical Hypnosis* **20**(1):69-75.

Edmonston, W. E., Jr. (1977c). Body morphology and the capacity for hypnosis. *Annals of New York Academy of Sciences* **296**:105-118.

Edmonston, W. E., Jr. (1981). *Hypnosis and Relaxation: Modern Verification of an Old Equation*. New York: John Wiley.

Edmonston, W. E., Jr., and Grotevant, W. R. (1975). Hypnosis and alpha density. *American J. of Clinical Hypnosis* **17**(4):221-232.

Edmonston, W. E., Jr., and Robertson, T. G., Jr. (1967). A comparison of the effects of task motivational and hypnotic induction instructions on responsiveness to hypnotic suggestibility scales. *American J. of Clinical Hypnosis* **9**(3):184-187.

Eisele, G., and Higgins, J. J. (1962). Hypnosis in educational and moral problems. *American J. of Clinical Hypnosis* **4**:259-263.

Eisen, M. R., and Fromm, E. (1983). The clinical use of self-hypnosis in hypnotherapy: Tapping the functions of imagery and adaptive regression. *International J. of Clinical and Experimental Hypnosis* **31**(4):243-255.

Eisenberg, H. (1978). Parapsychological perspectives on deep trance states: Invited address to the annual meeting of the Ontario Society of Clinical Hypnosis on May 23rd of 1976. *J. of the American Society of Psychosomatic Dentistry and Medicine* **25**(3):97-101.

Eli, I., and Kleinhauz, M. (1985). Hypnosis: A tool for an integrative approach in the treatment of the gagging reflex. *International J. of Clinical and Experimental Hypnosis* **33**(2):99-108.

Eliseo, T. S. (1975). The hypnotic treatment of sleepwalking in an adult. *American J. of Clinical Hypnosis* **17**(4):272-276.

Elkins, G. R. (1984). Hypnosis in the treatment of myofibrositis and anxiety: A case report. *American J. of Clinical Hypnosis* **27**(1):26-30.

Elkins, G. R., and Carter, B. D. (1981). Use of a science fiction-based imagery technique in child hypnosis. *American J. of Clinical Hypnosis* **23**(4):274-277.

Ellenberger, H. F. (1970). *The Discovery of the Unconscious: The History and Evolution of Dynamic Psychiatry*. New York: Basic Books

Ellis, A. (1962). *Reason and Emotion in Psychotherapy*. New York: Lyle Stuart.

Epstein, S. J., and Deyoub, P. L. (1981). Hypnotherapy for fear of choking: Treatment implications of a case report. *International J. of Clinical and Experimental Hypnosis* **29**(2):117-127.

Epstein, S. J., and Deyoub, P. L. (1983). Hypnotherapeutic control of exhibitionism: A brief communication. *International J. of Clinical and Experimental Hypnosis* **31**(2):63-66.

Erickson, M. H. (1938a). A study of clinical and experimental findings on hypnotic deafness. I. Clinical experimentation and findings. *J. of General Psychology* **19**:127-150.

Erickson, M. H. (1938b). A study of clinical and experimental findings on hypnotic deafness. II. Experimental findings with a conditioned response technique. *J. of General Psychology* **19**:151-167.

Erickson, M. H. (1939a). An experimental investigation of the possible antisocial use of hypnosis. *Psychiatry* **2**:391-414.

Erickson, M. H. (1939b). The induction of color-blindness by a technique of hypnotic suggestion. *J. of General Psychology* **20**:61-89.

Erickson, M. H. (1944). An experimental investigation of the hypnotic subject's apparent ability to become unaware of stimuli. *J. of General Psychology* **31**:191-212.

Erickson, M. H. (1954). Pseudo-orientation as a hypnotherapeutic procedure. *J. of Clinical and Experimental Hypnosis* **2**:261-283.

Erickson, M. H. (1966). Experiential knowledge of hypnotic phenomena employed for hypnotherapy. *American J. of Clinical Hypnosis* **8**:299-309.

Erickson, M. H. (1977a). Hypnotic approaches to therapy. *American J. of Clinical Hypnosis* **20**(1):20-35.

Erickson, M. H. (1977b). Control of physiological functions by hypnosis. *American J. of Clinical Hypnosis* **20**(1):8-19.

Erickson, M. H., and Erickson, E. M. (1941). Concerning the nature and character of post-hypnotic behavior. *J. of General Psychology* **24**:95-133.

Erickson, M. H., and Rossi, E. L. (1975). Varieties of double bind. *American J. of Clinical Hypnosis* **17**(3):143-157.

Erickson, M. H., and Rossi, E. L. (1976). Two level communication and the microdynamics of trance and suggestion. *American J. of Clinical Hypnosis* **18**(3):153-171.

Erickson, M. H., and Rossi, E. L. (1977). Autohypnotic experiences of Milton H. Erickson. *American J. of Clinical Hypnosis* **20**(1):36-54.

Erickson, M. H. and Rossi, E. L. (1980). *Experiencing Hypnosis: Therapeutic Approaches to Altered States*. New York: Ivrington Publishers.

Erickson, M. H.; Rossi, E. L.; and Rossi, S. I. (1976). *Hypnotic Realities: The Induction of Clinical Hypnosis and Forms of Indirect Suggestion*. New York: Irvington Publishers.

Estabrooks, G. H. (1951). The possible antisocial use of hypnotism. *Personality: Symposia on Topical Issues* **1**:294-299.

Estabrooks, G. H. (1957). *Hypnotism*. New York: E. P. Dutton.

Evans, F. J. (1977). Hypnosis and sleep: The control of altered states of awareness. *Annals of New York Academy of Sciences* **296**:162-174.

Evans, F. J. (1979). Contextual forgetting: Posthypnotic source amnesia. *J. of Abnormal Psychology* **88**(5):556-563.

Evans, F. J. (1982). Hypnosis and sleep. *Research Communications in Psychology, Psychiatry and Behavior* **7**(2):241-256.

Evans, F. J. (1983). Conflict resolution during hypnosis:A commentary on McConkey's analysis. *British J. of Experimental and Clinical Hypnosis* **1**(1):21-23.

Evans, F. J., and Kihlstrom, J. F. (1973). Posthypnotic amnesia as disturbed retrieval. *J. of Abnormal Psychology* **82**(2):317-323.

Evans, F. J.; Kihlstrom, J. F.; and Orne, E. C. (1973). Quantifying subjective reports during posthypnotic amnesia. In *Proceedings of the 81st Annual Convention of the American Psychological Association.*

Evans, F. J., and Orne, M. T. (1971). The disappearing hypnotist: The use of simulating subjects to evaluate how subjects perceive experimental procedures. *International J. of Clinical and Experimental Hypnosis* **19**(4):277-296.

Evans, J. M. (1982). The intuitive process: An investigation of personal and transpersonal aspects using hypnosis. *Dissertation Abstracts International* **43**(2-B):507.

Evers, J. (1983). The effectiveness of a nonauthoritarian rapid hypnotic induction in individuals of high and low hypnotic susceptibility. *Dissertation Abstracts International* **43**(9-B):3027.

Ewin, D. M. (1974). Condyloma acuminatum: Successful treatment of four cases by hypnosis. *American J. of Clinical Hypnosis* **17**(2):73-78.

Ewin, D. M. (1983). Emergency room hypnosis for the burned patient. *American J. of Clinical Hypnosis* **26**(1):5-8.

Ewin, D. M. (1984). Hypnosis in surgery and anesthesia. In W. C. Wester II and A. H. Smith Jr. (Eds.), *Clinical Hypnosis: A Multidisciplinary Approach* (pp. 210-235). Philadelphia: J. B. Lippincott.

Ewin, D. M. (1986). The effect of hypnosis and mental set on major surgery and burns. *Psychiatric Annals* **16**(2):115-118.

Eysenck, H. J. (1961). Classification and the problem of diagnosis. In H. J. Eysenck (Ed.). *Handbook of Abnormal Psychology.* New York: Basic Books.

Eysenck, H. J. (1963). Behavior therapy, spontaneous remission and transference in neurotics. *American J. of Psychiatry* **119**:867-871.

Eysenck, H. J., and Rees, W. L. (1945). States of heightened suggestibility: Narcosis. *J. of Mental Science* **91**:301-310.

Fabbri, R., Jr. (1976). Hypnosis and behavior therapy: A coordinated approach to the treatment of sexual disorders. *American J. of Clinical Hypnosis* **19**(1):4-8.

Falick, P. (1968). The lie detector and the right to privacy. *New York State Bar J.* **40**(2):102-110.

Farabollini, F.; di Prisco, C. L.; and Carli, G. (1981). Neuroendocrine changes following habituation of animal hypnosis in male rabbits. *Behavioral Brain Research* **2**(3):363-372.

Farthing, G. W.; Brown, S. W.; and Venturino, M. (1982). Effects of hypnotizability and mental imagery on signal detection sensitivity and response bias. *International J. of Clinical and Experimental Hypnosis* **30**(3):289-305.

Farthing, G. W.; Brown, S. W.; and Venturino, M. (1983). Involuntariness of response on the Harvard Group Scale of Hypnotic Susceptibility. *International J. of Clinical and Experimental Hypnosis* **31**(3):170-181.

Farthing, G. W.; Venturino, M.; and Brown, S. W. (1983). Relationship between two different types of imagery vividness questionnaire items and three hypnotic susceptibility scale factors: A brief communication. *International J. of Clinical and Experimental Hypnosis* **31**(1):8-13.

Farthing, G. W.; Venturino, M.; and Brown, S. W. (1984). Suggestion and distraction in the control of pain: Test of two hypotheses. *J. of Abnormal Psychology* **93**(3):266-276.

Faw, V., and Wilcox, W. W. (1958). Personality characteristics of susceptible and unsusceptible hypnotic subjects. *J. of Clinical and Experimental Hypnosis* **6**:83-94.

Faw, V.; Sellers, D. J.; and Wilcox, W. W. (1968). Psychopathological effects of hypnosis. *International J. of Clinical and Experimental Hypnosis* **16**:26-37.

Feamster, J. H., and Brown, J. E. (1963). Hypnotic aversion to alcohol: Three-year follow up of one patient. *American J. of Clinical Hypnosis* **6**:164-166.

Fee, A. F., and Reilley, R. R. (1982). Hypnosis in obstetrics: A review of techniques. *J. of American Society of Psychosomatic Dentistry and Medicine* **29**(1):17-29.

Feldman, B. E. (1977). A phenomenological and clinical inquiry into deep hypnosis. *Dissertation Abstracts International* **37**(12-B):6323.

Fellows, B. J. (1982). Neglected issues in the debate over the use of hypnosis in criminal investigations. *Bulletin of the British Society of Experimental and Clinical Hypnosis* **1982**(5):85-89.

Fellows, B. J. (1984). Preliminary report on the use of hypnotic and imaginative procedures during pregnancy and childbirth in Hungary. *British J. of Experimental and Clinical Hypnosis* **1**(2):53-54.

Fellows, B. J., and Armstrong, V. (1977). An experimental investigation of the relationship between hypnotic susceptibility and reading involvement. *American J. of Clinical Hypnosis* **20**(2):101-105.

Fellows, B. J., and Creamer, M. (1978). An investigation of the role of hypnosis, hypnotic susceptibility and hypnotic induction in the production of age regression. *British J. of Social and Clinical Psychology* **17**(2):165-171.

Fernandez, G. R. (1955). Hypnotism in the treatment of the stress factor in dermatological conditions. *British J. of Medical Hypnosis* **7**(2):21-24.

Ferrera, S. J., and Wade, N. L. (1982). Hypnotic testimony: To be or not to be? *Medical Hypnoanalysis* **3**(3):112-117.

Field, P. B., and Kline, M. V. (1974). Previous psychotherapy among hypnotherapy applicants. *American J. of Clinical Hypnosis* **17**(2):125-130.

Field, P. B.; Evans, F. J.; and Orne, M. T. (1965). Order of difficulty of suggestions during hypnosis. *International J. of Clinical and Experimental Hypnosis* **13**(3):183-192.

Finke, R. A., and MacDonald, H. (1978). Two personality measures relating hypnotic susceptibility to absorption. *International J. of Clinical and Experimental Hypnosis* **26**(3):178-183.

Finkelstein, S. (1982). Re-establishment of traumatically disrupted finger flexor function: A brief communication. *International J. of Clinical and Experimental Hypnosis* **30**(1):1-3.

Finkelstein, S., and Howard, M. G. (1982-1983). Cancer prevention: A three year pilot study. *American J. of Clinical Hypnosis* **25**(2-3):177-187.

Fischer, R. (1977). On flashback and hypnotic recall. *International J. of Clinical and Experimental Hypnosis* **25**(4):217-235.

Fisher, C. (1953). Studies on the nature of suggestion. I. Experimental induction of dreams by direct suggestion. *J. of American Psychological Association* **1:**222.

Fisher, S. (1954). The role of expectancy in the performance of posthypnotic behavior. *J. of Abnormal and Social Psychology* **49:**503-507.

Fisher, S. (1955). An investigation of alleged conditioning phenomena under hypnosis. *J. of Clinical and Experimental Hypnosis* **3:**71.

Fogel, B. S. (1984). The "sympathetic ear": Case reports of a self-hypnotic approach to chronic pain. *American J. of Clinical Hypnosis* **27**(2):103-106.

Fogel, S. (1976). Psychogenic tremor and asomatognosia. *American J. of Clinical Hypnosis* **19**(1):57-61.

Fogelman, M. J., and Crasilneck, H. B. (1956). Food intake and hypnosis. *J. American Diet Association* **32:**519.

Ford, L. F., and Yeager, C. L. (1948). Changes in the electroencephalogram in subjects under hypnosis. *Diseases of the Nervous System* **9:**190-192.

Fourie, D. P. (1980). Relationship aspects of hypnotic susceptibility. *Perceptual and Motor Skills* **51**(3, part 2):1032-1034.

Fourie, D. P. (1981). Hypnosis and psi: Taking stock. *Parapsychological J. of South Africa* **3**(1):17-27.

Fourie, D. P. (1983). Width of the hypnotic relationship: An interactional view of hypnotic susceptibility and hypnotic depth. *Australian J. of Clinical and Experimental Hypnosis* **11**(1):1-14.

Fowler, W. L. (1961). Hypnosis and learning. *International J. of Clinical and Experimental Hypnosis* **9:**223-232.

Francis, J. G. (1984). Stopping stuttering with hypnosis. *Australian J. of Clinical and Experimental Hypnosis* **12**(1):9-21.

Frankel, F. H. (1973). The effects of brief hypnotherapy in a series of psychosomatic problems. *Psychotherapy and Psychosomatics* **22:**269-275.

Frankel, F. H. (1974). Trance capacity and the genesis of phobic behavior. *Archives of General Psychiatry* **31**(2):261-263.

Frankel, F. H. (1975). Hypnosis as a treatment method in psychosomatic medicine. *International J. of Psychiatry in Medicine* **6**(1-2):75-85.

Frankel, F. H. (1976). *Hypnosis: Trance as a Coping Mechanism.* New York: Plenum Press.

Frankel, F. H. (1978). The relationship between research and clinical practice: Bridging the gap. *Australian J. of Clinical and Experimental Hypnosis* **6**(1):7-15.

Frankel, F. H. (1978-1979). Scales measuring hypnotic responsivity: A clinical perspective. *American J. of Clinical Hypnosis* **21**(2-3):208-217.

Frankel, F. H. (1981). Reporting hypnosis in the medical context: A brief communication. *International J. of Clinical and Experimental Hypnosis* **29**(1):10-14.

Frankel, F. H. (1982). Hypnosis and hypnotizability scales: A reply. *International J. of Clinical and Experimental Hypnosis* **30**(4):377-392.

Frankel, F. H.; Apfel, R. J.; Kelly, S. F.; Benson, H.; Quinn, T.; Newmark, J.; and Malmaud, R. (1979). The use of hypnotizability scales in the clinic: A review after six years. *International J. of Clinical and Experimental Hypnosis* **27**(2): 63-73.

Frankel, F. H., and Misch, R. C. (1973). Hypnosis in a case of long-standing psoriasis in a person with character problems. *International J. of Clinical and Experimental Hypnosis* **21**(3):121-130.

Frankel, F. H., and Orne, M. T. (1976). Hypnotizability and phobic behavior. *Archives of General Psychiatry* **33**(10):1259-1261.

Frankel, F. H., and Zamansky, H. S. (Eds.) (1978). *Hypnosis at Its Bicentennial, Selected Papers.* New York: Plenum Press.

Franklin, L. M. (1957). Hypnosis in general practice. *Med World* **87**:514-518.

Franks, C. M. (1966). Conditioning and conditioned aversion therapies in the treatment of the alcoholic. *International J. of the Addictions* **1**:61-98.

Franzini, L. R., and McDonald, R. D. (1973). Marijuana usage and hypnotic susceptibility. *J. of Consulting and Clinical Psychology* **40**(2):176-180.

Fredericks, L. E. (1978). Teaching of hypnosis in the overall approach to the surgical patient. *American J. of Clinical Hypnosis* **20**(3):175-183.

Fredericks, L. E. (1980). The value of teaching hypnosis in the practice of anesthesiology. *International J. of Clinical and Experimental Hypnosis* **28**(1):6-15.

French, A. P., and Tupin, J. P. (1974). Therapeutic application of a simple relaxation method. *American J. of Psychotherapy* **28**(2):282-287.

Fricton, J. R., and Roth, P. (1985). The effects of direct and indirect hypnotic suggestions for analgesia in high and low susceptible subjects. *American J. of Clinical Hypnosis* **27**(4):226-231.

Frid, M., and Singer, G. (1979). Hypnotic analgesia in conditions of stress is partially reversed by naloxone. *Psychopharmacology* **63**(3):211-215.

Friedman, H., and Taub, H. A. (1977). The use of hypnosis and biofeedback procedures for essential hypertension. *International J. of Clinical and Experimental Hypnosis* **25**(4):335-347.

Friedman, H., and Taub, H. A. (1978). A six-month follow-up of the use of hypnosis and biofeedback procedures in essential hypertension. *American J. of Clinical Hypnosis* **20**(3):184-188.

Friedman, H., and Taub, H. A. (1982). Accessibility—a necessary control for studies of essential hypertension: A brief communication. *International J. of Clinical and Experimental Hypnosis* **30**(1):4-8.

Friedman, H., and Taub, H. A. (1984). Brief psychological training procedures in migraine treatment. *American J. of Clinical Hypnosis* **26**(3):187-200.

Friedman, H., and Taub, H. A. (1985). Extended follow-up study of the effects of brief psychological procedures in migraine therapy. *American J. of Clinical Hypnosis* **28**(1):27-33.

Friedman, H.; Taub, H. A.; and Syracuse Veterans Administration Medical Center. (1982). An evaluation of hypnotic susceptibility and peripheral temperature elevation in the treatment of migraine. *American J. of Clinical Hypnosis* **24**(3):172-182.

Frischholz, E. J.; Blumstein, R.; and Spiegel, D. (1982). Comparative efficacy of hypnotic behavioral training and sleep/trance hypnotic induction: Comment on Katz. *J. of Consulting and Clinical Psychology* **50**(5):766-769.

Frischholz, E. J., and Spiegel, D. (1986). Adjunctive uses of hypnosis in the treatment of smoking. *Psychiatric Annals* **16**(2):87-90.

Frischholz, E. J.; Spiegel, H.; and Spiegel, D. (1981). Hypnosis and the unhypnotizable: A reply to Barber. *American J. of Clinical Hypnosis* **24**(1):55-58.

Frischholz, E. J.; Spiegel, H.; Tryon, W. W.; and Fisher, S. (1981). The relationship between the Hypnotic Induction Profile and the Stanford Hypnotic Susceptibility Scale, Form C: revisited. *American J. of Clinical Hypnosis* **24**(2):98-105.

Frischholz, E. J., and Tryon, W. W. (1980). Hypnotizability in relation to the ability to learn thermal biofeedback. *American J. of Clinical Hypnosis* **23**(1):53-56.

Frischholz, E. J.; Tryon, W. W.; Fisher, S.; Maruffi, B. L.; Vellios, A. T.; and Spiegel, H. (1980). The relationship between the Hypnotic Induction Profile and the Stanford Hypnotic Susceptibility Scale, Form C: A replication. *American J. of Clinical Hypnosis* **22**(4):185-196.

Fromm, E. (1972). Ego activity and ego passivity in hypnosis. *International J. of Clinical and Experimental Hypnosis* **20**(4):238-251.

Fromm, E. (1975). Self-hypnosis: A new area of research. *Psychotherapy: Theory, Research and Practice* **12**(3):295-301.

Fromm, E. (1977a). Altered states of consciousness and hypnosis: A discussion. *International J. of Clinical and Experimental Hypnosis* **25**(4):325-334.

Fromm, E. (1977b). An ego-psychological theory of altered states of consciousness. *International J. of Clinical and Experimental Hypnosis* **25**(4):372-387.

Fromm, E.; Brown, D. P.; Hurt, S. W.; Oberlander, J. Z.; Boxer, A. M.; and Pfeifer, G. (1981). The phenomena and characteristics of self-hypnosis. *International J. of Clinical and Experimental Hypnosis* **29**(3):189-246.

Fromm, E., and Eisen, M. (1982). Self-hypnosis as a therapeutic aid in the mourning process. *American J. of Clinical Hypnosis* **25**(1):3-14.

Fromm, E., and Shor, R. E. (1972). *Hypnosis: Research Developments and Perspectives.* Chicago: Aldine.

Fromm, E., and Shor, R. E. (Eds.). (1979). *Hypnosis, Developments in Research and New Perspectives* (2d ed.). New York: Aldine.

Frost, E. A. (1978). Acupuncture and hypnosis: Apples and oranges. *New York State J. of Medicine* **78**(11):1768-1772.

Frumkin, L. R.; Ripley, H. S.; and Cox, G. B. (1978). Changes in cerebral hemispheric lateralization with hypnosis. *Biological Psychiatry* **13**(6):741-750.

Frutiger, A. D. (1981). Treatment of penetration phobia through the combined use of systematic desensitization and hypnosis: A case study. *American J. of Clinical Hypnosis* **23**(4):269-273.

Fuchs, K.; Hoch, Z.; Paldi, E.; Abramovici, H.; Brandes, J. M.; Timor-Tritsch, I.; and Kleinhaus, M. (1973). Hypno-desensitization therapy of vaginismus. Part I. "In vitro" method. Part II. "In vivo" method. *International J. of Clinical and Experimental Hypnosis* **21**(3):144-156.

Fuchs, K.; Paldi, E.; Abramovici, H.; and Peretz, B. A. (1980). Treatment of hyperemesis gravidarum by hypnosis. *International J. of Clinical and Experimental Hypnosis* **28**(4):313-323.

Fung, E. H., and Lazar, B. S. (1983). Hypnosis as an adjunct in the treatment of von Willebrand's disease. *International J. of Clinical and Experimental Hypnosis* **31**(4):256-265.

Furst, A. (1973). *Post-Hypnotic Instructions.* Hollywood: Wilshire Book Co.

Galski, T. J. (1981). The adjunctive use of hypnosis in the treatment of trichotillomania: A case report. *American J. of Clinical Hypnosis* **23**(3):198-201.

Gard, B., and Kurtz, R. M. (1979). Hypnotic age regression and cognitive perceptual tasks. *American J. of Clinical Hypnosis* **21**(4):270-277.

Gardner, G. G. (1976a). Hypnosis and mastery: Clinical contributions and directions for research. *International J. of Clinical and Experimental Hypnosis* **24**(3):202-214.

Gardner, G. G. (1976b). Attitudes of child health professionals toward hypnosis: Implications for training. *International J. of Clinical and Experimental Hypnosis* **24**(2):63-73.

Gardner, G. G. (1977). Hypnosis with infants and preschool children. *American J. of Clinical Hypnosis* **19**(3):158-162.

Gardner, G. G. (1980). Hypnosis with children: Selected readings. *International J. of Clinical and Experimental Hypnosis* **28**(3):289-293.

Gardner, G. G. (1981). Teaching self-hypnosis to children. *International J. of Clinical and Experimental Hypnosis* **29**(3):300-312.

Gardner, G. G., and Lubman, A. (1982-1983). Hypnotherapy for children with cancer: Some current issues. *American J. of Clinical Hypnosis* **25**(2-3):135-142.

Gardner, G. G., and Olness, K. (1981). *Hypnosis and Hypnotherapy with Children*. New York: Grune and Stratton.

Gardner, G. G., and Tarnow, J. D. (1980). Adjunctive hypnotherapy with an autistic boy. *American J. of Clinical Hypnosis* **22**(3):173-179.

Garrett, J. B., and Wallace, B. (1975). A novel test of hypnotic anesthesia. *International J. of Clinical and Experimental Hypnosis* **23**(2):139-147.

Garver, R. B. (1977). The enhancement of human performance with hypnosis through neuromotor facilitation and control of arousal level. *American J. of Clinical Hypnosis* **19**(3):177-181.

Garver, R. B. (1984). Eight steps to self-hypnosis. *American J. of Clinical Hypnosis* **26**(4):232-235.

Garver, R. B.; Fuselier, G. D.; and Booth, T. B. (1981). The hypnotic treatment of amnesia in an air force basic trainee. *American J. of Clinical Hypnosis* **24**(1):3-6.

Gaston, C. D., and Hutzell, R. R. (1976). Hypnosis to reduce smoking in a deaf patient. *American J. of Clinical Hypnosis* **19**(2):125-127.

Gaunitz, S. C. B.; Nystrom-Bonnier, E.; and Skalin, M. (1980). Posthypnotic suggestions and behavior change: Highly hypnotizables compared with simulators. *Scandinavian J. of Psychology* **21**(4):269-273.

Geiselman, R. E.; Bjork, R. A.; and Fishman, D. L. (1983). Disrupted retrieval in directed forgetting: A link with posthypnotic amnesia. *J. of Experimental Psychology: General* **112**(1):58-72.

Geiselman, R. E.; MacKinnon, D. P.; Fishman, D. L.; Jaenicke, C.; Larner, B. R.; Schoenberg, S.; and Swartz, S. (1983). Mechanisms of hypnotic and nonhypnotic forgetting. *J. of Experimental Psychology: Learning, Memory and Cognition* **9**(4):626-635.

George, F. R. (1983). The role of prostaglandins in mediating the behavioral, physiological and biochemical effects of alcohol. *Dissertation Abstracts International* **43**(7-B):2383.

George, F. R.; Howerton, T. C.; Elmer, G. I.; and Collins, A. C. (1983). Antagonism of alcohol hypnosis by blockade of prostaglandin synthesis and activity: Genotype and time course effects. *Pharmacology, Biochemistry and Behavior* **19**(1):131-136.   .

Getzels, J. W., and Jackson, P. W. (1962). *Creativity and Intelligence*. New York: John Wiley.

Gheorghiu, V., and Holdevici, I. (1980). Attempt to test suggestibility by "indirect," "direct" and "indirect-direct" approaches following hypnotic induction. *Revue roumaine des sciences sociales—Sèrie de psychologie* **24**(2):161-173.

Gheorghiu, V. A., and Orleanu, P. (1982). Dental implant under hypnosis. *American J. of Clinical Hypnosis* **25**(1):68-70.

Gheorghiu, V. A., and Reyher, J. (1982). The effect of different types of influence on an "indirect-direct" form of a scale of sensory suggestibility. *American J. of Clinical Hypnosis* **24**(3):191-199.

Giacalone, A. V. (1981). Hysterical dysphonia: Hypnotic treatment of a ten-year-old female. *American J. of Clinical Hypnosis* **23**(4):289-293.

Gibbons, D. (1974). Hyperempiria, a new "altered state of consciousness" induced by suggestion. *Perceptual and Motor Skills* **39**:47-53.

Gibbons, D. E. (1976). Hypnotic vs. hyperempiric induction procedures: An experimental comparison. *Perceptual and Motor Skills* **42**(3):834.

Gibbons, D. E. (1979). *Applied Hypnosis and Hyperempiria*. New York: Plenum Press.

Gibbons, D. E. (1982a). Hypnosis as a trance state: The future of a shared delusion. *Bulletin of the British Society of Experimental and Clinical Hypnosis* **1982**(5):1-4.

Gibbons, D. E. (1982b). A reply to the comments of Wagstaff and Vingoe. *Bulletin of the British Society of Experimental and Clinical Hypnosis* **1982**(5):12-13.

Gibson, H. B. (1977). Animal hypnosis and human hypnosis: New experimental evidence relating to an old controversy. *Psychologia: An International J. of Psychology in the Orient* **20**(3):136-144.

Gibson, H. B. (1982). The use of hypnosis in police investigations. *Bulletin of the British Psychological Society* **35**:138-142.

Gibson, H. B., and Corcoran, M. E. (1975). Personality and differential susceptibility to hypnosis: Further replication and sex differences. *British J. of Psychology* **66**(4):513-520.

Gibson, H. B.; Corcoran, M. E.; and Curran, J. D. (1977). Hypnotic susceptibility and personality: The consequences of diazepam and the sex of the subject. *British J. of Psychology* **68**(1):51-59.

Gibson, M. (1984a). Hypnosis with children. *British J. of Experimental and Clinical Hypnosis* **2**(1):31-34.

Gibson, M. (1984b). Hypnosis with children: A reply to Cowell's comments. *British J. of Experimental and Clinical Hypnosis* **2**(1):41-42.

Gidro, F. L., and Bowersbuch, M. K. (1948). A study of the plantar response in hypnotic age regression. *J. of Nervous and Mental Disease* **107**:443-458.

Gilbert, J. E., and Barber, T. X. (1972). Effects of hypnotic induction, motivational suggestions, and level of suggestibility on cognitive performance. *International J. of Clinical and Experimental Hypnosis* **20**(3):156-168.

Gill, M. M. (1972). Hypnosis as an altered and regressed state. *International J. of Clinical and Experimental Hypnosis* **20**(4):224-237.

Gillett, P. L., and Coe, W. C. (1984). The effects of rapid induction analgesia (RIA), hypnotic susceptibility and the severity of discomfort on reducing dental pain. *American J. of Clinical Hypnosis* **27**(2):81-90.

Gillispie, C. C. (Ed.). (1974). *Dictionary of Scientific Biography.* New York: Charles Scribner's Sons.

Gindes, B. C. (1979). *New Concepts of Hypnosis.* Hollywood: Wilshire Book Co.

Gindhart, L. R. (1981a). The use of a metamorphic story in therapy: A case report. *American J. of Clinical Hypnosis* **23**(3):202-206.

Gindhart, L. R. (1981b). Untying a "not." *American J. of Clinical Hypnosis* **24**(2):117-123.

Gindhart, L. R. (1983). The use of a symbolic hand posture in trance induction. *Australian J. of Clinical Hypnotherapy and Hypnosis* **4**(2):69-73.

Girodo, M., and Wood, D. (1979) Talking yourself out of pain: The importance of believing that you can. *Cognitive Therapy and Research* **3**(1):23-33.

Glad, W. R.; Tyre, T. F.; and Adesso, V. J. (1976). A multidimensional model of cigarette smoking. *American J. of Clinical Hypnosis* **19**(2):82-90.

Glass, L. B., and Barber, T. X. (1961). A note on hypnotic behavior, the definition of the situation and the placebo effect. *J. of Nervous and Mental Disease* **132**(6):539-541.

Glenn, T. J., and Simonds, J. F. (1977). Hypnotherapy of a psychogenic seizure disorder in an adolescent. *American J. of Clinical Hypnosis* **19**(4):245-250.

Godec, C. J. (1979). Inhibition of hyperreflexic bladder during hypnosis: A case report. *American J. of Clinical Hypnosis* **22**(1):170-172.

Golan, H. P. (1975). Further case reports from the Boston City Hospital. *American J. of Clinical Hypnosis* **18**(1):55-59.

Goldberger, N. I., and Wachtel, P. L. (1973). Hypnotizability and cognitive controls. *International J. of Clinical and Experimental Hypnosis* **21**(4):298-304.

Goldfarb, D. A., and O'Brien, R. M. (1985). Classical conditioning as a means of increasing hypnotic susceptibility. Paper presented to The Association for the Advancement of Behavior Therapy Houston, November.

Goldstein, L. (1982). Some recent advances in research on hypnosis: Introductory remarks. *Research Communications in Psychology, Psychiatry, and Behavior* **7**(2):145-147.

Goldstein, Y. (1981). The effect of demonstrating to a subject that she is in a hypnotic trance as a variable in hypnotic interventions with obese women. *International J. of Clinical and Experimental Hypnosis* **29**(1):15-23.

Gordon, J. E. (1967). *Handbook of Clinical and Experimental Hypnosis.* New York: Macmillan.

Gordon, M. C. (1972). Age and performance differences of male patients on modified Stanford Hypnotic Susceptibility Scales. *International J. of Clinical and Experimental Hypnosis* **20**(3):152-155.

Gordon, M. C. (1973). Suggestibility of chronic schizophrenic and normal males matched for age. *International J. of Clinical and Experimental Hypnosis* **21**(4):284-288.

Gorsky, B. H. (1980). The computer as an aid in teaching hypnosis. *American J. of Clinical Hypnosis.* **23**(2):132-134.

Gorsky, B. H., and Gorsky, S. R. (1981). *Introduction to Medical Hypnosis* New York: Medical Examination Publishing Co.

Gorton, B. E. (1949a). The physiology of hypnosis. I. A review of the literature. *Psychiatric Quarterly* **23**:317-343.

Gorton, B. E. (1949b). The physiology of hypnosis. II. A review of the literature. *Psychiatric Quarterly* **23**:375-385.

Gottesfeld, M. L. (1978). Treatment of vaginismus by psychotherapy with adjunctive hypnosis. *American J. of Clinical Hypnosis* **20**(4):272-275.

Gouch, D. A., and Fross, G. H. (1976). *What Every Subject Should Know about Hypnosis and Self Hypnosis.* South Orange, NJ: Power Pub.

Gould, S. S., and Tissler, D. M. (1984). The use of hypnosis in the treatment of Herpes Simplex II. *American J. of Clinical Hypnosis* **26**(3):171-174.

Graham, C., and Leibowitz, H. W. (1972). The effect of suggestion on visual acuity. *International J. of Clinical and Experimental Hypnosis* **20**(3):169-186.

Graham, K. R. (1977). Perceptual processes and hypnosis: Support for a cognitive-state theory based on laterality. *Annals of New York Academy of Sciences* **296**:274-283.

Graham, K. R. (1978). Laterality theory of hypnosis. Paper presented at First European Congress of Hypnosis in Psychology and Psychosomatic Medicine, Malmo, Sweden, June 1-4.

Graham, K. R., and Greene, L. D. (1981). Hypnotic susceptibility related to an independent measure of compliance—alumni annual giving: A brief communication. *International J. of Clinical and Experimental Hypnosis* **29**(4):351-354.

Graham, K. R., and Patton, A. (1968). Retroactive inhibition, hypnosis and hypnotic amnesia. *International J. of Clinical and Experimental Hypnosis* **16**:68-74.

Graham, K. R., and Pernicano, K. (1979). Laterality, hypnosis, and the autokinetic effect. *American J. of Clinical Hypnosis* **22**(2):79-84.

Graham, K. R.; Wright, G. W.; Toman, W. J.; and Mark, C. B. (1975). Relaxation and hypnosis in the treatment of insomnia. *American J. of Clinical Hypnosis* **18**(1):39-42.

Grahs, C. E. (1979). Bilateral alpha activity as a function of hypnosis, math and spatial mental tasks and a part-whole tactile matching task. *Dissertation Abstracts International* **39**(8-A):4820-4821.

Grant, D. H. (1982). The use of hypnosis and suggestions to improve study habits, study attitudes, self-concept, and reduction of test anxiety. *Dissertation Abstracts International* **43**(6-B):1980.

Gravitz, M. A. (1971). Psychodynamics of resistance to hypnotic induction. *Psychotherapy: Theory, Research and Practice* **8**(2):185-187.

Gravitz, M. A. (1978). Seminar on hypnotic treatment of pain at Adelphi University, December.

Gravitz, M. A. (1979). Hypnotherapeutic management of epileptic behavior. *American J. of Clinical Hypnosis* **21**(4):282-284.

Gravitz, M. A. (1980). Discussion. *American J. of Clinical Hypnosis* **23** (2):103-111.

Gravitz, M. A. (1981*a*). Non-verbal hypnotic techniques in a centrally deaf brain-damaged patient. *International J. of Clinical and Experimental Hypnosis* **29**(2):110-116.

Gravitz, M. A. (1981*b*). Bibliographic sources of nineteenth century hypnosis literature. *American J. of Clinical Hypnosis* **23**(3):217-219.

Gravitz, M. A. (1981*c*). The production of warts by suggestion as a cultural phenomenon. *American J. of Clinical Hypnosis* **23**(4):281-283.

Gravitz, M. A. (1983*a*). Early uses of the telephone and recordings in hypnosis. *American J. of Clinical Hypnosis* **25**(4):280-282.

Gravitz, M. A. (1983*b*). An early case of investigative hypnosis: A brief communication. *International J. of Clinical and Experimental Hypnosis* **21**(4):224-226.

Gravitz, M. A. (1985*a*). A case of forensic hypnosis. In E. T. Dowd and J. M. Healy (Eds.). *Case Studies in Hypnotherapy.* New York: Guilford Press.

Gravitz, M.A. (1985*b*). Resistance in investigative hypnosis: Determinants and management. *American J. of Clinical Hypnosis* **28**(2):76-83.

Gravitz, M. A. (1985*c*). An 1846 report of tumor remission associated with hypnosis. *American J. of Clinical Hypnosis* **28**(1):16-19.

Gravitz, M. A. (1985d). The Moll hypnosis collection: Historical background. *Bulletin of the Medical Library Association* **73**(3):292-293.

Gravitz, M. A., and Gerton, M. I. (1982). Polgar as Freud's hypnotist? Contrary evidence. *American J. of Clinical Hypnosis* **24**(4):272-276.

Gravitz, M. A., and Gerton, M. I. (1984a). Origins of the term hypnotism prior to Braid. *American J. of Clinical Hypnosis* **27**(2):107-110.

Gravitz, M. A., and Gerton, M. I., (1984b). Hypnosis in the historical development of psychoanalytic psychotherapy. In W. C. Wester II and A. H. Smith, *Clinical Hypnosis: A Multidisciplinary Approach* (pp. 1-17). Philadelphia: Lippincott.

Gravitz, M. A., and Gravitz, R. F. (1977). The collected writings of Milton H. Erickson: A complete bibliography 1929-1977. *American J. of Clinical Hypnosis* **20**(1):84-93.

Greene, R. J. (1973). Combining rational-emotive and hypnotic techniques: Treating depression. *Psychotherapy: Theory, Research and Practice* **10**(1):71-73.

Gregg, V. H. (1982). Posthypnotic amnesia for recently learned material: A comment on the paper by J. F. Kihlstrom (1980). *Bulletin of the British Society of Experimental and Clinical Hypnosis* **1982**(5):27-30.

Grisanti, G.; Cusimano, F.; and Traina, F. (1980). Cortical evoked response audiometry (CERA) under hypnosis. *J. of Auditory Research* **20**(4):253-262.

Gross, M. (1980). Hypnosis as a diagnostic tool. *American J. of Clinical Hypnosis* **23**(1):47-52.

Gross, M. (1984). Hypnosis in the therapy of anorexia nervosa. *American J. of Clinical Hypnosis* **26**(3):175-181.

Gross, M. A., and Morse, D. R. (1976). Acupuncture and endodontics: A review and preliminary study. *J. of Endodontics* **2**(8):236-243.

Gruber, L. N. (1983). Hypnotherapeutic techniques in patients with affective instability. *American J. of Clinical Hypnosis* **25**(4):263-266.

Gruen, W. (1972). A successful application of systematic self-relaxation and self-suggestions about postoperative reactions in a case of cardiac surgery. *International J. of Clinical and Experimental Hypnosis* **20**(3):143-151.

Gruenewald, D. (1978). Analogues of multiple personality in psychosis. *International J. of Clinical and Experimental Hypnosis* **26**(1):1-8.

Gruenewald, D. (1981). Failures in hypnotherapy: A brief communication. *International J. of Clinical and Experimental Hypnosis* **29**(4):345-350.

Gruenewald, D. (1982a). Problems of relevance in the application of laboratory data to clinical situations. *International J. of Clinical and Experimental Hypnosis* **30**(4):345-353.

Gruenewald, D. (1982b). A psychoanalytic view of hypnosis. *American J. of Clinical Hypnosis* **24**(3):185-190.

Greunewald, D. (1982c). Some thoughts on the distinction between the hypnotic situation and the hypnotic condition. *American J. of Clinical Hypnosis* **25**(1):46-51.

Gruenewald, D. (1984). On the nature of multiple personality: Comparisons with hypnosis. *International J. of Clinical and Experimental Hypnosis* **32**(2):170-190.

Gruzelier, J.; Brow, T.; Perry, A.; Rhonder, J.; and Thomas, M. (1984). Hypnotic susceptibility: A lateral predisposition and altered cerebral asymmetry under hypnosis. *International J. of Psychophysiology* **2**(2):131-139.

Gur, R., and Reyher, J. (1973). Relationship between style of hypnotic induction and direction of lateral eye movements. *J. of Abnormal Psychology* **82**(3):499-505.

Gur, R. C., and Reyher, J. (1976). Enhancement of creativity via free-imagery and hypnosis. *American J. of Clinical Hypnosis* **18**(4):237-249.

Gustavson, J. L., and Weight, D. G. (1981). Hypnotherapy for a phobia of slugs: A case report. *American J. of Clinical Hypnosis* **23**(4):258-262.

Gwynne, P. H.; Tosi, D. J.; and Howard, L. (1978). Treatment of nonassertion through rational stage directed hypnotherapy (RSDH) and behavioral rehearsal. *American J. of Clinical Hypnosis* **20**(4):263-271.

Hall, C. S. (1953). A cognitive theory of dream symbols. *J. of General Psychology* **48**:169-185.

Hall, C. S., and Lindzey, G. (1957). *Theories of Personality.* New York: John Wiley.

Hall, H. R. (1982-1983). Hypnosis and the immune system: A review with implications for cancer and the psychology of healing. *American J. of Clinical Hypnosis* **25**(2-3):92-103.

Hall, J. A. (1984). Toward a psycho-structural theory: Hypnosis and the structure of dreams. *American J. of Clinical Hypnosis* **26**(3):159-165.

Hall, M. D. (1982-1983). Using relaxation imagery with children with malignancies: A developmental perspective. *American J. of Clinical Hypnosis* **25**(2-3):143-149.

Hall, W. D. (1978). Psychological processes in pain perception: The prospects of a signal detection theory analysis. *Dissertation Abstracts International* **38**(10-B):5083-5084.

Ham, M. L. (1981). Hypnotic amnesia: A phenomenological and quantitative analysis. *Dissertation Abstracts International* **42**(6-B): 2600.

Ham, M. W., and Spanos, N. P. (1974). Suggested auditory and visual hallucinations in task-motivated and hypnotic subjects. *American J. of Clinical Hypnosis* **17**(2):94-101.

Ham, M. W.; Spanos, N. P.; and Barber, T. X. (1976). Suggestibility in hospitalized schizophrenics. *J. of Abnormal Psychology* **85**(6):550-557.

Hammer, E. F. (1954). Posthypnotic suggestion and test performance. *J. of Clinical and Experimental Hypnosis* **2**:178-185.

Hammerschlag, H. E. (1957). *Hypnotism and Crime.* Hollywood: Wilshire Book Co.

Hammond, D. C. (1984). Myths about Erickson and Ericksonian hypnosis. *American J. of Clinical Hypnosis* **26**(4):236-245.

Hammond, D. C.; Keye, W. R.; and Grant, C. W., Jr., (1983). Hypnotic analgesia with burns: An initial Study. *American J. of Clinical Hypnosis* **26**(1):56-59.

Handelsman, M. M. (1984). Self-hypnosis as a facilitator of self-efficacy: A case example. *Psychotherapy* **21**(4):550-553.

Hariman, J. (1979). Case notes and hypnotic techniques: Existential spiritual exercises. *Australian J. of Clinical and Experimental Hypnosis* **7**(3):279-281.

Hariman, J. (1980). What is hypnotism? A proposal. *Australian J. of Clinical Hypnotherapy* **1**(1):2-11.

Hariman, J. (1981). *How to Use the Power of Self-Hypnosis.* Wellingborough: Thorsons.

Hariman, J. (1982). The bearing of the "concentration" theory of hypnosis on the Freudian conception of the unconscious. *Australian J. of Clinical Hypnotherapy* **3**(2):85-90.

Hart, M. M. (1981). Memory for details of an aggressive interpersonal interchange as a function of hypnotic induction. *Dissertation Abstracts International* **41**(11-B):4292.

Hart, R. R. (1980). The influence of a taped hypnotic induction treatment procedure on the recovery of surgery patients. *International J. of Clinical and Experimental Hypnosis* **28**(4):324-332.

Harvey, M. A. (1979). An experimental analogue of hypnotic hypermnesia. *Dissertation Abstracts International* **39**(9-B):4616.

Harvey, M. A., and Sipprelle, C. N. (1978). Color blindness, perceptual interference, and hypnosis. *American J. of Clinical Hypnosis* **20**(3):189-193.

Havens, R. A. (1977). Using modeling and information to modify hypnotizability. *International J. of Clinical and Experimental Hypnosis* **25**(3):167-174.

Haward, L. (1984). Forensic hypnosis: A continuing debate. *Australian J. of Clinical Hypnotherapy and Hypnosis* **5**(2):82-86.

Hebert, S. W. (1984). A simple hypnotic approach to treat test anxiety in medical students and residents. *J. of Medical Education* **59**(10):841-842.

Hedberg, A. G. (1974). The effect of certain examiner and subject characteristics on responsiveness to suggestion. *International J. of Clinical and Experimental Hypnosis* **22**(4):354-364.

Heide, F. J.; Wadlington, W. L.; and Lundy, R. M. (1980). Hypnotic responsivity as a predictor of outcome in meditation. *International J. of Clinical and Experimental Hypnosis* **28**(4):358-366.

Helwig, C. V. (1978). A comparison of the effectiveness of hypnotic-motivational, task-motivational, and relaxation instructions in eliciting the recall of anxiety-inducing material. *Dissertation Abstracts International* **38**(10-A):6013.

Herod, J. W. (1984). Dream your impossible dream: A taped suggestion. *Medical Hypnoanalysis* **5**(4):157-158.

Heron, W. T. (1952). Hypnosis as a factor in the production and detection of crime. *British J. of Medical Hypnotism* **3**(3):15-29.

Herzog, A. (1984). On multiple personality: Comments on diagnosis, etiology, and treatment. *International J. of Clinical and Experimental Hypnosis* **32**(2):210-221.

Hibbard, W. S., and Worring, R. W. (1981). *Forensic Hypnosis: The Practical Application of Hypnosis in Criminal Investigation.* Springfield, IL: Charles C. Thomas.

Hibler, N. S. (1979). The use of hypnosis in United States Air Force investigations. Paper presented at American Psychological Association 87th Annual Convention, New York City, September.

Hibler, N. S. (1984a). Forensic hypnosis: To hypnotize, or not to hypnotize, that is the question! *American J. of Clinical Hypnosis* **27**(1):52-57.

Hibler, N. S. (1984b). Investigative aspects of forensic hypnosis. In W. C. Wester II and A. H. Smith (Eds.), *Comprehensive Clinical Hypnosis* (pp. 525-527). Philadelphia: J. B. Lippincott.

Hiland, D. N., and Dzieszkowski, P. A. (1984). Hypnosis in the investigation of aviation accidents. *Aviation, Space, and Environmental Medicine* **55**(12):1136-1142.

Hilgard, E. R. (1965) *Hypnotic Susceptibility.* New York: Harcourt, Brace and World.

Hilgard, E. R. (1968). *The Experience of Hypnosis.* New York: Harcourt, Brace and World.

Hilgard, E. R. (1973a). The domain of hypnosis: With some comments on alternative paradigms. *American Psychologist* **23**:972-982.

Hilgard, E. R. (1973b). Dissociation revisited. In M. Henle, J. James, and J. Sullivan (Eds.). *Historical Conceptions of Psychology* (pp. 205-219.). New York, Springer.

Hilgard, E. R. (1974a). Toward a neo-dissociation theory: Multiple cognitive controls in human functioning. *Perspectives in Biology and Medicine* **17**:301-316.

Hilgard, E. R. (1974b). Hypnosis is no mirage. *Psychology Today* **8**(6):120-128.

Hilgard, E. R. (1975). Hypnosis. *Annual Review of Psychology* **26**:19-44.

Hilgard, E. R. (1977a). Hypnotic reduction of pain in laboratory and clinic. *Australian J. of Clinical Hypnosis* **5**(1):3-11.

Hilgard, E. R. (1977b). The problem of divided consciousness: A neodissociation interpretation. *Annals of New York Academy of Sciences* **296:** 48-59.

Hilgard, E. R. (1978). A neo-dissociation interpretation of pain reduction in hypnosis. *Psychological Review* **80:**396-411.

Hilgard, E. R. (1978-1979). The Stanford Hypnotic Susceptibility Scales as related to other measures of hypnotic responsiveness. *American J. of Clinical Hypnosis* **21**(2-3):68-83.

Hilgard, E. R. (1979). Consciousness and control: Lessons from hypnosis. *Australian J. of Clinical and Experimental Hypnosis* **7**(2):103-115.

Hilgard, E. R. (1981a). Hypnotic susceptibility scales under attack: An examination of Weitzenhoffer's criticisms. *International J. of Clinical and Experimental Hypnosis* **29**(1):24-41.

Hilgard, E. R. (1981b). Further discussion of the HIP and the Stanford Form C: A reply to a reply by Frischholz, Spiegel, Tryon and Fisher. *American J. of Clinical Hypnosis* **24**(2):106-108.

Hilgard, E. R. (1981c). The eye roll sign and other scores of the Hypnotic Induction Profile (HIP) as related to the Stanford Hypnotic Susceptibility Scale, Form C (SHSS:C): A critical discussion of a study by Frischholz and others. *American J. of Clinical Hypnosis* **24**(2):89-97.

Hilgard, E. R. (1982). Hypnotic susceptibility and implications for measurement. *International J. of Clinical and Experimental Hypnosis* **30**(4):394-403.

Hilgard, E. R. (1984). The hidden observer and multiple personality. *International J. of Clinical and Experimental Hypnosis* **32**(2):248-253.

Hilgard, E. R., and Bentler, P. M. (1963). Predicting hypnotizability from the Maudsley Personality Inventory. *British J. of Psychology* **54:**63-69.

Hilgard, E. R.; Crawford, H. J.; Bowers, P.; and Kihlstrom, J. F. (1979). A tailored SHSS:C, permitting user modification for special purposes. *International J. of Clinical and Experimental Hypnosis* **27:**(2):125-133.

Hilgard, E. R.; Crawford, H. J.; and Wert, A. (1979). The Stanford Hypnotic Arm Levitation Induction and Test (SHALIT): A six minute hypnotic induction and measurement scale. International J. of Clinical and Experimental Hypnosis **27**(2):111-124.

Hilgard, E. R., and Hilgard, J. R. (1975). *Hypnosis in the Relief of Pain.* Los Altos: William Kaufmann.

Hilgard, E. R.; Hilgard, J. R.; MacDonald, H.; Morgan, A. H.; and Johnson, L. S. (1978). Covert pain in hypnotic analgesia: Its reality as tested by the real-simulator design. *J. of Abnormal Psychology* **87**(6):655-663.

Hilgard, E. R., and Hommel, L. S. (1961). Selective amnesia for events within hypnosis in relation to repression. *J. of Personality* **29:**205-216.

Hilgard, E. R., and Loftus, E. F. (1979). Effective interrogation of the eyewitness. *International J. of Clinical and Experimental Hypnosis* **27**(4):342-357.

Hilgard, E. R., and Morgan, A. H. (1975). Heart rate and blood pressure in the study of laboratory pain in man under normal conditions and as influenced by hypnosis. *Acta Neurobiologiae Experimentalis* **35**:741-759.

Hilgard, E. R.; Morgan, A. H.; Lange, A. F.; Lenox, J. R.; MacDonald, H.; Marshall, G. D.; and Sachs, L. B. (1974). Heart rate changes in pain and hypnosis. *Psychophysiology* **11**(6):692-702.

Hilgard, E. R.; Morgan, A. H.; and MacDonald, H. (1975). Pain and dissociation in the cold pressor test: A study of hypnotic analgesia with "hidden reports" through automatic key pressing and automatic talking. *J. of Abnormal Psychology* **84**(3):280-289.

Hilgard, E. R.; Sheehan, P. W.; Monteiro, K. P.; and MacDonald, H. (1981). Factorial structure of the Creative Imagination Scale as a measure of hypnotic responsiveness: An international comparative study. *International J. of Clinical and Experimental Hypnosis* **29**(1):66-76.

Hilgard, E. R., and Tart, C. T. (1966). Responsiveness to suggestions following waking and imagination instructions and following induction of hypnosis. *J. of Abnormal Psychology* **71**(3):196-208.

Hilgard, J. R. (1965). Personality and hypnotizability: Inferences from case studies. In E. R. Hilgard, *Hypnotic Susceptibility* (pp. 343-374). New York: Harcourt, Brace and World.

Hilgard, J. R. (1974). Sequelae to hypnosis. *International J. of Clinical and Experimental Hypnosis* **22**(4):281-298.

Hilgard, J. R. (1979). *Personality and Hypnosis: A Study of Imaginative Involvement* (2d ed.). Chicago: University of Chicago Press.

Hilgard, J. R., and Hilgard, E. R. (1979). Assessing hypnotic responsiveness in a clinical setting: A multi-item clinical scale and its advantages over single-item scales. *International J. of Clinical and Experimental Hypnosis* **27**(2):134-150.

Hilgard, J. R.; Hilgard, E. R.; and Newman, M. F. (1961). Sequelae to hypnotic induction with special reference to earlier chemical anesthesia. *J. of Nervous and Mental Disease* **133**:461-478.

Hilgard, J. R., and LeBaron, S. (1982). Relief of anxiety and pain in children and adolescents with cancer: Quantitative measures and clinical observations. *International J. of Clinical and Experimental Hypnosis* **30**(4):417-442.

Hilton, J. (1967) *Dying*. New York: Penguin Books.

Hodge, J. R. (1959). The management of dissociative reactions with hypnosis. *International J. of Clinical and Experimental Hypnosis* **7**(4):217-221.

Hodge, J. R. (1972). Hypnosis as a deterrent to suicide. *American J. of Clinical Hypnosis* **15**(1):20-24.

Hodge, J. R. (1976). Contractual aspects of hypnosis. *International J. of Clinical and Experimental Hypnosis* **24**(4):391-399.

Hodge, J. R. (1977). Advanced course in hypnotherapy and hypnoanalysis at the Institute for Research in Hypnosis in New York City, April.

Hodge, J. R. and Wagner, E. E. (1964). The validity of hypnotically induced emotional states. *American J. of Clinical Hypnosis* **7**(1):37-41.

Hodge, J. R., and Wagner, E. E. (1969a). The effect of trance depth on Rorschach responses. *American J. of Clinical Hypnosis* **11**(4):234-238.

Hodge, J. R., and Wagner, E. E. (1969b). An exploration of psychodynamics with hypnosis. *American J. of Clinical Hypnosis* **12**(2):91-94.

Hodge, J. R.; Wagner, E. E.; and Schreiner, F. (1966a). Hypnotic validation of two Hand Test scoring categories. *J. of Projective Techniques and Personality Assessment* **30**(4):385-386.

Hodge, J. R.; Wagner, E. E.; and Schreiner, F. (1966b). The validity of hypnotically induced emotional states: Part II. *American J. of Clinical Hypnosis* **9**(2):129-134.

Hoen, P. T. (1978). Effects of hypnotizability and visualizing ability on imagery-mediated learning. *International J. of Clinical and Experimental Hypnosis* **26**(1):45-54.

Hoffman, M. L. (1982-1983). Hypnotic desensitization for the management of anticipatory emesis in chemotherapy. *American J. of Clinical Hypnosis* **25**(2-3):173-176.

Hoffman, W. F. (1985). Hypnosis as a diagnostic tool. *American J. of Psychiatry* **142**(2):272-273.

Hogan, M.; MacDonald, J.; and Olness, K. (1984). Voluntary control of auditory evoked responses by children with and without hypnosis. *American J. of Clinical Hypnosis* **27**(2):91-94.

Hollander, B. (1976). *Methods and Uses of Hypnosis and Self Hypnosis.* Hollywood: Wilshire Book Co.

Holloway, E. L., and Donald, K. M. (1982). Self-hypnosis to self-improvement: A group approach. *J. for Specialists in Group Work* **7**(3):199-208.

Holmes, P. A., and Delprato, D. J. (1978). Classical conditioning of "hypnotic" arm movement. *Psychological Record* **28**(2):305-313.

Holombo, L. K. (1979). Unilateral hypnotic deafness. *Dissertation Abstracts International* **39**(11B):5613.

Holroyd, J. (1980). Hypnosis treatment for smoking: An evaluative Review. *International J. of Clinical and Experimental Hypnosis* **28**(4):341-357.

Holroyd, J. C.; Nuechterlein, K. H.; and Shapiro, D. (1982). Individual differences in hypnotizability and effectiveness of hypnosis or biofeedback. *International J. of Clinical and Experimental Hypnosis* **30**(1):45-65.

Hong, G. K. (1982). The hypnotic enhancement of creativity. *Dissertation Abstracts International* **43**(6-B):1983-1984.

Hong, G. K.; Skiba, A. H.; Yepes, E.; and O'Brien, R. M. (1982). Effects of ethnicity of hypnotist and subject on hypnotic susceptibility. *International J. of Clinical and Experimental Hypnosis* **30**(1):23-31.

Hood, R. W. (1973). Hypnotic susceptibility and reported religious experience. *Psychological Reports* **33**(2):549-550.

Horevitz, R. (1983). Hypnosis for multiple personality disorder: A framework for beginning. *American J. of Clinical Hypnosis* **26**(2):138-145.

Horsley, I. A. (1982). Hypnosis and self-hypnosis in the treatment of psychogenic dysphonia: A case report. *American J. of Clinical Hypnosis* **24**(4):277-283.

Howard, L.; Reardon, J. P.; and Tosi, D. (1982). Modifying migraine headache through rational stage directed hypnotherapy: A cognitive-experiential perspective. *International J. of Clinical and Experimental Hypnosis* **30**(3):257-269.

Howard, M. L. (1979). The effects of changes in the contextual demands on the verbal report of posthypnotic amnesia. *Dissertation Abstracts International* **40**(2-A):755.

Howard, M. L., and Coe, W. C. (1980). The effects of context and subjects' perceived control in breaching posthypnotic amnesia. *J. of Personality* **48**(3):342-359.

Howland, J. S. (1975). The use of hypnosis in the treatment of a case of multiple personality. *J. of Nervous and Mental Disease* **161**(2):138-142.

Huff, D. (1954). *How to Lie with Statistics.* New York: W. W. Norton.

Huff, P. M. (1980). The use of hypnosis in remediating reading in children diagnosed learning disabled. *Dissertation Abstracts International* **40**(8-A):4491.

Hull, C. L. (1968). *Hypnosis and Suggestibility: An Experimental Approach.* 1933 Reprint. New York: Appleton-Century-Crofts.

Hunchak, J. F. (1980). Hypnotic induction by entopic phenomena. *American J. of Clinical Hypnosis* **22**(4):223-224.

Hurley, J. D. (1980). Differential effects of hypnosis, biofeedback training, and trophotropic responses on anxiety, ego strength, and locus of control. *J. of Clinical Psychology* **36**(2):503-507.

Huse, B. (1930). Does the hypnotic trance favor the recall of faint memories? *J. of Experimental Psychology* **13**:519-529.

Hynes, J. V. (1982). Hypnotic treatment of five adult cases of trichotillomania. *Australian J. of Clinical and Experimental Hypnosis* **10**(2):109-115.

Ikemi, Y., and Nakagawa, S. (1962). A psychosomatic study of contageous dermatitis. *Kyushu J. of Medical Science* **13**:335-350.

Illovsky, J. (1963). An experience with group hypnosis in reading disability in primary behavior disorders. *J. Genetic Psychology* **102**:61-67.

Ingram, R. E.; Saccuzzo, D. P.; McNeill, B. W.; and MacDonald, R. (1979). Speed of information processing in high and low susceptible subjects: A preliminary study. *International J. of Clinical and Experimental Hypnosis* **27**(1):42-47.

Jackson, J. A. (1979). Hypnosis in the treatment of a hypertensive patient: A longitudinal study. *Australian J. of Clinical and Experimental Hypnosis* **7**(3):199-206.

Jackson, J. A.; Gass, G. C.; and Camp, E. M. (1979). The relationship between posthypnotic suggestion and endurance in physically trained subjects. *International J. of Clinical and Experimental Hypnosis* **27**(3):278-293.

Jackson, T. L., Jr., and Barkley, R. A. (1976). The effects of hypnotic induction versus high motivation on oral temperature. *International J. of Clinical and Experimental Hypnosis* **24**(1):22-28.

Jackson, T. L., Jr., and Hastings, J. E. (1981). Hypnosis and oral temperature: Not correlated. *American J. of Clinical Hypnosis* **23**(4):278-280.

Jacobson, E. (1938). *Progressive Relaxation*. Chicago: University of Chicago Press.

Jacobson, E. (1962). *You Must Relax*. New York: McGraw-Hill.

Janet, P. (1925). *Psychological Healing. Vol. 1*. New York: Macmillan.

Janis, I. L., and Feshbach, S. (1965). Effects of fear-arousing communications. In H. Proshansky and B. Seidenberg (Eds.), *Basic Studies in Social Psychology* (pp. 157-174). New York: Holt, Rinehart & Winston.

Jansen, R. D. (1981). Attentional alterations of slant-specific interference between line segments in eccentric vision. *Dissertation Abstracts International* **41**(11-B):4293.

Jeffrey, T. B.; Jeffrey, L. K.; Greuling, J. W.; and Gentry, W. R. (1985). Evaluation of a brief group treatment package including hypnotic induction for maintenance of smoking cessation: A brief communication. *International J. of Clinical and Experimental Hypnosis* **33**(2):95-98.

Johnson, G. M., and Hallenbeck, C. E. (1985). A case of obsessional fears treated by brief hypno-imagery intervention. *American J. of Clinical Hypnosis* **27**(4):232-236.

Johnson, L. S. (1979). Self-hypnosis: Behavioral and phenomenological comparisons with heterohypnosis. *International J. of Clinical and Experimental Hypnosis* **27**(3):240-264.

Johnson, L. S. (1981). Current research in self-hypnotic phenomenology: The Chicago paradigm. *International J. of Clinical and Experimental Hypnosis* **29**(3):247-258.

Johnson, L. S.; Dawson, S. L.; Clark, J. L.; and Sikorsky, C. (1983). Self-hypnosis versus hetero-hypnosis: Order effects and sex differences in behavioral and experimental impact. *International J. of Clinical and Experimental Hypnosis* **31**(3):139-154.

Johnson, L. S., and Weight, D. G. (1976). Self-hypnosis versus heterohypnosis: Experiential and behavioral comparisons. *J. of Abnormal Psychology* **85**(5):523-526.

Johnson, L. S., and Wiese, K. F. (1979). Live versus tape-recorded assessments of hypnotic responsiveness in pain-control patients. *International J. of Clinical and Experimental Hypnosis* **27**(2):74-84.

Johnson, R. F. Q. (1976). Hypnotic time distortion and the enhancement of learning: New data pertinent to the Krauss-Katzell-Krauss experiment. *American J. of Clinical Hypnosis* **19**(2):98-102.

Johnson, R. F. Q., and Barber, T. X. (1976). Hypnotic suggestions for blister formation: Subjective and physiological effects. *American J. of Clinical Hypnosis* **18**(3):172-181.

Johnson, R. F., and Barber, T. X. (1978). Hypnosis, suggestions, and warts: An experimental investigation implicating the importance of "believed-in efficacy." *American J. of Clinical Hypnosis* **20**(3):165-174.

Jones, B., and Spanos, N. P. (1982). Suggestions for altered auditory sensitivity, the negative subject effect and hypnotic susceptibility: A signal detection analysis. *J. of Personality and Social Psychology* **43**(3):637-647.

Jones, C. W. (1977). Hypnosis and spinal fusion by Harrington Instrumentation. *American J. of Clinical Hypnosis* **19**(3):155-157.

Jordan-Viola, E. P. (1982). Attitudes toward hypnosis, absorption in naturally-occurring hypnotic-like experiences, and hypnotic susceptibility of chronic alcoholics and heroin addicts. *Dissertation Abstracts International* **43**(1-B):232.

Joseph, L. M. (1978). Maximization of hypnotic suggestibility through subject characteristic and environmental matching. *Dissertation Abstracts International* **38**(7-A):4048.

Juhasz, J. B. (1979). Theories of hypnosis and theories of imagining. *Academic Psychology Bulletin* **1**(2):119-128.

Jupp, J. J.; Collins, J. K.; and McCabe, M. P. (1985). Estimates of hypnotizability: Standard group scale versus subjective impression in clinical populations. *International J. of Clinical and Experimental Hypnosis* **33**(2):140-149.

Kaplan, J. M., and Deabler, H. L. (1975). Hypnotherapy with a severe dissociative hysterical disorder. *American J. of Clinical Hypnosis* **18**(2):83-89.

Karlin, R. A. (1983). Forensic hypnosis—two case reports: A brief communication. *International J. of Clinical and Experimental Hypnosis* **31**(4):227-234.

Karlin, R.; Morgan, D.; and Goldstein, L. (1980). Hypnotic analgesia: A preliminary investigation of quantitated hemispheric electroencephalographic and attentional correlates. *J. of Abnormal Psychology* **89**(4):591-594.

Karlin, R.; Weinapple, M.; Rochford, J.; and Goldstein, L. (1979). Quantitated EEG features of negative affective states: Report of some hypnotic studies. *Research Communications in Psychology, Psychiatry and Behavior* **4**(4):397-413.

Katcher, A.; Segal, H.; and Beck, A. (1984). Comparison of contemplation and hypnosis for the reduction of anxiety and discomfort during dental surgery. *American J. of Clinical Hypnosis* **27**(1):14-21.

Katz, N. W. (1978). Hypnotic inductions as training in cognitive self-control. *Cognitive Therapy and Research* **2**(4):365-369.

Katz, N. W. (1980). Hypnosis and the addictions: A critical review. *Addictive Behaviors* **5**(1):41-47.

Kaye, J. M. (1984). Hypnotherapy and family therapy for the cancer patient: A case study. *American J. of Clinical Hypnosis* **27**(1):38-41.

Kearns, J. S., and Zamansky, H. S. (1984). Synthetic versus analytic imaging ability as correlates of hypnotizability. *International J. of Clinical and Experimental Hypnosis* **32**(1):41-50.

Kellerman, J. (1981). Hypnosis as an adjunct to thought-stopping and covert reinforcement in the treatment of homicidal obsessions in a twelve-year-old boy. *International J. of Clinical and Experimental Hypnosis* **29**(2):128-135.

Kellogg, E. R. (1929). Duration of the effects of posthypnotic suggestion. *J. of Experimental Psychology* **12**:502.

Kelly, S. F. (1980). Hypnotizability and the inadvertent experience of pain: A brief communication. *International J. of Clinical and Experimental Hypnosis* **28**(3):189-191.

Kelly, S. F. (1984). Measured hypnotic response and phobic behavior: A brief communication. *International J. of Clinical and Experimental Hypnosis* **32**(1):1-5.

Kelly, S. F.; Fisher, S.; and Kelly, R. J. (1978). Effects of cannabis intoxication on primary suggestibility. *Psychopharmacology* **56**(2):217-219.

Kennedy, S. (1977). Seminar on hypnosis in clinical practice at N. Y. U. Postgraduate School of Medicine, October.

Khatami, M. (1978). Creativity and altered states of consciousness. *Psychiatric Annals* **8**(3):57-64.

Kiesler, C. A. (1977). The training of psychiatrists and psychologists. *American Psychologist* **32**(2):107-108.

Kihlstrom, J. F. (1977). Models of posthypnotic amnesia. *Annals of New York Academy of Sciences* **296**:284-301.

Kihlstrom, J. F. (1978). Context and cognition in posthypnotic amnesia. *International J. of Clinical and Experimental Hypnosis* **26**(4):246-267.

Kihlstrom, J. F. (1979). Hypnosis and psychopathology: Retrospect and prospect. *J. of Abnormal Psychology* **88**(5):459-473.

Kihlstrom, J. F. (1980). Posthypnotic amnesia for recently learned material: interactions with"episodic" and "semantic" memory. *Cognitive Psychology* **12**(2):227-251.

Kihlstrom, J. F. (1982). Hypnosis and the dissociation of memory, with special reference to posthypnotic amnesia. *Research Communications in Psychology, Psychiatry and Behavior* **7**(2):181-197.

Kihlstrom, J. F. (1983). Instructed forgetting: Hypnotic and nonhypnotic. *J. of Experimental Psychology: General* **112**(1):73-79.

Kihlstrom, J. F. (1985). Hypnosis. *Annual Review of Psychology* **36**:385-418.

Kihlstrom, J. F.; Diaz, W. A.; McClellan, G. E.; Ruskin, P. M.; Pistole, D. D.; and Shor, R. E. (1980). Personality correlates of hypnotic susceptibility: Needs for achievement and autonomy, self-monitoring, and masculinity-femininity. *American J. of Clinical Hypnosis* **22**(4):225-230.

Kihlstrom, J. F.; Easton, R. D.; and Shor, R. E. (1983). Spontaneous recovery of memory during posthypnotic amnesia. *International J. of Clinical and Experimental Hypnosis* **31**(4):309-323.

Kihlstrom, J. F., and Edmonston, W. E., Jr. (1971). Alterations in consciousness in neutral hypnosis: Distortions in semantic space. *American J. of Clinical Hypnosis* **13**(4):243-248.

Kihlstrom, J. F., and Evans, F. J. (1976). Recovery of memory after posthypnotic amnesia. *J. of Abnormal Psychology* **85**(6):564-569.

Kihlstrom, J. F., and Evans, F. J. (1977). Residual effect of suggestions for posthypnotic amnesia: A re-examination. *J. of Abnormal Psychology* **86**(4):327-333.

Kihlstrom, J. F., and Evans, F. J. (1978). Generic recall during posthypnotic amnesia. *Bulletin of the Psychonomic Society* **12**(1):57-60.

Kihlstrom, J. F.; Evans, F. J.; Orne, E. C.; and Orne, M. T. (1980). Attempting to breach posthypnotic amnesia. *J. of Abnormal Psychology* **89**(5):603-616.

Kihlstrom, J. F., and Register, P. A. (1984). Optimal scoring of amnesia on the Harvard Group Scale of Hypnotic Susceptibility, Form A. *International J. of Clinical and Experimental Hypnosis* **32**(1):51-57.

Kihlstrom, J. F., and Shor, R. E. (1978). Recall and recognition during posthypnotic amnesia. *International J. of Clinical and Experimental Hypnosis* **26**(4):330-349.

Kihlstrom, J. F., and Twersky, M. (1978). Relationship of posthypnotic amnesia to waking memory performance. *International J. of Clinical and Experimental Hypnosis* **26**(4):292-306.

Kihlstrom, J. F., and Wilson, L. (1984). Temporal organization of recall during posthypnotic amnesia. *J. of Abnormal Psychology* **93**(2):200-208.

Kim, S. C. (1983). Ericksonian hypnotic framework for Asian-Americans. *American J. of Clinical Hypnosis* **25**(4):235-241.

King, D. L., and Lummis, G. (1974). Effects of visual sensory-restriction and recent experience with the imagined stimulus on a suggestibility measure. *International J. of Clinical and Experimental Hypnosis* **22**(3):239-248.

Kingsbury, G. C. (1957). *The Practice of Hypnotic Suggestion.* Hollywood: Wilshire Book Co.

Kirsch, I.; Council, J. R.; and Vickery, A. R. (1984). The role of expectancy in eliciting hypnotic responses as a function of type of induction. *J. of Consulting and Clinical Psychology* **52**(4):708-709.

Kir-Stimon, W. (1978). Hypnosis as a tool for termination of therapy. *International J. of Clinical and Experimental Hypnosis* **26**(3):134-142.

Klatzky, R. L., and Erdelyi, M. H. (1985). The response criterion problem in tests of hypnosis and memory. *International J. of Clinical and Experimental Hypnosis* **33**(3):246-257.

Kleinhauz, M., and Beran, B. (1981). Misuses of hypnosis: A medical emergency and its treatment. *International J. of Clinical and Experimental Hypnosis* **29**(2):148-161.

Kleinhauz, M., and Beran, B. (1984). Misuse of hypnosis: A factor in psychopathology. *American J. of Clinical Hypnosis* **26**(3):283-290.

Kleinhauz, M.; Dreyfuss, D. A.; Beran, B.; Goldberg, T.; and Azikri, D. (1979). Some after-effects of stage hypnosis: A case study of psychopathological manifestations. *International J. of Clinical and Experimental Hypnosis* **27**(3):219-226.

Kleinhauz, M.; Eli, I.; and Rubinstein, Z. (1985). Treatment of dental and dental-related behavioral dysfunctions in a consultative outpatient clinic: A preliminary report. *American J. of Clinical Hypnosis* **28**(1):4-9.

Kleinmuntz, B. (1974). *Essentials of Abnormal Psychology.* New York: Harper & Row.

Kline, M. V. (1950). Hypnotic age regression and intelligence. *J. Genetic Psychology* **77**:129.

Kline, M. V. (1957). Hypnosis in dental medicine: Educational and clinical considerations. *J. of the American Dental Association* **54**:797-807.

Kline, M. V. (1958a). The dynamics of hypnotically induced antisocial behavior. *J. Psychology* **45**:239-245.

Kline, M. V. (1958b). *Freud and Hypnosis.* New York: Julian Press.

Kline, M. V. (1958c). Clinical and experimental hypnosis in contemporary behavioral sciences. In M. K. Bowers (Ed.), *Introductory Lecture in Medical Hypnosis* (pp. 1-9). New York: Institute for Research in Hypnosis.

Kline, M. V. (1966). Hypnotic amnesia in psychotherapy. *International J. of Clinical and Experimental Hypnosis* **14**(2):112-120.

Kline, M. V. (1972a). Freud and hypnosis: A reevaluation. *International J. of Clinical and Experimental Hypnosis* **20**(4):252-263.

Kline, M. V. (1972b). The production of antisocial behavior through hypnosis: New clinical data. *International J. of Clinical and Experimental Hypnosis* **20**(2):80-94.

Kline, M. V. (1975). Sensory hypnotherapy and regression during psychological stress. *Clinical Social Work J.* **3**(4):298-308.

Kline, M. V. (1976). Dangerous aspects of the practice of hypnosis and the need for legislative regulation. *Clinical Psychologist* **29**(2):3-6.

Kline, M. V. (1977). Advanced course in hypnotherapy and hypnoanalysis at the Institute for Research in Hypnosis, New York City, April.

Kline, M. V. (1978). Seminar on hypnotic treatment of pain at Adelphi University, December.

Kline, M. V. (1979a). Hypnosis with specific relation to biofeedback and behavior therapy: Theoretical and clinical considerations. *Psychotherapy and Psychosomatics* **31**(1-4):294-300.

Kline, M. V. (1979b). Defending the mentally ill: The insanity defense and the role of forensic hypnosis. *International J. of Clinical and Experimental Hypnosis* **27**(4):375-401.

Kline, M. V. (1984). Multiple personality: Facts and artifacts in relation to hypnotherapy. *International J. of Clinical and Experimental Hypnosis* **32**(2):198-209.

Kluft, R. P. (1982). Varieties of hypnotic interventions in the treatment of multiple personality. *American J. of Clinical Hypnosis* **24**(4):230-240.

Kluft, R. P. (1983). Hypnotherapeutic crisis intervention in multiple personality. *American J. of Clinical Hypnosis* **26**(2):73-83.

Kluft, R. P. (1985a). Using hypnotic inquiry protocols to monitor treatment progress and stability in multiple personality disorder. *American J. of Clinical Hypnosis* **28**(2):63-75.

Kluft, R. P. (1985b). Hypnotherapy of childhood multiple personality disorder. *American J. of Clinical Hypnosis* **27**(4):201-210.

Kluft, R. P. (1986). Hypnosis in the treatment of phobias. *Psychiatric Annals* **16**(2):96-101.

Knox, V. J.; Crutchfield, L.; and Hilgard, E. R. (1975). The nature of task interference in hypnotic dissociation: An investigation of hypnotic behavior. *International J. of Clinical and Experimental Hypnosis* **23**(4):305-323.

Knox, V. J.; Gekoski, W. L.; Shum, K.; and McLaughlin, D. M. (1981). Analgesia for experimentally induced pain: Multiple sessions of acupuncture compared to hypnosis in high- and low-susceptible subjects. *J. of Abnormal Psychology* **90**(1):28-34.

Knox, V. J.; Morgan, A. H.; and Hilgard, E. R. (1974). Pain and suffering in ischemia: The paradox of hypnotically suggested anesthesia as contradicted by reports from the "hidden observer." *Archives of General Psychiatry* **30**:840-847.

Knutsen, E. S. (1977). A study and further analysis of personality changes after the Silva Mind Control Course. *Dissertation Abstracts International* **37**(9-B):4687-4688.

Koadlow, E. (1979). Contraindications and indications to the use of hypnosis in psychosexual dysfunction. *Australian J. of Clinical and Experimental Hypnosis* **7**(3):253-259.

Koe, G. G. (1982). An experimental investigation of the effects of hypnotically induced suggestions on self concept and reading performance. *Dissertation Abstracts International* **43**(2-A):403.

Kohen, D. P.; Olness, K. N.; Colwell, S. O.; and Heimel, A. (1984). The use of relaxation-mental imagery (self-hypnosis) in the management of 505 pediatric behavioral encounters. *Developmental and Behavioral Pediatrics* **5**(1):21-25.

Kondreck, J. G. (1963). Hypnosis in photography. *Hypnosis Quarterly* **8**(3):22-25.

Kornfeld, A. D. (1984). Hypnosis and behavior therapy: Historical relationships. *International J. of Psychosomatics* **31**(2):22-26.

Kornfeld, A. D. (1985a). A spontaneous catatonic-like reaction associated with hypnotic regression: A brief case report. *American J. of Clinical Hypnosis* **27**(3):180-182.

Kornfeld, A. D. (1985b). Hypnosis and behavior therapy II: Contemporary developments. *International J. of Psychosomatics* **34**(4):13-17.

Koster, S. (1950). Remarkable patients to whom hypnosis brought relief. *Acta Psychiat.* **25**:393-400.

Kraft, W. A., and Rodolfa, E. R. (1982). The use of hypnosis among psychologists. *American J. of Clinical Hypnosis* **24**(4):249-257.

Kraft, W. A.; Rodolfa, E. R.; and Reilley, R. R. (1985). Current trends in hypnosis and hypnotherapy. *American J. of Clinical Hypnosis* **28** (1):20-26.

Krauss, H. H.; Katzell, R.; and Krauss, B. J. (1974). Effect of hypnotic time distortion upon free recall learning. *J. of Abnormal Psychology* **83**:140-144.

Krebs, S. L. (1957). *The Fundamental Principles of Hypnosis.* 1906. Reprint. New York: Julian Press.

Krenz, E. W. (1984). Improving competitive performance with hypnotic suggestions and modified autogenic training: Case reports. *American J. of Clinical Hypnosis* **27**(1):58-63.

Krippner, S. (1963). Hypnosis and reading improvement among university students. *American J. of Clinical Hypnosis* **5**:187-193.

Krippner, S. (1966). The use of hypnosis with elementary and secondary school children in a summer reading clinic. *American J. of Clinical Hypnosis* **8**:261-266.

Krippner, S. (1977). Research in creativity and psychedelic drugs. *International J. of Clinical and Experimental Hypnosis* **25**(4):274-308.

Kroger, W. S. (1960). Techniques of hypnosis. *J. of American Medical Association* **172**(7):131/675-136/680.

Kroger, W. S. (1977a). *Clinical and Experimental Hypnosis in Medicine, Dentistry and Psychology* (2d ed.). Los Angeles: J. B. Lippincott.

Kroger, W. S. (1977b). Advanced course in hypnotherapy and hypnoanalysis at the Institute for Research in Hypnosis in New York City, April.

Kroger, W. S. (1977c). *Childbirth with Hypnosis.* Hollywood: Wilshire Book Co.

Kroger, W. S., and DeLee, S. T. (1957). Use of hypnoanesthesia for caesarean section and hysterectomy. *J. of American Medical Association* **163**(6):442-444.

Kroger, W. S., and Douce, R. (1979). Hypnosis in criminal investigation. *International J. of Clinical and Experimental Hypnosis* **27**(4):358-374.

Kroger, W. S., and Douce, R. G. (1980). Forensic uses of hypnosis. *American J. of Clinical Hypnosis* **23**(2):86-93.

Kroger, W. S., and Fezler, W. D. (1976). *Hypnosis and Behavior Modification: Imagery conditioning.* Philadelphia: J. B. Lippincott Co.

Kubiak, R. V. (1983). Hypnosis: Anesthetic agent in major surgery: A case report. *Medical Hypnoanalysis* **4**(1):46-48.

Kubie, L. S. (1972). Illusion and reality in the study of sleep, hypnosis, psychosis and arousal. *International J. of Clinical and Experimental Hypnosis* **20**(4):205-223.

Kubler, R. E. (1969). *On Death and Dying.* New York: Macmillan.

Kuhn, L., and Russo, S. (1977). *Modern Hypnosis.* Hollywood: Wilshire Book Co.

Kupper, H. I. (1945). Psychic concomitants in wartime injuries. *Psychosomatic Medicine* **7**:15-21.

Kurokawa, N.; Suematsu, H.; Tamai, H.; Esaki, M.; Aoki, H.; and Ikemi, Y. (1977). Effect of emotional stress on human growth hormone secretion. *J. of Psychosomatic Research* **21**(3):231-235.

LaBaw, W.; Holton, C.; Tewell, K.; and Eccles, D. (1975). The use of self-hypnosis by children with cancer. *American J. of Clinical Hypnosis* **17**(4):233-238.

Laguaite, J. K. (1976). The use of hypnosis with children with deviant voices. *International J. of Clinical and Experimental Hypnosis* **24**(2):98-104.

Lake, D. (1984). The use of an initial handout for patients. *Australian J. of Clinical and Experimental Hypnosis* **12**(1):62-64.

Lamb, C. S. (1982). Negative hypnotic imagery/fantasy: Application to two cases of "unfinished business." *American J. of Clinical Hypnosis* **24**(4):266-271.

Lamb, C. S. (1985). Hypnotically-induced deconditioning: Reconstruction of memories in the treatment of phobias. *American J. of Clinical Hypnosis* **28**(2):56-62.

Lane, B. (1948). A validation test of the Rorschach movement interpretation. *American J. of Orthopsychiatry* **18**:292-296.

Lang, P. J.; Lazovik, A. D.; and Reynolds, D. J. (1965). Desensitization, suggestibility and pseudo-therapy. *J. of Abnormal Psychology* **70**:395-402.

Laurence, J. R., and Perry, C. (1981). The "hidden observer" phenomenon in hypnosis: Some additional findings. *J. of Abnormal Psychology* **90**(4):334-344.

Laurence, J. R., and Perry, C. (1982). Montreal norms for the Harvard Group Scale of Hypnotic Susceptibility, Form A. *International J. of Clinical and Experimental Hypnosis* **30**(2):167-176.

Laurence, J. R., and Perry, C. (1983a). Forensic hypnosis in the late nineteenth century. *International J. of Clinical and Experimental Hypnosis* **31**(4):266-283.

Laurence, J. R., and Perry, C. (1983b). Hypnotically created memory among highly hypnotizable subjects. *Science* **222**(4623):523-524.

Laurence, J. R.; Perry, C.; and Kihlstrom, J. (1983). "Hidden observer" phenomena in hypnosis: An experimental creation? *J. of Personality and Social Psychology* **44**(1):163-169.

Lavoie, G.; Sabourin, M.; and Langlois, J. (1973). Hypnotic susceptibility, amnesia and IQ in chronic schizophrenia. *International J. of Clinical and Experimental Hypnosis* **21**(3):157-168.

Lazar, B. S. (1977). Hypnotic imagery as a tool in working with a cerebral palsied child. *International J. of Clinical and Experimental Hypnosis* **25**(2):78-87.

Lazar, B. S., and Dempster, C. R. (1981). Failures in hypnosis and hypnotherapy: A review. *American J. of Clinical Hypnosis* **24**(1):48-54.

Lazar, B. S., and Dempster, C. R. (1984). Operator variables in successful hypnotherapy. *International J. of Clinical and Experimental Hypnosis* **32**(1):28-40.

Lazar, B. S., and Jedliczka, Z. T. (1979). Utilization of manipulative behavior in a retarded asthmatic child. *American J. of Clinical Hypnosis* **21**(4):287-292.

Lazarus, A. A. (1973). "Hypnosis" as a facilitator in behavior therapy. *International J. of Clinical and Experimental Hypnosis* **21**(1):25-31.

LeBaron, S., and Zeltzer, L. K. (1984). Research on hypnosis in hemophilia—Preliminary success and problems: A brief communication. *International J. of Clinical and Experimental Hypnosis* **32**(3):290-295.

LeCron, L. M. (1952). The loss during hypnotic age regression of an established conditioned reflex. *Psychiatric Quarterly* **26**:657.

LeCron, L. M. (1964). *Self Hypnotism: The Technique and Its Use in Daily Living.* New York: Signet Books.

LeCron, L. M. (1969). Breast development through hypnotic suggestion. *J. of American Society of Psychosomatic Dentistry and Medicine* **16**(2):58-61.

LeCron, L. M. (1971). *The Complete Guide to Hypnosis.* New York: Harper & Row.

LeCron, L. M. (1974). *How to Stop Smoking through Self Hypnosis.* Hollywood: Wilshire Book Co.

LeCron, L. M., and Bordeaux, J. (1949). *Hypnotism Today.* New York: Grune & Stratton.

Lehman, R. E. (1978). Brief hypnotherapy of neurodermatitis: A case with four-year followup. *American J. of Clinical Hypnosis* **21**(1):48-51.

Leibowitz, H. W.; Lundy, R. M.; and Guez, J. R. (1980). The effect of testing distance on suggestion-induced visual field narrowing. *International J. of Clinical and Experimental Hypnosis* **28**(4):409-420.

Leibowitz, H. W.; Post, R. B.; Rodemer, C. S.; Wadlington, W. L.; and Lundy, R. M. (1980). Roll vection analysis of suggestion-induced visual field narrowing. *Perception and Psychophysics* **28**(2):173-176.

Lert, A. S. (1979). The effects of hypnosis, hypnotizability, and instructions on the free-recall learning of nonsense syllables: An extension of the London-Fuhrer design. *Dissertation Abstracts International* **40**(4-B):1900.

Leva, R. A. (1974). Performance of low susceptible S's on Stanford Profile Scales after sensory deprivation. *Psychological Reports* **34**(3):835-838.

Leva, R. A. (1975). Correlation between Rotter's I-E Scale and the Harvard Group Scale of Hypnotic Susceptibility under three sets of instructions. *Perceptual and Motor Skills* **41**(2):614.

Leva, R. A., and Rywick, T. (1979). HIP eye-roll: High scoring by untrained raters. *American J. of Clinical Hypnosis* **22**(2):91-94.

Levine, E. S. (1980). Indirect suggestions through personalized fairy tales for treatment of childhood insomnia. *American J. of Clinical Hypnosis* **23**(1):57-63.

Levine, J. L.; Kurtz, R. M.; and Lauter, J. L. (1984). Hypnosis and its effects on left and right hemisphere activity. *Biological Psychiatry* **19**(10):1461-1475.

Levine, K. N.; Grassi, J. R.; and Gerson, M. J. (1943). Hypnotically induced mood changes in the verbal and graphic Rorschach. A case study. *Rorschach Research Exchange* **7**:130-144.

Levitan, A. A. (1985). Hypnotic death rehearsal. *American J. of Clinical Hypnosis* **27**(4):211-215.

Levitt, E. E. (1977). Research strategies in evaluating the coercive power of hypnosis. *Annals of New York Academy of Sciences* **296**:86-89.

Levitt, E. E.; Aronoff, G.; and Morgan, C. D. (1974). A note on possible limitations on the use of the Harvard Group Scale of Hypnotic Susceptibility, Form A. *International J. of Clinical and Experimental Hypnosis* **22**(3):234-238.

Levitt, E. E.; Aronoff, G.; Morgan, C. D.; Overley, T. M.; and Parrish, M.

J. (1975). Testing the coercive power of hypnosis: Objectionable acts. *International J. of Clinical and Experimental Hypnosis* **23**(1):59-67.

Levitt, E. E., and Baker, E. L. (1983). The hypnotic relationship—another look at coercion, compliance and resistance: A brief communication. *International J. of Clinical and Experimental Hypnosis* **31**(3):125-131.

Levitt, E. E., and Hershman, S. (1961). The clinical practice of hypnosis in the U.S.: A survey. Paper read at 14th International Congress of Applied Psychology, Copenhagen, August.

Levitt, E. E., and Hershman, S. (1963). Clinical practice of hypnosis in the United States: A preliminary survey. *International J. of Clinical and Experimental Hypnosis* **11**:55-65.

Levitt, E. E.; Overley, T. M.; and Rubinstein, D. (1975). The objectionable act as a mechanism for testing the coercive power of the hypnotic state. *American J. of Clinical Hypnosis* **17**(4):263-266.

Lewis, B. J. (1979). Treatment of a schizoid personality using hypno-operant therapy. *American J. of Clinical Hypnosis* **22**(1):42-46.

Li, C. L.; Ahlberg, D.; Lansdell, H.; Gravitz, M. A.; Chen, T. C.; Ting, C. Y.; Bak, A. F.; and Blessing, D. (1975). Acupuncture and hypnosis: Effects on induced pain. *Experimental Neurology* **49**:272-280.

Lieberman, J.; Lavoie, G.; and Brisson, A. (1978). Suggested amnesia and order of recall as a function of hypnotic susceptibility and learning conditions in chronic schizophrenic patients. *International J. of Clinical and Experimental Hypnosis* **26**(4):268-280.

Lieberman, L. R. (1977). Hypnosis research and the limitations of the experimental method. *Annals of New York Academy of Sciences* **296**:60-68.

Lindner, H. (1973). Psychogenic seizure states: A psychodynamic study. *International J. of Clinical and Experimental Hypnosis* **21**(4):261-271.

Lindner, H. (1977). Hypnotherapy: Patient-therapist relationship. *Annals of New York Academy of Sciences* **296**: 238-249.

Lindner, H. (1984). Therapist and patient reactions to life-threatening crises in the therapist's life. *International J. of Clinical and Experimental Hypnosis* **32**(1):12-27..

Lindner, H., and Frank, R. A. (1973). Hypnotherapy: Patient-therapist reactions. *Psychotherapy: Theory, Research and Practice* **10**(1):66-70.

Linton, P. H.; Travis, R. P.; Kuechenmeister, C. A.; and White, H. (1977). Correlation between heart rate covariation, personality and hypnotic state. *American J. of Clinical Hypnosis* **19**(3):148-151.

Loftus, E. F., and Loftus, G. R. (1980). On the permanence of stored information in the human brain. *American Psychologist* **35**(5):409-420.

London, P. (1961). Subject characteristics in hypnosis research: Part I. A survey of experience, interest and opinion. *International J. of Clinical and Experimental Hypnosis* **9**:151-161.

London, P. (1962). *The Children's Hypnotic Susceptibility Scale*. Palo Alto: Consulting Psychologists Press.

London, P. (1965). Developmental experiments in hypnosis. *J. of Projective Techniques and Personality Assessment* **29**:189-199.

London, P.; Convant, M.; and Davison, G. C. (1966). More hypnosis in the unhypnotizable: Effects of hypnosis and exhortation on rote learning. *J. of Personality* **34**:71-79.

London, R. T., and Forman, L. M. (1979). Seminar on hypnosis in clinical practice at N. Y. U. Post-graduate School of Medicine, October.

London, R. T., and Forman, L. M. (Eds.). (1982). *Hypnosis in Clinical Practice*. New York: New York University Post Graduate Medical School, 1977.

London, R. W. (1982). Hypnosis: A review and re-evaluation. *Australian J. of Clinical Hypnotherapy and Hypnosis* **3**(1):5-19.

Lovett, D. J. W. (1953a). Studies on the physiology of awareness. *American J. of Clinical Hypnosis* **110**:205.

Lovett, D. J. W. (1953b). Studies on the physiology of awareness: Axiometric analysis of emotion and the differential planes of consciousness seen in hypnosis. *J. of Clinical and Experimental Psychopathology* **14**:113-126.

Ludwig, A. M. (1983). The psychobiological functions of dissociation. *American J. of Clinical Hypnosis* **26**(2):93-99.

Ludwig, A. M., and Lyle, W. H., Jr. (1964). Tension induction and the hyperalert trance. *J. of Abnormal and Social Psychology* **69**(1):70-76.

Lundy, R. M.; Geselowitz, L.; and Shertzer, C. L. (1985). Role-played and hypnotically induced simulation of psychopathology on the MMPI: A partial replication. *International J. of Clinical and Experimental Hypnosis* **33**(4):302-309.

Lupica, V. P. (1976). Hypnosis therapy for ciliary spasm. *J. of American Optometric Association* **47**(1):102.

Lynn, S. J.; Nash, M. R.; Rhue, J. W.; Frauman, D.; and Stanley, S. (1983). Hypnosis and the experience of nonvolotion. *International J. of Clinical and Experimental Hypnosis* **31**(4):293-308.

Lynn, S. J. Nash, M. R.; Rhue, J. W.; Frauman, D. C.; and Sweeney, C. A. (1984). Nonvolition, expectancies, and hypnotic rapport. *J. of Abnormal Psychology* **93**(3):295-303.

McCabe, M. P.; Collins, J. K.; and Burns, A. M. (1978). Hypnosis as an altered state of consciousness. I: A review of traditional theories. *Australian J. of Clinical and Experimental Hypnosis* **6**(1):39-54.

McCabe, M. P.; Collins, J. K.; and Burns, A. M. (1979). Hypnosis as an altered state of consciousness: II. A review of contemporary theories and empirical evidence. *Australian J. of Clinical and Experimental Hypnosis* **7**(1):7-25.

McConkey, K. M. (1980). Creatively imagined "amnesia." *American J. of Clinical Hypnosis* **22**(4):197-205.

McConkey, K. M. (1983a). The impact of conflicting communications on response to hypnotic suggestion. *J. of Abnormal Psychology* **92**(3):351-358.

McConkey, K. M. (1983b). Challenging hypnotic effects: The impact of conflicting influences on response to hypnotic suggestion. *British J. of Experimental and Clinical Hypnosis* **1**(1):3-10.

McConkey, K. M. (1983c). Social and cognitive preparedness: Response to Wagstaff. *British J. of Experimental and Clinical Hypnosis* **1**(1):17-19.

McConkey, K. M. (1983d). Behavior, experience, and effort in hypnosis. *Australian J. of Clinical and Experimental Hypnosis* **11**(2):73-81.

McConkey, K. M. (1983e). Conflict, consistency, and conviction in hypnosis: Response to Evans. *British J. of Experimental and Clinical Hypnosis* **1**(1):25-26.

McConkey, K. M. (1984). The impact of an indirect suggestion. *International J. of Clinical and Experimental Hypnosis* **32**(3):307-314.

McConkey, K. M., and Nogrady, H. (1984). Hypnosis, hypnotizability and story recall. *Australian J. of Clinical and Experimental Hypnosis* **12**(2):93-98.

McConkey, K. M., and Perry, C. (1985). Benjamin Franklin and Mesmerism. *International J. of Clinical and Experimental Hypnosis* **33**(2):122-130.

McConkey, K., and Sheehan, P. W. (1976). Contrasting interpersonal orientations in hypnosis: Collaborative versus contractual modes of response. *J. of Abnormal Psychology* **85**(4):390-397.

McConkey, K. M. and Sheehan, P. W. (1980). Inconsistency in hypnotic age regression and cue structure as supplied by the hypnotist. *International J. of Clinical and Experimental Hypnosis* **28**(4):394-408.

McConkey, K. M., and Sheehan, P. W. (1981). The impact of videotape playback of hypnotic events on posthypnotic amnesia. *J. of Abnormal Psychology* **90**(1):46-54.

McConkey, K. M., and Sheehan, P. W. (1982a). Effort and experience on the Creative Imagination Scale. *International J. of Clinical and Experimental Hypnosis* **30**(3):280-288.

McConkey, K. M., and Sheehan, P. W. (1982b). Rating analysis of the hypnotist's interaction with real and simulating subjects. *Australian J. of Clinical and Experimental Hypnosis* **10**(2):79-88.

McConkey, K. M.; Sheehan, P. W.; and Cross, D. G. (1980). Post-hypnotic amnesia: Seeing is not remembering. *British J. of Social and Clinical Psychology* **19**(1):99-107.

McConkey, K. M.; Sheehan, P. W.; and Law, H. G. (1980). Structural analysis of the Harvard Group Scale of Hypnotic Susceptibility, Form A. *International J. of Clinical and Experimental Hypnosis* **28**(2):164-175.

McConkey, K. M.; Sheehan, P. W.; and White, K. D. (1979). Comparison of the Creative Imagination Scale and the Harvard Group Scale of Hypnotic Susceptibility, Form A. *International J. of Clinical and Experimental Hypnosis* **27**(3):265-277.

McCord, H. (1956). Hypnosis as an aid to the teaching of a severely mentally retarded teenage boy. *J. of Clinical and Experimental Hypnosis* **4**:21-25.

McCord, H., and Sherrill, C. J. (1961). A note on increased ability to do calculus posthypnotically. *American J. of Clinical Hypnosis* **4**:124.

McCranie, E. J., and Crasilneck, H. B. (1955). The conditioned reflex in hypnotic age regression. *J. of Clinical and Experimental Psychopathology* **16**:120.

McCranie, E. J.; Crasilneck, H. B.; and Teter, H. R. (1955). The electroencephalogram in hypnotic age regression. *Psychiatric Quarterly* **29**:85-88.

McCue, P. A. (1982). Hypnotic time distortion: Experimental work, clinical applications and theoretical considerations. *Bulletin of the British Society of Experimental and Clinical Hypnosis* **1982**(5):14-20.

McDermott, D., and Sheehan, P. W. (1976). Interpersonal orientations in hypnosis: Toward egalitarian interaction in the hypnotic test situation. *American J. of Clinical Hypnosis* **19**(2):108-115.

McDonald, R. D., and Smith, J. R. (1975). Trance logic in tranceable and simulating subjects. *International J. of Clinical and Experimental Hypnosis* **23**(1):80-89.

McDowell, M. (1949). Juvenile warts removed with the use of hypnotic suggestion. *Bulletin of the Menninger Clinic* **13**:124-126.

McDowell, M. (1953). Hypnosis in dermatology. In J. M. Schneck, *Hypnosis in Modern Medicine.* Springfield, IL: Charles C. Thomas.

McGill, O. (1947). *Encyclopedia of Stage Hypnotism.* Colon, MI: Abbotts Magic Novelty Co.

McGraw, M. B. (1941). Development of the plantar response in young infants. *American J. of Diseases of Children* **61**:1215-1221.

McGuinness, T. P. (1984). Hypnosis in the treatment of phobias: A review of the literature. *American J. of Clinical Hypnosis* **26**(4):261-272.

McIntosh, I. B., and Hawney, M. (1983). Patient attitudes to hypnotherapy in a general medical practice: A brief communication. *International J. of Clinical and Experimental Hypnosis* **31**(4):219-223.

McKimmie, J. (1984). Mental spring cleaning: Guided imagery in the primary school. *Australian J. of Clinical and Experimental Hypnosis* **12**(1):55-58.

MacCraken, P. J.; Gogel, W. C.; and Blum, G. S. (1980). Effects of posthypnotic suggestion on perceived egocentric distance. *Perception* **9**(5):561-568.

MacHovec, F. J. (1976). The evil eye: Superstition or phenomenon? *American J. of Clinical Hypnosis* **19**(2):74-79.

MacHovec, F. J. (1979). The cult of Asklipios. *American J. of Clinical Hypnosis* **22**(2):85-90.

MacHovec, F. J. (1981a). Hypnosis to facilitate recall in psychogenic amnesia and fugue states: Treatment variables. *American J. of Clinical Hypnosis* **24**(1):7-13.

MacHovec, F. J. (1981b). Shakespeare on hypnosis: The Tempest. *American J. of Clinical Hypnosis* **24**(2):73-78.

MacHovec, F. J. (1985). Treatment variables and the use of hypnosis in the brief therapy of post-traumatic stress disorders. *International J. of Clinical and Experimental Hypnosis* **33** (1):6-14.

MacHovec, F. J., and Man, S. C. (1978). Acupuncture and hypnosis compared: Fifty-eight cases. *American J. of Clinical Hypnosis* **21**(1):45-47.

MacLeod-Morgan, C. (1982). EEG lateralization in hypnosis: A preliminary report. *Australian J. of Clinical and Experimental Hypnosis* **10**(2):99-102.

MacMillan, M. B. (1977). The cathartic method and the expectancies of Breuer and Anna O. *International J. of Clinical and Experimental Hypnosis* **25**(2):106-118.

Maher-Loughnan, G. P. (1975). Intensive hypno-autohypnosis in resistant psychosomatic disorders. *J. of Psychosomatic Research* **19**:361-365.

Malott, J. M. (1984). Active-alert hypnosis: Replication and extension of previous research. *J. of Abnormal Psychology* **93**(2):246-249.

Manganiello, A. J. (1984). A comparative study of hypnotherapy and psychotherapy in the treatment of Methadone addicts. *American J. of Clinical Hypnosis* **26**(4):273-279.

Marcus, F. L.; Hill, A.; and Keegan, M. (1945). Identification of posthypnotic signals and responses. *J. of Experimental Psychology* **35:**163.

Marcuse, F. L. (1953). Antisocial behavior and hypnosis. *J. of Clinical and Experimental Hypnosis* **1:**18-20.

Marcuse, F. L. (1976). *Hypnosis—Fact and Fiction.* New York: Penguin Books.

Margolis, C. G. (1982-1983). Hypnotic imagery with cancer patients. *American J. of Clinical Hypnosis* **25**(2-3):128-134.

Margolis, C. G.; Domangue, B. B.; Ehleben, C.; and Shrier, L. (1983). Hypnosis in the early treatment of burns: A pilot study. *American J. of Clinical Hypnosis* **26**(1):9-15.

Margolis, J., and Margolis, C. G. (1979). The theory of hypnosis and the concept of persons. *Behaviorism* **7**(2):97-111.

Marmer, M. J. (1956). The role of hypnosis in anesthesiology. *J. of American Medical Association* **162**(5):441-443.

Maslach, C. (1979). Negative emotional biasing of unexplained arousal. *J. of Personality and Social Psychology* **37**(6):953-969.

Maslach, C.; Marshall, C.; and Zimbardo, P. G. (1972). Hypnotic control of peripheral skin temperature: A case report. *Psychophysiology* **9**(6):600-605.

Mason, A. A. (1952). Case of congenital ichthyosiform erythroderma of Broeg treated by hypnosis. *British Medical J.* **2**:422-423.

Mason, A. A. (1955). Surgery under hypnosis. *Anesthesia* **10**(3):295-299.

Matheson, G. (1979a). Modification of depressive symptoms through posthypnotic suggestion. *American J. of Clinical Hypnosis* **22**(1):61-64.

Matheson, G. (1979b). Hypnotic aspect of religious experiences. *J. of Psychology and Theology* **7**(1):13-21.

Matheson, G., and Grehan, J. F. (1979). A rapid induction technique. *American J. of Clinical Hypnosis* **21**(4):297-299.

Matthews, W. J. (1981). Posthypnotic conflict and psychopathology: Evidence for repression or inadequate methodology? *Dissertation Abstracts International* **41**:(8-B):3188.

Matthews, W. J.; Bennett, H.; Bean, W.; and Gallagher, M. (1985). Indirect versus direct hypnotic suggestions—An initial investigation: A brief communication. *International J. of Clinical and Experimental Hypnosis* **33**(3):219-223.

Matthews, W. J., Jr.; Kirsch, I.; and Allen, G. J. (1984). Posthypnotic conflict and psychopathology—controlling for the effects of posthypnotic suggestions: A brief communication. *International J. of Clinical and Experimental Hypnosis* **32**(4):362-365.

Matthews, W. J.; Kirsch, I.; and Mosher, D. (1985). Double hypnotic induction: An initial empirical test. *J. of Abnormal Psychology* **94**(1):92-95.

Maultsby, M. C. (1971). Systematic, written homework in psychotherapy. *Psychotherapy: Theory, Research and Practice* **8**:195-198.

Mead, S., and Roush, E. S. (1949). Study of the effect of hypnotic suggestions on physiologic performance. *Arch. Phys. Med.* **30**:700-706.

Meares, A. (1960a). *A System of Medical Hypnosis.* Philadelphia: W. B. Saunders Co.

Meares, A. (1960b). *Shapes of Sanity. A Study in the Therapeutic Use of Modelling in the Waking and Hypnotic State.* Springfield, IL: Charles C. Thomas.

Meares, A. (1982-1983). A form of intensive meditation associated with the regression of cancer. *American J. of Clinical Hypnosis* **25**(2-3):114-121.

Meek, V. (1982). An obstetric anecdote. *Australian J. of Clinical and Experimental Hypnosis* **10**(2):119-120.

Meeker, W. B., and Barber, T. X. (1971). Toward an explanation of stage hypnosis. *J. of Abnormal Psychology* **77**(1):61-70.

Megas, J. C., and Coe, W. C. (1975). Hypnosis as role enactment: The effect of positive information about hypnosis on self-role congruence. *American J. of Clinical Hypnosis* **18**(2):132-137.

Melzack, R., and Perry, C. (1975). Self-regulation of pain: The use of alpha-feedback and hypnotic training for the control of chronic pain. *Experimental Neurology* **46**:452-469.

Mercer, M., and Gibson, R. W. (1950). Rorschach content analysis in hypnosis: Chronological age regression. *J. of Clinical Psychology* **6**:352-358.

Merkur, D. (1984). The nature of the hypnotic state: A psychoanalytic approach. *International Review of Psycho-Analysis* **11**(3):345-354.

Meyers, S. (1977). Response to authority and the effects on suggestibility of defining the situation as an imagination test or as hypnosis. *Dissertation Abstracts International* **38**(3-B):1411-1412.

Migliore, E. T. (1979). The effect of hypnotic procedures on the creative thinking of five and six year olds. *Dissertation Abstracts International* **40**(1-B):432.

Milgram, S. (1963). Behavioral study of obedience. *J. of Abnormal and Social Psychology* **67**:371-378.

Milgram, S. (1969). *Obedience to Authority.* New York: Harper Row.

Miller, A. (1986). Hypnotherapy in a case of dissociated incest. *International J. of Clinical and Experimental Hypnosis* **34**(1):13-28.

Miller, D. E. (1979). The structure and processes of authority relations: Hypnosis. *Dissertation Abstracts International* **40**(5-A):2937.

Miller, H. R. (1983). Psychogenic seizures treated by hypnosis. *American J. of Clinical Hypnosis* **25**(4):248-252.

Miller, J. (1983). "Spontaneous" age regression: A clinical report. *American J. of Clinical Hypnosis* **26**(1):53-55.

Miller, J. A. (1980). Hypnosis in a boy with leukemia. *American J. of Clinical Hypnosis* **22**(4):231-235.

Miller, L. S., and Cross, H. J. (1985). Hypnotic susceptibility, hypnosis, and EMG feedback in the reduction of frontalis muscle tension. *International J. of Clinical and Experimental Hypnosis* **33**(3):258-272.

Miller, M. (1976). *Therapeutic Hypnosis.* New York: Human Sciences Press.

Miller, R. D. (1984). The possible use of auto-hypnosis as a resistance during hypnotherapy. *International J. of Clinical and Experimental Hypnosis* **32**(2):236-247.

Miller, R. J. (1980). The Harvard Group Scale of Hypnotic Susceptibility as a predictor of nonhypnotic suggestibility. *International J. of Clinical and Experimental Hypnosis* **28**(1):46-52.

Miller, R. J., and Leibowitz, H. W. (1976). A signal detection analysis of hypnotically induced narrowing of the peripheral visual field. *J. of Abnormal Psychology* **85**(5):446-454.

Miller, R. J.; Hennessy, R. T.; and Leibowitz, H. W. (1973). The effect of hypnotic ablation of the background on the magnitude of the Ponzo perspective illusion. *International J. of Clinical and Experimental Hypnosis* **21**(3):180-191.

Milne, G. (1982). Hypnotic treatment of a cancer patient. *Australian J. of Clinical and Experimental Hypnosis* **10**(2):123-124.

Miner, J. P. (1984). Cognitive functioning in hypnosis: The effect of hypnotic susceptibility and capacity for trance. *Dissertation Abstracts International* **45**(2-B):680.

Mitchell, M. B. (1932). Retroactive inhibition and hypnosis. *J. of General Psychology* **7**:343-359.

Moldawsky, R. J. (1984). Hypnosis as an adjunctive treatment in Huntington's disease. *American J. of Clinical Hypnosis* **26**(4):229-231.

Moll, A. (1958). *The Study of Hypnosis.* 1889. Reprint. New York: Julian Press.

Montgomery, G. T., and Crowder, J. E. (1972). The symptom substitution hypothesis and the evidence. *Psychotherapy: Theory, Research and Practice* **9**(2):98-102.

Monzen, S. (1977). Error performance and awareness in the process of task achievement in calculation tasks. *Japanese J. of Psychology* **47** (6):301-307.

Monzen, S. (1980). Conflicts of will motives (3): Effect of attention and the development of the maintenance mechanism of subconscious motives. *Japanese Psychological Research* **22**(2):55-63.

Moon, H., and Moon, T. (1984). Hypnosis and childbirth: Self-report and comment. *British J. of Experimental and Clinical Hypnosis* **1**(2):49-52.

Moon, T. (1982). Does this "hypnosis" really exist? Another look at Gibbon's "Hypnosis as a trance state: The future of a shared delusion." *Bulletin of the British Society of Experimental and Clinical Hypnosis* **1982**(5):80-84.

Moore, C. L. (1981). Hypnosis: An adjunct to pediatric consultation. *American J. of Clinical Hypnosis* **23**(3):211-216.

Moore, L. E., and Kaplan, J. Z. (1983). Hypnotically accelerated burn wound healing. *American J. of Clinical Hypnosis* **26**(1):16-19.

Moore, M. R. (1982). Ericksonian theories of hypnosis. *American J. of Clinical Hypnosis* **24**(3):183-184.

Morgan, A. H., and Hilgard, E. R. (1973). Age differences in susceptibility to hypnosis. *International J. of Clinical and Experimental Hypnosis* **21**(2):78-85.

Morgan, A. H., and Hilgard, J. R. (1978-1979a). The Stanford Hypnotic Clinical Scale for Children. *American J. of Clinical Hypnosis* **21**(2-3)148-169.

Morgan, A. H., and Hilgard, J. R. (1978-1979b). The Stanford Hypnotic Clinical Scale for Adults. *American J. of Clinical Hypnosis* **21**(2-3):134-147.

Morgan, A. H.; Johnson, D. L.; and Hilgard, E. R. (1974). The stability of hypnotic susceptibility: A longitudinal study. *International J. of Clinical and Experimental Hypnosis* **22**(3):249-257.

Morgan, A. H.; MacDonald, H.; and Hilgard, E. R. (1974). EEG alpha: Lateral asymmetry related to task and hypnotizability. *Psychophysiology* **11**(3):275-282.

Morgan, D. C. (1980). Hypnotic analgesia and quantitated hemispheric EEG. *Dissertation Abstracts International* **41**(1-B):361.

Morgan, G. (1980). *Hypnosis in Ophthalmology.* Birmingham, AL: Aesculapius Publishing Co.

Morgan, W. P.; Hirota, K.; Weitz, G. A.; and Balke, B. (1976). Hypnotic perturbation of perceived exertion: Ventilatory consequences. *American J. of Clinical Hypnosis* **18**(3):182-190.

Morgan, W. P.; Raven, P. B.; Drinkwater, B. L.; and Horvath, S. M. (1973). Perceptual and metabolic responsivity to standard bicycle ergometry following various hypnotic suggestions. *International J. of Clinical and Experimental Hypnosis* **21**(2):86-101.

Morris, B. A. P. (1985). Hypnotherapy of warts using the Simonton visualization technique: A case report. *American J. of Clinical Hypnosis* **27**(4):237-240.

Morris, F. (1975). *Self Hypnosis in Two Days.* New York: E. P. Dutton.

Morse, D. R. (1975). Hypnosis in the practice of endodontics. *J. of American Society of Psychosomatic Dentistry and Medicine* **22**(1):17-22.

Morse, D. R. (1976). Use of a meditative state for hypnotic induction in the practice of endodontics. *Oral Surgery* **41**(5):664-672.

Morse, D. R. (1977a). Overcoming "practice stress" via meditation and hypnosis. *Dental Survey* 32-34, 36.

Morse, D. R. (1977b). An exploratory study of the use of meditation alone and in combination with hypnosis in clinical dentistry. *J. of American Society of Psychosomatic Dentistry and Medicine* **24**(4):113-120.

Morse, D. R. (1978). The practice-building spell. *Dental Survey* **20**:24-26.

Morse, D. R.; Martin, J. S.; Furst, M. L.; and Dubin, L. L. (1977). A physiological and subjective evaluation of meditation, hypnosis and relaxation. *Psychosomatic Medicine* **39**(5):304-324.

Morse, D. R.; Schacterle, G. R.; Esposito, J. V.; Furst, M. L.; and Bose, K. (1981). Stress, relaxation and saliva: A follow-up study involving clinical endodontic patients. *J. of Human Stress* **7**(3):19-26.

Morse, D. R.; Schoor, R. S.; and Cohen, B. B. (1984). Surgical and non-surgical dental treatments for a multi-allergic patient with mediation-hypnosis as the sole anesthetic: Case report. *International J. of Psychosomatics* **31**(2):27-33.

Morse, D. R., and Wilcko, J. M. (1979). Nonsurgical endodontic therapy for a vital tooth with meditation-hypnosis as the sole anesthetic: A case report. *American J. of Clinical Hypnosis* **21**(4):258-262.

Moss, C. S., and Bremer, B. (1973). Exposure of a "medical modeler" to behavior modification. *International J. of Clinical and Experimental Hypnosis* **21**(1):1-12.

Mott, T., Jr. (1979). The clinical importance of hypnotizability. *American J. of Clinical Hypnosis* **21**(4):263-269.

Mott, T., Jr. (1982). The role of hypnosis in psychotherapy. *American J. of Clinical Hypnosis* **24**(4):241-248.

Mott, T., Jr., and Roberts, J. (1979). Obesity and hypnosis: A review of the literature. *American J. of Clinical Hypnosis* **22**(1):3-7.

Mount, G. R.; Walters, S. R.; Rowland, R. W.; Barnes, P. R.; and Payton, T. I. (1978). The effects of relaxation techniques on normal blood pressure. *Behavioral Engineering* **5**(1):1-4

Moyer, W. W. (1976). Countercontrol in hypnotic control groups. *Psychological Reports* **39**(3):1083-1089.

Mozdzierz, G. J. (1985). The use of hypnosis and paradox in the treatment of a case of chronic urinary retention/"bashful bladder." *American J. of Clinical Hypnosis* **28**(1):43-47.

Muehleman, T. (1978). Age regression as a possible enhancement to conception: A case report. *American J. of Clinical Hypnosis* **20**(4):282-283.

Mullins, J. G. (1981). An investigation of communication in hypnosis. *Dissertation Abstracts International* **41**(10-B):3900.

Murphy, J. K., and Fuller, A. K. (1984). Hypnosis and biofeedback as adjunctive therapy in blepharospasm: A case report. *American J. of Clinical Hypnosis* **27**(1):31-37.

Murray-Jobsis, J. (1985). Exploring the schizophrenic experience with the use of hypnosis. *American J. of Clinical Hypnosis* **28**(1):34-42.

Mutter, C. B. (1979). Regressive hypnosis and the polygraph: A case study. *American J. of Clinical Hypnosis* **22**(1):47-50.

Mutter, C. B. (1980). Critique of videotape presentation on forensic hypnotic regression: "The case of Dora." *American J. of Clinical Hypnosis* **23**(2):99-101.

Mutter, C. B. (1981). I. A hypnotherapeutic approach to exhibitionism: Outpatient therapeutic strategy. *J. of Forensic Science* **26**(1):129-133.

Mutter, C. B. (1984). The use of hypnosis with defendants. *American J. of Clinical Hypnosis* **27**(1):42-51.

Mutter, C. B. (1985). American Board of Medical Hypnosis: Current update. *American J. of Clinical Hypnosis* **27**(4):245-246.

Myers, S. A. (1983a). Vivid fantasy and imaginative abilities as related to hypnotic responsiveness. *American J. of Clinical Hypnosis* **26**(1):45-52.

Myers, S. A. (1983b). The Creative Imagination Scale: Group norms for children and adolescents. *International J. of Clinical and Experimental Hypnosis* **31**(1):28-36.

Nace, E. P., and Orne, M. T. (1970). Fate of an uncompleted posthypnotic suggestion. *J. of Abnormal Psychology* **75**(3):278-285.

Nace, E. P.; Orne, M. T.; and Hammer, A. G. (1974). Posthypnotic amnesia as an active psychic process. *Archives of General Psychiatry* **31**(2):257-260.

Nallapa, J. S. (1952). Hypnosis in intermittent Claudication. *Case Indian. M. Gaz.* **87**:43-45.

Nardi, T. J. (1981). Treating sleep paralysis with hypnosis. *International J. of Clinical and Experimental Hypnosis* **29**(4):358-365.

Nash, C. B. (1982). Hypnosis and transcendental meditation as inducers of ESP. *Parapsychology Review* **13**(1):19-20.

Nash, M. R.; Johnson, L. S.; and Tipton, R. D. (1979). Hypnotic age regression and the occurrence of transitional object relationships. *J. of Abnormal Psychology* **88**(5):547-555.

Nash, M. R.; Lynn, S. J.; and Givens, D.L. (1984). Adult hypnotic susceptibility, childhood punishment, and child abuse: A brief communication. *International J. of Clinical and Experimental Hypnosis* **32**(1):6-11.

Nash, M. R.; Lynn, S. J.; and Stanley, S. M. (1984). The direct hypnotic suggestion of altered mind/body perception. *American J. of Clinical Hypnosis* **27**(2):95-102.

Nash, M. R.; Lynn, S. J.; Stanley, S.; Frauman, D.; and Rhue, J. (1985). Hypnotic age regression and the importance of assessing interpersonally relevant affect. *International J. of Clinical and Experimental Hypnosis* **33**(3):224-235.

Nathan, P. E., and Harris, S. L. (1975). *Psychopathology and Society.* New York: McGraw-Hill.

Navradszky, L. I. (1980). Mechanism of defense: A tachistoscopic demonstration of perceptual defense against an hypnotically intensified unconscious conflict. *Dissertation Abstracts International* **40**(7-B):3411.

Nelson, J. (1980). Investigation of effects of hypnosis, relaxation, and mental rehearsal on performance scores of golfers and runners. *Dissertation Abstracts International* **41**(4-B):1484.

Newman, M. (1974). Hypnotic handling of a suicidal patient in the fugue state: A case report. *American J. of Clinical Hypnosis* **17**(2):131-133.

Newman, R. (1979). A note on posture in hypnotic induction. *Australian J. of Clinical and Experimental Hypnosis* **7**(3):287-288.

Newton, B. W. (1982-1983). The use of hypnosis in the treatment of cancer patients. *American J. of Clinical Hypnosis* **25**(2-3):104-113.

New York Times. (1979). Cautious use of investigative hypnosis is growing. August 19: 49.

Nogrady, H.; McConkey, K. M.; Laurence, J. R.; and Perry, C. (1983).

Dissociation, duality and demand characteristics in hypnosis. *J. of Abnormal Psychology* **92**(2):223-235.

Nugent, W. R. (1985). A methodological review of case studies published in the American Journal of Clinical Hypnosis. *American J. of Clinical Hypnosis* **27**(4):191-200.

Nugent, W. R.; Carden, N. A.; and Montgomery, D. J. (1984). Utilizing the creative unconscious in the treatment of hypodermic phobias and sleep disturbances. *American J. of Clinical Hypnosis* **26**(3):201-205.

O'Brien, C. P., and Weisbrot, M. M. (1983). Behavioral and psychological components of pain management. *National Institute on Drug Abuse: Research Monograph Series* Mono **45**:36-45.

O'Brien, R. M. (1977). Hypnosis and task-motivation instructions for "post-experimental" posthypnotic suggestions. *Perceptual and Motor Skills* **45**:1274.

O'Brien, R. M.; Cooley, L. E.; Ciotti, J.; and Henninger, K. M. (1981). Augmentation of systematic desensitization of snake phobia through posthypnotic dream suggestion. *American J. of Clinical Hypnosis* **23**(3):231-238.

O'Brien, R. M.; Kramer, C. E.; Chiglinsky, M. A.; Stevens, G. E.; Nunan, L. J.; and Fritzo, J. A. (1977). Moral development examined through hypnotic and task motivated age regression. *American J. of Clinical Hypnosis* **19**(4):209-213.

O'Brien, R. M., and Rabuck, S. J. (1976). Experimentally produced self-repugnant behavior as a function of hypnosis and waking suggestion: A pilot study. *American J. of Clinical Hypnosis* **18**(4):272-276.

O'Brien, R. M., and Rabuck, S. J. (1977). A failure to hypnotically produce nocturnal emissions. *American J. of Clinical Hypnosis* **19**(3):182-184.

Obstoj, I., and Sheehan, P. W. (1977). Aptitude for trance, task generalizability, and incongruity response in hypnosis. *J. of Abnormal Psychology* **86**(5):543-552.

Obstoj, I., and Sheehan, P. W. (1983). Posthypnotic amnesia and the cognitive efficiency of schizophrenics. *International J. of Clinical and Experimental Hypnosis* **31**(3):155-169.

O'Connell, D. N., and Orne, M. T. (1962). Bioelectric correlates of hypnosis: An experimental re-evaluation. *J. of Psychiatric Research* **1**:201-213.

O'Connell, D. N., and Orne, M. T. (1966). A comparison of hypnotic susceptibility as assessed by diagnostic ratings and initial standardized test scores. *International J. of Clinical and Experimental Hypnosis* **14**(4):324-332.

O'Connell, D. N., and Orne, M. T. (1968). Endosomatic electrodermal correlates of hypnotic depth and susceptibility. *J. of Psychiatric Research* **6**:1-12.

O'Connell, D. N.; Shor, R. E.; and Orne, M. T. (1970). Hypnotic age regression: An empirical and methodological analysis. *J. of Abnormal Psychology* Monograph **76**(3 part 2):1-32.

O'Grady, K. E. (1980). The absorption scale: A factor-analytic assessment. *International J. of Clinical and Experimental Hypnosis* **28**(3):281-288.

O'Hare, C.; White, G.; Lunden, B.; and MacPhillamy, D. (1975). An experiment in "step-wise" mutual hypnosis and shared guided fantasy. *American J. of Clinical Hypnosis* **17**(4):239-246.

Oker-Blom, N.; Cedercreutz, C.; von Willebrandt, E.; Hayry, P.; Kiistala, U.; and Mustakallio, K. (1981). Psychical factors in infectious disease and immunological response. *Psychiatria Fennica 1981* Suppl. 195-196.

Okhowat, V. O. (1985). An eclectic hypno-emotive approach to psychotherapy. *International J. of Clinical and Experimental Hypnosis* **33**(2):109-121.

Oliver, G. W. (1977). Symbolic aspects of hypnagogic imagery associated with theta EEG feedback. *Dissertation Abstracts International* **37**(8-B):4159.

Oliver, G. W. (1982-1983). A cancer patient and her family: A case study. *American J. of Clinical Hypnosis* **25**(2-3): 156-160.

Olness, K. (1975). The use of self-hypnosis in the treatment of childhood nocturnal enuresis. *Clinical Pediatrics* **14**(3):273-279.

Olness, K. (1976). Autohypnosis in functional megacolon in children. *American J. of Clinical Hypnosis* **19**(1):28-32.

Olness, K. (1977). In-service hypnosis education in a children's hospital. *American J. of Clinical Hypnosis* **20**(1):80-83.

Olness, K. (1981). Imagery (self-hypnosis) as adjunct therapy in childhood cancer. Clinical experience with 25 patients. *American J. of Pediatric Hematology/Oncology* **3**(3):313-321.

Olness, K. N. (1985). Little people, images, and child health. *American J. of Clinical Hypnosis* **27**(3):169-174.

Olness, K. N., and Conroy, M. M. (1985). A pilot study of voluntary control of transcutaneous PO_2 by children: A brief communication. *International J. of Clinical and Experimental Hypnosis* **33**(1):1-5.

Orme, G. C. (1981). Hypnosis, pain control and personality change in rheumatoid arthritic patients. *Dissertation Abstracts International* **41**(8-B):3192.

Orne, M. T. (1951). The mechanisms of hypnotic age regression: An experimental study. *J. of Abnormal and Social Psychology* **46**(2):213-225.

Orne, M. T. (1959). The nature of hypnosis: Artifact and essence. *J. of Abnormal and Social Psychology* **58**(3):277-299.

Orne, M. T. (1962a). Psychotherapy and Hypnosis: Implications from research. In J. Masserman (Ed.), *Current Psychiatric Therapies Volume II* (p. 75-86). New York: Grune & Stratton.

Orne, M. T. (1962b). On the social psychology of the psychological experiment: With particular reference to demand characteristics and their implications. *American Psychologist* **17**(11):776-783.

Orne, M. T. (1962c). Antisocial behavior and hypnosis: Problems of control and validation in empirical studies. In G. H. Estabrooks (Ed.), *Hypnosis: Current Problems* (pp. 137-192. New York: Harper & Row.

Orne, M. T. (1962d). Hypnotically induced hallucinations. In L. J. West (Ed.), *Hallucinations* (pp. 211-219). New York: Grune & Stratton.

Orne, M. T. (1964). A note on the occurrence of hypnosis without conscious intent. *International J. of Clinical and Experimental Hypnosis* **12**(2):75-77.

Orne, M. T. (1965a). Undesirable effects of hypnosis: The determinants and management. *International J. of Clinical and Experimental Hypnosis* **13**(4):226-237.

Orne, M. T. (1965b). Psychological factors maximizing resistance to stress: With special reference to hypnosis. In S. Z. Klausner (Ed.), *The Quest for Self Control* (pp. 286-328). New York: Macmillan.

Orne, M. T. (1966a). Hypnosis, motivation and compliance. *American J. of Psychiatry* **122**(7):721-726.

Orne, M. T. (1966b). On the mechanisms of posthypnotic amnesia. *International J. of Clinical and Experimental Hypnosis* **14**(2):121-134.

Orne, M. T. (1967). What must a satisfactory theory of hypnosis explain? *International J. of Psychiatry* **3**(1):206-211.

Orne, M. T. (1970). Hypnosis, motivation, and the ecological validity of the psychological experiment. In W. J. Arnold and M. M. Page (Eds.), *Nebraska Symposium on Motivation* (pp. 187-265). Lincoln: University of Nebraska Press.

Orne, M. T. (1971). The simulation of hypnosis: Why, how and what it means. *International J. of Clinical and Experimental Hypnosis* **19**(4):183-210.

Orne, M. T. (1972). Can a hypnotized subject be compelled to carry out otherwise unacceptable behavior? *International J. of Clinical and Experimental Hypnosis* **20**(2):101-117.

Orne, M. T. (1976). Mechanisms of hypnotic pain control. In J. J. Bonica and D. Albe-Fessard (Eds.) *Advances in Pain Research and Therapy: Volume 1* (pp. 717-726). New York: Raven Press.

Orne, M. T. (1977). The construct of hypnosis: Implications of the definition for research and practice. *Annals of New York Academy of Sciences* **296**:14-33.

Orne, M. T. (1979). The use and misuse of hypnosis in court. *International J. of Clinical and Experimental Hypnosis* **27**(4):311-341.

Orne, M. T. (1982). Seminar on the use of hypnosis in treatment at the Institute of the Pennsylvania Hospital, January.

Orne, M. T.; Dinges, D. F.; and Orne, E. C. (1984). On the differential diagnosis of multiple personality in the forensic context. *International J. of Clinical and Experimental Hypnosis* **32**(2):118-169.

Orne, M. T., and Evans, F. J. (1965). Social control in the psychological experiment: Antisocial behavior and hypnosis. *J. of Personality and Social Psychology* **1**(3):189-200.

Orne, M. T., and Evans, F. J. (1966). Inadvertent termination of hypnosis with hypnotized and simulating subjects. *International J. of Clinical and Experimental Hypnosis* **14**(1):61-78.

Orne, M. T., and Hammer, A. G. (1974). Hypnosis. In *Encyclopedia Britannica* (pp. 133-140) (15th ed.). Chicago: Encyclopedia Britannica.

Orne, M. T.; Hilgard, E. R.; Spiegel, H.; Spiegel, D.; Crawford, H. J.; Evans, F. J.; Orne, E. C.; and Frischholz, E. J. (1979). The relation between the Hypnotic Induction Profile and the Stanford Hypnotic Susceptibility Scales, Forms A and C. *International J. of Clinical and Experimental Hypnosis* **27**(2):85-102.

Orne, M. T., and McConkey, K. M. (1981). Toward convergent inquiry into self-hypnosis. *International J. of Clinical and Experimental Hypnosis* **29**(3):313-323.

Orne, M. T., and O'Connell, D. N. (1967). Diagnostic ratings of hypnotizability. *International J. of Clinical and Experimental Hypnosis* **15**(3):125-133.

Orne, M. T.; Sheehan, P. W.; and Evans, F. J. (1968). Occurrence of posthypnotic behavior outside the experimental setting. *J. of Personality and Social Psychology* **9**(2):189-196.

Ortega, D. F. (1984). Hypnosis in the treatment of hypnopompic hallucinations. *American J. of Clinical Hypnosis* **27**(2):111-113.

Ousby, W. J. (1977). *Self Hypnosis and Scientific Self Suggestion.* New York: Arco.

Overlade, D. C. (1976). The production of fasiculations by suggestion. *American J. of Clinical Hypnosis* **19**(1):50-56.

Owens, D. (1980). A study in the viability of the hypnotic process with institutionalized adult mentally retarded males. *Dissertation Abstracts International* **41**(4-B):1519-1520.

Packard, V. (1958). *The Hidden Persuaders.* New York: Pocket Books.

Packer, E. (1979). A study of the expert opinion of a panel of hypnotherapists on the use of hypnosis in the courts. *Dissertation Abstracts International* **40**(4-B):1907.

Page, J. D. (1975). *Psychopathology* (2d ed.). Chicago: Aldine.

Pajntar, M.; Jeglic, A.; Stefancic, M.; and Vodovnik, L. (1980). Improvements of motor response by means of hypnosis in patients with peripheral nerve lesions. *International J. of Clinical and Experimental Hypnosis* **28**(1):16-26.

Parker, J. L. (1979). The use of hypnosis to reinstate a child's impaired writing performance resulting from neurological damage. *Australian J. of Clinical and Experimental Hypnosis* **7**(3):225-230.

Parker, P. D., and Barber, T. X. (1964). Hypnosis, task-motivating instructions and learning performance. *J. of Abnormal and Social Psychology* **69**:499-504.

Parrish, M. J. (1974). Moral predisposition and hypnotic influence of "immoral" behavior: An exploratory study. *American J. of Clinical Hypnosis* **17**(2):115-124.

Parrish, M.; Lundy, R. M.; and Leibowitz, H. W. (1969). Effect of hypnotic age regression on the magnitude of the Ponzo and Poggendorff illusion. *J. of Abnormal Psychology* **74**:693-698.

Paskewitz, D. A. (1977). EEG alpha activity and its relationship to altered states of consciousness. *Annals of New York Academy of Sciences* **296**:154-161.

Paterson, A. S. (1974). Hypnosis as an adjunct to the treatment of alcoholics and drug addicts. *International J. of Offender Therapy and Comparative Criminology* **18**(1):40-45.

Patten, E. F. (1930). The duration of posthypnotic suggestions. *J. of Abnormal and Social Psychology* **25**:319.

Patterson, R. B. (1980). Hypnotherapy of hysterical monocular blindness: A case report. *American J. of Clinical Hypnosis* **23**(2):119-121.

Pattie, F. A. (1935). A report of attempts to produce uniocular blindness by hypnotic suggestion. *British J. of Medical Psychology* **15**:230-241.

Pattie, F. A. (1941). The production of blisters by hypnotic suggestions: A review. *J. of Abnormal and Social Psychology* **36**:62-72.

Pattie, F. A. (1950). The genuineness of unilateral deafness produced by hypnosis. *American J. of Psychology* **63**:84-86.

Pattie, F. A. (1956). Methods of induction, susceptibility of subjects and criteria of hypnosis. Chapter 2 in R. M. Dorcus (Ed.), *Hypnosis and Its Therapeutic Applications.* New York: McGraw-Hill.

Pattie, F. A. (1979). A Mesmer-Paradis myth dispelled. *American J. of Clinical Hypnosis* **22**(1):29-31.

Paul, G. L. (1966). *Insight vs. Desensitization in Psychotherapy: An Experiment in Anxiety Reduction.* Stanford, CA: Stanford University Press.

Paul, G. L. (1967). Inhibition of physiological response to stressful imagery by relaxation training and hypnotically suggested relaxation. *Behavior Research and Therapy* **7**:249-256.

Pearson, P. (1982). Effects of post-hypnotic suggestion on the performance of a fine motor skill. *Australian J. of Clinical Hypnotherapy and Hypnosis* **3**(2):75-84.

Pederson, L. L.; Scrimgeour, W. G.; and Lefcoe, N. M. (1975). Comparison of hypnosis plus counseling, counseling alone, and hypnosis alone in a community service smoking withdrawal program. *J. of Consulting and Clinical Psychology* **43**(6):920.

Pederson, L. L.; Scrimgeour, W. G.; and Lefcoe, N. M. (1979). Variables of hypnosis which are related to success in a smoking withdrawal program. *International J. of Clinical and Experimental Hypnosis* **27**(1):14-20.

Pekala, R. J., and Kumar, V. K. (1984). Predicting hypnotic susceptibility by a self-report phenomenological state instrument. *American J. of Clinical Hypnosis* **27**(2):114-121.

Pelletier, A. M. (1977). Hysterical aphonia: A case report. *American J. of Clinical Hypnosis* **20**(2):149-153.

Pelletier, A. M. (1979). Three uses of guided imagery in hypnosis. *American J. of Clinical Hypnosis* **22**(1):32-36.

Pelletier, K. R., and Peper, E. (1977). Developing a biofeedback model: Alpha EEG feedback as a means for pain control. *International J. of Clinical and Experimental Hypnosis* **25**(4):361-371.

Pereira, M., and Austrin, H. R. (1980). Locus of control and status of the experimenter as predictors of suggestibility. *International J. of Clinical and Experimental Hypnosis* **28**(4):367-374.

Perry, B. J. (1980). Control of physiological phenomena via hypnosis with special reference to contraception. *Australian J. of Clinical Hypnotherapy* **1**(2):73-77.

Perry, C. (1973). Imagery, fantasy and hypnotic susceptibility. *J. of Personality and Social Psychology* **26**(2):217-221.

Perry, C. (1977a). Is hypnotizability modifiable? *International J. of Clinical and Experimental Hypnosis* **25**(3):125-146.

Perry, C. (1977b). Uncanceled hypnotic suggestions: The effects of hypnotic depth and hypnotic skill on their posthypnotic persistence. *American J. of Abnormal Psychology* **86**(5):570-574.

Perry, C. (1977c). Variables influencing the posthypnotic persistence of an uncanceled hypnotic suggestion. *Annals of New York Academy of Sciences* **296**:264-273.

Perry, C. (1979). Hypnotic coercion and compliance to it: A review of evidence presented in a legal case. *International J. of Clinical and Experimental Hypnosis* **27**(3):187-218.

Perry, C. (1984). Dissociative phenomena of hypnosis. *Australian J. of Clinical and Experimental Hypnosis* **12**(2):71-84.

Perry, C., and Chisholm, W. (1973). Hypnotic age regression and the Ponzo and Poggendorff illusions. *International J. of Clinical and Experimental Hypnosis* **21**(3):192-204.

Perry, C., and Laurence, J. R. (1980). Hypnotic depth and hypnotic susceptibility: A replicated finding. *International J. of Clinical and Experimental Hypnosis* **28**(3):272-280.

Perry, C., and Laurence, J. R. (1983a). The enhancement of memory by hypnosis in the legal investigative situation. *Canadian Psychology* **24**(3):155-167.

Perry, C., and Laurence, J. R. (1983b). Hypnosis, surgery, and mind-body interaction: An historical evaluation. *Canadian J. of Behavioural Science* **15**(4):351-372.

Perry, C., and Mullen, G. (1975). The effects of hypnotic susceptibility on reducing smoking behavior treated by an hypnotic technique. *J. of Clinical Psychology* **31**(3):498-505.

Perry, C. W., and Sheehan, P. W. (1978). Aptitude for trance and situational effects of varying the interpersonal nature of the hypnotic setting. *American J. of Clinical Hypnosis* **20**(4):256-262.

Perry, C., and Walsh, B. (1978). Inconsistencies and anomalies of response as a defining characteristic of hypnosis. *J. of Abnormal Psychology* **87**(5):574-577.

Peters, J. E.; Dhanens, T. P.; Lundy, R. M.; and Landy, F. J. (1974). A factor analytic investigation of the Harvard Group Scale of Hypnotic Susceptibility, Form A. *International J. of Clinical and Experimental Hypnosis* **22**(4):377-387.

Peters, J. E.; Lundy, R. M.; and Stern, R. M. (1973). Peripheral skin temperature responses to hot and cold suggestions. *International J. of Clinical and Experimental Hypnosis* **21**(3):205-212.

Peters, J. E., and Stern, R. M. (1973). Peripheral skin temperature and vasomotor responses during hypnotic induction. *International J. of Clinical and Experimental Hypnosis* **21**(2):102-108.

Pettigrew, C. G. (1978). Experimental manipulation of death anxiety. *Dissertation Abstracts International* **38**(7-B):3411.

Pettigrew, C. G., and Dawson, J. G. (1979). Death anxiety: State or trait? *J. of Clinical Psychology* **35**(1):154-158.

Pettinati, H. M. (1982). Measuring hypnotizability in psychotic patients. *International J. of Clinical and Experimental Hypnosis* **30**(4):404-416.

Pettinati, H. M. R. (1979). Selectivity in memory during posthypnotic amnesia. *Dissertation Abstracts International* **40**(2-B):898-899.

Pettinati, H. M., and Evans, F. J. (1978). Posthypnotic amnesia: Evaluation of selective recall of successful experiences. *International J. of Clinical and Experimental Hypnosis* **26**(4):317-329.

Pettinati, H. M.; Evans, F. J.; Orne, E. C.; and Orne, M. T. (1981). Restricted use of success cues in retrieval during posthypnotic amnesia. *J. of Abnormal Psychology* **90**(4):345-353.

Pettitt, G. A. (1982). Retarded ejaculation; Adjunctive treatment by hypnotically induced dreams in the context of sex therapy. *Australian J. of Clinical and Experimental Hypnosis* **10**(2):89-98.

Petty, G. L. (1976). Desensitization of parents to tantrum behavior. *American J. of Clinical Hypnosis* **19**(2):95-97.

Petty, G. L. (1978). The effects of hypnosis on visual imagery. *Dissertation Abstracts International* **38**(11-B):5586-5587.

Phillips, A. (1981). *Transformational Psychotherapy: An Approach to Creative Hypnotic Communication*. New York: Elsevier.

Piedmont, R. L. (1981). Effects of hypnosis and biofeedback upon the regulation of peripheral skin temperature. *Perceptual and Motor Skills* **53**(3):855-862.

Pistole, D. D. (1979). A multivariate assessment of hypnotic susceptibility as a function of locus of control, method of induction, and sex of subject. *Dissertation Abstracts International* **40**(3-B):1403-1404.

Place, M. (1984). Hypnosis and the child. *J. of Child Psychology and Psychiatry and Allied Disciplines* **25**(3):339-347.

Plapp, J. M. (1976). Experimental hypnosis in a clinical setting: A report of the atypical use of hypnosis in the treatment of a disturbed adolescent. *American J. of Clinical Hypnosis* **18**(3):145-152.

Platonow, K. I. (1933). On the objective proof of the experimental personality age regression. *J. of General Psychology* **9**:190.

Player, W. O. (1982). Effects of hypnosis on thermal biofeedback. *Dissertation Abstracts International* **42**(7-B):2999-3000.

Plotkin, W. B., and Schwartz, W. R. (1982). A conceptualization of hypnosis: Exploring the place of appraisal and anomaly in behavior and experience. *Advances in Descriptive Psychology* **1982**(2):139-199.

Podmore, F. (1963). *From Mesmer to Christian Science*. New Hyde Park, NY: University Books.

Polk, W. M. (1983). Treatment of exhibitionism in a 38-year-old male by hypnotically assisted covert sensitization. *International J. of Clinical and Experimental Hypnosis* **31**(3):132-138.

Porter, J. (1978). Suggestions and success imagery for study problems. *International J. of Clinical and Experimental Hypnosis* **26**(2):63-75.

Powell, D. H. (1980). Helping habitual smokers using flooding and hypnotic desensitization technique: A brief communication. *International J. of Clinical and Experimental Hypnosis* **28**(3):192-196.

Powers, M. (1960). *Advanced Techniques of Hypnosis*. Hollywood: Wilshire Book Co.

Powers, M. (1977a). *Self Hypnosis*. Hollywood: Wilshire Book Co.

Powers, M. (1977b) *A Practical Guide to Self Hypnosis*. Hollywood: Wilshire Book Co.

Price, J. (Ed.). (1972). *Abnormal Psychology: Current Perspectives*. Del Mar, CA: CRM Books.

Pulos, L. (1980). Mesmerism revisited: The effectiveness of Esdaile's techniques in the production of deep hypnosis and total body hypnoanaesthesia. *American J. of Clinical Hypnosis* **22**(4):206-211.

Pulver, S. E., and Pulver, M. P. (1975). Hypnosis in medical and dental practice: A survey. *International J. of Clinical and Experimental Hypnosis* **22**(1):28-47.

Pulver, S. E., and Smith, L. H. (1965). Physicians studying hypnosis. *Archives of General Psychiatry* **12**:557-561.

Putnam, W. H. (1979). Hypnosis, and distortions in eyewitness memory. *International J. of Clinical and Experimental Hypnosis* **27**(4):437-448.

Query, W. T. (1981). Family size, birth order and hypnotizability: A brief communication. *International J. of Clinical and Experimental Hypnosis* **29**(2):107-109.

Radtke, H. L., and Spanos, N. P. (1981a). Was I hypnotized? A social psychological analysis of hypnotic depth reports. *Psychiatry* **44**(4):359-376.

Radtke, H. L., and Spanos, N. P. (1981b). Temporal sequencing during posthypnotic amnesia: A methodological critique. *J. of Abnormal Psychology* **90**(5):476-485.

Radtke, H. L., and Spanos, N. P. (1982). The effect of rating scale descriptors on hypnotic depth reports. *J. of Psychology* **111**(2):235-245.

Radtke, H. L.; Spanos, N. P.; Armstrong, L. A.; Dillman, N.; and Boisvenue, M. E. (1983). Effects of electromyographic feedback and progressive relaxation training on hypnotic susceptibility: Disconfirming results. *International J. of Clinical and Experimental Hypnosis* **31**(2):98-106.

Radtke, H. L.; Spanos, N. P.: Malva, C. L. D.; and Stam, H. J. (1985). Temporal organization and hypnotic amnesia using a modification of the Harvard Group Scale of Hypnotic Susceptibility. *International J. of Clinical and Experimental Hypnosis* **34**(1):41-54.

Radtke-Bodorik, H. L.; Planas, M.; and Spanos, N. P. (1980). Suggested amnesia, verbal inhibition, and disorganized recall for a long word list. *Canadian J. of Behavioural Science* **12**(1):87-97.

Radtke-Bodorik, H. L.; Spanos, N. P.: and Haddad, M. G. (1979). The effects of spoken versus written recall on suggested amnesia in hypnotic and task-motivated subjects. *American J. of Clinical Hypnosis* **22**(1):8-16.

Rafky, D. M., and Bernstein, J. (1984). Forensic hypnosis and witness recall: The effect of trance depth. *J. of Police Science and Administration* **12**(3):277-286.

Raginsky, B. B. (1951). Use of hypnosis in anesthesiology. *Personality* **1**:340-348.

Raginsky, B. B. (1953). Hypnosis in internal medicine. In J. M. Schneck (Ed.), *Hypnosis in Modern Medicine*. Springfield. IL: Charles C. Thomas.

Raginsky, B. B. (1959). Temporary cardiac arrest induced under hypnosis. *International J. of Clinical and Experimental Hypnosis* **7**(1):53-68.

Raginsky, B. B. (1962). Sensory hypnoplasty with case illustrations. *International J. of Clinical and Experimental Hypnosis* **10**:205-219.

Raginsky, B. B. (1967). Rapid regression to the oral and anal levels through sensory hypnoplasty. *International J. of Clinical and Experimental Hypnosis* **15**(1):19-30.

Raginsky, B. B. (1969). Hypnotic recall of aircrash cause. *International J. of Clinical and Experimental Hypnosis* **17**(1):1-19.

Raikov, V. L. (1975). Theoretical substantiation of deep hypnosis. *American J. of Clinical Hypnosis* **18**(1):23-27.

Raikov, V. L. (1976). The possibility of creativity in the active stages of hypnosis. *International J. of Clinical and Experimental Hypnosis* **24**(3):258-268.

Raikov, V. L. (1977). Theoretical analysis of deep hypnosis: Creative activity of hypnotized subjects into transformed self-consciousness. *American J. of Clinical Hypnosis* **19**(4):214-220.

Raikov, V. L. (1978). Specific features of suggested anesthesia in some forms of hypnosis in which the subject is active. *International J. of Clinical and Experimental Hypnosis* **26**(3):158-166.

Raikov, V. L. (1980). Age regression to infancy by adult subjects in deep hypnosis. *American J. of Clinical Hypnosis* **22**(3):156-163.

Raikov, V. L. (1982). Hypnotic age regression to the neonatal period: Comparisons with role playing. *International J. of Clinical and Experimental Hypnosis* **30**(2):108-116.

Raikov, V. L. (1983-1984). EEG recordings of experiments in hypnotic age regression. *Imagination, Cognition and Personality* **3**(2):115-132.

Rainer, D. D. (1984). Eyewitness testimony: Does hypnosis enhance accuracy, distortion, and confidence? *Dissertation Abstracts International* **45**(1-B):340.

Rappaport, A. (1977) Pain control through hypnosis. In A. R. Guerra (Ed.), *Modern Anesthesia in Dentistry* (pp. 17-23). Philadelphia: Franklin Institute Press.

Raskin, R. H. (1979). The addition of self-hypnosis training to the standard medical treatment of essential hypertension. *Dissertation Abstracts International* **40**(5-B):2383-2384.

Rausch, V. (1980). Cholecystectomy with self-hypnosis. *American J. of Clinical Hypnosis* **22**(3):124-129.

Ravitz, L. J. (1982). EEG correlates of hypnotically-revivified seizures. *J. of the American Society of Psychosomatic Dentistry and Medicine* **29**(4):128-140.

Raynaud, J.; Michaux, D.; Bleirad, G.; Capderou, A.; Bordachar, J.; and Durand, J. (1984). Changes in rectal and mean skin temperature in response to suggested heat during hypnosis in man. *Psychology and Behavior* **33**(2):221-226.

Redd, W. H.; Rosenberger, P. H.; and Hendler, C. S. (1982-1983). Controlling chemotherapy side effects. *American J. of Clinical Hypnosis* **25**(2-3):161-172.

Register, P. A., and Kihlstrom, J. F. (1986). Finding the hypnotic virtuoso. *International J. of Clinical and Experimental Hypnosis* **34**(2):84-97.

Reid, W. H. (1975). Treatment of somnambulism in military trainees. *American J. of Psychotherapy* **29**(1):101-106.

Reiff, R., and Scheerer, M. (1959). *Memory and Hypnotic Age Regression: Developmental Aspects of Cognitive Function Explored through Hypnosis.* New York: International Universities Press.

Reilley, R. R.; Parisher, D. W.; Carona, A.; and Dobrovolsky, N. W. (1980). Modifying hypnotic susceptibility by practice and instruction. *International J. of Clinical and Experimental Hypnosis* **28**(1):39-45.

Reilley, R. R., and Rodolfa, E. R. (1981). Concentration, attention, and hypnosis. *Psychological Reports* **48**(3):811-814.

Reis, H. T.; Wheeler, L.; and Wolff, E. (1975). Multiple pathways to hypnotic susceptibility: A new scheme for predicting the depth of hypnosis. *American J. of Clinical Hypnosis* **17**(3):175-184.

Reiser, M. (1980). Handbook of Investigative Hypnosis. Los Angeles: LEHI Publishing Co.

Reiser, M. (1984). Police use of investigative hypnosis: Scientism, ethics and power games. *American J. of Forensic Psychology* **2**(3):115-143.

Reiser, M., and Nielson, M. (1980). Investigative hypnosis: A developing specialty. *American J. of Clinical Hypnosis* **23**(2):75-84.

Reiss, S.; Peterson, R. A.; Eron, L. D.; and Reiss, M. M. (1977). *Abnormality—Experimental and Clinical Approaches.* New York: Macmillan.

Reiter, P. J. (1956). The influence of hypnosis on somatic fields of function. In L. M. LeCron (Ed.), *Experimental Hypnosis* (pp. 241-263). New York: Macmillan.

Reiter, P. J. (1958). *Antisocial or Criminal Acts and Hypnosis: A case Study.* Springfield, IL: Charles C. Thomas.

Relinger, H. (1984). Hypnotic hypermnesia: A critical review. *American J. of Clinical Hypnosis* **26**(3):212-225.

Reyher, J. (1968). Hypnosis. In J. Vernon (Ed.), *Introduction to Psychology: A Self-Selection Textbook.* Dubuque: Wm. C. Brown Co.

Reyher, J. (1969). Comment on "Artificial induction of posthypnotic conflict." *J. of Abnormal Psychology* **74** (4):420-422.

Reyher, J. (1973). Can hypnotized subjects simulate waking behavior: *American J. of Clinical Hypnosis* **16**(1):31-36.

Reyher, J. (1977a). Clinical and experimental hypnosis: Implications for theory and methodology. *Annals of the New York Academy of Sciences* **296**:69-85.

Reyher, J. (1977b). Spontaneous visual imagery: Implications for psychoanalysis, psychopathology and psychotherapy. *J. of Mental Imagery* **2**:253-274.

Reyher, J., and Pottinger, J. (1976). The significance of the interpersonal relationship in the induction of hypnosis. *American J. of Clinical Hypnosis* **19**(2):103-107.

Reyher, J., and Smyth, L. (1971). Suggestibility during the execution of a posthypnotic suggestion. *J. of Abnormal Psychology* **78**(3):258-265.

Reyher, J.; Wilson, J. G.; and Hughes, R. P. (1979). Suggestibility and type of interpersonal relationship: Special implications for the patient-practitioner relationship. *J. of Research in Personality* **13**(2):175-186.

Rhodes, R. H. (1975). *Therapy through Hypnosis.* Hollywood: Wilshire Book Co.

Richman, D. N. (1965). A critique of two recent theories of hypnosis: The psychoanalytic theory of Gill and Brenman contrasted with the behavioral theory of Barber. *Psychiatric Quarterly* **39**:278-292.

Rios, R. J. (1980). The effect of hypnosis and meditation on state and trait anxiety and locus of control. *Dissertation Abstracts International* **40**(12-A, part 1):6209-6210.

Ritow, J. K. (1979). Brief treatment of a vomiting phobia. *American J. of Clinical Hypnosis* **21**(4):293-296.

Rivers, S. M. (1981). Suggested amnesia in the context of directed forgetting. *Dissertation Abstracts International* **41**(10-B):3875-3876.

Roberts, A. C. (1982). The abuse of hypnosis in the legal system. *American J. of Forensic Psychiatry* **3**(2):67-86, 100.

Roberts, A. H.; Schuler, J.; Bacon, J. G.; Zimmerman, R. L.; and Patterson, R. (1975). Individual differences and automatic control: Absorption, hypnotic susceptibility, and the unilateral control of skin temperature. *J. of Abnormal Psychology* **84**(3):272-279.

Roberts, A. H., and Tellegen, A. (1973). Ratings of "trust" and hypnotic susceptibility. *International J. of Clinical and Experimental Hypnosis* **21**(4):289-297.

Robitscher, J. B. (1974). Psychosurgery and other somatic means of altering behavior. *Bulletin of American Academy of Psychiatry and the Law* **2**(1):7-33.

Rockey, E. E. (1977) Seminar on hypnosis in clinical practice at N.Y.U. Postgraduate School of Medicine, October.

Roden, R. G. (1979). Psychoanalytically oriented hypnotic treatment of autoerythrocytic sensitization and blindness. *American J. of Clinical Hypnosis* **21**(4):278-281.

Roden, R. G. (1980). Hypnotherapy of one-eyed subjects. *American J. of Clinical Hypnosis* **22**(4):236-237.

Rodgers, C. W. (1974). Prediction of hypnotic susceptibility from the Edwards Personal Preference Schedule: Negative finding. *Psychological Reports* **34**(2):406.

Rodolfa, E. R.; Kraft, W. A.; and Reilley, R. R. (1985). Current trends in hypnosis and hypnotherapy: An interdisciplinary assessment. *American J. of Clinical Hypnosis* **28**(1):20-26.

Rodolfa, E. R.; Kraft, W. A.; Reilley, R. R.; and Blackmore, S. H. (1982). Hypnosis training in APA- and non-APA-approved clinical/counseling doctoral programs. *Professional Psychology* **13**(5):670-673.

Rodolfa, E. R.; Kraft, W. A.; Reilley, R. R.; and Blackmore, S. H. (1983). The status of research and training in hypnosis in APA accredited clinical/counseling psychology internship sites: A national survey. *International J. of Clinical and Experimental Hypnosis* **31**(4):284-292.

Rogers, B. M. (1982). Electrophysiological and experiential correlates of hypnosis. *Dissertation Abstracts International* **43**(1-B):262.

Rosen, H. (1941). The hypnotic and hypnotherapeutic control of severe pain. *American J. of Psychiatry* **107**:917-925.

Rosen, H. (1959). Hypnosis in medical practice: Uses and abuses. *Chicago Medical Society Bulletin* **62**:428-436.

Rosen, H. (1960a). Hypnosis—applications and misapplications. *J. of American Medical Association* **172**(7):139/683-143/687.

Rosen, H. (1960b). *Hypnotherapy in Clinical Psychiatry*. New York: Julian Press.

Rosen, S. (1982). *My Voice Will Go with You: The Teaching Tales of Milton H. Erickson*. New York: Norton.

Rosenberg, S. W. (1982-1983). Hypnosis in cancer care: Imagery to enhance the control of the physiological and psychological "side-effects" of cancer therapy. *American J. of Clinical Hypnosis* **25**(2-3):122-127.

Rosenhan, D., and London, P. (1963). Hypnosis in the unhypnotizable: A study in rote learning. *J. of Experimental Psychology* **65**:30-34.

Rosenthal, B. G. (1944). Hypnotic recall of material learned under anxiety and non-anxiety producing conditions. *J. of Experimental Psychology* **34**:369-389.

Ross, C. A. (1984). Diagnosis of multiple personality during hypnosis: A case report. *International J. of Clinical and Experimental Hypnosis* **32**(2):222-235.

Ross, P. J. (1981). Hypnosis as a counseling tool. *British J. of Guidance and Counseling* **9**(2):173-179.

Rossi, E. L. (Ed.). (1980). *The Collected Papers of Milton H. Erickson. Volume I. The Nature of Hypnosis and Suggestion. Volume II. Hypnotic Alterations of Sensory, Perceptual and Psychophysical Processes*. New York: Irvington Publishers.

Rossi, E. L. (1982). Hypnosis and ultradian cycles: A new state(s) theory of hypnosis? *American J. of Clinical Hypnosis* **25**(1):21-32.

Rowen, R. (1981). Hypnotic age regression in the treatment of a self-destructive habit: Trichotillomania. *American J. of Clinical Hypnosis* **23**(3):195-197.

Rowland, L. W. (1939). Will hypnotized persons try to harm themselves or others? *J. of Abnormal and Social Psychology* **34**:114-117.

Ruch, J. C. (1975). Self-hypnosis: The result of heterohypnosis or vice-versa. *International J. of Clinical and Experimental Hypnosis* **23**(4):282-304.

Ruch, J. C.; Morgan, A. H.; and Hilgard, E. R. (1974). Measuring hypnotic responsiveness: A comparison of the Barber Suggestibility Scale and the Stanford Hypnotic Susceptibility Scale, Form A. *International J. of Clinical and Experimental Hypnosis* **22**(4):365-376.

Russell, R. J. (1980). The effects of hypnosis and mastery imagery on task performance. *Dissertation Abstracts International* **41**(6-B):2368.

Ryan, M. L., and Sheehan, P. W. (1977). Reality testing in hypnosis: Subjective versus objective effects. *International J. of Clinical and Experimental Hypnosis* **25**(1):37-51.

Ryken, K., and Coe, W. C. (1977). Sequelae to hypnosis in perspective. Paper presented to the annual convention of the American Psychological Association, San Francisco, August.

Saavedra, R. L., and Miller, R. J. (1983). The influence of experimentally induced expectations on responses to the Harvard Group Scale of Hypnotic Susceptibility, Form A. *International J. of Clinical and Experimental Hypnosis* **31**(1):37-46.

Sabourin, M. (1982). Hypnosis and brain function: EEG correlates of state-trait differences. *Research Communications in Psychology, Psychiatry and Behavior* **7**(2):149-168.

Sabourin, M.; Brisson, M. A.; and Deschambault, A. (1980). Evaluation of hypnotically-suggested selective deafness by heart-rate conditioning and reaction time. *Psychological Reports* **47**(3, part 1):995-1002.

Saccuzzo, D. P.; Safran, D.; Anderson, V.; and McNeil, B. (1982). Visual information processing in high and low susceptible subjects. *International J. of Clinical and Experimental Hypnosis* **30**(1):32-44.

Sacerdote, P. (1972). Some individualized hypnotherapeutic techniques. *International J. of Clinical and Experimental Hypnosis* **20**(1):1-14.

Sacerdote, P. (1977). Applications of hypnotically elicited mystical states to the treatment of physical and emotional pain. *International J. of Clinical and Experimental Hypnosis* **25**(4):309-324.

Sacerdote, P. (1978). Teaching self-hypnosis to patients with chronic pain. *J. of Human Stress* **4**(2):18-21.

Sacerdote, P. (1981). Teaching self-hypnosis to adults. *International J. of Clinical and Experimental Hypnosis* **29**(3):282-299.

Sacerdote, P. (1982a). A non-statistical dissertation about hypnotizability scales and clinical goals: Comparison with individualized induction and deepening procedures. *International J. of Clinical and Experimental Hypnosis* **30**(4):354-376.

Sacerdote, P. (1982*b*). Further reflections on the hypnotizability scales: A comment. *International J. of Clinical and Experimental Hypnosis* **30**(4):393.

Sachs, B. C. (1986). Stress and self-hypnosis. *Psychiatric Annals* **16**(2):110-114.

Sachs, L. B.; Feuerstein, M.; and Vitale, J. H. (1977). Hypnotic self-regulation of chronic pain. *American J. of Clinical Hypnosis* **20**(2):106-113.

Sackeim, H. A. (1982). Lateral asymmetry in bodily response to hypnotic suggestions. *Biological Psychiatry* **17**(4):437-447.

Sackeim, H. A., and Nordlie, J. W. (1979). A model of hysterical and hypnotic blindness: Cognition, motivation, and awareness. *J. of Abnormal Psychology* **88**(5):474-489.

Saletu, B.; Saletu, M.; Brown, M.; Stern, J; Sletten, I.; and Ulett, G. (1975). Hypno-analgesia and acupuncture analgesia: A neurophysiological reality. *Neuropsychobiology* **1**(4):218-242.

Salter, A. (1973). *What is Hypnosis?* (4th ed.). New York: Farrar, Straus & Giroux.

Salzberg, H. C. (1960). The effects of hypnotic, posthypnotic and waking suggestions on performance using tasks varied in complexity. *International J. of Clinical and Experimental Hypnosis* **8**:251-258.

Salzberg, H. C. (1977). The hypnotic interview in crime detection. *American J. of Clinical Hypnosis* **19**(4):255-258.

Salzberg, H. C., and DePiano, F. A. (1980). Hypnotizability and task motivating suggestions: A further look at how they affect performance. *International J. of Clinical and Experimental Hypnosis* **28**(3):261-271.

Sampimon, R. L. H., and Woodruff, M. F. A. (1946). Some observations concerning the use of hypnosis as a substitute for anesthesia *Medical J. of Australia* **1**:393-395.

Sanders, B. L. (1979). An examination of the relationship between hypnosis and functional brain asymmetry in dichotic listening tasks. *Dissertation Abstracts International* **40**(4-B):1912-1913.

Sanders, G. S., and Simmons, W. L. (1983). Use of hypnosis to enhance eyewitness accuracy: Does it work? *J. of Applied Psychology* **68**(1):70-77.

Sanders, S. (1976). Mutual group hypnosis as a catalyst in fostering creative problem solving. *American J. of Clinical Hypnosis* **19**(1):62-66.

Sanders, S. (1977*a*). Mutual group hypnosis and smoking. *American J. of Clinical Hypnosis* **20**(2):131-135.

Sanders, S. (1977*b*). An exploration of utilization techniques in short-term hypnotherapy. *American J. of Clinical Hypnosis* **20**(1):76-79.

Sanders, S. (1978). Creative problem-solving and psychotherapy. *International J. of Clinical and Experimental Hypnosis* **26**(1):15-21.

Sanders, S. (1982). Hypnotic dream utilization in hypnotherapy. *American J. of Clinical Hypnosis* **25**(1):62-67.

Sarbin, T. R. (1939). Rorschach patterns under hypnosis. *American J. Orthopsychiatry* **9**:315-318.

Sarbin, T. R. (1950a). Contributions to role-taking theory. I. Hypnotic behavior. *Psychological Review* **57**(5):255-270.

Sarbin, T. R. (1950b). Mental changes in experimental regression. *J. of Personality* **19**:221.

Sarbin, T. R. (1984). Nonvolition in hypnosis: A semiotic analysis. *Psychological Record* **34**(4):537-549.

Sarbin, T. R., and Coe, W. C. (1972). *Hypnosis: A Social Psychological Analysis of Influence Communication*. New York: Holt, Rinehart and Winston.

Sarbin, T. R., and Coe, W. C. (1979). Hypnosis and psychopathology: Replacing old myths with fresh metaphors. *J. of Abnormal Psychology* **88**(5):506-526.

Sarbin, T. R., and Farberow, N. L. (1952). Contributions to role taking theory: A clinical study of self and role. *J. of Abnormal and Social Psychology* **47**:117.

Sargent, C. L. (1978). Hypnosis as a psi-conducive state: A controlled replication study. *J. of Parapsychology* **42**(4):257-275.

Sarles, R. M. (1975). The use of hypnosis with hospitalized children. *J. of Clinical Child Psychology* **4**(3):36-38.

Saunders, C. (1969). The amount of truth. In L. Pearson (Ed.), *Death and Dying: Current Issues in the Treatment of the Dying Person*. Cleveland: Press of Case Western Reserve University.

Scagnelli, J. (1976). Hypnotherapy with schizophrenic and borderline patients: Summary of therapy with eight patients. *American J. of Clinical Hypnosis* **19**(1):33-38.

Scagnelli, J. (1977). Hypnotic dream therapy with a borderline schizophrenic: A case study. *American J. of Clinical Hypnosis* **20**(2):136-145.

Scagnelli, J. (1980). Hypnotherapy with psychotic and borderline patients: The use of trance by patient and therapist. *American J. of Clinical Hypnosis* **22**(3):164-169.

Scagnelli-Jobsis, J. (1982). Hypnosis with psychotic patients: A review of the literature and presentation of a theoretical framework. *American J. of Clinical Hypnosis* **25**(1):33-45.

Scagnelli-Jobsis, J. (1983). Hypnosis with psychotic patients: Response to Spiegel. *American J. of Clinical Hypnosis* **25**(4):295-298.

Schafer, D. W. (1975). Hypnosis use on a burn unit. *International J. of Clinical and Experimental Hypnosis* **23**(1):1-14.

Schafer, D. W. (1981). The recognition and hypnotherapy of patients with unrecognized altered states. *American J. of Clinical Hypnosis* **23**(3):176-183.

Schafer, D. W., and Hernandez, A. (1978). Hypnosis, pain and the context of therapy. *International J. of Clinical and Experimental Hypnosis* **26**(3):143-153.

Schafer, D. W., and Rubio, R. (1978). Hypnosis to aid the recall of witnesses. *International J. of Clinical and Experimental Hypnosis* **26**(2):81-91.

Schathin, A. J. (1978). Admissibility of polygraph evidence in the state of New York. *Nassau Lawyer* **25**(7):331-343.

Schell, R. E. (Ed.). (1975). *Developmental Psychology Today.* New York: Random House.

Schilder, P. (1956). *The Nature of Hypnosis.* New York: International Universities Press.

Schirado, W. C. (1979). The effects of standardized and personalized hypnotic induction techniques on depth of trance. *Dissertation Abstracts International* **40**(6-B):2856.

Schlutter, L. C. (1979). A comparison of treatments for prefrontal muscle contraction headache. *Dissertation Abstracts International* **39**(10-B):5086.

Schneck, J. M. (1954). Ichthyosis treated with hypnosis. *Dis. Nerv. Sys.* **15**:211-214.

Schneck, J. M. (1965). A reevaluation of Freud's abandonment of hypnosis. *J. of the History of the Behavioral Sciences* **1**(2):191-195.

Schneck, J. M. (1975). Prehypnotic suggestion in psychotherapy. *American J. of Clinical Hypnosis* **17**(3):158-159.

Schneck, J. M. (1976). Freud's "medical hypnotist." *American J. of Clinical Hypnosis* **19**(2):80-81.

Schneck, J. M. (1977*a*). Hypnotherapy for ptyalism. *International J. of Clinical and Experimental Hypnosis* **25**(1):1-3.

Schneck, J. M. (1977*b*). Sleep paralysis and microsomatognosia with special reference to hypnotherapy. *International J. of Clinical and Experimental Hypnosis* **25**(2):72-77.

Schneck, J. M. (1978*a*). Benjamin Rush and animal magnetism, 1789 and 1812. *International J. of Clinical and Experimental Hypnosis* **26**(1):9-14.

Schneck, J. M. (1978*b*). Henry James, George Du Maurier, and Mesmerism. *International J. of Clinical and Experimental Hypnosis* **26**(2):76-80.

Schneck, J. M. (1980). Hypnotherapy for narcolepsy. *International J. of Clinical and Experimental Hypnosis* **28**(2):95-100.

Schneck, J. M. (1985). A history of the founding of the American Board of Medical Hypnosis. *American J. of Clinical Hypnosis* **27**(4):241-244.

Schofield, L. J., and Platoni, K. (1976). Manipulation of visual imagery under various hypnosis conditions. *American J. of Clinical Hypnosis* **18**(3):191-199.

Schofield, L. J., and Reyher, J. (1974). Thematic productions under hypnotically aroused conflict in age regressed and waking states using the real-simulator design. *J. of Abnormal Psychology* **83**(2):130-139.

Scholder, M. H. (1982). The argument against the use of hypnosis to improve or enhance the memory of courtroom witnesses. *Law and Psychology Review* **7**:71-86.

Schraa, J. C., and Dirks, J. F. (1981). Hypnotic treatment of the alexithymic patient: A case report. *American J. of Clinical Hypnosis* **23**(3):207-210.

Schulman, R. E., and London, P. (1963). Hypnosis and verbal learning. *J. of Abnormal and Social Psychology* **67**:363-370.

Schuyler, B. A., and Coe, W. C. (1981). A physiological investigation of volitional and nonvolitional experience during posthypnotic amnesia. *J. of Personality and Social Psychology* **40**(6):1160-1169.

Schwarz, B. E.; Bickford, R. G.; and Rasmussen, W. C. (1955). Hypnotic phenomena including hypnotically activated seizures studied with the electroencephalogram. *J. of Nervous and Mental Disease* **122**:564.

Schwartz, W. (1978a). Time and context during hypnotic involvement. *International J. of Clinical and Experimental Hypnosis* **26**(4):307-316.

Schwartz, W. R. (1978b). Time and context in the hypnotic state: An examination of some state specific effects. *Dissertation Abstracts International* **38**(7-B):3415.

Schwartz, W. (1980). Hypnosis and episodic memory. *International J. of Clinical and Experimental Hypnosis* **28**(4):375-385.

Scott, D. L. (1974). *Modern Hospital Hypnosis: Especially for Anaesthetists.* London: Lloyd-Luke.

Scott, D. L. (1975). Hypnosis in plastic surgery. *American J. of Clinical Hypnosis* **18**(2):98-104.

Scott, E. M. (1977). Hypnosis in the courtroom. *American J. of Clinical Hypnosis* **19**(3):163-165.

Scott, E. M. (1978). Hypnosis with an alleged blackout. *American J. of Clinical Hypnosis* **20**(3):209-212.

Scrignar, C. B. (1981). Rapid treatment of contamination phobia with handwashing compulsion by flooding with hypnosis. *American J. of Clinical Hypnosis* **23**(4):252-257.

Sears, A. B. (1954). A comparison of hypnotic and waking recall. *J. of Clinical and Experimental Hypnosis* **2**:296-304.

Sears, A. B. (1955). A comparison of hypnotic and waking learning of the International Morse Code. *J. of Clinical and Experimental Hypnosis* **3**:215-221.

Sears, R. R. (1932). An experimental study of hypnotic anesthesia. *J. of Experimental Psychology* **15**(1):1-22.

Segall, M. M. (1975). *The Questions They Ask about Hypnosis.* South Orange, NJ: Power Pub.

Seif, B. (1982). Hypnosis in a man with fear of voiding in public facilities. *American J. of Clinical Hypnosis* **24**(4):288-289.

Seif, B. (1985). Clinical hypnosis and recurring nightmares: A case report. *American J. of Clinical Hypnosis* **27**(3):166-168.

Selavan, A. (1975). Hypnosis and transactional analysis theory. *American J. of Clinical Hypnosis* **17**(4):260-262.

Sellars, R. W. (1979). In search of hypnotic hypermnesia for contextual material under conditions of retroactive interference.*Dissertation Abstracts International* **40**(3-B):1385.

Sexton, R. O., and Maddock, R. C. (1979). Age regression and age progression in psychotic and neurotic depression. *American J. of Clinical Hypnosis* **22**(1):37-41.

Sextus, C. (1957). *Hypnotism.* 1893. Reprint. Hollywood: Wilshire Book Co.

Shapiro, A. (1982-1983). Psychotherapy as adjunct treatment for cancer patients. *American J. of Clinical Hypnosis* **25**(2-3):150-155.

Shaposhnikov, A. (1982). Some paranormal properties of the human mind: Proceedings of the Third World Congress of psychotronic research. *PSI Research* **1**(2):93-100.

Sharma, A. (1981). Was Ramakrishna a hypnotist? *J. of Psychological Researches* **25**(2):105-107.

Shaul, R. D. (1978). Eyewitness testimony and hypnotic hypermnesia. *Dissertation Abstracts International* **39**(5-B):2521.

Shaw, L. H. (1978). Hypnosis and drama: A note on a novel use of self-hypnosis. *International J. of Clinical and Experimental Hypnosis* **26**(3):154-157.

Sheehan, D. V. (1978). Influence of psychosocial factors on wart remission. *American J. of Clinical Hypnosis* **20**(3):160-164.

Sheehan, D. V.; Latta, W. D.; Regina, E. G.; and Smith, G. M. (1979). Empirical assessment of Spiegel's Hypnotic Induction Profile and eye-roll hypothesis. *International J. of Clinical and Experimental Hypnosis* **27**(2):103-110.

Sheehan, E. P.; Smith, H. V.; and Forrest, D. W. (1982). A signal detection study of the effects of suggested improvement on the monocular visual acuity of myopes. *International J. of Clinical and Experimental Hypnosis* **30**(2):138-146.

Sheehan, P. W. (1973). Analysis of the heterogeneity of "faking" and "simulating" performance in the hypnotic setting. *International J. of Clinical and Experimental Hypnosis* **21**(3):213-225.

Sheehan, P. W. (1977). Incongruity in trance behavior: A defining property of hypnosis? Annals of New York Academy of Sciences **296**:194-207.

Sheehan, P. W. (1979). Clinical and research hypnosis: Toward rapprochement. *Australian J. of Clinical and Experimental Hypnosis* **7**(2):135-146.

Sheehan, P. W. (1980). Factors influencing rapport in hypnosis. *J. of Abnormal Psychology* **89**(2):263-281.

Sheehan, P. W. (1982). Imagery and hypnosis—Forging a link, at least in part. *Research Communications in Psychology, Psychiatry and Behavior* **7**(2):257-272.

Sheehan, P. W., and Dolby, R. M. (1975). Hypnosis and the influence of most recently perceived events. *J. of Abnormal Psychology* **84**(4):331-345.

Sheehan, P. W., and Dolby, R. M. (1979). Motivated involvement in hypnosis: The illustration of clinical rapport through hypnotic dreams. *J. of Abnormal Psychology* **88**(5):573-583.

Sheehan, P. W.; Grigg, L.; and McCann, T. (1984). Memory distortion following exposure to false information in hypnosis. *J. of Abnormal Psychology* **93**(3):259-265.

Sheehan, P. W., and McConkey, K. M. (1979). Australian norms for the Harvard Group Scale of Hypnotic Susceptibility, Form A. *International J. of Clinical and Experimental Hypnosis* **27**(3):294-304.

Sheehan, P. W., and McConkey, K. M. (1982). *Hypnosis and Experience: The Exploration of Phenomena and Process.* Hillsdale, NJ: Erlbaum.

Sheehan, P. W.; McConkey, K. M.; and Cross, D. (1978). Experimental analysis of hypnosis: Some new observations on hypnotic phenomena. *J. of Abnormal Psychology* **87**(5):570-573.

Sheehan, P. W.; Obstoj, I.; and McConkey, K. (1976). Trance logic and cue structure as supplied by the hypnotist. *J. of Abnormal Psychology* **85**(5):459-472.

Sheehan, P. W., and Orne, M. T. (1968). Some comments on the nature of posthypnotic behavior. *J. of Nervous and Mental Disease* **146**(3):209-220.

Sheehan, P. W., and Perry, C. W. (1976). *Methodologies of Hypnosis: A Critical Appraisal of Contemporary Paradigms of Hypnosis.* Hillsdale, NJ: Erlbaum.

Sheehan, P. W., and Tilden, J. (1983). Effects of suggestibility and hypnosis on accurate and distorted retrieval from memory. *J. of Experimental Psychology: Learning, Memory, and Cognition* **9**(2):283-293.

Sheehan, P. W., and Tilden, J. (1984). Real and simulated occurrences of memory distortion in hypnosis. *J. of Abnormal Psychology* **93**(1):47-57.

Sheldon, W. H. (1954). *Atlas of Men.* New York: Harper & Brothers.

Shepperson, V. L., and Henslin, E. R. (1984). Hypnosis and metaphor in Christian context: History, abuse and use. *J. of Psychology and Theology* **12**(2):100-108.

Shiel, R. C. (1982). Hypnosis and verbal functioning. *Dissertation Abstracts International* **43**(6-B):2003.

Shor, R. E. (1970). *The Inventory of Self-Hypnosis. (Form A): Breaths Version.* Durham, NH: Symbolic Process Laboratory.

Shor, R. E., and Easton, R. D. (1973). A preliminary report on research comparing self- and hetero-hypnosis. *American J. of Clinical Hypnosis* **16**:37-44.

Shor, R. E., and Orne, E. C. (1962). *Manual: Harvard Group Scale of Hypnotic Susceptibility, Form A.* Palo Alto: Consulting Psychologists Press.

Shor, R. E.; Orne, M. T.; and O'Connell, D. N. (1962). Validation and cross-validation of a scale of self-reported personal experiences which predicts hypnotizability. *J. of Psychology* **53**:55-75.

Shor, R. E.; Orne, M. T.; and O'Connell, D. N. (1966). Psychological correlates of plateau hypnotizability in a special volunteer sample. *J. of Personality and Social Psychology* **3**(1):80-95.

Shor, R. E.; Pistole, D. D.; Easton, R. D.; and Kihlstrom, J. F. (1984). Relation of predicted to actual hypnotic responsiveness, with special reference to posthypnotic amnesia. *International J. of Clinical and Experimental Hypnosis* **32**(4):376-387.

Shulik, A. M. (1979). Right versus left hemispheric communication styles in hypnotic inductions and the facilitation of hypnotic trance. *Dissertation Abstracts International* **40**(6-B):2826.

Siegel, E. F. (1979). Control of phantom limb pain by hypnosis. *American J. of Clinical Hypnosis* **21**(4):285-286.

Silber, S. (1973). Fairy tales and symbols in hypnotherapy of children with certain speech disorders. *International J. of Clinical and Experimental Hypnosis* **21**(4):272-283.

Silber, S. (1980). Induction of hypnosis by poetic hypnogram. *American J. of Clinical Hypnosis* **22**(4):212-216.

Silberner, J. (1986). Hypnotism under the knife. *Science News* **129**(12):186-187.

Silver, M. J. (1974). Hypnotizability as a function of repression, adaptive regression, and mood. *J. of Consulting and Clinical Psychology* **42**(1):41-46.

Simek, T. C., and O'Brien, R. M. (1981). *Total Golf.* Garden City, NY: Doubleday.

Simon, J. (1977). Creativity and altered states of consciousness. *American J. of Psychoanalysis* **37**(1):3-12.

Simon, M. J. (1983). The effect of manipulated expectancies on posthypnotic amnesia. *Dissertation Abstracts International* **43** (7-B):2358.

Simon, M. J., and Salzberg, H. C. (1981). Electromyographic feedback and taped relaxation instructions to modify hypnotic susceptibility and amnesia. *American J. of Clinical Hypnosis* **24**(1):14-21.

Simon, M. J., and Salzberg, H. C. (1985). The effect of manipulated expectancies on posthypnotic amnesia. *International J. of Clinical and Experimental Hypnosis* **33**(1):40-51.

Singer, J. L., and Pope, K. S. (1981). Daydreaming and imagery skills as predisposing capacities for self-hypnosis. *International J. of Clinical and Experimental Hypnosis* **29**(3):271-281.

Skiba, A. H. (1983). The comparative efficacy of traditional hypnotic and rapid induction analgesia. *Dissertation Abstracts International* **43**(12B):4161.

Slavin, R. J. (1977). Differences in the subjective experience of hypnosis: A comparison of female field-independent and female field-dependent subjects at three depths of hypnosis. *Dissertation Abstracts International* **37**(8-B):4168.

Sloane, M. C. (1981). A comparison of hypnosis vs. waking state and visual vs. non-visual recall instructions for witness/victim memory retrieval in actual major crimes. *Dissertation Abstracts International* **42**(6-B):2551.

Smigielski, J. S. (1982). Imagery enhancement: An investigation of the effects of hypnosis and practice. *Dissertation Abstracts International* **43**(6-B):2004.

Smith, D. E. (1980). Hypnotic susceptibility and eye movement during rest. *American J. of Clinical Hypnosis* **22**(3):147-155.

Smith, H. D. (1975). The use of hypnosis in treating inorgasmic sexual response in women. *J. of American Institute of Hypnosis* **16**(3):119-125.

Smith, H. V.; Forrest, D. W.; and Sheehan, E. P. (1983). Suggested improvement, music and the visual acuity of myopes: A reply. *International J. of Clinical and Experimental Hypnosis* **31**(4):241-242.

Smith, M. C. (1983). Hypnotic memory enhancement of witnesses: Does it work? *Psychological Bulletin* **94**(3):387-407.

Smith, M. S., and Kamitsuka, M. (1984). Self-hypnosis misinterpreted as CNS deterioration in an adolescent with leukemia and vincristine toxicity. *American J. of Clinical Hypnosis* **26**(4):280-282.

Smith, S. J., and Balaban, A. B. (1983). A multidimensional approach to pain relief: Case report of a patient with systemic lupus erythematosus. *International J. of Clinical and Experimental Hypnosis* **31**(2):72-81.

Smyth, L. D. (1981a). Towards a social learning theory of hypnosis: I. Hypnotic suggestibility. *American J. of Clinical Hypnosis* **23**(3):147-168.

Smyth, L. D. (1981b). An experimental hypnotic approach to teaching the psychoanalytic theory of the neurosis. *International J. of Clinical and Experimental Hypnosis* **29**(2):101-106.

Smyth, L. D. (1982). Psychopathology as a function of neuroticism and a hypnotically implanted aggressive conflict. *J. of Personality and Social Psychology* **43**(3);555-564.

Smyth, L. D., and Lowy, D. (1983). Auditory vigilance during hypnosis: A brief communication. *International J. of Clinical and Experimental Hypnosis* **31**(2):67-71.

Snyder, E. D., and Shor, R. E. (1983). Trance-inductive poetry: A brief communication. *International J. of Clinical and Experimental Hypnosis* **31**(1):1-7.

Sochevanov, N. (1984). The influence of certain factors on the intensity of the biophysical effect. *PSI Research* **3**(1):16-20.

Solovey, G., and Milechnin, A. (1957). Concerning the nature of hypnotic phenomena. *J. of Clinical and Experimental Hypnosis* **5**:67-76.

Sommerschield, H., and Reyher, J. (1973). Posthypnotic conflict, repression and psychopathology. *J. of Abnormal Psychology* **82**(2):278-290.

Soper, P. H., and L'Abate, L. (1977). Paradox as a therapeutic technique: A review. *International J. of Family Counseling* **5**(1):10-21.

Spanos, N. P. (1970). Barber's reconceptualization of hypnosis: An evaluation of criticisms. *J. of Experimental Research in Personality* **4**:241-258.

Spanos, N. P. (1971). Goal directed fantasy and the performance of hypnotic test suggestions. *Psychiatry* **34**:86-96.

Spanos, N. P. (1982). Hypnotic behavior: A cognitive, social psychological perspective. *Research Communications in Psychology, Psychiatry and Behavior* **7**(2):199-213.

Spanos, N. P. (1983). The hidden observer as an experimental creation. *J. of Personality and Social Psychology* **44**(1):170-176.

Spanos, N. P.; Ansari, F.; and Stam, H. J. (1979). Hypnotic age regression and eidetic imagery: A failure to replicate. *J. of Abnormal Psychology* **88**(1):88-91.

Spanos, N. P., and Barber, T. X. (1968). "Hypnotic" experiences as inferred from subjective reports: Auditory and visual hallucinations. *J. of Experimental Research in Personality* **3**(2):136-150.

Spanos, N. P., and Barber, T. X. (1974). Toward a convergence in hypnotic research. *American Psychologist* **29**(7):500-511.

Spanos, N. P., and Barber,T. X. (1976). Behavior modification and hypnosis. In M. Hersen et al (Ed.), *Progress in Behavior Modification: Vol 3.* (pp. 1-44). New York: Academic Press.

Spanos, N. P., and Bertrand, L. D. (1985). EMG biofeedback, attained relaxation and hypnotic susceptibility: Is there a relationship? *American J. of Clinical Hypnosis* **27**(4):219-225.

Spanos, N. P., and Bodorik, H. L. (1977). Suggested amnesia and disorganized recall in hypnotic and task-motivated subjects. *J. of Abnormal Psychology* **86**(3):295-305.

Spanos, N. P.; Churchill, N.; and McPeake, J. D. (1976). Experimental response to auditory and visual hallucination suggestions in hypnotic subjects. *J. of Consulting and Clinical Psychology* **44**(5):729-738.

Spanos, N. P., and De Groh, M. (1983). Structure of communication and reports of involuntariness by hypnotic and nonhypnotic subjects. *Perceptual and Motor Skills* **57**(3, part 2):1179-1186.

Spanos, N. P.; De Groh, M.; and Weekes, J. R. (1984). Involuntariness and attributions: A reply to Zamansky and Bartis. *British J. of Experimental and Clinical Hypnosis* **2**(1):53-54.

Spanos, N. P., and D'Eon, J. L. (1980). Hypnotic amnesia, disorganized recall, and inattention. *J. of Abnormal Psychology* **89**(6):744-750.

Spanos, N. P.; Dubreuil, D. L.; Saad, C. L.; and Gorassini, D. (1983). Hypnotic elimination of prism-induced aftereffects: Perceptual effect or responses to experimental demands? *J. of Abnormal Psychology* **92**(2):216-222.

Spanos, N. P., and Gorassini, D. R. (1984). Structure of hypnotic test suggestions and attributions of responding involuntarily. *J. of Personality and Social Psychology* **46**(3):688-696.

Spanos, N. P.; Gorassini, D. R.; and Petrusic, W. (1981). Hypnotically induced limb anesthesia and adaptation to displacing prisms: A failure to confirm. *J. of Abnormal Psychology* **90**(4):329-333.

Spanos, N. P., and Gottlieb, J. (1979). Demonic possession, mesmerism, and hysteria: A social psychological perspective on their historical interrelations. *J. of Abnormal Psychology* **88**(5):527-546.

Spanos, N., and Ham, M. W. (1975). Involvement in suggestion-related imagings and the "hypnotic dream." *American J. of Clinical Hypnosis* **18**(1):43-51.

Spanos, N. P., and Hewitt, E.C. (1980). The hidden observer in hypnotic analgesia: Discovery or experimental creation? *J. of Personality and Social Psychology* **39**(6):1201-1214.

Spanos, N. P.; Horton, C.; and Chaves, J. F. (1975). The effects of two cognitive strategies on pain threshold. *J. of Abnormal Psychology* **84**(6):677-681.

Spanos, N. P.; Jones, B.; and Malfara, A. (1982). Hypnotic deafness: Now you hear it—now you still hear it. *J. of Abnormal Psychology* **91**(1):75-77.

Spanos, N. P.; Kennedy, S. K.; and Gwynn, M. I. (1984). Moderating effects of contextual variables on the relationship between hypnotic susceptibility and suggested analgesia. *J. of Abnormal Psychology* **93**(3):285-294.

Spanos, N. P.; McNeil, C.; Gwynn, M. I.; and Stam, H. J. (1984). Effects of suggestion and distraction on reported pain in subjects high and low on hypnotic susceptibility. *J. of Abnormal Psychology* **93**(3):277-284.

Spanos, N. P.; McNeil, C.; and Stam, H. J. (1982). Hypnotically "reliving" a prior burn: Effects on blister formation and localized skin temperature. *J. of Abnormal Psychology* **91**(4):303-305.

Spanos, N. P., and McPeake, J. D. (1975a). Involvement in everyday imaginative activities, attitudes toward hypnosis and hypnotic suggestibility. *J. of Personality and Social Psychology* **31**(3):594-598.

Spanos, N. P. and McPeake, J. D. (1975*b*). The interaction of attitudes toward hypnosis and involvement in everyday imaginative activities on hypnotic suggestibility. *American J. of Clinical Hypnosis* **17**(4):247-252.

Spanos, N. P., and McPeake, J. D. (1977). Cognitive strategies, reported goal-directed fantasy, and response to suggestion in hypnotic subjects. *American J. of Clinical Hypnosis* **20**(2):114-123.

Spanos, N. P.; McPeake, J. D.; and Carter, W. (1973). Effects of pretesting on response to a visual hallucination suggestion in hypnotic subjects. *J. of Personality and Social Psychology* **28**(3):293-297.

Spanos, N. P.; McPeake, J. D.; and Churchill, N. (1976). Relationships between imaginative ability variables and the Barber Suggestibility Scale. *American J. of Clinical Hypnosis* **19**(1):39-46.

Spanos, N. P.; Mullens, D.; and Rivers, S. M. (1979). The effects of suggestion structure and hypnotic vs. task-motivation instructions on response to hallucination suggestions. *J. of Research in Personality* **13**(1):59-70.

Spanos, N. P.; Nightingale, M. E.; Radtke, H. L.; and Stam, H. J. (1980). The stuff hypnotic "dreams" are made of. *J. of Mental Imagery* **4**(2):99-110.

Spanos, N. P., and Radtke, H. L. (1982). Hypnotic amnesia as strategic enactment: A cognitive, social-psychological perspective. *Research Communications in Psychology, Psychiatry and Behavior* **7**(2):215-231.

Spanos, N. P.; Radtke, H. L.; Bertrand, L. D.; Addie, D. L.; and Drummond, J. (1982). Disorganized recall, hypnotic amnesia and subjects' faking: More disconfirmatory evidence. *Psychological Reports* **50**(2):383-389.

Spanos, N. P.; Radtke, H. L.; and Dubreuil, D. L. (1982). Episodic and semantic memory in posthypnotic amnesia: A reevaluation. *J. of Personality and Social Psychology* **43**(3):565-573.

Spanos, N. P.; Radtke-Bodorik, H. L.; Ferguson, J. D.; and Jones, B. (1979). The effects of hypnotic susceptibility, suggestions for analgesia, and the utilization of cognitive strategies on the reduction of pain. *J. of Abnormal Psychology* **88**(3):282-292.

Spanos, N. P.; Radtke-Bodorik, H. L.; and Shabinsky, M. A. (1980). Amnesia, subjective organization and learning of a list of unrelated words in hypnotic and task-motivated subjects. *International J. of Clinical and Experimental Hypnosis* **28**(2):126-139.

Spanos, N. P.; Radtke-Bodorik, H. L.; and Stam, H. J. (1980). Disorganized recall during suggested amnesia: Fact not artifact. *J. of Abnormal Psychology* **89**(1):1-19.

Spanos, N. P.; Rivers, S. M.; and Gottlieb, J. (1978). Hypnotic responsivity, meditation, and laterality of eye movements. *J. of Abnormal Psychology* **87**(5):566-569.

Spanos, N. P.; Rivers, S. M.; and Ross, S. (1977). Experienced involuntariness and response to hypnotic suggestions. *Annals of New York Academy of Sciences* **296**:208-221.

Spanos, N. P.; Spillane, J.; and McPeake, J. D. (1976). Cognitive strategies and response to suggestion in hypnotic and task-motivated subjects. *American J. of Clinical Hypnosis* **18**(4):254-262.

Spanos, N. P.; Stam, H. J.; D'Eon, J. L.; Pawlak, A. E.; and Radtke-Bodorik, H. L. (1980b).Effects of social-psychological variables on hypnotic amnesia. *J. of Personality and Social Psychology* **39**(4):737-750.

Spanos, N. P.; Stam, H. J.; Rivers, S. M.; and Radtke, H. L. (1980). Meditation, expectation and performance on indices of nonanalytic attending. *International J. of Clinical and Experimental Hypnosis* **28**(3):244-251.

Spanos, N. P.; Tkachyk, M. E.; Bertrand, L. D.; and Weekes, J. R. (1984). The dissipation hypothesis of hypnotic amnesia: More disconfirming evidence. *Psychological Reports* **55**(1):191-196.

Sparks, L. (1962). *Self Hypnosis.* New York: Grune & Stratton.

Spiegel, D. (1980). Hypnotizability and psychoactive medication. *American J. of Clinical Hypnosis* **22**(4):217-222.

Spiegel, D. (1981). Vietnam grief work using hypnosis. *American J. of Clinical Hypnosis* **24**(1):33-40.

Spiegel, D. (1983). Hypnosis with psychotic patients: Comment on Scagnelli-Jobsis. *American J. of Clinical Hypnosis* **25**(4):289-294.

Spiegel, D. (1985). The use of hypnosis in controlling cancer pain. *Ca-A Cancer J. for Clinicians* **35**(4):221-231.

Spiegel, D.; Frischholz, E. J.; Maruffi, B.; and Spiegel, H. (1981). Hypnotic responsivity and the treatment of flying phobia. *American J. of Clinical Hypnosis* **23**(4):239-247.

Spiegel, D., and Rosenfeld, A. (1984). Spontaneous hypnotic age regression: Case report. *J. of Clinical Psychiatry* **45**(12):522-524.

Spiegel, D., and Spiegel, H. (1984). Uses of hypnosis in evaluating malingering and deception. *Behavioral Sciences and the Law* **2**(1):51-65.

Spiegel, H. (1974a). *Manual for Hypnotic Induction Profile—Eye Roll Levitation Method.* New York: Soni Medica.

Spiegel, H. (1974b). The grade 5 syndrome: The highly hypnotizable person. *International J. of Clinical and Experimental Hypnosis* **22**(4):303-319.

Spiegel, H. (1977). The Hypnotic Induction Profile (HIP): A review of its development. *Annals of New York Academy of Sciences* **296**:129-142.

Spiegel, H.; Aronson, M.; Fleiss, J. L.; and Haber, J. (1976). Psychometric analysis of the Hypnotic Induction Profile. *International J. of Clinical and Experimental Hypnosis* **24**(3):300-315.

Spiegel, H., and Linn, L. (1969). The "ripple effect" following adjunct hypnosis in analytic psychotherapy. *American J. of Psychiatry* **126**:53-58.

Spiegel, H.; Samuelly, I.; and McPherson, D. (1982). Comments on the ISH code of ethics and resolution. *Bulletin of the British Society of Experimental and Clinical Hypnosis* **1982**(5):77-79.

Spiegel, H.; Shor, J.; and Fishman, S. (1945). An hypnotic ablation technique for the study of personality development. *Psychosomatic Medicine* **7**:273.

Spiegel, H., and Spiegel, D. (1978). *Trance and Treatment: Clinical Uses of Hypnosis*. New York: Basic Books.

Spies, G. (1979). Desensitization of test anxiety: Hypnosis compared with biofeedback. *American J. of Clinical Hypnosis* **22**(2):108-111.

Spithill, A. C. (1974). Treatment of a monosymptomatic tic by hypnosis: A case study. *American J. of Clinical Hypnosis* **17**(2):88-93.

Springer, C. J.; Sach, L. B.; and Morrow, J. E. (1977). Group methods of increasing hypnotic susceptibility. *International J. of Clinical and Experimental Hypnosis* **25**(3):184-191.

Stacher, G.; Schuster, P.; Bauer, P.; Lahoda, R.; and Shulze, D. (1975). Effects of suggestion of relaxation or analgesia on pain threshold and pain tolerance in the waking and in the hypnotic state. *J. of Psychosomatic Research* **19**:259-265.

Stager, G. L., and Lundy, R. M. (1985). Hypnosis and the learning and recall of visually presented material. *International J. of Clinical and Experimental Hypnosis* **33**(1):27-39.

Staib, A. R., and Logan, D. R. (1977). Hypnotic stimulation of breast growth. *American J. of Clinical Hypnosis* **19**(4):201-208.

Stalnaker, J. M., and Riddle, E. E. (1932). The effect of hypnosis on long delayed recall. *J. of General Psychology* **6**:429-440.

Stam, H. J., Petrusic, W. M.; and Spanos, N. P. (1981). Magnitude scales for cold pressor pain. *Perception and Psychophysics* **29**(6):612-617.

Stam, H. J.; Radtke-Bodorik, H. L.; and Spanos, N. P. (1980). Repression and hypnotic amnesia: A failure to replicate and an alternative formulation. *J. of Abnormal Psychology* **89**(4):551-559.

Stam, H. J., and Spanos, N. P. (1980). Experimental designs, expectancy effects, and hypnotic analgesia. *J. of Abnormal Psychology* **89**(6):751-762.

Stam, H. J., and Spanos, N. P. (1982). The Asclepian dream healings and hypnosis: A critique. *International J. of Clinical and Experimental Hypnosis* **30**(1):9-22.

Stambaugh, E. E. (1977). Hypnotic treatment of depression in the Parkinsonian patient: A case study. *American J. of Clinical Hypnosis* **19**(3):185-186.

Stambaugh II, E. E., and House, A. E. (1977). Multimodality treatment of migraine headache: A case study utilizing biofeedback, relaxation, auto-genic and hypnotic treatments. *American J. of Clinical Hypnosis* **19**(4):235-240.

Stanley, R. O. (1984). Exhibitionism: A three phase intervention. *Australian J. of Clinical and Experimental Hypnosis* **12**(1):31-36.

Stanton, H. E. (1975a). Weight loss through hypnosis. *American J. of Clinical Hypnosis* **18**(1):34-38.

Stanton, H. E. (1975b). Weight loss through hypnosis. *American J. of Clinical Hypnosis* **18**(2):94-97.

Stanton, H. E. (1976a). Hypnosis and encounter group volunteers: A validation study of the Sensation-Seeking Scale. *J. of Counseling and Clinical Psychology* **44**(4):692.

Stanton, H. E. (1976b). Fee-paying and weight loss: Evidence for an interesting interaction. *American J. of Clinical Hypnosis* 19(1)47-49.

Stanton, H. E. (1977). The utilization of suggestions derived from rational-emotive therapy. *International J. of Clinical and Experimental Hypnosis* **25**(1):18-26.

Stanton, H. E. (1978a Hypnotherapy at a distance through use of the telephone. *American J. of Clinical Hypnosis* **20**(4):278-281.

Stanton, H. E. (1978b). A one-session hypnotic approach to modifying smoking behavior. *International J. of Clinical and Experimental Hypnosis* **26**(1):22-29.

Stanton, H. E. (1979a). Short-term treatment of enuresis. *American J. of Clinical Hypnosis* **22**(2):103-107.

Stanton, H. E. (1979b). Increasing internal control through hypnotic ego-enhancement. *Australian J. of Clinical and Experimental Hypnosis* **7**(3):219-223.

Stanton, H. E. (1979c). Elaborations on Elton's "secret room." *Australian J. of Clinical and Experimental Hypnosis* **7**(3):283-285.

Stanton, H. E. (1981). Enuresis, homoeopathy, and enhancement of the placebo effect. *American J. of Clinical Hypnosis* **24**(1):59-61.

Stanton, H. E. (1982). Changing the personal history of the bed-wetting child. *Australian J. of Clinical and Experimental Hypnosis* **10**(2):103-107.

Starker, S. (1973). Hysterical reactions to hypnotic induction. *Psychotherapy: Theory, Research and Practice* **10**(2):141-144.

Starker, S. (1975). Implications of the behavioral approach to hypnosis. *American J. of Psychotherapy* **29**(3):402-408.

Stava, L. (1984). The use of hypnotic uncovering techniques in the treatment of pedophilia: A brief communication. *International J. of Clinical and Experimental Hypnosis* **32**(4):350-355.

Stein, C. (1975). Brief hypnotherapy for conversion cephalgia (repression headache). *American J. of Clinical Hypnosis* **17**(3):198-201.

Stein, V. T. (1980). Hypnotherapy of involuntary movements in an 82-year-old male. *American J. of Clinical Hypnosis* **23**(2):128-131.

Stein, V. T. (1982). The effect of traditional hypnosis, alert hypnosis and task motivation suggestions on the recall of contextual material by college students. *Dissertation Abstracts International* **42**(10-B):4176-4177.

Stern, D. A. (1982). The effect of a Ganzfeld and an experimentally induced demand upon free association. *Dissertation Abstracts International* **43**(3-B):887.

Stern, D. B.; Spiegel, H.; and Nee, J. C. M. (1978-1979). The Hypnotic Induction Profile: Normative observations, reliability and validity. *American J. of Clinical Hypnosis* **21**(2-3):109-133.

Stern, J. A.; Brown, M.; Ulett, G. A.; and Sletten, I. (1977). A comparison of hypnosis, acupuncture, morphine, Valium, aspirin, and placebo in the management of experimentally induced pain. *Annals of New York Academy of Sciences* **296**:175-193.

Sternbach, R. A. (1982). On strategies for identifying neurochemical correlates of hypnotic analgesia: A brief communication. *International J. of Clinical and Experimental Hypnosis* **30**(3):251-256.

Sternlicht, M., and Wanderer, Z. W. (1963). Hypnotic susceptibility and mental deficiency. *International J. of Clinical and Experimental Hypnosis* **11**:104-111.

Stevenson, J. H. (1973). *The effect of hypnotic and post hypnotic dissociation on the performance of interfering tasks.* Doctoral Dissertation, Stanford University, Ann Arbor, MI: University Microfilms. No. 73-4601.

Stevenson, J. H. (1976). Effect of posthypnotic dissociation on the performance of interfering tasks. *J. of Abnormal Psychology* **85**(4):398-407.

Stevenson, R. (1978). Self-hypnosis for the athlete. *Hypnosis Quarterly* **21**(3):11-16.

St. Jean, R. (1978). Posthypnotic behavior as a function of experimental surveillance. *American J. of Clinical Hypnosis* **20**(4):250-255.

St. Jean, R. (1980). Hypnotic time distortion and learning: Another look. *J. of Abnormal Psychology* **89**(1):20-24.

St. Jean, R., and Coe, W. C. (1981). Recall and recognition memory during posthypnotic amnesia: A failure to confirm the disrupted-search hypothesis and the memory disorganization hypothesis. *J. of Abnormal Psychology* **90**(3):231-241.

St. Jean, R., and MacLeod, C. (1983). Hypnosis, absorption, and time perception. *J. of Abnormal Psychology* **92**(1):81-86.

St. Jean, R.; MacLeod, C.; Coe, W. C.; and Howard, M. (1982). Amnesia and hypnotic time estimation. *International J. of Clinical and Experimental Hypnosis* **30**(2):127-137.

Stolzenberg, J., and Kroger, W. S. (1961). *Dental Hypnosis.* Hollywood: Wilshire Book Co.

Stone, H. (1977). Pain, fear and stress phenomena in dental patients. In A. R. Guerra, *Modern Anesthesia in Dentistry* (pp. 1-4). Philadelphia: Franklin Institute Press.

Stone, J. A. (1981). Direct and indirect suggestions with hypnotized and nonhypnotized subjects. *Dissertation Abstracts International* **41**(10-B):3903.

Stratton, J. G. (1977). The use of hypnosis in law enforcement criminal investigations: A pilot program. *J. of Police Science and Administration* ·**5**(4):399-406.

Straus, R. A. (1977). The life change process: Weight loss and other enterprises of personal transformation, with particular emphasis on hypnosis, behavior modification, and scientology. *Dissertation Abstracts International* **38**(6-A):3767.

Straus, R. A. (1980). A naturalistic experiment investigating the effects of hypnotic induction upon Creative Imagination Scale performance in a clinical setting. *International J. of Clinical and Experimental Hypnosis* **28**(3):218-224.

Stricherz, M. E. (1982). Social influence, Ericksonian strategies and hypnotic phenomena in the treatment of sexual dysfunction. *American J. of Clinical Hypnosis* **24**(3):211-218.

Stromberg, B. V. (1975). The use of subjective questioning in hypnotic psychotherapy. *J. of Clinical Psychology* **31**(1):110-115.

Surman, O. S. (1979). Postnoxious desensitization: Some clinical notes on the combined use of hypnosis and systematic desensitization. *American J. of Clinical Hypnosis* **22**(1):54-60.

Surman, O. S.; Hackett, T. P.; Silverberg, E. L.; and Behrendt, D. M. (1974). Usefulness of psychiatric intervention in patients undergoing cardiac surgery. *Archives of General Psychiatry* **30**(6):830-835.

Sutcliffe, J. P. (1960). "Credulous" and "skeptical" view of hypnotic phenomena: A review of certain evidence and methodology. *International J. of Clinical and Experimental Hypnosis* **8**:73-101.

Sutcliffe, J. P. (1961). "Credulous" and "skeptical" views of hypnotic phenomena: Experiments in (an)esthesia, hallucination and delusion. *J. of Abnormal and Social Psychology* **62**:189-200.

Sutherland, E. B. (1984). The effects of hypnosis upon cerebral hemispheric lateralization. *Dissertation Abstracts International* **44**(11-B):3545.

Swartz, C. M. (1982). Review of G. Ambrose and G. Newbold *Handbook of Medical Hypnosis* and R. Udolf *Handbook of Hypnosis for Professionals* *American J. of Psychiatry* **139**(2):251-252.

Sweeney, C. A.; Lynn, S. J.; and Bellezza, F. S. (1985). Hypnosis, hypnotizability, and imagery-mediated learning. *International J. of Clinical and Experimental Hypnosis* **34**(1):29-40.

Swezey, R. W. (1977-1978). Future directions in simulation and training. *J. of Educational Technology Systems* **6**(4):285-292.

Swiercinsky, D., and Coe, W. C. (1970). Hypnosis, hypnotic responsiveness, and learning meaningful material. *International J. of Clinical and Experimental Hypnosis* **18**(3):217-222.

Swiercinsky, D., and Coe, W. C. (1971). The effect of "alert" hypnosis and hypnotic responsiveness on reading comprehension. *International J. of Clinical and Experimental Hypnosis* **19**(3):146-153.

Taboada, E. L. (1975). Night terrors in a child treated with hypnosis. *American J. of Clinical Hypnosis* **17**(4):270-271.

Tappeiner, D. A. (1977). A psychological paradigm for the interpretation of the charismatic phenomenon of prophecy. *J. of Psychology and Theology* **5**(1):23-29.

Tarasoff v. Regents of University of California. 529 P.2d 553 (1974); 131 Cal. Rptr. 14; 551 P.2d 334 (1976).

Tart, C. T. (1970). Self-report scales of hypnotic depth. *International J. of Clinical and Experimental Hypnosis* **18**(2):105-125.

Tart, C. T. (1978-1979). Quick and convenient assessment of hypnotic depth: self-report scales. *American J. of Clinical Hypnosis* **21**(2-3):186-207.

Tart, C. T., and Hilgard, E. R. (1966). Responsiveness to suggestions under "hypnosis" and "waking-imagination" conditions: A methodological observation. *International J. of Clinical and Experimental Hypnosis* **14**(3):247-256.

Tasini, M. F., and Hackett, T. P. (1977). Hypnosis in the treatment of warts in immunodeficient children. *American J. of Clinical Hypnosis* **19**(3):152-154.

Taub-Bynum, E. B., and House, J. J. (1983). The teaching of hypnosis: Outline and method. *J. of American College Health* **32**(2):82-85.

Taylor, R. E. (1985) Imagery for the treatment of obsessional behavior: A case study. *American J. of Clinical Hypnosis* **27**(3):175-179.

Tebecis, A. K., and Provins, K. A. (1975). Hypnosis and eye movements. *Biological Psychology* **3**:31-47.

Tebecis, A. K., and Provins, K. A. (1976). Further studies of physiological concomitants of hypnosis: Skin temperature, heart rate and skin resistance. *Biological Psychology* **4**:249-257.

Tebecis, A. K.; Provins, K. A.; Farnbach, R. W.; and Pentony, P. (1975). Hypnosis and the EEG. *J. of Nervous and Mental Disease* **161**(1):1-17.

Tellegen, A. (1978-1979). On measures and conceptions of hypnosis. *American J. of Clinical Hypnosis* **21**(2-3):219-237.

Tellegen, A., and Atkinson, G. (1976). Complexity and measurement of hypnotic susceptibility: A comment on Coe and Sarbin's alternative interpretation. *J. of Personality and Social Psychology* **33**(2):142-148.

Teltscher, H. O. (1983). Hypnosis and the patient-therapist relationship. *J. of the American Society of Psychosomatic Dentistry and Medicine* **30**(4):127-134.

Teten, H. D. (1979). A discussion of the precepts surrounding the use of hypnosis as an investigative aid by the Federal Bureau of Investigation. Paper presented at the American Psychological Association 87th Annual Convention in New York City, September.

Thigpen, C. H., and Cleckley, H. M. (1984). On the incidence of multiple personality disorder: A brief communication. *International J. of Clinical and Experimental Hypnosis* **32**(2):63-66.

Thorne, D. E. (1969). Amnesia and hypnosis. *International J. of Clinical and Experimental Hypnosis* **17**(4):225-241.

Thorne, D. E., and Beier, E. G. (1968). Hypnotist and manner of presentation effects on a standardized hypnotic susceptibility test. *J. of Consulting and Clinical Psychology* **32**(5):610-612.

Thorne, D. E., and Fisher, A. G. (1978). Hypnotically suggested asthma. *International J. of Clinical and Experimental Hypnosis* **26**(2):92-103.

Thorne, D. E., and Hall, H. V. (1974). Hypnotic amnesia revisited. *International J. of Clinical and Experimental Hypnosis* **22**(2):167-178.

Thorne, D. E.; Rasmus, C.; and Fisher, A. G. (1976). Are "fat girls" more hypnotically susceptible? *Psychological Reports* **38**(1):267-270.

Tilton, P. (1980). Hypnotic treatment of a child with thumb-sucking, enuresis and encopresis. *American J. of Clinical Hypnosis* **22**(4):238-240.

Tilton, P. (1983). Pseudo-orientation in time in the treatment of agoraphobia. *American J. of Clinical Hypnosis* **25**(4):267-269.

Tilton, P. (1984). The hypnotic hero: A technique for hypnosis with children. *International J. of Clinical and Experimental Hypnosis* **32**(4):366-375.

Time. (1976). Svengali squad: L.A. police. **108**:76 (Sept. 13).

Timm, H. W. (1983). The factors theoretically affecting the impact of forensic hypnosis techniques on eyewitness recall. *J. of Police Science and Administration* **11**(4):442-450.

Timney, B. N., and Barber, T. X. (1969). Hypnotic induction and oral temperature. *International J. of Clinical and Experimental Hypnosis* **17**(2):121-132.

Tinterow, M. M. (1970). *Foundations of Hypnosis.* Springfield, IL: Charles C. Thomas.

Tomlinson, W. K., and Perret, J. J. (1974). Mesmerism in New Orleans, 1845-1861. *American J. of Psychiatry* **131**(12):1402-1404.

Toomey, T. C., and Sanders, S. (1983). Group hypnotherapy as an active control strategy in chronic pain. *American J. of Clinical Hypnosis* **26**(1):20-25.

Torda, C. (1975). Observations on the effects of anxiety and anger on the content of concurrent dreams. *American J. of Clinical Hypnosis* **17**(4):253-259.

Tosi, D. J., and Henderson, G. W. (1983). Rational stage-directed therapy: A cognitive experimental system using hypnosis, imagery, cognitive restructuring, and developmental staging. *J. of Rational-Emotive Therapy* **1**(1):15-19.

Towe, D. H. (1984). Control of electromyographic activity in subjects demon'strating high and low levels of hypnotizability. *Dissertation Abstracts International* **44**(11-B):3545.

Tracy, D. F. (1952). *Hypnosis.* New York: Sterling Publishing Co.

Trenerry, M. R., and Jackson, T. L. (1983). Hysterical dystonia successfully treated with post-hypnotic suggestion. *American J. of Clinical Hypnosis* **26**(1):42-44.

Trevan, W. (1979). Effects of hypnotic age regression on Piagetian cognitive developmental tasks. *Dissertation Abstracts International* **40**(4-B):1919.

Triplet, R. G. (1982). The relationship of Clark L. Hull's hypnosis research to his later learning theory: The continuity of his life's work. *J. of the History of the Behavioral Sciences* **18**(1):22-31.

True, R. M. (1949). Experimental control in hypnotic age regression states. *Science* **110**:583-584.

True, R. M., and Stephenson, C. W. (1951). Controlled experiments correlating electroencephalogram pulse and plantar reflexes with hypnotic age regression and induced emotional states. *Personality* **1**:252-263.

Trustman, R.; Dubovsky, S.; and Titley, R. (1977). Auditory perception during general anesthesia—myth or fact? *International J. of Clinical and Experimental Hypnosis* **25**(2):88-105.

Tuite, P. A.; Braun, B. G.; and Frischholz, E. J. (1986). Hypnosis and eyewitness testimony. *Psychiatric Annals* **16**(2):91-95.

Turco, R. N. (1981). Regrief treatment facilitated by hypnosis. *American J. of Clinical Hypnosis* **24**(1):62-64.

Turco, R. N., and Scott, E. M. (1982). Hypnosis: Complications—An illustrative clinical example. *International J. of Offender Therapy and Comparative Criminology* **26**(2):133-137.

Turin, A. C. (1977). Biofeedback, suggestion, and biofeedback plus suggestion in the induction of voluntary digital hyperthermia: An experimental comparison. *Dissertation Abstracts International* **38**(2-B):920.

Twerski, A. J., and Naar, R. (1976). Guilt clarification via age regression. *American J. of Clinical Hypnosis* **18**(3):204-206.

Udolf, R. (1983). *Forensic Hypnosis—Psychological and Legal Aspects.* Lexington, MA: Lexington Books.

Uherik, A., and Sebej, F. (1979). Effect of hypnotic suggestion on bilateral asymmetry of bioelectrical skin reactivity. *Studia Psychologica* **21**(2):91-97.

Ulett, G. A.; Akpinar, S.; and Itil, T. M. (1972). Hypnosis by video tape. *International J. of Clinical and Experimental Hypnosis* **20**(1):46-51.

Uribe-de-Fazzano, C. (1980). Effectiveness of hypnosis in the treatment of migraine: The role of hypnotizability. *Dissertation Abstracts International* **41**(2-B):703.

U.S. News & World Report. (1978). Hypnotic detectives. Oct. 2:75.

Vacchiano, R. B., and Strauss, P. S. (1975). Dogmatism, authority and hypnotic susceptibility. *American J. of Clinical Hypnosis* **17**(3):185-189.

Van Der Hart, O. (1981). Treatment of a phobia for dead birds: A case report. *American J. of Clinical Hypnosis* **23**(4):263-265.

Van Der Hart, O. (1985). Metaphoric hypnotic imagery in the treatment of functional amenorrhea. *American J. of Clinical Hypnosis* **27**(3):159-165.

Van Dyke, P., and Harris, R. B. (1982). Phobia: A case report. *American J. of Clinical Hypnosis* **24**(4):284-287.

Van Ginneken, J. (1984). The killing of the father: The background of Freud's group psychology. *Political Psychology* **5**(3):391-414.

Van Gorp, W. G.; Meyer, R. G.; and Dunbar, K. D. (1985). The efficacy of direct versus indirect hypnotic induction techniques on reduction of experimental pain. *International J. of Clinical and Experimental Hypnosis* **33**(4):319-328.

Van Nuys, D. W. (1972). Drug use and hypnotic susceptibility. *International J. of Clinical and Experimental Hypnosis* **20**(1):31-37.

Van Nuys, D. W. (1973). Meditation, attention, and hypnotic susceptibility: A correlational study. *International J. of Clinical and Experimental Hypnosis* **21**(2):59-69.

Van Nuys, D. (1975). On the phrasing of hypnotic suggestions: A brief case report. *Psychotherapy: Theory, Research and Practice* **12**(3):302-304.

Van Nuys, D. (1977). Successful treatment of sacroiliac pain by telephone. *J. of American Society of Psychosomatic Dentistry and Medicine* **24**(3):73-75.

Van Pelt, S. J. (1952). Some dangers of stage hypnotism. *British J. of Medical Hypnosis* **3**(2):30-38.

Van Pelt, S. J. (1953). Asthma? Is there any such disease? *British J. of Medical Hypnosis* **4**(3):17-25.

Van Pelt, S. J. (1975a). Hypnosis and space travel. *J. of American Institute of Hypnosis* **16**(6):17-21.

Van Pelt, S. J. (1975b). Hypnosis in business. *J. of American Institute of Hypnosis* **16**(6):42-43.

Van Pelt, S. J. (1975c). Hypnosis and anxiety. *J. of American Institute of Hypnosis* **16**(6):10-15, 45.

Van Pelt, S. J. (1975d). The role of hypnotic suggestion in the aetiology and treatment of the psychoneurotic. *J. of American Institute of Hypnosis* **16**(6):27-33.

Van Pelt, S. J.; Ambrose, G.; and Newbold, G. (1957). *Medical Hypnosis Handbook*. Hollywood: Wilshire Book Co.

Van Rooyen, E. J. (1981). Hypnotherapy of a neurotic reading problem. *American J. of Clinical Hypnosis* **24**(2):124-127.

Venn, J. (1984). The spiral technique of hypnotic induction: A brief communication. *International J. of Clinical and Experimental Hypnosis* **32**(3):287-289.

Vilenskaya, L. (1984). Microphenomena or macrophenomena? Meeting greater challenges. *PSI Research* **3**(1):98-112.

Vingoe, F. J. (1973). Comparison of the Harvard Group Scale of Hypnotic Susceptibility, Form A and the Group Alert Trance Scale in a university population. *International J. of Clinical and Experimental Hypnosis* **21**(3):169-179.

Vingoe, F. J. (1982a). Attitudes of clinical and educational psychologists towards hypnosis training and treatment. *Bulletin of the British Society of Experimental and Clinical Hypnosis* **1982**(5):37-41.

Vingoe, F. J. (1982b). A comment on Gibbons' "Hypnosis as a trance state: The future of a shared delusion." *Bulletin of the British Society of Experimental and Clinical Hypnosis* **1982**(5):8-11.

Vodovnik, L.; Roskar, E.; Pajntar, M.; and Gros, N. (1979). Modeling the voluntary hypnosis-induced motor performance of hemiparetic patients. *IEEE Transactions on Systems, Man, and Cybernetics* **9**(12):850-855.

Wadden, T. A., and Flaxman, J. (1981). Hypnosis and weight loss: A preliminary study. *International J. of Clinical and Experimental Hypnosis* **29**(2):162-173.

Wadden, T. A., and Penrod, J. H. (1981). Hypnosis in the treatment of alcoholism: A review and appraisal. *American J. of Clinical Hypnosis* **24**(1):41-47.

Wagenfeld, J., and Carlson, W. A. (1979). Use of hypnosis in the alleviation of reading problems. *American J. of Clinical Hypnosis* **22**(1):51-53.

Wagstaff, G. F. (1977a). Post-hypnotic amnesia as disrupted retrieval: A role-playing paradigm. *Quarterly J. of Experimental Psychology* **29**(3):499-504.

Wagstaff, G. F. (1977b). An experimental study of compliance and post-hypnotic amnesia. *British J. of Social and Clinical Psychology* **16**(3):225-228.

Wagstaff, G. F. (1977c). Goal-directed fantasy, the experience of nonvolition, and compliance. *Social Behavior and Personality* **5**(2):389-393.

Wagstaff, G. F. (1981). *Hypnosis, Compliance and Belief*. New York: St. Martin.

Wagstaff, G. F. (1982a). Hypnosis and recognition of a face. *Perceptual and Motor Skills* **55**(3, part 1):816-818.

Wagstaff, G. F. (1982b). Amnesia, compliance and men of straw: A tailpiece.

Bulletin of the British Society of Experimental and Clinical Hypnosis **1982**(5):42-45.

Wagstaff, G. F. (1982c). Comment on Gibbons' "Hypnosis as a trance state: The future of a shared delusion." *Bulletin of the British Society of Experimental and Clinical Hypnosis* **1982**(5):5-7.

Wagstaff, G. F. (1983a). A comment on McConkey's "Challenging hypnotic effects: The impact of conflicting influences on response to hypnotic suggestion." *British J. of Experimental and Clinical Hypnosis* **1**(1):11-15.

Wagstaff, G. F. (1983b). Suggested improvement of visual acuity: A statistical reevaluation. *International J. of Clinical and Experimental Hypnosis* **31**(4):239-240.

Wagstaff, G. F. (1984). The enhancement of witness memory by "hypnosis": A review and methodological critique of the experimental literature. *British J. of Experimental and Clinical Hypnosis* **2**(1):3-12.

Wagstaff, G. F., and Ovenden, M. (1979). Hypnotic time distortion and free-recall learning—An attempted replication. *Psychological Research* **40**(3):291-298.

Wagstaff, G. F., and Sykes, C. T. (1984). Hypnosis and the recall of emotionally-toned material. *IRCS Medical Science: Psychology and Psychiatry* **12**(1-2):137-138.

Wain, H. J. (1980a). *Clinical Hypnosis in Medicine.* Miami, FL: Symposia Specialists.

Wain, H. J. (1980b). Pain control through use of hypnosis. *American J. of Clinical Hypnosis* **23**(1):41-46.

Wain, H. J. (Ed.). (1981). *Theoretical and Clinical Aspects of Hypnosis.* Miami, FL: Symposia Specialists.

Wain, H. J. (1986). Pain control with hypnosis in consultation and liaison psychiatry. *Psychiatric Annals* **16**(2):106-109

Wain, H. J.; Amen, D. G.; and Oetgen, W. J. (1983). Cardiac arrhythmias and hypnotic intervention: Advantages, disadvantages, precautions, and theoretical considerations. *American J. of Clinical Hypnosis* **26**(1):1-8.

Wain, H.; Amen, D. G.; and Oetgen, W. J. (1984). Hypnotic intervention in cardiac arrhythmias: Advantages, disadvantages, precautions, and theoretical considerations. *American J. of Clinical Hypnosis* **27**(1):70-75.

Wakeman, R. J., and Kaplan, J. Z. (1978). An experimental study of hypnosis in painful burns. *American J. of Clinical Hypnosis* **21**(1):3-12.

Walker, D. L. (1984). Hypnosis and religion. *Australian J. of Clinical Hypnotherapy and Hypnosis* **5**(2):87-96.

Walker, N. S.; Garrett, J. B.; and Wallace, B. (1976). Restoration of eidetic imagery via hypnotic age regression: A preliminary report. *J. of Abnormal Psychology* **85**(3):335-337.

Walker, W. L. (1979). A modification of the eye fixation technique. *Australian J. of Clinical and Experimental Hypnosis* **7**(3):289-292.

Walker, W. L.; Collins, J. K.; and Krass, J. (1982). Four hypnosis scripts from the Macquarie weight control programme. *Australian J. of Clinical and Experimental Hypnosis* **10**(2):125-133.

Walker, W. L., and Diment, A. D. (1979). Music as a deepening technique. *Australian J. of Clinical and Experimental Hypnosis* **7**(1):35-36.

Wall, J. A. (1984). Toward a psycho-structural theory: Hypnosis and the structure of dreams. *American J. of Clinical Hypnosis* **26**(3):159-165.

Wall, P. D., and Lieberman, L. R. (1976). Effects of task motivation and hypnotic induction on hypermnesia. *American J. of Clinical Hypnosis* **18**(4):250-253.

Wallace, B. (1976). Immediate proprioception decrement with hypnotic anesthesia: A preliminary report. *Perceptual and Motor Skills* **42**(3):801-802.

Wallace, B. (1978). Restoration of eidetic imagery via hypnotic age regression: More evidence. *J. of Abnormal Psychology* **87**(6):673-675.

Wallace, B. (1979). *Applied Hypnosis: An Overview.* Chicago: Nelson-Hall.

Wallace, B. (1980). Autokinetic movement of an imagined and an hypnotically hallucinated stimulus. *International J. of Clinical and Experimental Hypnosis* **28**(4):386-393.

Wallace, B., and Fisher, L. E. (1979). Proprioception and the production of adaptation and intermanual transfer to prismatic displacement. *Perception and Psychophysics* **26**(2):113-117.

Wallace, B., and Fisher, L. E. (1982). Hypnotically induced limb anesthesia and adaptation to displacing prisms: Replication requires adherence to critical procedures. *J. of Abnormal Psychology* **91**(5):390-391.

Wallace, B., and Fisher, L. E. (1984). Prism adaptation with hypnotically induced limb anesthesia: The critical roles of head position and prism type. *Perception and Psychophysics* **36**(3):303-306.

Wallace, B., and Garrett, J. B. (1975). Perceptual adaptation with selective reductions of felt sensation. *Perception* **4**:437-445.

Wallace, B., and Hoyenga, K. B. (1980). Production of proprioceptive errors with induced hypnotic anesthesia. *International J. of Clinical and Experimental Hypnosis* **28**(2):140-147.

Wallace, B., and Hoyenga, K. B. (1981). Performance of fine motor coordination activities with an hypnotically anesthetized limb. *International J. of Clinical and Experimental Hypnosis* **29**(1):54-65.

Wallace, B.; Knight, T. A.; and Garrett, J. B. (1976). Hypnotic susceptibility and frequency reports to illusory stimuli. *J. of Abnormal Psychology* **85**(6):558-563.

Wallace, E. R., IV, and Rothstein, W. (1975). Symptom substitution in a male hysteric. *American J. of Psychoanalysis* **35**(4):355-357.

Wallach, M. A., and Kogan, N. (1965). *Modes of Thinking in Young Children.* New York: Holt, Rinehart & Winston.

Wallis, G. G., (1951). Metabolic rate, hypnosis and theopentone. *J. Royal Nav. Med. Ser.* **37**:48-50.

Walrath, L. C., and Hamilton, D. W. (1975). Autonomic correlates of meditation and hypnosis. *American J. of Clinical Hypnosis* **17**(3):190-197.

Warner, K. E. (1979). The use of hypnosis in the defense of criminal cases. *International J. of Clinical and Experimental Hypnosis* **27**(4):417-436.

Watkins, A. L. (1949). Discussion of Mead, S. and Rouch, E. S. Study of effect of hypnotic suggestions on physiologic performance. *Arch. Phys. Med.* **30**:700-706.

Watkins, H. H. (1976). Hypnosis and smoking: A five session approach. *International J. of Clinical and Experimental Hypnosis* **24**(4):381-390.

Watkins, H. H. (1980). The silent abreaction. *International J. of Clinical and Experimental Hypnosis* **28**(2):101-113.

Watkins, J. G. (1947). Antisocial compulsions induced under hypnotic trance. *J. of Abnormal and Social Psychology* **42**:256-259.

Watkins, J. G. (1951). A case of hypnotic trance induced in a resistant subject in spite of active opposition. *British J. of Medical Hypnotism* **2**:26-31.

Watkins, J. G. (1972). Antisocial behavior under hypnosis: Possible or impossible? *International J. of Clinical and Experimental Hypnosis* **20**(2):95-100.

Watkins, J. G. (1984). The Bianchi (L.A. hillside strangler) case: Sociopath or multiple personality? *International J. of Clinical and Experimental Hypnosis* **32**(2):67-101.

Waxman, D. (1981). *Hypnosis: A Guide for Patients and Practitioners.* London: George Allan & Unwin.

Weber, A. M., (1981). Facilitation of dissociation in relation to mental relaxation and hypnosis. *Australian J. of Clinical and Experimental Hypnosis* **9**(2):101-102.

Wedemeyer, C., and Coe, W. C. (1978). Contextual effects on state reports of hypnotic depth. Paper presented at the Annual Meeting of the Western Psychological Association at San Francisco, April 21.

Wedemeyer, C., and Coe, W. C. (1981). Hypnotic state reports: Contextual variation and phenomenological criteria. *J. of Mental Imagery* **5**(2):107-116.

Wein, A.; Golubev, V.; and Yakhno, N. (1979). Polygraphic analysis of sleep and wakefulness in patients with Parkinson's syndrome. *Waking and Sleeping* **3**(1):31-40.

Weisberg, J. (1979). Effect of hypnosis on manual dexterity in susceptible female college students. *Dissertation Abstracts International* **39**(8-B):3744.

Weitz, R. D. (1983). Psychological factors in the prevention and treatment of cancer. *Psychotherapy in Private Practice* **1**(4):69-76.

Weitzenhoffer, A. M. (1949). The production of antisocial acts under hypnosis. *J. of Abnormal and Social Psychology* **44**:420-422.

Weitzenhoffer, A. M. (1951). The transcendence of normal voluntary capacities in hypnosis: An evaluation. *Personality* **1**:272-282.

Weitzenhoffer, A. M. (1953). *Hypnotism: An Objective Study in Suggestibility.* New York: John Wiley.

Weitzenhoffer, A. M. (1957). *General Techniques of Hypnotism.* New York: Grune & Stratton.

Weitzenhoffer, A. M. (1972). The postural sway test: A historical note. *International J. of Clinical and Experimental Hypnosis* **20**(1):17-24.

Weitzenhoffer, A. M. (1974). When is an "instruction" an "Instruction." *International J. of Clinical and Experimental Hypnosis* **22**(3):258-269.

Weitzenhoffer, A. M. (1980a). What did he (Bernheim) say? A postscript and an addendum. *International J. of Clinical and Experimental Hypnosis* **28**(3):252-260.

Weitzenhoffer, A. M. (1980b). Hypnotic susceptibility revisited. *American J. of Clinical Hypnosis* **22**(3):130-146.

Weitzenhoffer, A. M., and Hilgard, E. R. (1959). *Stanford Hypnotic Susceptibility Scale, Forms A and B.* Palo Alto: Consulting Psychologists Press.

Weitzenhoffer, A. M., and Hilgard, E. R. (1962). *Stanford Hypnotic Susceptibility Scale, Form C.* Palo Alto: Consulting Psychologists Press.

Weitzenhoffer, A. M., and Hilgard, E. R. (1967). *Stanford Profile Scales of Hypnotic Susceptibility, Forms I and II.* Palo Alto: Consulting Psychologists Press.

Weitzenhoffer, A. M., and Weitzenhoffer, G. B. (1958). Sex, transference and susceptibility to hypnosis. *American J. of Clinical Hypnosis* **1**:15-24.

Wells, W. R. (1940). The extent and duration of posthypnotic amnesia. *J. of Psychology* **2**:137.

Wells, W. R. (1941). Experiments in the hypnotic production of crime. *J. of Psychology* **11**:63-102.

Welsh, D. K. (1978). Hypnotic control of blushing: A case study. *American J. of Clinical Hypnosis* **20**(3):213-215.

Werner, W. E. F.; Schauble, P. G.; and Knudson, M. S. (1982). An argument for the revival of hypnosis in obstetrics. *American J. of Clinical Hypnosis* **24**(3):149-171.

West, L. J. (1960). Psychophysiology of hypnosis. *J. of American Medical Association* **172**(7):128/672-131/675.

West, L. J., and Deckert, G. H. (1965). Dangers of hypnosis. *J. of American Medical Association* **192**:9-12.

West, L. J.; Niell, K. C.; and Hardy, J. D. (1952). Effects of hypnotic suggestion on pain perception and galvanic skin response. *Archives of Neurology and Psychiatry* **68**:549-560.

Wester, W. C., II, and Smith, A. H., Jr. (Eds.). (1984). *Clinical Hypnosis — A Multidisciplinary Approach.* Philadelphia: J. B. Lippincott Co.

Weyandt, J. A., (1976). Hypnosis in a dental patient with allergies. *American J. of Clinical Hypnosis* **19**(2):123-125.

Wheeler, L.; Reis, H. T.; Wolff, E.; Grupsmith, E.; and Mordkoff, A. M. (1974). Eye-roll and hypnotic susceptibility. *International J. of Clinical and Experimental Hypnosis* **22**(4):327-334.

White, R. W. (1941). A preface to the theory of hypnotism. *J. of Abnormal and Social Psychology* **36:**477-505.

White, R. W.; Fox, G. F.; and Harris, W. W. (1940). Hypnotic hypermnesia for recently learned material. *J. of Abnormal and Social Psychology* **35:**88-103.

Whitehorn, J. C.; Lundholm, H.; Fox, E. J.; and Benedict, F. G. (1932). Metabolic rate in "hypnotic sleep." *New England J. of Medicine* **206:**777-781.

Wickramasekera, I. (Ed.). (1976). *Biofeedback, Behavior Therapy and Hypnosis: Potentiating the Verbal Control of Behavior for Clinicians.* Chicago: Nelson-Hall.

Wickramasekera, I. E. (1977). On attempts to modify hypnotic susceptibility: Some psychophysiological procedures and promising directions. *Annals of New York Academy of Sciences* **296:**143-153.

Wicks, G. R. (1982). A rapid induction technique, mechanics and rationale. *Australian J. of Clinical and Experimental Hypnosis* **10**(2):117-119.

Widdifield, D. A. (1975). TA and hypnosis. *Transactional Analysis J.* **5**(2):131-132.

Wijesinghe, B. (1977). A case of frigidity treated by short-term hypnotherapy. *International J. of Clinical and Experimental Hypnosis* **25**(2):63-67.

Wilbur, C. B. (1984). Treatment of multiple personality. *Psychiatric Annals* **14**(1):27-31.

Wilcox, P., and Dawson, J. G. (1977). Role-played and hypnotically induced simulation of psychopathology on the MMPI. *J. of Clinical Psychology* **33**(3):743-745.

Willard, R. D. (1977). Breast enlargement through visual imagery and hypnosis. *American J. of Clinical Hypnosis* **19**(4):195-200.

Williams, J. E. (1974). Stimulation of breast growth by hypnosis. *J. of Sex Research* **10**(4):316-326.

Williams, J. A. (1983). Ericksonian hypnotherapy of intractable shoulder pain. *American J. of Clinical Hypnosis* **26**(1):26-29.

Williams, J. A. (1985). Indirect hypnotic therapy of nyctophobia: A case report. *American J. of Clinical Hypnosis* **28**(1):10-15.

Williams, S. (1984). Neo-dissociation theory and co-consciousness. *Interfaces* **11**(2):28-40.

Williamsen, J. A.; Johnson, H. J.; and Ericksen, C. W. (1965). Some characteristics of posthypnotic amnesia. *J. of Abnormal Psychology* **70:**123-131.

Wilson, L.; Greene, E.; and Loftus, E. F. (1986). Beliefs about forensic hypnosis. *International J. of Clinical and Experimental Hypnosis* **34**(2):110-121.

Wilson, S. C., and Barber, T. X., (1978). The Creative Imagination Scale as a measure of hypnotic responsiveness: Applications to experimental and clinical hypnosis. *American J. of Clinical Hypnosis* **20**(4):235-249.

Wineburg, E. N., and Straker, N. (1973). An episode of acute, self-limiting depersonalization following a first session of hypnosis. *American J. of Psychiatry* **130**(1):98-100.

Winn, R. B. (1965). *Dictionary of Hypnosis*. New York: Citadel Press.

Wiseman, R. J., and Reyher, J. (1973). Hypnotically induced dreams. Using the Rorschach inkblots as stimuli: A test of Freud's theory of dreams. *J. of Personality and Social Psychology* **27**(3):329-336.

Wladyslaw, M. (1981). *Understanding Hypnosis: A Brief Guide*. Washington, DC: Hypno Press.

Wolberg, L. M. (1948). *Medical Hypnosis. Volume 1. The Principles of Hypnotherapy*. New York: Grune & Stratton.

Wollman, L. (1978). Self-confidence achieved by hypnotic techniques. *J. of the American Society of Psychosomatic Dentistry and Medicine* **25**(2): 44.

Wolpe, J. (1982). *The Practice of Behavior Therapy*. (3d ed.).New York: Pergamon Press.

Wood, H. M. (1984). Journey to the mountains and lakes of Switzerland to discover lost years. *Australian J. of Clinical and Experimental Hypnosis* **12**(2):134-137.

Worthington, T. S. (1979). The use in court of hypnotically enhanced testimony. *International J. of Clinical and Experimental Hypnosis* **27**(4):402-416.

Wright, R. C. (1982). Trance and confusion in Gestalt therapy. *J. of Contemporary Psychotherapy* **13**(1):70-76.

Yamauchi, K. T. (1981). Dental fear in a chronic schizophrenic: A case report. *American J. of Clinical Hypnosis* **24**(2):128-131.

Yanchar, R. J., and Johnson, H. J. (1981). Absorption and attitude towards hypnosis: A moderator analysis. *International J. of Clinical and Experimental Hypnosis* **29**(4):375-382.

Yapko, M. D. (1981a). The effect of matching primary representational system predicates on hypnotic relaxation. *American J. of Clinical Hypnosis* **23**(3):169-175.

Yapko, M. D. (1981b). Neuro-linguistic programming, hypnosis, and interpersonal influence. *Dissertation Abstracts International* **41**(8-B):3204.

Yapko, M. D. (1983). A comparative analysis of direct and indirect hypnotic communication styles. *American J. of Clinical Hypnosis* **25**(4):270-276.

Yapko, M. D. (1984). Implications of the Ericksonian and neurolinguistic programming approaches for responsibility of therapeutic outcomes. *American J. of Clinical Hypnosis* **27**(2):137-143.

Yoder, N. S. (1982). Changes in suggestibility following alert hypnosis and concentrative meditation. *Dissertation Abstracts International* **43**(6-B):2013-2014.

Young, J., and Cooper, L. M. (1972). Hypnotic recall amnesia as a function of manipulated expectancy. *Proceedings of 80th Annual Convention of American Psychological Association* **7**:857-858.

Young, P. C. (1925). An experimental study of mental and physical functions in the normal and hypnotic states. *American J. of Psychology* **36**:214-232.

Young, P. C. (1928). The nature of hypnosis: As indicated by the presence or absence of post-hypnotic amnesia and rapport. *J. of Abnormal and Social Psychology* **22**:372-382.

Young, P. C. (1940). Hypnotic regression—fact or artifact? *J. of Abnormal and Social Psychology* **35**:273.

Young, P. C. (1952). Antisocial uses of hypnosis. In L. M. LeCron (Ed.), *Experimental Hypnosis*. New York: Macmillan.

Zakrzewski, K., and Szelenberger, W. (1981). Visual evoked potentials in hypnosis: A longitudinal approach. *International J. of Clinical and Experimental Hypnosis* **29**(1):77-86.

Zamansky, H. S. (1977). Suggestion and countersuggestion in hypnotic behavior. *J. of Abnormal Psychology* **86**(4):346-351.

Zamansky, H. S., and Bartis, S. P. (1984). Hypnosis as dissociation: Methodological considerations and preliminary findings. *American J. of Clinical Hypnosis* **26**(4):246-251.

Zeig, J. K. (1978). Tympanic temperature, hypnosis and laterality. *Dissertation Abstracts International* **39**(1-B):423-424.

Zeig, J. K. (1980a). Symptom prescription techniques: Clinical applications using elements of communication. *American J. of Clinical Hypnosis* **23**(1):23-33.

Zeig, J. K. (1980b). Symptom prescription and Ericksonian principles of hypnosis and psychotherapy. *American J. of Clinical Hypnosis* **23**(1):16-22.

Zeig, J. K. (Ed.). (1981). *A Teaching Seminar with Milton Erickson*. New York: Brunner-Mazel.

Zelig, M., and Beidleman, W. B. (1981). The investigative use of hypnosis: A word of caution. *International J. of Clinical and Experimental Hypnosis* **29**(4):401-412.

Zilbergeld, B.; Edelstien, M. G.; and Araoz, D. L. (Eds.). (1986). *Hypnosis—Questions and Answers*. New York; W. W. Norton.

Zlotogorski, Z., and Anixter, W. L. (1983). The use of hypnosis in the treatment of reflux esophagitis: A case report. *American J. of Clinical Hypnosis* **25**(4):232-234.

Name Index

Abramovici, H., 253, 402
Abrams, S., 273, 274, 365
Abramson, M., 98, 365
Acosta, E., Jr., 365
Adams, P., 365
Addie, D. L., 136, 461
Adesso, V. J., 185, 206, 405
Adler, A., 196, 216
Adrian, C., 369
Ahlberg, D., 120, 426
Aja, J. H., 183, 211, 365
Akpinar, S., 69, 470
Akstein, D., 365
Albe-Fessard, D., 439
Albert, I., 365
Albert, I. B., 97, 177, 365
Allen, B. P., 365
Allen, G. J., 171, 431
Allen, J. L., 91, 385
Allen, S. N., 142, 388
Allison, R. B., 274, 366
Alman, B. M., 172, 366
Ambrose, G., 466, 471
Amen, D. G., 238, 472
Andersen, M. S., 183, 211, 366
Anderson, J. A. D., 183, 230, 366
Anderson, J. W., 214, 366
Anderson, O., 366
Anderson, V., 450
Andreychuk, T., 389
Andrick, J. M., 292, 366 ˊ
Angelos, J. S., 366
Anixter, W. L., 238, 478
Ansari, F., 157, 459
Ansel, E. L., 183, 366
Aoki, H., 423
Apfel, R. J., 400
Appelbaum, P. S., 282, 366
Araoz, D. L., 184, 366, 367, 478
Armstrong, L. A., 445
Armstrong, V., 40, 398
Arnold, M. B., 376
Arnold, W. J., 439
Arns, P. A., 80, 377
Aronoff, G., 425
Arons, H., 38, 39, 74, 93, 275, 276, 277, 278, 367

Aronson, M., 462
As, A., 43, 44, 142, 367
Ascher, L. M., 226, 367
Aserinsky, E., 97
Asher, R., 95, 367
Ashford, B., 122, 367
Ashton, M. A., 151, 367
Astor, M. H., 212, 226, 228, 229, 236, 367
Astrup, C., 230, 367
Atkinson, G., 467
August, R. V., 238, 266, 367
Augustynek, A., 145, 367
Ault, R. L., 280, 367
Austrin, H. R., 367, 442
Avampato, J. J., 238, 368
Averill, J. R., 45, 392
Azikri, D., 420

Bacon, J. G., 448
Baer, L., 162, 368
Bak, A. F., 426
Bakal, P. A., 184, 368
Baker, E. L., 42, 184, 212, 221, 304, 321, 368, 426
Baker, R. A., 147, 159, 368
Baker, S. R., 184, 233, 368
Balaam, M., 182, 368
Balaban, A. B., 248, 458
Balaschak, B., 39, 368
Baldwin, B. A., 183, 368
Balke, B., 434
Ballinger, S. E., 368
Balson, P. M., 283, 368
Bandler, R., 369
Banyai, E. I., 57, 369
Barabasz, A. F., 46, 230, 369
Barabasz, M., 369
Barber, J., 119, 120, 172, 255, 369
Barber, T. X., 3, 6, 10, 11, 21, 22, 31, 32, 33, 37, 40, 41, 43, 44, 45, 46, 47, 55, 56, 68, 78, 85, 89, 92, 93, 94, 95, 96, 97, 98, 101, 103, 104, 106, 107, 110, 111, 112, 122, 127, 128, 133, 134, 136, 141, 142, 143, 144, 145, 146, 152, 154, 155, 156, 157, 161, 164, 165, 166, 167, 170, 175,

Barber, T. X. (*cont.*)
176, 204, 208, 209, 217, 227, 238, 244, 251, 252, 254, 266, 277, 320, 324, 336, 343, 344, 345, 363, 370, 371, 372, 373, 374, 375, 383, 387, 389, 401, 405, 409, 417, 431, 441, 448, 450, 459, 461, 468, 477
Barbour, J. S., 53, 105, 275, 378
Barkley, R. A., 184, 204, 375, 416
Barmark, S. M., 10, 375
Barnes, P. R., 435
Barnett, E. A., 375
Barrett, D. L., 176, 375
Barrios, A. A., 169, 170, 227, 375
Bartis, S. P., 174, 460, 478
Basden, B., 130, 386
Basden, D., 130, 386
Basker, M. A., 183, 230, 366
Bateman, W., 282, 375
Bauer, H., 376
Bauer, K. E., 92, 183, 376
Bauer, P., 463
Baugher, R. J., 133, 386
Baum, D., 40, 376
Baum, J., xvii
Beahrs, J. O., 174, 376
Bean, B. W., 376
Bean, W., 90, 431
Beary, J. F., 226, 377
Beck, A., 258, 418
Beecher, H. K., 110, 245, 376
Behrendt, D. M., 466
Beidleman, W. B., 279, 478
Beier, E. G., 468
Beigel, H. G., 376
Bell, G. K., 212, 218, 220, 221, 376
Bellezza, F. S., 143, 466
Bender, V. L., 376
Benedict, B. A., 380
Benedict, F. G., 183, 218, 476
Bennett, H., 90, 431
Bennett, L., 93, 376
Benson, G., 182, 368, 376
Benson, H., 10, 80, 226, 377, 400
Bentler, P. M., 41, 412
Beran, B., 307, 311, 420
Bergerone, C., 44, 377
Bergman, A. R., 377
Bergmann, M. S., 98, 377
Berman, R., 93, 377
Berner, P., 376
Bernhardt, R., 377
Bernheim, H., 7, 8, 10, 84, 358, 377
Bernstein, J., 279, 445
Bernstien, A. E., 377
Berry, G. C., 377
Bertrand, L. D., 136, 139, 377, 394, 459, 461, 462
Berwick, P. R., 183, 222, 377

Best, H. L., 155, 377
Biasiotto, J. L., 377
Bickford, R. G., 454
Binet, A., 9
Bishay, E..G., 259, 377
Bjork, R. A., 135, 403
Black, S., 104
Blackmore, S. H., 350, 449
Blair, P., 288
Bleirad, G., 446
Blessing, D., 426
Bliss, E. L., 183, 274, 378
Blocker, K., 368
Blum, G. S., 105, 106, 238, 275, 378, 389, 429
Blumstein, R., 63, 401
Boaz, D., 184, 233, 368
Bodorik, H. L., 121, 135, 136, 459
Boisvenue, M. E., 445
Bolocofsky, D. N., 183, 211, 378
Bond, J., 282
Bongartz, W., 29, 378
Bonica, J. J., 439
Boone, D., 177, 365
Booth, T. B., 13, 183, 403
Bordachar, J., 446
Bordeaux, J., 84, 165, 425
Boring, E. G., 378
Bornstein, P. H., 183, 211, 378
Bose, K., 434
Boswell, L. K., Jr., 273, 378
Botto, R. W., 378, 379
Bourne, P. G., 233, 379
Boutin, G. E., 184, 228, 290, 379
Bowen, B., 375
Bower, G. H., 275, 379
Bowers, K. S., 27, 160, 173, 266, 279, 379, 380, 394
Bowers, M. K., 420
Bowers, P., 27, 28, 152, 268, 380, 412
Bowersbuch, M. K., 154, 405
Boxer, A. M., 402
Bozick, B. J., 380
Brabender, V., 143, 380
Braid, J., 5, 6, 7, 8, 10, 63, 65, 352, 358, 380
Bramwell, J. M., 380
Brandes, J. M., 402
Brassfield, P. A., 183, 380
Brattberg, G., 259, 380
Braun, B. G., 183, 201, 234, 380, 469
Bremer, B., 195, 199, 219, 221, 435
Brende, J. O., 183, 218, 380
Brenman, M., 318, 320, 381
Brenneman, H. A., 160, 379
Brink, N. E., 224, 381
Brisson, A., 426
Brisson, M. A., 104, 450
Brodsky, A. M., 47, 381

Broen, W. E., Jr., 387
Brooks, F. R., 283, 368
Brow, T., 409
Brown, D. P., 184, 282, 381, 402
Brown, J. E., 232, 398
Brown, J. M., 184, 381
Brown, M., 121, 451, 465
Brown, R. J., 381
Brown, S. W., 27, 113, 397, 398
Browning, C. H., 381
Bruhn, R. A., 381
Brumley, W., 184, 381
Bryan, W. J., Jr., 275, 278, 381
Bubeck, M. F. H., 367
Buckner, L. G., 381, 386
Burger, J. M., 41, 386
Burns, A., 381
Burns, A. M., 10, 427
Burns, B., 171, 381
Burrows, G. D., 184, 350, 382, 391, 392
Bushnell, J. A., 382
Butler, B., 182, 241, 252, 258, 260, 261, 262, 382
Byers, A. P., 183, 338, 382
Bynum, E. B., 382

Caldwell, T. A., 184, 216, 382
Call, J. D., 382
Callen, K. E., 287, 288, 382
Calverley, D. S., 37, 40, 43, 46, 68, 97, 101, 104, 122, 127, 128, 133, 134, 144, 146, 161, 165, 170, 372, 373, 374, 375
Camp, E. M., 97, 416
Capderou, A., 446
Carasso, R. L., 183, 382
Carden, N. A., 184, 185, 437
Carew, R., 288
Carli, G., 352, 382, 397
Carlson, D., 63, 388
Carlson, W. A., 184, 471
Carney, R. E., 172, 366
Carol, M. P., 226, 377
Carona, A. J., 34, 382, 447
Carter, B. D., 222, 382, 395
Carter, W., 461
Case, D. B., 11, 271, 382
Cautela, J. R., 199, 227, 228, 231, 232, 233, 382, 383
Cedercreutz, C., 438
Cei, A., 44, 377
Cerio, J. E., 383
Cescato, M., 10, 22, 383
Channon, L. D., 12, 86, 183, 210, 383
Chapman, C. R., 116, 383
Charcot, J., 7, 8, 9, 11, 357, 359, 362, 384
Charlesworth, E. A., 383

Chaves, J. F., 22, 111, 184, 372, 375, 381, 383, 460
Cheek, D. B., 119, 183, 213, 216, 252, 269, 383, 384
Chen, T. C., 426
Chertok, L., 7, 8, 118, 384
Chiglinsky, M. A., 437
Chiofalo, L. C., 384
Chisholm, W., 157, 442
Christenson, J. A., 384
Christie, B., 384
Chubb, H., 384
Churchill, N., 103, 459, 461
Cioppa, F. J., 269, 385
Ciotti, J., 184, 437
Citrenbaum, C. M., 385
Clark, B. D., 350, 385
Clark, J. L., 297, 416
Clarke, J. C., 385
Clawson, T. A., 238, 252, 260, 265, 266, 385
Cleckley, H. M., 468
Cleveland, C. T., 385
Coe, W. C., 10, 41, 85, 91, 119, 130, 131, 133, 135, 137, 138, 139, 141, 145, 160, 167, 168, 314, 321, 326, 335, 345, 381, 384, 385, 386, 405, 415, 431, 450, 452, 454, 465, 467, 474
Cohen, B. B., 258, 434
Cohen, S. B., 184, 386
Cohen, W. I., 290, 385, 387
Cohn, A., xvii, 199, 330, 335, 387
Cole, R. D., 290, 387
Coleman, J. C., 387
Collins, A. C., 404
Collins, J. K., 10, 84, 183, 206, 417, 427, 473
Collison, D., 387
Colomb, C., 238, 239, 256, 387
Colwell, S. O., 304, 422
Comins, J. R., 387
Conn, J. H., 307, 310, 311, 316; 320, 323, 325, 326, 328, 372, 387
Conn, L., 238, 387
Conn, R. H., 372, 387
Connors, J. R., 387
Conroy, M. M., 96, 438
Convant, M., 142, 427
Cooley, L. E., 184, 437
Cooper, L. M., 31, 122, 141, 143, 145, 160, 161, 387, 478
Cooperman, S., 388
Cooperman, S. B., 76, 387
Copemann, C. D., 183, 231, 388
Corcoran, M. E., 404
Coules, J., 95, 374
Coulthard-Morris, L., 183, 211, 378
Council, J. R., 63, 388, 420

Counts, D. K., 183, 391
Counts, R. M., 98, 275, 388
Cowell, D., 388
Cox, G. B., 11, 402
Cox, T. H., 184, 388
Crasilneck, H. B., 92, 93, 95, 96, 98, 154,
    156, 165, 183, 240, 245, 246, 247,
    248, 249, 250, 388, 399, 429
Crawford, F. T., 352, 388
Crawford, H. J., 11, 28, 31, 104, 142,
    314, 365, 388, 389, 412, 440
Crawford, K., 11, 389
Creamer, M., 398
Cross, D. G., 139, 428, 456
Cross, H. J., 432
Crosson, B. A., 94, 389
Crosswell, G. L., 389
Crouse, E., 34, 389
Crowder, J. E., 183, 202, 433
Crowley, R. J., 389
Crutchfield, L., 172, 173, 421
Cummings, C. P., 389
Cunningham, P. V., 106, 389
Cupples, D. E., 389
Curran, J. D., 404
Cusimano, F., 408
Cutcomb, S. D., 389

Dalal, A. S., 22, 375, 389
Dalton, R., 183, 230, 366
Dampier, (Sir) W. C., 390
Daniels, L. K., 183, 184, 229, 230, 234,
    239, 257, 390
Das, J. P., 142, 143, 390
Dash, J., 184, 390
Dauven, J., 390
Dave, R. P., 176, 390
Davidson, R. J., 390
Davis, S., 40, 390
Davison, G. C., 142, 427
Dawson, J. G., 40, 100, 390, 443, 476
Dawson, S. L., 297, 416
Deabler, H. L., 183, 211, 215, 391, 417
Debetz, B., 391
Deckert, G. H., 307, 315, 475
Deeley, D. C., 106, 374
Deforest, F. D., 391
De Groh, M., 81, 459, 460
Degun, G., 185, 391
Degun, M. D., 185, 391
Deiker, T. E., 183, 184, 229, 391
DeLee, S. T., 248, 251, 252, 253, 254,
    423
Delmonte, M. M., 121, 391
Delprato, D. J., 391, 414
Dement, W. C., 291, 391
DeMers, G. E., 391
De Moor, W., 374
Dempsey, G. L., 185, 391

Dempster, C. R., 237, 283, 368, 424
Dengrove, E., 226, 228, 229, 232, 234,
    391
Dennerstein, L., 184, 350, 382, 391, 392
Denver, D. R., 69, 392
D'Eon, J. L., 136, 460, 462
DePiano, F. A., 149, 392, 451
de Puységur, A., 4
Deschambault, A., 104, 450
De Shazer, S., 184, 224, 392
DeStefano, R. F., 392
De Varennes, S., 392
Devine, D. A., 183, 211, 378
DeVoge, J. T., 392
DeVoge, S., 228, 236, 392
DeWitt, G. W., 45, 392
Deyoub, P. L., 53, 183, 184, 211, 330,
    392, 395
De Zulueta, F. I. S., 142, 392
Dhanens, T. P., 141, 145, 393, 443
Diamond, M. J., 34, 58, 63, 223, 393
Diaz, W. A., 419
Dickhaus, R. C., 143, 380
Dillman, N., 445
Dillon, R. F., 131, 393
Diment, A. D., 86, 383, 393, 473
Dimond, R. E., 259, 393
Dinges, D. F., 274, 439
di Prisco, C. L., 397
Dirks, J. F., 184, 201, 454
Dobrovolsky, N. W., 34, 447
Dolby, R. M., 178, 393, 456
Dollard, J., 189, 193, 194, 342, 393
Domangue, B. B., 430
Donald, K. M., 305, 414
Dorcus, R. M., 105, 393, 394, 441
Douce, R. G., 275, 423
Dougherty, R. E., 394
Doughtie, E. B., 383
Douglas, R. R., 183, 222, 377
Douglass, V. L., 394
Dowd, E. T., 407
Dreyfuss, D. A., 420
Drinkwater, B. L., 434
Droin, M. C., 118, 384
Drummond, J., 136, 461
Dubin, L. L., 239, 394, 434
Dubovsky, S., 469
Dubreuil, D. L., 115, 134, 139, 394, 460,
    461
Duff, J. L., 376, 394
Dull, R. A., 394
Dumas, L., 70, 394
Dumas, R. A., 394
Du Maurier, G., 17, 453
Dunbar, K. D., 119, 470
Duncan, B., 169, 394
Durand, J., 446
Dynes, J. B., 97, 394

Dywan, J., 279, 394
Dzieszkowski, P. A., 281, 411

Easton, R. D., 139, 293, 294, 295, 419, 457
Ebbinghaus, H., 129
Eccles, D., 264, 423
Edelstien, M. G., 221, 394, 478
Edmonds, G. M., 394
Edmonston, W. E., Jr., 44, 91, 157, 394, 395, 419
Ehleben, C., 430
Einstein, A., 349
Eisele, G., 142, 143, 395
Eisen, M., 402
Eisen, M. R., 303, 395
Eisenberg, H., 289, 395
Eli, I., 249, 356, 395, 420
Eliseo, T. S., 185, 395
Elkins, G. R., 11, 222, 382, 395
Ellenberger, H. F., 395
Elliotson, J., 5
Ellis, A., 195, 196, 395
Elmer, G. I., 404
Epstein, S. J., 184, 392, 395
Erdelyi, M. H., 148, 420
Erickson, E. M., 163, 164, 165, 167, 171, 396
Erickson, M. H., 89, 90, 96, 103, 106, 107, 160, 161, 163, 164, 165, 167, 171, 208, 213, 220, 221, 222, 223, 224, 229, 285, 297, 307, 320, 321, 325, 360, 369, 387, 395, 396, 408, 410, 419, 433, 449, 466, 476, 477, 478
Eriksen, C. W., 126, 128, 133, 476
Eron, L. D., 447
Esaki, M., 423
Esdaile, J., 5
Esposito, J. V., 434
Estabrooks, G. H., 124, 282, 283, 396, 439
Evans, F. J., 16, 18, 56, 121, 122, 123, 124, 126, 133, 134, 135, 137, 138, 139, 140, 167, 321, 396, 397, 399, 419, 440, 443
Evans, J. M., 397
Evers, J., 397
Ewin, D. M., 238, 245, 247, 265, 397
Eysenck, H. J., 190, 397

Fabbri, R., Jr., 184, 235, 397
Falick, P., 276, 397
Farabollini, F., 397
Farberow, N. L., 153, 452
Farnbach, R. W., 467
Farthing, G. W., 27, 113, 397, 398
Faw, V., 101, 314, 398
Feamster, J. H., 232, 398
Feather, B. W., 116, 383

Fee, A. F., 253, 398
Feldman, B. E., 398
Fellows, B. J., 40, 254, 398
Féré, C., 9
Ferguson, J. D., 112, 461
Fernandez, G. R., 95, 398
Ferrera, S. J., 398
Feshbach, S., 205, 416
Feuerstein, M., 241, 251
Fezler, W. D., 66, 423
Field, P. B., 56, 201, 202, 398, 399
Finke, R. A., 40, 399
Finkelstein, S., 259, 267, 399
Fischer, R., 399
Fisher, A. G., 96, 468
Fisher, C., 165, 399
Fisher, L. E., 115, 473
Fisher, S., 47, 166, 379, 399, 401, 412, 418
Fishman, D. L., 135, 403
Fishman, S., 155, 463
Flaxman, J., 183, 211, 471
Fleiss, J. L., 462
Fogel, B. S., 303, 399
Fogel, D. H., 271, 382
Fogel, S., 184, 221, 399
Fogelman, M. J., 165, 388, 399
Ford, L. F., 154, 399
Forgione, A., 375
Forman, L. M., 74, 185, 204, 244, 427
Forrest, D. W., 238, 455, 458
Fosshage, J. L., 372
Fourie, D. P., 46, 289, 399
Fowler, W. L., 143, 144, 399
Fox, E. J., 476
Fox, G. F., 141, 144, 476
Francis, J. G., 399
Frank, R. A., 261, 262, 426
Frankel, F. H., 23, 42, 53, 54, 182, 203, 238, 268, 269, 297, 347, 399, 400
Franklin, B., 4, 428
Franklin, L. M., 96, 400
Franks, C. M., 400
Franzini, L. R., 400
Frauman, D. C., 159, 427, 436
Fredericks, L. E., 239, 400
Frenader, G., 382
French, A. P., 226, 400
Freud, S., 3, 8, 9, 177, 186, 187, 188, 189, 190, 191, 193, 198, 218, 342, 354, 356, 359, 360, 366, 384, 410, 420, 453, 470, 477
Fricton, J. R., 120, 400
Frid, M., 114, 401
Friedman, H., 183, 271, 272, 401
Friesen, D. D., 381
Frischholz, E. J., 30, 53, 63, 184, 401, 412, 440, 462, 469
Fritzo, J. A., 437

Fromm, E., 10, 40, 295, 296, 297, 299, 303, 381, 395, 401, 402
Fross, G. H., 406
Frost, E. A., 121, 402
Frumkin, L. R., 11, 402
Frutiger, A. D., 184, 228, 402
Fuchs, K., 238, 253, 269, 402
Fullam, F., 387
Fuller, A. K., 259, 435
Fung, E. H., 259, 402
Furst, A., 402
Furst, M. L., 434
Fuselier, G. D., 12, 183, 403

Gagnon, F., 69, 392
Gallagher, M., 90, 431
Galski, T. J., 185, 402
Gard, B., 156, 402
Gardner, G. G., 71, 207, 260, 264, 295, 299, 303, 402, 403
Garrett, J. B., 115, 157, 403, 472, 473
Garver, R. B., 12, 183, 302, 403
Gass, G. C., 97, 416
Gaston, C. D., 185, 403
Gaunitz, S. C. B., 10, 100, 375, 403
Geiselman, R. E., 135, 140, 403
Geiwitz, P. J., 378
Gekoski, W. L., 121, 421
Gentry, W. R., 185, 206, 416
George, F. R., 403, 404
Gerson, M. J., 98, 275, 425
Gerton, M. I., 6, 408
Geselowitz, L., 100, 427
Getzels, J. W., 149, 404
Gheorghiu, V. A., 257, 404
Giacalone, A. V., 183, 404
Gibbons, D. E., 21, 57, 91, 344, 404, 471, 472
Gibson, H. B., 282, 352, 404
Gibson, M., 404, 405
Gibson, R. W., 98, 432
Gidro, F. L., 154, 405
Gilbert, J. E., 145, 405
Gill, M. M., 405
Gillett, P. L., 119, 405
Gilligan, S. G., 275, 379
Gillispie, C. C., 405
Gindes, B. C., 405
Gindhart, L. R., 224, 405
Girodo, M., 405
Gitelson, J., 369
Givens, D. L., 39, 436
Glad, W. R., 185, 206, 405
Glass, L. B., 43, 165, 374, 405
Glenn, T. J., 184, 405
Godec, C. J., 238, 405
Gogel, W. C., 429

Golan, H. P., 239, 255, 256, 405
Goldberg, T., 420
Goldberger, N. I., 405
Goldfarb, D. A., 34, 406
Goldstein, L., 15, 406, 417
Goldstein, Y., 82, 183, 406
Goleman, D. J., 390
Golubev, V., 474
Gorassini, D., 27, 115, 460
Gordon, J. E., 371, 406
Gordon, M. C., 406
Gorsky, B. H., 406
Gorsky, S. R., 406
Gorton, B. E., 92, 406
Gottesfeld, M. L., 185, 406
Gottlieb, J., 45, 460, 461
Gouch, D. A., 406
Gould, S. S., 268, 406
Graham, C., 130, 386, 406
Graham, H., 98, 377
Graham, K. R., 11, 130, 183, 226, 343, 406, 407
Grahs, C. E., 407
Granich, M., 185, 391
Grant, C. W., Jr., 247, 410
Grant, D. H., 407
Grassi, J. R., 98, 275, 425
Gravitz, M. A., 6, 7, 76, 238, 241, 244, 254, 267, 275, 407, 408, 426
Gravitz, R. F., 408
Greatrakes, V., 3
Green, M., 275, 378
Green, R. J., 227
Greene, E., 476
Greene, L. D., 406
Greene, R. J., 183, 408
Gregg, V. H., 408
Gregory, J., 393
Grehan, J. F., 77, 431
Greuling, J. W., 185, 206, 416
Grigg, L., 147, 456
Grinder, J., 369
Grisanti, G., 408
Gros, N., 259, 471
Gross, M., 183, 273, 408
Gross, M. A., 408
Grove, R. N., 69, 392
Gruber, L. N., 182, 408
Gruen, W., 252, 254, 408
Gruenewald, D., 54, 237, 408, 409
Grupsmith, E., 476
Gruzelier, J., 11, 409
Guerra, A. R., 446, 466
Guez, J. R., 105, 425
Guillotin, J. I., 4
Gur, R., 409
Gur, R. C., 151
Gustavson, J. L., 184, 409

Gwynn, M. I., 112, 113, 460
Gwynne, P. H., 227, 409

Haber, J., 462
Hackett, T. P., 238, 265, 466, 467
Haddad, M. G., 136, 445
Hahn, K. W., Jr., 112, 374
Hall, C. S., 177, 178, 341, 343, 409
Hall, H. R., 266, 267, 409
Hall, H. V., 134, 468
Hall, J. A., 92, 93, 95, 96, 98, 312, 388,
   409
Hall, M. D., 260, 266, 409
Hall, W. D., 409
Hallenbeck, G. E., 183, 416
Ham, M. L., 409
Ham, M. W., 103, 177, 409, 460
Hamilton, D. W., 474
Hammer, A. G., 121, 122, 124, 132, 138,
   367, 393, 436, 440
Hammer, E. F., 141, 143, 409
Hammerschlag, H. E., 410
Hammond, D. C., 247, 410
Handelsman, M. M., 303, 410
Hardy, J. D., 114, 475
Hariman, J., 410
Harris, R. B., 184, 470
Harris, S. L., 436
Harris, W. W., 141, 144, 476
Hart, M. M., 410
Hart, R. R., 254, 255, 410
Harvey, M. A., 106, 410
Hastings, J. E., 94, 184, 204, 375, 416
Havens, R. A., 36, 410
Haward, L., 275, 410
Hawney, M., 12, 429
Haynes, B., 147, 368
Hayry, P., 438
Healy, J. M., 407
Hebert, S. W., 184, 290, 410
Hedberg, A. G., 410
Heide, F. J., 121, 410
Heimel, A., 304, 422
Hell, (Rev.) M., 3
Helwig, C. V., 411
Henderson, G. W., 228, 469
Hendler, C. S., 261, 446
Henle, M., 411
Hennessy, R. T., 104, 432
Henninger, K. M., 184, 437
Henslin, E. R., 292, 456
Hernandez, A., 240, 453
Herod, J. W., 411
Heron, W. T., 93, 98, 365, 377, 411
Hersen, M., 459
Hershman, S., 310, 426
Herzog, A., 183, 411
Hewitt, E. C., 118, 460

Hibbard, W. S., 411
Hibler, N. S., 277, 280, 411
Higgins, J. J., 142, 143, 395
Hiland, D. N., 281, 411
Hilgard, E. R., 9, 25, 27, 28, 30, 31, 33,
   35, 37, 39, 40, 41, 43, 53, 57, 84,
   85, 93, 101, 104, 107, 110, 113,
   115, 116, 117, 118, 121, 126, 131,
   133, 138, 172, 173, 182, 279, 313,
   356, 359, 367, 369, 374, 375, 389,
   411, 412, 413, 421, 433, 434, 440,
   450, 467, 475
Hilgard, J. R., xiii, 31, 40, 260, 294, 309,
   310, 312, 313, 314, 375, 389, 412,
   413, 433
Hilton, J., 413
Hirota, K., 434
Hoch, Z., 402
Hodge, J. R., 98, 99, 185, 219, 220, 225,
   244, 275, 319, 413, 414
Hoen, P. T., 414
Hoffman, J. W., 80, 377
Hoffman, M. L., 260, 414
Hoffman, W. F., 273, 414
Hogan, M., 414
Holdevici, I., 404
Hollander, B., 414
Holloway, E. L., 305, 414
Holmes, P. A., 391, 414
Holombo, L. K., 414
Holroyd, J., 93, 185, 205, 414
Holroyd, J. C., 414
Holton, C., 264, 423
Hommel, L. S., 126, 133, 412
Hong, G. K., 39, 152, 414
Hood, R. W., 415
Horevitz, R. P., 183, 201, 380, 415
Horsley, I. A., 415
Horton, C., 111, 460
Horvath, S. M., 434
House, A. E., 183, 463
House, J. J., 350, 467
Howard, L., 183, 227, 409, 415
Howard, M., 160
Howard, M. G., 267, 399
Howard, M. L., 138, 321, 326, 386, 415
Howerton, T. C., 404
Howland, J. S., 183, 215, 415
Hoyenga, K. B., 115, 473
Huff, D., 415
Huff, P. M., 415
Hughes, R. P., 46, 448
Hull, C. L., xiii, 9, 23, 32, 37, 47, 129,
   172, 374, 415, 469
Hunchak, J. F., 64, 415
Hungerford, L. E., 350, 385
Hurley, J. D., 415
Hurt, S. W., 402

Huse, B., 141, 143, 415
Hutzell, R. R., 185, 403
Hyde, Mr., 291
Hynes, J. V., 185, 415

Ikemi, Y., 96, 415, 423
Illovsky, J., 143, 415
Ingram, R. E., 415
Itil, T. M., 69, 470

Jackson, J. A., 97, 270, 385, 416
Jackson, P. W., 149, 404
Jackson, T. L., Jr., 94, 183, 184, 204, 375, 416, 469
Jacobson, E., 15, 66, 197, 272, 416
Jaenicke, C., 403
James, H., 453
James, J., 411
Janet, P., 8, 10, 323, 416
Janis, I. L., 416
Jansen, R. D., 105, 378, 416
Jedliczka, Z. T., 259, 424
Jeffrey, L. K., 185, 206, 416
Jeffrey, T. B., 185, 206, 416
Jeglic, A., 259, 440
Jekyll, Dr., 291
Jenkins, M. T., 248, 249, 250, 388
Johnson, D. L., 433
Johnson, G. M., 183, 416
Johnson, H. J., 40, 126, 128, 135, 476, 477
Johnson, L. S., 69, 158, 293, 294, 295, 296, 297, 391, 412, 416, 436
Johnson, R. F. Q., 95, 162, 238, 417
Johnson, W. R., 376
Jones, B., 104, 112, 417, 460, 461
Jones, C. W., 252, 417
Jordan-Viola, E. P., 417
Joseph, L. M., 417
Juhasz, J. B., 417
Jupp, J. J., 85, 417

Kamitsuka, M., 304, 458
Kaplan, J. M., 183, 215, 417
Kaplan, J. Z., 247, 472
Karlin, R., 282
Karlin, R. A., 417
Katcher, A., 258, 418
Katz, N. W., 63, 183, 234, 401, 418
Katzell, R., 162, 417, 422
Kaye, J. M., 260, 418
Kearns, J. S., 418
Keegan, M., 430
Kellerman, J., 183, 418
Kellogg, E. R., 165, 418
Kelly, P., 266, 380
Kelly, R. J., 47, 418
Kelly, S. F., 42, 47, 184, 203, 400, 418
Kennedy, S., 241, 418

Kennedy, S. K., 112, 460
Keye, W. R., 247, 410
Khatami, M., 151, 418
Kiesler, C. A., 418
Kihlstrom, J. F., 28, 29, 37, 114, 118, 121, 122, 123, 124, 126, 129, 131, 132, 133, 134, 135, 137, 138, 139, 140, 275, 397, 408, 412, 418, 419, 424, 447, 457
Kiistala, U., 438
Kim, S. C., 201, 419
King, D. L., 419
King, M. E., 385
Kingsbury, G. C., 420
Kirsch, I., 63, 171, 388, 420, 431
Kir-Stimon, W., 224, 420
Klatzky, R. L., 147, 420
Klausner, S. Z., 439
Kleinhauz, M., 249, 256, 307, 311, 382, 395, 402, 420
Kleinmuntz, B., 420
Kleitman, N., 97
Kline, M. V., 9, 19, 71, 94, 116, 123, 156, 168, 182, 183, 201, 202, 215, 216, 217, 226, 240, 241, 244, 283, 314, 315, 324, 326, 335, 336, 398, 420, 421
Kluft, R. P., 183, 184, 421
Knight, T. A., 473
Knox, V. J., 117, 118, 121, 172, 173, 421
Knudson, M. S., 252, 253, 475
Knutsen, E. S., 421
Koadlow, E., 184, 421
Kobayashi, K., 321, 326, 386
Koe, G. G., 422
Kogan, N., 149, 473
Kohen, D. P., 238, 304, 422
Kohlberg, L., 158
Kondreck, J. G., 291, 422
Koperski, B. J., 11, 389
Kornfeld, A. D., 312, 422
Koster, S., 422
Kraft, S. P., 11, 382
Kraft, W. A., 12, 349, 350, 422, 449
Kramer, C. E., 437
Krass, J., 183, 206, 473
Krauss, B. J., 162, 417, 422
Krauss, H. H., 162, 417, 422
Krebs, S. L., 422
Krenz, E. W., 287, 422
Krimm, W. R., 133, 386
Krippner, S., 142, 143, 422
Kroger, W. S., 14, 53, 66, 74, 207, 238, 248, 250, 251, 252, 253, 254, 275, 279, 287, 295, 422, 423, 465
Krug, W. M., 91, 385
Kubiak, R. V., 252, 423
Kubie, L. S., 423
Kubler, R. E., 423

Kuechenmeister, C. A., 426
Kuhn, L., 423
Kumar, V. K., 442
Kupper, H. I., 154, 423
Kurokawa, N., 423
Kurtz, R., 34, 389
Kurtz, R. M., 11, 156, 402, 425

L'Abate, L., 224, 459
LaBaw, W., 260, 263, 264, 423
Lafontaine, J., 6
Laguaite, J. K., 238, 263, 269, 423
Lahoda, R., 463
Lake, D., 423
Lamb, C. S., 40, 184, 233, 423
Landy, F. J., 443
Lane, B., 98, 423
Lang, P. J., 228, 424
Lange, A. F., 413
Langlois, J., 424
Lansdell, H., 426
Larner, B. R., 403
Latta, W. D., 455
Laur, E., 389
Laurence, J. R., 4, 29, 85, 118, 275, 279,
    424, 436, 442, 443
Lauter, J. L., 11, 425
Lavoie, G., 424, 426
Lavoisier, A. L., 4
Law, H. G., 29, 428
Lazar, B. S., 237, 238, 259, 402, 424
Lazarus, A. A., 208, 424
Lazovik, A. D., 228, 424
Leavitt, H. D., 98, 377
LeBaron, S., 259, 260, 413, 424
LeCron, L. M., 84, 156, 165, 295, 384,
    424, 425, 447, 478
Lee, C., 259, 377
Lefcoe, N. M., 185, 205, 441, 442
Lehman, R. E., 238, 425
Leibowitz, H. W., 104, 105, 157, 406, 425,
    432, 441
Lenny, E., 393
Lenox, J. R., 413
Lert, A. S., 425
Leva, R. A., 425
Levine, E. S., 183, 425
Levine, J. L., 11, 425
Levine, K. N., 98, 275, 425
Levitan, A. A., 263, 425
Levitt, E. E., 310, 321, 322, 327, 425, 426
Lewis, B. J., 184, 232, 426
Li, C. L., 426
Liébeault, A. A., 6, 7, 37, 84
Lieberman, J., 426
Lieberman, L. R., 147, 385, 426, 473
Lindner, H., 184, 216, 261, 316, 426
Lindzey, G., 341, 343, 409
Linn, L., 268, 463

Linton, P. H., 92, 426
Loftus, E. F., 279, 412, 426, 476
Loftus, G. R., 279, 426
Logan, D. R., 96, 463
London, P., 29, 31, 36, 141, 142, 143,
    145, 387, 426, 427, 449, 454
London, R. T., 11, 74, 185, 204, 244, 427
Lonsdale, C., 369
Lovett, D. J. W., 96, 427
Lowy, D., 458
Lubman, A., 260, 264, 403
Ludwig, A. M., 174, 427
Lugosi, Bela, 14
Lummis, G., 419
Lunden, B., 438
Lundholm, H., 476
Lundy, R. M., 100, 105, 121, 141, 145,
    147, 157, 393, 410, 425, 427, 441,
    443, 463
Lupica, V. P., 238, 427
Lyle, W. H., Jr., 427
Lynn, S. J., 39, 40, 143, 159, 376, 427,
    436, 466

McCabe, M. P., 10, 85, 417, 427
McCann, T., 147, 456
McCanne, T. R., 92, 183, 376
McClellan, G. E., 419
McConkey, K. M., 4, 29, 33, 46, 58, 90,
    109, 139, 153, 296, 396, 428, 429,
    436, 440, 456, 472
McCord, H., 142, 143, 429
McCranie, E. J., 154, 156, 248, 249, 250,
    388, 429
McCue, P. A., 163, 429
McDermott, D., 429
McDonald, R. D., 109, 151, 367, 400, 429
McDowell, M., 94, 95, 429
McFall, M. E., 378
McGeorge, C. M., 230, 369
McGill, O., 429
McGraw, M. B., 154, 429
McGuinness, T. P., 184, 429
McIntosh, I. B., 12, 429
McKimmie, J., 429
McLaughlin, D. M., 121, 421
McNeil, B., 450
McNeil, B. W., 415
McNeil, C., 95, 113, 460
McNeil, D. W., 47, 381
McPeake, J. D., 91, 103, 375, 459, 460,
    461, 462
McPherson, D., 463
MacCraken, P. J., 429
MacDonald, H., 33, 40, 104, 107, 117,
    118, 314, 389, 399, 412, 413, 434
MacDonald, J., 414
MacDonald, R., 415
Machiavelli, N., 326, 358

MacHovec, F. J., 2, 121, 183, 218, 429, 430
MacKinnon, D. P., 403
MacLeod, C., 160, 465
MacLeod-Morgan, C., 11, 430
MacMillan, M. B., 430
MacPhillamy, D., 438
Maddock, R. C., 183, 216, 455
Maher-Loughnan, G. P., 238, 268, 298, 299, 430
Malfara, A., 104, 460
Malin, A. H., 255, 369
Malmaud, R., 400
Malott, J. M., 56, 430
Malva, C. L. D., 445
Man, S. C., 121, 430
Manganiello, A. J., 183, 233, 430
Marcus, F. L., 430
Marcuse, F. L., 430
Margolis, C. G., 247, 260, 430
Margolis, J., 430
Mark, C. B., 183, 407
Marmer, M. J., 248, 250, 251, 252, 253, 430
Marshall, C., 94, 430
Marshall, G. D., 413
Martin, D., 377
Martin, J. S., 434
Maruffi, B. L., 184, 401, 460
Maslach, C., 94, 275, 430
Mason, A. A., 95, 240, 250, 251, 252, 253, 431
Masserman, J., 438
Matheson, G., 77, 183, 291, 431
Matthews, W. J., Jr., 90, 171, 431
Maultsby, M. C., 231, 431
Mead, S., 97, 431, 474
Mear, 272
Meares, A., 215, 267, 431
Meek, V., 431
Meeker, W. B., 431
Megas, J. C., 431
Meinz, R., 389
Melzack, R., 120, 432
Mensh, I. N., 98, 275, 388
Mercer, M., 98, 432
Merkur, D., 432
Mesmer, F. A., ix, 3, 4, 5, 11, 344, 352, 354, 428, 441, 444, 453, 468
Meyer, R. G., 119, 470
Meyers, S., 432
Michael, C. M., 156, 388
Michaels, R. M., 155, 377
Michaux, D., 118, 384, 446
Migliore, E. T., 432
Milechnin, A., 96, 459
Milgram, S., 10, 132, 320, 432
Miller, A., 184, 432
Miller, D. E., 432

Miller, H. R., 184, 216, 432
Miller, J., 312, 432
Miller, J. A., 260, 432
Miller, L. S., 432
Miller, M., 432
Miller, N. E., 189, 193, 194, 342, 393
Miller, R. D., 304, 432
Miller, R. J., 29, 34, 104, 105, 432, 450
Milne, G., 260, 433
Miner, J. P., 433
Misch, R. C., 238, 268, 400
Mitchell, M. B., 141, 433
M'Naghten, 330, 331
Moldawsky, R. J., 259, 433
Moll, A., 35, 433
Monteiro, K. P., 33, 275, 379, 413
Montgomery, D. J., 184, 185, 437
Montgomery, G. T., 183, 202, 433
Monzen, S., 433
Moon, H., 433
Moon, T., 21, 433
Moore, C. L., 263, 433
Moore, L. E., 247, 433
Moore, M. R., 433
Mordkoff, A. M., 476
Morgan, A. H., 31, 107, 116, 117, 118, 172, 375, 412, 413, 421, 433, 434, 450
Morgan, C. D., 425
Morgan, D., 417
Morgan, D. C., 434
Morgan, G., 434
Morgan, W. P., 93, 434
Morris, B. A. P., 238, 434
Morris, F., 434
Morrow, J. E., 463
Morse, D. R., 121, 239, 252, 256, 257, 258, 408, 434
Mosher, D., 431
Moss, C. S., 195, 199, 219, 221, 435
Mott, T., Jr., 53, 183, 185, 211, 238, 387, 435
Mount, G. R., 272, 435
Moyer, W. W., 435
Mozdzierz, G. J., 184, 435
Muehleman, T., 272, 435
Mullen, G., 185, 205, 443
Mullens, D., 103, 461
Mullin, C. S., 369
Mullins, J. G., 435
Murphy, J. K., 259, 435
Murray-Jobsis, J., 184, 435
Mustakallio, K., 438
Mutter, C. B., 10, 184, 435
Myers, S. A., 33, 40, 435

Naar, R., 159, 469
Nace, E. P., 121, 122, 124, 132, 138, 168, 436

Nakagawa, S., 96, 415
Nallapa, J. S., 94, 436
Nardi, T. J., 238, 436
Nash, C. B., 289, 436
Nash, J. K., 105, 378
Nash, M. R., 39, 158, 159, 427, 436
Nathan, P. E., 436
Navarrete, F. J., 376
Navradszky, L. I., 436
Nee, J. C., 31, 375, 463
Nelson, J., 436
Newbold, G., 466, 471
Newman, M., 185, 313, 436
Newman, M. F., 413
Newman, R., 436
Newmark, J., 400
Newton, B. W., 260, 267, 436
Niell, K. C., 114, 475
Nielson, M., 275, 447
Nightingale, M. E., 178, 461
Nogrady, H., 174, 428, 436
Nordlie, J. W., 451
Norton, K., 287
Nuechterlein, K. H., 93, 414
Nugent, W. R., 184, 185, 347, 437
Nunan, L. J., 437
Nuttman, D., 376
Nygard, J. W., 94
Nystrom-Bonnier, E., 100, 403

Oberlander, J. Z., 402
O'Brien, C. P., 239, 437
O'Brien, R. M., xvii, 34, 39, 41, 158, 170,
    178, 184, 234, 235, 288, 326, 406,
    414, 437, 457
Obstoj, I., 109, 437, 456
O'Connell, D. N., 157, 437, 440
Oetgen, W. J., 238, 472
O'Grady, K. E., 40, 438
O'Hare, C., 438
Oker-Blom, N., 438
Okhowat, V. O., 226, 438
Oliver, G. W., 260, 438
Olness, K. N., 96, 183, 222, 238, 239,
    241, 270, 304, 403, 414, 422, 438
Olsen, P. T., 372
Orleanu, P., 257, 404
Orme, G. C., 438
Orne, E. C., 28, 29, 139, 274, 397, 419,
    439, 440, 443, 457
Orne, M. T., 8, 10, 18, 30, 42, 56, 57, 69,
    101, 102, 108, 110, 111, 113, 114,
    116, 121, 122, 123, 124, 125, 126,
    132, 133, 134, 138, 139, 140, 152,
    153, 157, 166, 167, 168, 170, 203,
    207, 208, 248, 274, 277, 279, 296,
    309, 310, 311, 312, 313, 314, 315,
    316, 320, 321, 323, 324, 325, 331,
    344, 345, 346, 379, 399, 400, 419,

Orne, M. T. (*cont.*)
    436, 437, 438, 439, 440, 443, 456,
    457
Ortega, D. F., 183, 440
Ousby, W. J., 440
Ovenden, M., 162
Overlade, D. C., 440
Overley, T. M., 425, 426
Owens, D., 440

Packard, V., 286, 440
Packer, E., 440
Page, J. D., 440
Page, M. M., 439
Pajntar, M., 259, 440, 471
Paldi, E., 253, 402
Paracelsus (AKA: Von Hohenheim,
    T. P. A. B.), 2, 3
Paris, D. A., 378
Parisher, D. W., 34, 447
Parker, J. L., 259, 440
Parker, P. D., 143, 144, 441
Parkinson, B., 139, 377
Parrish, M. J., 157, 322, 425, 441
Paskewitz, D. A., 441
Paterson, A. S., 441
Patrick, B. S., 147, 368
Patten, E. F., 165, 441
Patterson, R., 448
Patterson, R. B., 183, 441
Pattie, F. A., 95, 104, 441
Patton, A., 130, 407
Paul, G. L., 228, 441
Pavlov, I., 94, 353
Pawlak, A. E., 462
Payton, T. I., 435
Pearson, P., 98, 441
Peded, O., 382
Pederson, L. L., 185, 205, 441, 442
Pekala, R. J., 442
Pelletier, A. M., 183, 442
Pelletier, K. R., 442
Penrod, J. H., 183, 234, 471
Pentony, P., 467
Peper, E., 442
Pereira, M., 442
Pereira, M. J., 367
Peretz, B. A., 253, 402
Perin, C. T., 368
Perls, F., 192, 305
Pernicano, K., 11, 407
Perret, J. J., 468
Perry, A., 409
Perry, B. J., 273, 442
Perry, C., 4, 29, 46, 81, 85, 108, 118,
    120, 157, 169, 185, 205, 275, 279,
    394, 424, 428, 432, 436, 442, 443,
    456
Peters, J. E., 81, 443

Peterson, R. A., 447
Petrusic, W. M., 115, 460, 463
Pettigrew, C. G., 443
Pettinati, H. M., 42, 133, 443
Pettitt, G. A., 184, 443
Petty, G. L., 183, 234, 443, 444
Pfeifer, G., 402
Phillips, A., 444
Piaget, J., 469
Piedmont, R. L., 94, 444
Pistole, D. D., 419, 444, 457
Place, M., 238, 264, 444
Planas, M., 136, 445
Plapp, J. M., 184, 222, 444
Platoni, K., 453
Platonow, K. I., 155, 444
Player, W. O., 444
Plotkin, W. B., 444
Podmore, F., 444
Polgar, F., 408
Polk, W. M., 184, 231, 444
Pollack, A. A., 271, 382
Pollock, D. H., 184, 229, 391
Pope, K. S., 294, 458
Porter, J., 290, 444
Porter, M. L., 378
Post, R. B., 105, 425
Pottinger, J., 448
Powell, D. H., 185, 206, 444
Powers, M., 444
Price, J., 261, 444
Prince, M., 8
Proshansky, H., 416
Provins, K. A., 467
Pulos, L., 5, 444
Pulver, M. P., 239, 244, 444
Pulver, S. E., 239, 244, 316, 444, 445
Putnam, W. H., 279, 445

Query, W. T., 39, 445
Quinn, T., 400

Rabuck, S. J., 178, 326, 437
Radtke, H. L., 35, 85, 134, 136, 139, 178,
    445, 461, 462
Radtke-Bodorik, H. L., 112, 136, 137, 445,
    461, 462, 463
Rafky, D. M., 279, 445
Raginsky, B. B., 92, 215, 248, 249, 251,
    252, 445, 446
Raikov, V. L., 154, 446
Rainer, D. D., 446
Rank, O., 216
Rappaport, A., 239, 256, 446
Raskin, R. H., 446
Rasmus, C., 468
Rasmussen, W. C., 454
Rausch, V., 303, 446
Raven, P. B., 434

Ravitz, L. J., 184, 446
Raynaud, J., 94, 446
Reardon, J. P., 183, 415
Redd, W. H., 261, 446
Rees, W. L., 397
Regina, E. G., 455
Register, P. A., 29, 419, 447
Reid, W. H., 185, 208, 447
Reiff, R., 155, 157, 447
Reilley, R. R., 34, 253, 349, 350, 385,
    398, 422, 447, 449
Reis, H. T., 447, 476
Reiser, M., 275, 282, 447
Reiss, M. M., 447
Reiss, S., 447
Reiter, P. J., 94, 95, 447
Relinger, H., 141, 447
Reyher, J., 11, 35, 46, 151, 166, 171,
    381, 404, 409, 447, 448, 454, 459,
    477
Reynolds, D. J., 228, 424
Rhodes, R. H., 448
Rhonder, J., 409
Rhue, J. W., 159, 427, 436
Richman, D. N., 448
Riddle, E. E., 141, 143, 463
Rios, R. J., 448
Ripley, H. S., 11, 402
Ritow, J. K., 184, 448
Rivers, S. M., 27, 45, 103, 448, 461, 462
Roberts, A. C., 282, 448
Roberts, A. H., 448
Roberts, J., 183, 211, 435
Robertson, T. G., Jr., 395
Robitscher, J. B., 448
Rochford, J., 417
Rockey, E. E., 46, 182, 448
Rodemer, C. S., 105, 425
Roden, R. G., 183, 448
Rodgers, C. W., 448
Rodolfa, E. R., 12, 349, 350, 422, 447,
    449
Rogers, B. M., 449
Rogers, C., 71, 185, 191, 208
Rosen, J., 201, 240, 307, 311, 316, 449
Rosen, S., 449
Rosenberg, S. W., 449
Rosenberger, P. H., 261, 446
Rosenfeld, A., 312, 462
Rosenhan, D., 142, 143, 449
Rosenthal, B. G., 141, 144, 146, 449
Rosenthal, R., 375
Roskar, E., 259, 471
Ross, C. A., 273, 449
Ross, P. J., 212, 449
Ross, S., 27, 462
Rossi, E. L., 213, 223, 297, 396, 449
Rossi, S. I., 297, 396
Rossiter, T., 368

Roth, P., 120, 400
Rothstein, W., 183, 201, 473
Roush, E. S., 97, 431, 474
Rowen, R., 185, 450
Rowland, L. W., 317, 318, 319, 321, 322, 450
Rowland, R. W., 435
Rubinstein, D., 426
Rubinstein, Z., 249, 420
Rubio, R., 280, 453
Ruch, J. C., 293, 294, 450
Ruggieri, V., 44, 377
Rush, B., 453
Ruskin, P. M., 419
Russell, R. J., 450
Russo, S., 423
Ryan, M. L., 81, 450
Rychtarik, R. C., 378
Ryken, K., 314, 335, 386, 450
Rywick, T., 425

Saad, C. L., 115, 460
Saavedra, R. L., 34, 450
Sabourin, M., 104, 424, 450
Saccuzzo, D. P., 415, 450
Sacerdote, P., 54, 207, 212, 215, 217, 244, 245, 295, 302, 303, 450, 451
Sachs, B. C., 451
Sachs, L. B., 241, 392, 413, 451, 463
Sackeim, H. A., 11, 451
Safran, D., 450
Saletu, B., 120, 451
Saletu, M., 451
Salter, A., 11, 34, 343, 451
Salzberg, H. C., 122, 140, 142, 144, 149, 275, 392, 451, 457
Sampimon, R. L. H., 250, 252, 451
Samuelly, I., 463
Sanders, B. L., 451
Sanders, G. S., 279, 451
Sanders, S., 151, 185, 206, 222, 237, 241, 451, 452, 468
Sarbin, T. R., 10, 98, 153, 156, 167, 386, 452, 467
Sargent, C. L., 289, 290, 452
Sarles, R. M., 263, 264, 452
Saunders, C., 452
Scagnelli, J., 184, 223, 452
Scagnelli-Jobsis, J., 41, 184, 452
Schacterle, G. R., 434
Schafer, D. W., 76, 182, 217, 240, 241, 246, 280, 388, 452, 453 .
Scharcoff, J. A., 386
Schathin, A. J., 276, 453
Schauble, P. G., 252, 253, 475
Scheerer, M., 155, 157, 447
Schell, R. E., 453
Schilder, P., 453
Schirado, W. C., 453

Schlutter, L. C., 453
Schneck, J. M., 10, 18, 95, 184, 207, 238, 372, 429, 453
Schoenberg, S., 403
Schofield, L. J., 453, 454
Scholder, M. H., 282, 454
Schoor, R. S., 258, 434
Schraa, J. C., 184, 201, 454
Schreiner, F., 99, 275, 414
Schuler, J., 448
Schulman, R. E., 142, 143, 454
Schuster, P., 463
Schuyler, B. A., 138, 454
Schwarz, B. E., 454
Schwartz, W., 444, 454
Scott, D. L., 250, 252, 261, 454
Scott, D. S., 56, 375
Scott, E. M., 281, 454, 469
Scott, N., 93, 376
Scrignar, C. B., 184, 230, 454
Scrimgeour, W. G., 185, 205, 441, 442
Sears, A. B., 141, 143, 146, 454
Sears, R. R., 454
Seay, B., 40, 390
Sebej, F., 469
Segal, H., 258, 418
Segall, M. M., 454
Seidenberg, B., 416
Seif, B., 183, 184, 455
Selavan, A., 455
Sellars, R. W., 455
Sellars, D. J., 314, 398
Sexton, R. O., 183, 216, 455
Sextus, C., 455
Shabinsky, M. A., 137, 461
Shapiro, A., 260, 267, 455
Shapiro, D., 93, 414
Shaposhnikov, A., 289, 455
Sharma, A., 455
Shaul, R. D., 455
Shaw, L. H., 283, 455
Sheehan, D. V., 30, 455
Sheehan, E. P., 238, 455, 458
Sheehan, P. W., 29, 33, 40, 46, 58, 81, 109, 139, 147, 153, 166, 167, 170, 178, 181, 238, 387, 393, 413, 428, 429, 437, 440, 443, 450, 455, 456
Sheldon, W. H., 44, 355, 358, 456
Shepperson, V. L., 292, 456
Sherrill, C. J., 429
Shertzer, C. L., 100, 427
Shiel, R. C., 456
Shor, J., 155, 463
Shor, R. E., 28, 40, 69, 129, 139, 157, 293, 294, 295, 402, 437, 457, 459
Shrier, L., 430
Shulik, A. M., 457
Shulze, D., 463
Shum, K., 121, 421

Siegel, E. F., 248, 457
Sikorsky, C., 297, 416
Silber, S., 69, 185, 222, 457
Silberner, J., 249, 457
Silver, M. J., 375, 457
Silverberg, E. L., 466
Simek, T. C., 288, 457
Simmons, W. L., 279, 451
Simon, J., 151, 457
Simon, M. J., 122, 140, 457
Simonds, J. F., 184, 405
Simonson, E., 93, 377
Singer, G., 114, 401
Singer, J. L., 294, 458
Sipprelle, C. N., 106, 410
Skalin, M., 100, 403
Skiba, A. H., 39, 119, 414, 458
Skinner, B. F., 194, 232, 343, 358
Slavin, R. J., 458
Sletten, I., 121, 451, 465
Sloane, M. C., 458
Smigielski, J. S., 458
Smith, A. H., 408
Smith, A. H., Jr., 397, 411, 475
Smith, D. E., 45, 458
Smith, E. W. L., 389
Smith, G. M., 455
Smith, H. D., 458
Smith, H. V., 238, 455, 458
Smith, J. A., 133, 386
Smith, J. R., 109, 429
Smith, L. H., 316, 445
Smith, M. C., 279, 458
Smith, M. S., 304, 458
Smith, S. J., 248, 458
Smyth, L. D., 11, 166, 171, 275, 315,
    448, 458
Snyder, E. D., 69, 459
Sochevanov, N., 459
Solderholm, E., 288
Solovey, G., 96, 459
Sommerschield, H., 171, 459
Soper, P. H., 224, 459
Soucy, G. P., 379
Spanos, N. P., 2, 22, 27, 45, 81, 85, 91,
    95, 101, 103, 104, 111, 112, 113,
    115, 118, 121, 131, 134, 135, 136,
    137, 139, 157, 177, 178, 372, 377,
    393, 394, 409, 417, 445, 459, 460,
    461, 462, 463
Sparks, L., 462
Spiegel, D., 42, 47, 53, 63, 183, 184, 185,
    218, 240, 274, 303, 312, 401, 440,
    452, 462, 463
Spiegel, H., 11, 30, 31, 40, 53, 155, 184,
    204, 205, 268, 271, 274, 302, 375,
    401, 412, 440, 462, 463, 465
Spies, G., 184, 290, 463
Spillane, J., 462

Spinler, D., 183, 211, 378
Spithill, A. C., 185, 214, 463
Springer, C. J., 463
Stacher, G., 114, 376, 463
Stager, G. L., 147, 463
Staib, A. R., 96, 463
Stalnaker, J. M., 141, 143, 463
Stam, H. J., 2, 95, 112, 113, 136, 157,
    178, 445, 459, 460, 462, 463
Stambaugh, E. E., II, 183, 463
Stanley, R. O., 464
Stanley, S., 159, 427, 436
Stanton, H. E., 75, 183, 185, 204, 207,
    210, 224, 464
Starker, S., 182, 207, 464
Stava, L., 184, 464
Steadman, C., 393
Steen, P., 386
Stefancic, M., 259, 440
Stein, C., 183, 220, 464
Stein, V. T., 238, 465
Steinringer, H., 376
Stephenson, C. W., 154, 469
Stern, D. A., 465
Stern, D. B., 30, 375, 391, 465
Stern, J. A., 121, 451, 465
Stern, R. M., 81, 443
Sternbach, R. A., 114, 465
Sternlicht, M., 36, 465
Stevens, G., 259, 377
Stevens, G. E., 437
Stevenson, J. H., 172, 173, 465
Stevenson, R., 287, 465
Stevenson, R. L., 291
Stewart, R. S., 184, 216, 382
Stirman, J. A., 388
St. Jean, R., 137, 160, 162, 167, 465
St. Jean, R. L., 41, 386
Stolzenberg, J., 465
Stone, H., 239, 252, 254, 256, 257, 466
Stone, J. A., 466
Straker, N., 310, 477
Stratton, J. G., 275, 280, 466
Straus, R. A., 151, 466
Strauss, P. S., 470
Stricherz, M. E., 184, 466
Strickler, C. B., 129
Stromberg, B. V., 213, 466
Suematsu, H., 423
Sullivan, H. S., 189, 191
Sullivan, J., 411
Surman, O. S., 226, 254, 466
Sutcliffe, J. P., 21, 466
Sutherland, E. B., 466
Svengali, 17, 18, 332, 468
Swade, R. H., 238, 252, 260, 265, 266,
    385
Swartz, C. M., 91, 160, 466
Swartz, S., 403

Sweeney, C. A., 143, 427, 466
Swezey, R. W., 467
Swiercinsky, D., 141, 145, 467
Sykes, C. T., 147, 472
Szelenberger, W., 478

Taboada, E. L., 183, 235, 467
Talone, J. M., 393
Tamai, H., 423
Tappeiner, D. A., 291, 467
Tarasoff, V., 225, 467
Tarnow, J. D., 71, 403
Tart, C. T., 85, 374, 413, 467
Tasini, M. F., 238, 265, 467
Taub, H. A., 183, 271, 272, 401
Taub-Bynum, E. B., 350, 467
Taul, J. H., 386
Taylor, R. E., 183, 467
Tebecis, A. K., 467
Tellegen, A., 448, 467
Teltscher, H. O., 468
Teten, H. D., 280, 281, 468
Teter, H. R., 154, 429
Tewell, K., 264, 423
Thal, A. D., 269, 385
Thigpen, C. H., 468
Thomas, M., 409
Thorndike, E. L., 150
Thorne, D. E., 96, 124, 133, 134, 468
Tilden, J., 147, 456
Tilton, P., 183, 184, 222, 229, 468
Timm, H. W., 279, 468
Timney, B. N., 94, 468
Timor-Tritsch, I., 402
Ting, C. Y., 426
Tinterow, M. M., 468
Tipton, R. D., 158, 436
Tissler, D. M., 268, 406
Titley, R., 469
Tkachyk, M. E., 139, 462
Toman, W. J., 183, 407
Tomlinson, W. K., 468
Toomey, T. C., 241, 468.
Torda, C., 177, 468
Tosi, D. J., 183, 227, 228, 379, 409, 415, 469
Towe, D. H., 469
Tracy, D. F., 469
Traina, F., 408
Travis, R. P., 426
Trenerry, M. R., 183, 469
Trevan, W., 469
Trilby, 17
Triplet, R. G., 9, 469
True, R. M., 141, 142, 154, 155, 469
Trustman, R., 469
Tryon, W. W., 401, 412
Tuite, P. A., 469
Tupin, J. P., 226, 400

Turco, R. N., 184, 218, 469
Turin, A. C., 469
Twerski, A. J., 159, 469
Twersky, M., 122, 419
Tyre, T. E., 185, 206, 405

Udolf, R., x, xi, 199, 278, 279, 282, 330, 335, 387, 466, 469
Uherik, A., 469
Ulett, G. A., 69, 121, 451, 465, 470
Uribe-de-Fazzano, C., 470

Vacchiano, R. B., 470
Van Der Hart, O., 184, 238, 470
Van Dyke, P., 184, 470
Van Ginneken, J., 470
Van Gorp, W. G., 119, 470
Van Helmont, J. B., 2
Van Nuys, D., 207, 247, 470
Van Pelt, S. J., 92, 96, 201, 203, 290, 314, 470, 471
Van Rooyen, E. J., 220, 471
Vellios, A. T., 401
Venn, J., 66, 471
Venturino, M., 27, 113, 397, 398
Vernon, J., 447
Vickery, A. R., 63, 388, 420
Vilenskaya, L., 471
Vingoe, F. J., 12, 21, 471
Vitale, J. H., 241, 451
Vodovnik, L., 259, 440, 471
Vogt, O., 35
Von Willebrandt, E., 438

Wachtel, P. L., 405
Wadden, T. A., 183, 211, 234, 471
Wade, N. L., 398
Wadlington, W. L., 105, 121, 410, 425
Wagenfeld, J., 184, 471
Wagner, E. E., 98, 99, 219, 220, 275, 414
Wagstaff, G. F., 21, 27, 135, 147, 162, 238, 279, 280, 471, 472
Wain, H. J., 238, 240, 472
Wakeman, R. J., 247, 472
Walker, D. L., 291, 472
Walker, N. S., 157, 472
Walker, W. L., 86, 183, 206, 393, 472, 473
Wall, J. A., 473
Wall, P. D., 147, 473
Wallace, B., 106, 115, 157, 158, 403, 472, 473
Wallace, E. R., IV, 183, 201, 473
Wallach, M. A., 149, 473
Wallis, G. G., 94, 474
Walrath, L. C., 474
Walsh, B., 81, 108, 443
Walters, S. R., 435
Wanderer, Z. W., 36, 465

Warner, K. E., 474
Watkins, A. L., 97, 474
Watkins, H. H., 205, 218, 474
Watkins, J. G., 274, 319, 320, 322, 323, 474
Waxman, D., 474
Weber, A. M., 474
Wedemeyer, C., 85, 474
Weekes, J. R., 139, 460, 462
Weight, D. G., 184, 293, 294, 296, 409, 416
Wein, A., 474
Weinapple, M., 417
Weisberg, J., 474
Weisbrot, M. M., 239, 437
Weitz, G. A., 434
Weitz, R. D., 267, 474
Weitzenhoffer, A. M., xiii, 7, 25, 27, 35, 37, 46, 97, 101, 104, 367, 474, 475
Weitzenhoffer, G. B., 37, 475
Wells, W. R., 165, 475
Welsh, D. K., 183, 475
Werner, W. E. F., 252, 253, 475
Wert, A., 31, 412
West, L. J., 114, 307, 315, 439, 475
Wester, W., 408
Wester, W. C., II, 397, 411, 475
Weyandt, J. A., 239, 243, 475
Wheeler, L., 447, 476
White, G., 438
White, H., 426
White, K. D., 33, 429
White, R. W., 141, 144, 476
Whitehorn, J. C., 94, 476
Wickramasekera, I. E., 34, 476
Wicks, G. R., 77, 476
Widdifield, D. A., 476
Wiese, K. F., 69, 416
Wigan, E. R., 104
Wijesinghe, B., 183, 476
Wilbur, C. B., 183, 476
Wilcko, J. M., 257, 434
Wilcox, P., 100, 476
Wilcox, W. W., 101, 314, 398
Wilkie, R., 53, 183, 211, 392
Willard, R. D., 96, 746
Williams, D., 389
Williams, J. A., 184, 248, 476
Williams, J. E., 96, 476

Williams, M. H., 97, 365
Williams, S., 118, 175, 476
Williamsen, J. A., 126, 128, 129, 133, 476
Wilson, B. J., 388
Wilson, J.·G., 46, 448
Wilson, L., 135, 419, 476
Wilson, S. C., 33, 56, 375, 477
Wineburg, E. N., 310, 477
Winegardner, J., 378
Winn, R. B., 477
Winnett, R. L., 378
Wiseman, R. J., 477
Wladyslaw, M., 477
Wolberg, L. M., 477
Wolff, E., 447, 476
Wollman, L., 290, 477
Wolpe, J., 195, 196, 199, 311, 477
Wood, D., 405
Wood, H. M., 477
Woodruff, M. F. A., 250, 252, 451
Worring, R. W., 411
Worthington, T. S., 279, 477
Wright, G. W., 183, 407
Wright, R. C., 477
Wurzmann, A. G., 91, 385

Yakhno, N., 474
Yamauchi, K. T., 256, 477
Yanchar, R. J., 40, 477
Yapko, M. D., 90, 477
Yeager, C. L., 154, 399
Yehuda, S., 382
Yepes, E., 39, 414
Yoder, N. S., 478
Young, J., 122, 478
Young, P. C., 141, 143, 155, 294, 318, 321, 322, 478

Zakrzewski, K., 478
Zamansky, H. S., 173, 174, 400, 418, 460, 478
Zeig, J. K., 221, 478
Zeigarnik, B., 166, 286, 364
Zelig, M., 279, 478
Zeltzer, L. K., 259, 424
Zilbergeld, B., 478
Zimbardo, P. G., 94, 430
Zimmerman, R. L., 448
Zlotogorski, Z., 238, 478

Subject Index

Ability, hypnotic, 13, 45. *See also* suscepti-
  bility; Trance capacity
Abreaction, 159, 190, 198, 201, 212,
  216-218, 250, 351
  silent, 218
  spontaneous, 212, 362
Academic major, 26, 38
Academic performance, 290
Acetylcholine, 114
Acquisition, 351
Acting out, 215
Acupuncture, 112, 120, 121
  placebo, 120, 121
Addiction, 183, 240, 351
Adolescents, 260
Adultery, 332
Advertising, 283-287
  subliminal, 286
Affect bridge, 217, 351
Afterimage, 64, 106, 107
  negative, 106, 358
  positive, 106, 360
Age
  mental, 36
  progression, 159, 217, 234, 351
  regression, 11, 24, 26, 30, 31, 111, 118,
    141, 142, 144, 146, 149, 152-159,
    181, 208, 212, 216, 217, 233, 234,
    244, 274, 280, 346, 347, 351
  drawings in, 153, 154
  duality effect in, 118
  to previous life, 159
  spelling under, 153
  spontaneous, 312
  -specific behaviors, 154
Aggression, displaced, 215
Agnosia, 28, 351
AIDS, 267
Aids, mechanical, 68, 69-71, 74
Alcohol, 47
Alcoholism, 183, 199, 227, 231, 232, 234,
  338
Alexithymia, 184, 351
Alienation, of part of self, 192
Allergies, 96
Alpha waves, 120
Amenorrhea, 238

American Law Institute, insanity test, 330
American Medical Association, 10
American Psychological Association, 10,
  174, 327
American Society of Clinical Hypnosis, 206,
  349
Amnesia, 29, 30, 84, 111, 119, 128, 133,
  183, 234, 351
  content, 124, 353
  posthypnotic, 26, 29, 31, 121-140, 160,
    166, 167, 172, 282, 294, 328, 360
  indirect measurement of, 131, 134
  lifting of, 138, 275
  models of, 129
  partial, 84, 123
  pseudo-, 126, 138, 360
  reversibility of, 121, 126, 132, 138
  selective, 358
  source, 124, 134, 362
  specific, 362
  spontaneous, 122, 123, 362
Amputation, psychological, 243
Analgesia, 28, 32, 84, 109-121, 172,
  239-248, 351
  hand, 169
  rapid induction, 119, 120, 172
Analysis, training, 189
Anal stage, 186, 216
Anesthesia, 351. *See also* Hypnoanesthesia
  balanced, 250
  chemical, hearing during, 119
  glove, 7, 243, 255, 257, 356
Anesthesiologists, 239, 249
Anesthetic, 238, 303
  chemical, 5, 46, 119, 250, 251, 256
  after-effects of, 251
Aneurysm, 255
Anorexia nervosa, 183, 209, 352
Anorgasmia, 235
Anosmia, 26, 28, 352
Anoxia, 209, 251
Anxiety, 41, 121, 171, 187, 192, 193, 197,
  198, 213, 214, 223, 224, 228, 249,
  251, 309, 310, 313, 352
  moral, 358. *See also* Guilt
  posthypnotic, 309, 310, 313
  preoperative, 251

Anxiety (*cont.*)
  reality, 355
  test, 290
Anxiety-producing material, 141, 148, 193,
    197, 212, 234
Aortic stenosis, 255
Apollonian, 40
Arm
  catalepsy, 22, 61, 75, 77, 78, 85, 126,
    163
  heaviness, 25, 26, 29, 49
  immobilization, 25, 26, 29
  levitation, 48, 49, 59-62, 72, 74, 85, 91,
    352
  lowering, 28
  rigidity, 25, 26, 29
Arousal conditions, 148, 149
Arrhythmia, 238
Arterial oxygen level, 96
Artifact, group, 23
As Questionnaire, 43, 44
Assassination, 283
Assertiveness training, 196-197, 235
Association, free, 8, 188
Asthma, 96-97, 238, 259
Astrology, 2
Attention, focusing of, 73
Attention-capturing devices, 69
Attenuation rates, patient, 231
Attitude, 362
  hypnotic, 44
Authority figure, 10
Autohypnosis, 268-269, 295-296,
    299-300, 352, 362. *See also* Self-
    hypnosis
Autokinetic movement, 106
Automatic talking, 116, 117, 131, 356
Automatic writing, 28, 113, 116, 131, 172,
    173, 352, 356
Awakening. *See also* Hypnosis, termination
    of; Trance, termination of
  difficulties in, 87, 88, 308, 309
  hypersuggestibility upon, 278

Babinski sign, 153, 352
Baquet, 3
Barber-Glass Questionnaire, 43
Barber Suggestibility Scale, 31-33, 37, 44,
    56, 144, 167
  objective score on, 33
  subjective score on, 33
Basal metabolism rate, 94
Basic trust, 44
Beat note, 352
Behavior
  antisocial, 317-327, 331
  criminal, 317-327, 330
  experimentally legitimized, 321, 355

Behavior (*cont.*)
  immoral, 317-327
  maladaptive, 194, 198, 221, 359, 363
  modification, 185, 193-199, 200, 201,
    202, 209, 358
  posthypnotic, 126, 127, 164-166
  self-injurious, 317-327
  shaping, 198
Bender-Gestalt Test, 153
Biofeedback, 35, 94, 259, 271-272, 352
Birth control, 272-273
Bleeding, control of, 93, 238, 256
Blindness
  hypnotic, 104, 106, 107
  hysterical, 155
Blind ratings, 140, 156, 283
Blind studies, 346, 352
Blisters, 95-96
Blood, distribution of, 93-94
Blood pressure, 93, 116, 120, 270-272
  diastolic, 93, 270, 271
  systolic, 93, 270, 271
Body language, 188
Bone conduction, 104
Borderline patients, 184, 221, 223
"Born again" Christians, 39
Braidism, 6, 61, 63-65, 352
Brainstorming, 150, 151, 206
Brawner case, 330
Breast, development, 96
British Medical Society, 10
Bruxism, 201, 352
Burger's disease, 94
Burn patients, 245-248

Calendar tearing, 220
California Psychological Inventory (CPI), 43
Cancer, 238, 241, 260-263, 266-269
  breast, 261, 266
    metastasized, 261, 262, 266
  remission of, 266-268
    spontaneous, 267
Cardiac arrest, 77
  block, 92
  rate, 92, 93
Carotid artery pressure "method," 77
Catalepsy, 7, 351, 352
Cataleptic state, 19, 312
Cattell 16 Personality Factors Questionnaire,
    43
Cerebral circulation, 94
Cerebral hemisphere
  dominant, 11
  nondominant, 11
Ceremonies, religious, 2
Certifying boards, in hypnosis, 10
Challenges, 51, 64, 352

Chaperone technique, 69, 208, 352
Character disorders, 190, 353
Chemotherapy, 260, 261, 266
Chevreul pendulum, 49, 70, 214, 353
Child abuse, 39, 325
Childbirth, 82, 248, 249, 251-254
Childhood experiences, 36, 39-40
  birth order, 39
  family size, 39
Children, 44, 64, 155, 157, 158, 203, 222,
    232, 259, 260, 263, 264, 269, 270,
    299, 304
  terminally ill, 264
Children's Hypnotic Susceptibility Scale,
    29-30
Chloroform, 5
Classic suggestion effect, 27
Client-centered therapy. *See* Therapy, Ro-
    gerian
Coercion, hypnotic, 328
Cognitive restructuring, 230
Cognitive strategies, 11, 111, 139
Cognitive tasks, 141, 145
Cold sores, 96
Color, complementary, 106
Color blindness, 106
Command, 353
Communication, 226, 227, 229
  of abstract ideas concretely, 285
  nonverbal, 69, 285
  of unconditional positive regard for pa-
    tient, 191
Compulsion, 230
Concentration, 59, 73, 79, 82, 143, 145
Conditioning, 231
  classical, 35, 198, 199, 353
  covert, 199, 231-232, 234
  higher order, 169
  instrumental, 193, 198, 357, 359
  operant, 193, 198-199, 231, 357, 359
  Pavlovian, 353
Confabulations, 279, 280, 282
Conference, preinduction, 65, 207
Confession, hypnotically obtained, 275,
    277-278
Confidence, in the integrity of the experi-
    menter, 320
Conflict
  hypnotic generation of, 165, 171, 174,
    275, 315
  internal, 200, 363
  sexual, hypnotic generation of, 171
  unconscious, 187, 354
Confounding variables, 353
Confusion, posthypnotic period of, 313
Confusion technique, 72
Congenital icthyosiform erythroderma, 95
Conscience, 186

Consciousness, 353
  altered states of, 10, 56, 57, 151, 363
Consent form, 334
Conspiracy, 328, 329
Constitutional rights, 275
Contact lenses, 58
Contraception. *See* Birth control
Control, loss of, 16-17, 35, 224
  group, 346, 353
  perceived locus of, 224, 360
  transfer of, 82
  variable, 353
Conversion reaction, 41
Convicts, 199
Convulsions, 3, 4
Couch, analytic, 179, 187, 188, 190
Counterconditioning, 361
Countertransference, 189, 207, 215, 223,
    258, 261, 312, 316, 354. *See also*
    Relationship
Couriers, hypnotized, 282, 283
Creative Imagination Scale, 33, 56, 151
  problem solving, 150
Creativity, 11, 149-152, 291
  effects of hypnosis on, 150
  factors inhibiting, 151
  tests of, 149-150
Credulous position, the, 21
Crime, mental capacity to commit. *See*
    M'Naghten Rule
Criminal attempt, 327
Criminal behavior. *See* Behavior, criminal
Criminal investigation
  FBI guidelines for use of hypnosis in, 280
  generation of leads in, 279
  U.S. Air Force guidelines for use of hyp-
    nosis in, 280
Criminal responsibility, 328-333
  solicitation, 328, 329
Crisis, 4, 354
Crisis intervention, 183
Cross-examination, 281
Crying, posthypnotic, 310
Crystal ball, imaginary, 220
Cue
  posthypnotic, 360
  for reinduction, 75
  word, embedded in a sentence, 166
Cultures, primitive, 2
Cure rate, 190
  spontaneous, 190

Davis-Husband Scale, 84
Daydreaming, 175, 294, 355. *See also* Fan-
    tasy
Day residue, 354
Deafness. *See* Hallucination, of deafness

Death, 261, 301
    intellectual, 261
    physical, 261
    rehearsal, hypnotic, 263
    social, 261
Debridements, 246
Deception, of subjects, 318, 319, 328
Decompensation, 309, 354
Defense mechanisms, 187, 212, 213, 262, 354
Delirium, postoperative, 254
Delta waves, 16, 154
Delusions, 183, 222, 354
Demand characteristics, 10, 11, 140, 168, 345, 354
Denial, 227, 264, 354
Dental procedures. *See also* Hypnosis, in dentistry
    drilling, 255
    implants, 257
Dentures, 256
Department of Health, Education and Welfare, 335
Department of Health and Human Services, 335
Dependent variable, 354
Depression, 159, 183, 227, 310, 354
    posthypnotic, 309, 310
    postpartum, 252
Depressive equivalent, 248
Dermatitis, 238
Desensitization, 234
    covert, 229
    systematic, 197-199, 226, 230, 232, 234, 235
Diagnosis, 195
Diagnostic and Statistical Manual, DSM III, 71
Digit-symbol substitution task, 143
Dionysian, 40
Disease. *See* Illness
Disease process, hypnotic intervention in, 264-272
Disorientation, 163, 296
Dissociation, 113, 117, 123, 164, 172-175, 212, 352, 354
    pathological, 215, 358
Dissociative state, 11
    reactions, 212
Divorce, 303
Doctoral dissertations, 350
Double bind, 223, 354
Double blind studies, 113, 354
Dramatizations, 285
Dream(s), 2, 108, 160, 188
    cognitive theory of, 177
    erotic, 178
    hypnotically induced, 26, 28, 30, 31,

Dream(s) *(cont.)*
    165, 175-179, 206, 212, 219, 220, 226, 234, 357
    uses of, 218-222
    hypnotic manipulation of, 176, 229
    incubation centers, 2
    interpretation of, 149, 177, 192, 212, 218-220, 265
    validity of, 219
    of knowledge, 358
    latent content of, 218
    lucid, 41, 219, 358
    manifest content of, 218, 354
    nocturnal, 41, 175-176, 355, 363
    NREM, 175
    posthypnotic, 175, 176
    suggesting theme of, 219
    symbolism, 177
    transference reflected in, 220
    verbal reports of, 102
    work, 176
Drowsiness, posthypnotic, 313
Drug abuse, 232, 233, 234. *See also* Addiction
Drug, analgesic, 120
Du Sommeil, 6
Dynamics, 354

Ectomorphy, 44, 355
Edwards Personal Preference Schedule, 43
EEG. *See* Electroencephalogram
Effortless experiencing, 152
Ego, 11, 186, 188, 354
    alien, 190, 353
    alter-, 192
    boundaries, 192, 223
    building, 190, 223, 255
    defenses, 221. *See also* Defense mechanisms
    distorting mechanisms, 244
    dystonic. *See* Ego, alien
    functions, 186
    ideal, 186, 191
    observing, 118, 219, 221, 258, 295, 328, 358, 359
    participating, 219, 295, 359
    splitting, 219, 295, 296, 355
    state, primative, 221
    strength, 212, 223
    strengthening, 120, 200, 223, 230, 234, 269, 330
    syntonic, 190, 321, 353
Ejaculation
    premature, 184, 235
    retarded, 184
EKG. *See* Electrocardiogram

Electrocardiogram, 120
Electroencephalogram, 16, 97, 110, 120, 153, 154, 160, 177, 250, 355
Electromyogram, 35, 355
Embedded Figures Test, 44
Emotion, 98-100, 355
  generation of, 217-218
  patient induced, 189, 258
Emotionally charged material, 212, 220
Emotional reactions, 212
Emotional state, hypnotically induced, 98-100, 220, 357
  spontaneous, 217
Empathy, 223
Encopresis, 183
Endomorphy, 44, 355
Endorphins, 114
Endurance, 97. *See also* Fatigue
Enuresis, 183, 202, 355
Environment, detachment from, 73
Epileptic seizures, 154, 238, 273
Eros, 186
Erythema, 95
ESP, 19, 245, 289-290, 355
Ether, 5
Ethical review boards, 335, 348
Ethics, 174, 210, 231, 287, 288, 299, 326, 327, 332, 333, 350. *See also* Hypnotist, misconduct by
Euphemistic expressions, 242
Euphoria, 221
Exhibitionism, 231
Exhortations for honesty in reports, 101, 132, 345
Exorcism, hypnotic, 222
Experiences
  birth, 216
  mystical, 39
  religious, 39, 226, 291
Experimental design
  counterbalanced, 353
  factorial, 355
  within-subjects, repeated-measures, 275, 364
Experimenter bias, 170, 346, 354, 355
Extinction, 157, 194, 197, 198, 355
  covert, 231, 233
  resistance to, 233
Eye
  blink, 157, 276
  catalepsy, 6, 26, 29, 84
  closure, 25, 26, 29, 60, 64, 73, 80, 82, 84, 144, 146
  fixation, 57, 61, 63-65
  flutter, 60, 64, 80
  movements, 105-106
    lateral, 45
    post-rotational, 105

Eye (*cont.*)
  muscles, fatigue of, 63
  roll, 12, 30

Fables, 149
Failure
  in induction, 72
  to meet challenge, passive, 51
  in therapy, 237
Fainting, posthypnotic, 310
Fairy tales, use of with children, 222
Faith healing, 2, 3
Faking, an effect, 345, 346
Fantasy, 40, 66, 149, 203, 212, 216, 221, 223, 236, 280, 295, 355. *See also* Daydreaming
  erotic, 244
  goal-directed, 61, 91, 356
  rape, 310
Fatigue, 97. *See also* Endurance
Fear, 15, 34, 57, 58, 60, 78, 82, 95, 195-198, 208, 217, 223, 236, 255, 355. *See also* Phobia
  of loss of control, 67
Feedback, delayed, auditory, 104
Feedback loop, 200, 240, 355, 363. *See also* Vicious cycle
Feelings
  of grandiosity and power, 207, 315
  of self-mastery and control, 207, 211
  subjective, 66, 79-82
Fictional finalisms, 196
Finger lock, 25, 29, 50-51
Fixation, 356
Flees box, 104, 356
Flooding, 198, 230, 356
  covert, 230
  hypnotic, 230
  in vivo, 230
Flower method, 67-69
Folie a deux, 208, 356
Follow-ups, 203-205, 211, 224, 232
Fractionation, 86, 356
Frame of reference, 195, 200, 210, 221
Free will, 187
French Academy of Science, 4
Frigidity, 183, 235, 356
Fugue, 183

G, 149, 356
Galvanic skin response, 80, 94-95, 114, 171, 276, 356
Gastric secretions, 98
Generality of findings, 356
Generalization, 193, 198, 356
Genital stage, 186
Government regulations, concerning hypnosis, 335-339

Grafting procedures, 246
Grief, pathological, 184
Group data, 23, 228
GSR. *See* Galvanic skin response
Guilford-Zimmerman Temperament Scale, 43
Guilt, 196, 356. *See also* Anxiety, moral
Guttman Scale, 84

Habit(s)
  maladaptive, 210, 353
  study, 142
Hallucinations, 32, 100-109, 111, 126, 165, 183, 212, 230, 243, 256, 355
  auditory, 29, 101, 103, 104
  of blindness, uniocular, 104, 106, 107
  of cold, 30
  of color, 106
  of deafness, 103, 104, 106, 107, 118
    unilateral, 104
  double, 108, 109
  of fly, 29, 101
  gustatory, 26, 30, 101, 108, 166
  illogical aspects of, 108
  of mosquito, 26
  multi-modality, 101
  of music, 28
  negative, 22, 26, 28, 101, 103, 107-109, 114, 296, 323, 358
  of normal people, 100
  olfactory, 28, 30, 101, 108
  of pain, 107
  psychotic, 100
  schizophrenic, 100
  tactile, 101, 107
  of thirst, 33
  of TV set, 220, 244, 269, 280
  visual, 26, 28, 30, 101-103, 109, 178
  vividness of, 107
  of voice, 26
  positive, 22, 101, 107, 108, 296, 360
  posthypnotic, 108
Hand
  attraction, 25, 51-52
  levitation. *See* Arm, levitation
  repulsion, 25, 26, 51-52
Hands Test, 99
Harvard Group Scale of Hypnotic Susceptibility (HGSHS), 25, 28-29, 33, 36, 44, 56, 106, 122, 125, 126, 146, 293-294
Harvey lecture, 5
Headache, 183, 227, 230. *See also* Migraine
  posthypnotic, 310, 313
Heart rate(s), 100, 116. *See also* Pulse rate
  concordance of, 92
Helium balloon technique, 204, 205, 244, 356

Hemophilia, 259
Hemorrhage
  gastrointestinal, 259
  retrobulbar, 255
Hernia, 20
Herpes simplex, 268
Heterohypnosis, 248-255, 293-295
Hidden observer, the, 104, 113, 117, 118, 131, 173, 174, 213, 356
Hierarchy
  covert, 228
  desensitization, 197, 198, 228
  in vivo, 228
Higher mental processes, 193
HIP. *See* Hypnotic Induction Profile
Historical records, 153
History taking, 273
Homosexuality, 199, 231
Honesty. *See* Exhortations for honesty in reports
Human engineering, 15
Huntington's disease, 259
Hyperemesis gravidarum, 253
Hypermnesia, 20, 140-149, 153, 357
Hypersuggestibility, 55, 56, 164, 165
Hypertension, essential, 270-272
Hypnoanalgesia, 113-115, 118. *See also* Pain control
Hypnoanalysis, 211, 212, 265, 357
Hypnoanesthesia, 2, 46, 111, 116, 182, 237, 239, 240, 243, 248-255. *See also* Anesthetic
  advantages of, 251-253
  in childbirth, 248
  indications for, 150
  reluctance to use, 248-249
Hypnoidal state, 357
Hypnomystical states, 244-245
Hypnosis, 357
  in acting, 283
  adjunctive, 259-260
  adverse reaction to. *See* Sequelae
  in advertising, 283-287
  "against will" of subject, 319
  aiding conception, 272-273
  in air-crash investigations, 280-281
  animal, 351
  applications of, 181-292
    nontherapeutic, 274-292
    therapeutic, 182-274. *See also* Hypnosis, clinical
  in behavior modification, 226-237
  in burn treatment, 245-248
  clinical, 42, 57, 58, 85, 179, 181, 182, 353. *See also* Hypnosis, therapeutic applications of
  contraindications for, 249
  in court, 281-282
  in daily life, 15, 292

Hypnosis (*cont.*)
"dangers" of, 17-19, 207-208. *See also*
　Sequelae
demonstrations of, 47, 62
in dentistry, 233, 237-245, 248-253,
　255-259
　advantages of, 256
　problems with, 256
depth of. *See* Trance, depth
in diagnosis, 273-274
effects on hypnotist, 207, 208, 258, 259,
　262
in entertainment, 291
episodic, 309
in espionage, 282-283
experimental, 85, 179, 181, 182, 355
fear of, 66, 67
forensic, 147, 233, 275-282, 356
government regulations concerning,
　335-339
group. *See* Hypnosis, induction of, group;
　Hypnotherapy, group
group training session, 249
highway, 15, 292, 356
history of, 2-10
inadvertent, 23
induction of, 32, 35, 55-79, 170,
　319-320. *See also* Hypnosis, meth-
　ods of induction
　authoritarian, 79
　with children, 270
　covert, 226, 257
　distractions during, 74
　during sleep, 78
　formal, 59, 208
　group, 62, 63
　initial, 79, 82
　mechanical aids to, 68-71
　nonverbal, 3
　rapid, 77-78. *See also* Hypnosis, in-
　　stant
　repeated. *See* Fractionation
　standardized, 23, 70, 83-84
"instant," 75-78
investigative uses of, 279-281
legal problems of, 307-308, 328-339
in law enforcement, 275-282
by letter, 76
in medicine, 237-274
methods of induction, 57, 59, 61, 66-68,
　70, 71
　arm levitation, 58-63
　Braidism, 63-65
　cognitive inductions, 65-66, 86, 353
　Flower method, 67-69
　new and combination methods, 71-74
　progressive relaxation, 66-67
　spiral technique, 66
military, 282-283

Hypnosis (*cont.*)
misconceptions about, 1, 12, 13-20, 57,
　254, 310, 316, 317
misuse of, 314
in modeling, 291
in movies and television, 15, 291, 292
naturally occurring, 15, 292
neutral, 38, 57, 63, 79-82, 91, 93-95,
　98, 100, 117, 136, 141-143, 359
in obstetrics, 248
patient requests for, 208
per se. *See* Hypnosis, neutral
physiological effects of, 91-98
positive after-effects of, 313
by prescription, 338, 339
psychological problems of, 307-317
in psychological research, 274-275
in psychotherapy, 182-185
in Rational-Emotive Therapy, 227-228
in religion, 291, 292
repeated, 35-36, 204
restrictive legislation concerning, 335-339
signs of, 79-83, 227
　objective, 80-81
　subjective, 81-82
in space travel, 291
in sports, 287-289
stage, 11, 75, 108, 312, 335, 336, 338,
　339, 345. *See also* Hypnotist, stage
in systematic desensitization, 228-229
by telephone, 76, 247
termination of, 18, 86-88. *See also*
　Awakening
Hypnotechnician, 338, 339, 357. *See also*
　Hypnotist, lay
　treating alcoholics, 338
Hypnotherapist, 316
Hypnotherapy, 7, 172, 182-185, 199,
　201-238, 270, 357
　adjunctive, 259, 260
　analytic, 211-226
　　miscellaneous techniques of, 222-224
　for cancer patients, 266-268
　group, 206, 236, 254
　palliative, 260-264
　sensory, 215, 216, 362
　to modify course of organic disease,
　　264-272
"Hypnotic eye," 65
Hypnotic Induction Profile, 25, 30-31, 42
Hypnotism, definition, 357
Hypnotist. *See also* Operator
　adverse reaction to hypnosis in, 316-
　　317
　amateur, 309, 310, 330
　death of, 18
　diction and accent of, 14
　illusory power of, 315
　immoral, 325

Hypnotist (cont.)
    lay, 311, 330, 334, 337, 339, 357. See
        also Hypnotechnician
    misconduct by, 324, 325, 332. See also
        Ethics
    nineteenth century, 6
    power fantasies of, 316
    role of, 13, 82
    stage, 50, 74-77, 108, 311, 312,
        335-337. See also Hypnosis, stage
    voice of, 32, 68, 69, 73-74, 82
Hypnotizability, 357. See also Susceptibility
Hypnus, 15
Hypochondriasis, 183
Hysteria, 41, 183, 274
Hysterics, 7

Id, 186, 354
Ideas
    abstract, 229
    "irrational," 195, 196
Idioms, 80, 308
Illness
    chronic, 260-264, 303
    organic, 359
    psychosomatic, 184, 216, 234, 238, 264,
        361
    terminal, 260-264
Illusion, 65, 222, 357
    Poggendorff, 157
    Ponzo, 105, 157
    Tatchner-Ebbinghaus, 105
Image, 357
    manipulation, hypnotic, 229-237
    multi-sensory, 65
    visual, 65
Imagery, 40, 45, 86, 151, 206, 215, 229,
        232, 294, 362
    concrete, 223
    eidetic, 148, 157, 158, 355
    hypnotically induced, uses of, 215, 226
    shift, 223, 357
Imagination, 13, 151-152.
Immune system, 266-267
Impotence, 183, 235, 357
Imprinting, 216
Impulsive acts. See Acting out
Incompetence, professional, 77
Independent variable, 357
Individual differences, 79
Induction procedures, 31, 44, 72-74, 78,
        83. See also Hypnosis, methods of
        induction
Induction ritual. See Hypnosis, induction of,
        formal
Infants, 154
Information retrieval, hypnotic, 212-217
Insanity, defense of, 329, 330

Insight, 190, 195, 201, 221, 222, 225, 357
Insomnia, 183, 226
Instructions, first-person, 294-296
    misunderstanding of, 308
Intelligence, 15, 150. See also IQ
Interference between simultaneous tasks,
        172, 173
Interpretations, 192, 214, 219, 357
    premature, 214
Interview, preinduction, 57, 207
Invasion of privacy, 276, 318
Inventory of Self-Hypnosis (ISH), 293, 294
In vivo procedures, 228
IQ, 34, 36-38, 153, 155, 156. See also In-
        telligence
Ishihara Plates, 106

Jacobson's relaxation method, 15, 66, 197
JND. See Just noticeable difference; Limen,
        difference
Just noticeable difference, 258, 352
Juvenile rheumatoid arthritis, 269

Ketamine, 120

Labor, premature, 252
    time in, 252
Lacrimation, 80
Lactation, postpartum, 252
Lancet, 5
Language, 13-14, 222
    body. See Communication, nonverbal
    foreign, 130, 142, 308
    slang, 177
Latency stage, 186
Law of parsimony, 342
Laying on of hands, 3
Layman, practice of psychotherapy by, 334,
        337-339
Learning, 140-149. See also Conditioning
    emotional, 198
    verbal, 162
Leary Interpersonal Checklist, 43
LeCron-Bordeaux Scale, 84
Lee's Hypnotic Characteristic Inventory, 44,
        46
Lethargy, 7, 357
Leukemia, 304
Libido, 186
Lie detection, 276-277. See also Polygraph
Limen, 362
    absolute, 358
    difference, 358
    time, 286
Listening, dichotic, 173, 354
Literalness of understanding, 80

Logic-tight compartments, 108
Lying, under hypnosis, 281

Machiavellianism, 358
Machiavellianism Scale, 326
Magic finger technique, 243
Magnetic fluid, 2, 3
Magnetic healers, 2, 3, 6
Magnetism, 4
    animal, 2, 9, 352
Magnetists, 74, 358
Magnets, 2, 4
Malingering, 274
Malpractice, 224, 331, 333-335, 348
    insurance, 333, 334
Mantra, 297, 358
Maudsley Personality Inventory, 43
McGill Pain Questionnaire, 120
Medical consultation, 209
Medical device, 335
Medical lobbying, 337, 339
Medical model, 191, 194, 358
Medicine, organized, 337
Meditation, 258. *See also* Transcendental
    meditation
Megacolon, functional, 238, 270
Memories, birth, 216
    pseudo-, 233
Memory, 129, 135, 147-149
    distortion, 281-282
    earliest, 216
    enhancement effect, 281
    episodic, 134
    hypnotically generated, 214
    indirect measurement of, 131, 134
    photographic. *See* Imagery, eidetic
    recording function of, 121
    residual deficit in, after posthypnotic am-
        nesia, 126
    retrieval function of, 121
    semantic, 134
    short-term, 145
    visual, 142
    waking, 57, 132
Mental age, 155, 156
Mental defectives, 37
Mental illness, 191, 194
Mesmerism, 5
Mesomorphy, 44, 358
Metaphors, use of, 86, 224
Methadone maintenance, 233-234
Metronome, 68
Migraine, 183, 216, 230-231. *See also*
    Headache
Minitrance, 163-165, 358
Minivacation, 243, 256
Minnesota Multiphasic Personality Inventory
    (MMPI), 41, 43, 100, 314

Miranda warning, 278, 358
Misconceptions about hypnosis. *See* Hypno-
    sis, misconceptions about
Misconduct, sexual, 324-326
MMPI. *See* Minnesota Multiphasic Personal-
    ity Inventory
M'Naghten Rule, 329-331
Modeling, 236
    covert, 211
Monoideism, 6, 10, 73, 358
Morphine, 120, 121
Mortality rates, surgical, 5
Motivation, 35, 222
    consumer, 284-286
    patient, 211, 223
    task, 10
    unconscious, 284
Motivational instructions. *See* Task motiva-
    tional instructions
Motor activity, spontaneous, 214
Motoric-Ideational Activity Preference Scale,
    43
Mourning process, 303
Muscle, capability of, 97-98
Music, background and mood, 71
Myers-Briggs Inventory, 43
Myopia, 238
Myths, about hypnosis. *See* Hypnosis, mis-
    conceptions about

Nail biting, 183
Naloxone, 114
Nancy School, 7, 358
Narcissism, 190, 221, 223, 304
Narcolepsy, 238
Nausea
    anticipatory, 261
    postoperative, 251, 253
Negativism
    active, 359
    passive, 359
Neglect hypothesis, the, 131
Negligence. *See* Malpractice
Neoplasms, 266. *See also* Cancer
"Nerve centers," hypnotic, 77
Nervous system, autonomic, 92, 93, 95, 98,
    104, 197, 230, 238, 264, 276, 287,
    352, 355
Neurohypnology, 6
Neurohypnosis, 6
Neurosis, 359
    spontaneous remission rate of, 190
Neurotics, 41, 193
Nicotine addiction, 182. *See also* Smoking
Nightmare, 183. *See also* Night terrors
Night terrors, 183, 235
Nitrous oxide, 5, 34-35
Nocturnal emissions, 178

Nonsense syllables, 129, 141, 142, 144-147, 161, 359, 362
Novocaine, 203

Obessions, 183
Odyssean, 40
Operator, 32, 62, 65, 67, 68, 73, 80, 85, 88. *See also* Hypnotist
Oral stage, 186
Ordinal scales, 22
Organismic variable, 359
Otis Self-Administering Test of Mental Ability, 156
Oxygen level, arterial, 96
Overeating, 183, 185, 200-211, 267. *See also* Weight control

Pain, 359
    acute, 237
    chronic, 120, 237, 239, 240, 246, 303, 304
    cold pressor, 112, 116, 119, 121, 353
    concentration on, 74
    dental, 119-120, 203
    etiology of, 202
    ischemic, 113, 116, 121, 357
    laboratory induced, 110
    low back, 248, 311
    mental correlates of, 110
    nonsurgical, 248
    objective indices of, 110
    organic, 120, 239
    physician induced, 237
    physiological indices of, 110, 111
    postoperative, 237, 253
    pre-operative, 251
    sacroiliac, 247
    sensation, 109
    threshold of, 114
Pain control, 104, 115, 116, 202-204, 242, 245
    by age regression, 244
    by analysis of pain, 243
    by direct suggestion, 242
    by dissociation, 243
    by distraction, 243
    magic finger, technique of, 243
    medication, 240
    posthypnotic, 237, 253
    by psychological amputation, 243
    red balloon technique, 204
    by relaxation, 242
    by time distortion, 244
    by transfer of pain, 242
    by transformation of pain, 242-243

Paired associates list, 133, 141, 142, 359
Panic, posthypnotic, 310
Paralysis, hysterical, 155, 202
Paramnesias, 171, 359
Paranoia, 310
Paranoid reaction, 312, 316
Paranoids, 41
Paris School, 7, 359
Passes, 74-75
Patients, 12, 13, 30, 87, 143, 189, 222, 224, 225, 246
    borderline, 184, 221, 223, 304
    cancer, 260-262, 266
    chronically ill, 237
    depressed, 225
    dialysis, 259
    gynecological, 262
    negativistic, 224
    suicidal, 224, 225
    terminally ill, 237, 261, 263
Pep talk, 289
Perceived self, 191. *See also* Self-image
Perception, 360, 362
Perceptual defense, 286
Perceptual distortion, 212, 227, 323
Perjury, 281
    subornation of, 278
Personality, 40-42, 353, 360
    apollonian, 40
    brittle, 18
    cancer, 260
    Dionysian, 40
    disorders, 184
    of hypnotist, 58
    hysterical, 41
    inventory, 42-43
    maladaptive, 190
    multiple, 172, 174, 183, 215, 223, 273, 274, 358
    odyssean, 40
    passive-aggressive, 235, 360
    schizoid, 184, 232
    of subject, 58
    tests of, 42-45
Phallic stage, 186
Phobia, 42, 184, 195-198, 200, 228, 230, 234, 356, 360
    cat, 195, 197
    dental, 203, 233, 255-257
    flying, 198
    injection, 229, 259
Phrenologists, 19
Physical contact, subject-hypnotist, 4, 74, 75
Placebo, 77, 79, 82, 111, 113, 114, 120, 121, 245, 352, 354
Placebo effect, 118, 360, 363
Polygraph, 80, 276. *See also* Lie detection

Postoperative tubes, catheters and needles, 253
Postural sway, 25, 29, 52, 53
Practice effect, 142
Preconscious, 187, 360
Prefrontal lobotomy, 110, 111, 116
Premature ejaculation, 184, 235
Primary familiar amyloidosis, 262
Primary processes, 212, 223, 355, 360
Proactive inhibition, 131
Projection, 227, 360
Projective technique, 42, 43
Pruritus, 311
Pseudo-orientation, 229
Psoriasis, 238, 268
Psychic connections. *See* Association, free
Psychic determinism, 186
Psychic energy, 356
    pain, 187. *See also* Anxiety
Psychoanalysis, 3, 7, 9, 186-191, 351, 355, 357, 363
    classical, 187, 188
Psychopath, 360
Psychosexual development, stages of, 186
Psychosis, 311, 361
Psychotherapy, 182-237. *See also* Therapy
    analytic, 191, 195, 201, 212, 215
    methods of, 71, 72, 185-201
    schools of, 185-201
Psychotic episode, 315
Psychotics, 42, 190, 193, 217, 221, 223, 304
Puberty, 36
Pulse rate, 120. *See also* Heart rate
Punishment, 359

Questions
    ideomotor, 216, 265, 272, 357
    leading, 213
Questioning
    hypnotic, 213-215
    ideomotor, 213, 214
    subjective, 213, 362

Random assignment, of subjects to treatment groups, 275
Random sample, 361
Random selection, of subjects, 275, 347
Rape, 332
Rapport, 14, 34, 36, 38, 58, 82, 223, 241, 270, 361
Rational-Emotive Therapy, 185, 195, 196, 227
Reactions. *See also* Response
    hysterical, 3, 4, 11
    to incest, 184

Reactive inhibition, 157
Reactive potential, 157
Reading disorders, 184
Reality testing, 212, 217
Real time, 160, 361
Recall, 127, 129, 137, 144-148, 361. *See also* Memory
    clustering of items in, 135, 136
    generic, 138
    semantic organization of, 133, 135, 137
Reciprocal inhibition, 361
Recognition, 129, 131, 137, 361
Redintegration, 124
Reflection, 192
Reflex
    gag, 238, 252
    Hering, 77, 356
Regression, 156, 212, 217, 218, 361, 362. *See also* Age, regression
    hypnotic, fostering of, 215-217
    in the service of the ego, 151
    spontaneous, 212, 215, 250
Reinforcement, 193, 200, 198-200, 210, 211, 232, 355, 358, 362
    covert, 226
        negative, 231, 232, 358
        positive, 227, 232, 234, 360
    negative, 232
    vicarious, 363
Reinforcement schedule, partial, 233, 359
    variable interval, 162, 363
Reinforcement Survey Schedule, 232
Relationships, 361. *See also* Countertransference; Transference
    dentist-patient, 256
    doctor-patient, 256, 325
    hypnotist-subject, 45, 46, 58, 76, 164, 167, 178, 323, 324, 326
    interpersonal, 69
    reality, 332
    therapeutic, 222, 224
    therapist-patient, 219, 221, 317
Relaxation, 62, 74, 84, 146, 198, 226, 230, 258
    progressive, 66, 67, 212, 226, 230
Relearning method, 129, 131, 361. *See also* Savings method
Release signal, 361
Reliability, 24, 361
    coefficient, 24
    equivalent forms, 24
    split-half, 24
    stability, 24
    test-retest, 24
Religion, 36, 39, 291, 292. *See also* Hypnosis, in religion
REM, 97, 100, 122, 160, 177. *See also* Sleep, REM

Reports
anecdotal, 348
clinical, 347-349
Repression, 132-134, 187, 193
Reputation, professional, 333
Research, 55, 78, 90, 95, 115, 128-130,
    144, 148, 159, 342, 349, 350
in hypnotherapy of cancer, 267
in marketing, 285, 291
replication of, 115, 289, 290
Resistance, 188, 221-224, 361
hypnotic overcoming of, 212, 221, 222
Respiration, rate of, 60, 62, 96, 120
Response, 361. See also Reactions
cognitive, 48
covert, 195
erotic, 199
ideomotor, 48, 60, 126, 213, 214, 357
Retarded ejaculation, 184
Retroactive inhibition, 130, 131, 133, 361
Revivification, 152-159, 346, 361
"Rhinocerous principle," 319, 320
Ripple effect, 268
Rod and frame test, 44
Rogerian therapy. See therapy, Rogerian
Role playing, 134, 135, 152, 192, 196
Role reversal, 192, 222, 223
Rorschach test, 42-44, 98, 99, 125, 153

Salivation, 238, 252, 256
Savings method, 129, 361. See also Re-
    learning method
Schizophrenia, 184
paranoid, 222, 256, 315
Schizophrenics, 41, 42, 100, 223, 272
Sciatica, 7
Secondary gains, 361
Secondary processes, 361
Secret messages, 282, 283
Secrets, 16
Seduction, hypnotic, 324-326, 331-333
Seizure. See also Epileptic seizures
psychogenic, 184, 216, 273
Self
ideal, 191
perceived, 360. See also Self-image
Self-acceptance, 222
Self-concept, 223, 232
Self-esteem, 208, 224
Self-hypnosis, 13, 96, 204, 207, 210, 223,
    234, 236, 241, 259, 262, 264, 271,
    272, 283, 291-305, 352, 362. See
    also Autohypnosis
advantages of, 298, 299, 302
with children, 264
contraindications for, 299
disadvantages of, 298, 299

Self-hypnosis (cont.)
induction rituals, 296, 299-303
problems with, 304, 305
spontaneous, 274, 297
training in, 299-301
Self-image, 191, 200, 236, 360, 362. See
    also Perceived self
Self-incrimination, right against, 267
Self-mastery, 223
Sensation, 362
Sensitization, covert, 227, 231, 232
Sensory deprivation, 46, 100
Sensory hypnoplasty, 215, 216, 362
Sequelae, 87, 309-315, 362
anxiety, 309, 310, 312, 313
in clinical setting, 310-313, 315
confusion, 313
crying, 310
dependency, 310
depersonalization, 310
depression, 310
dizziness, 310
drowsiness, 309, 313
fainting, 310
headache, 87, 309, 313
laboratory, 309, 310, 312-314
long-term reactions, 310-313
major, 309-313
minor, 309, 311, 313
muscle cramp, 87
nausea, 309, 310
numbness, 87
panic, 310
psychotic behavior, 310, 312
self-limited, 308, 310
sex difficulties, 310
short-term reactions, 309, 313, 314
vomiting, 310
Serial list, 362
Set, 362. See also Suggestions, prehypnotic
Sexual avoidance syndrome, 235
deviation, 184, 231
disorders, 216, 235, 357
dysfunction, 184
problems, 200
Shock, surgical, 251, 252
Shor Personal Experience Questionnaire, 43,
    44
"Shoulds," 196
"Sick person," self-concept, 212
Side effects
of chemical anesthetics, 251
of chemotherapy, 237, 260, 261
of hypnosis, 114
of medications, 245
of placebos, 245
of radiation, 260
"Significant others," 191

Simulation group, 362. *See also* Subjects, simulating
Skeptical position, the, 21
Skill induction, 63
Sleep,
  NREM, 177, 359
  paradoxical, 16
  REM, 359, 361. *See also* REM
  spindles, 16
  stages of, 16
Slips of speech, 188
Smoking, 42, 184, 185, 202, 203, 208-211, 231, 232, 235, 267, 302, 321. *See also* Suggestions, anti-smoking
  cessation of, 204-206
  criteria of success in treating, 205
  group treatment of, 205, 206
  nonhypnotic techniques, 204
  rate of, 204, 205
  single-session therapy for, 204
Social distance, 222, 223
Social roles, 10, 345
Social role theory, 362
Somatotype, 355, 358
Somnambulism, 5, 7, 11, 21, 122, 185, 208, 362
Sounds and Images Test, 151
Spasm, ciliary, 238
Speech, disorders, 185
Spontaneous recovery, 157, 362
Stanford-Binet Test, 155, 156
Stanford Hypnotic Arm Levitation Induction and Test (SHALIT), 31
Stanford Hypnotic Clinical Scale for Adults (SHCSA), 31
Stanford Hypnotic Clinical Scale for Children (SHCSC), 31
Stanford Hypnotic Susceptibility Scale (SHSS), 25-29, 34, 35, 42, 43, 116, 126, 173, 226, 313, 314
Stanford Profile Scales of Hypnotic Suscepti-bility (SPSHS), 27-28
Startle reaction, 103
Starvation cycle, in burn victims, 246
State reports, 85
Stereotypes, 39
Stimulus, 362
  ambiguous, 42
Stress, 114
  emotional, 203
  practice-induced, 258
  reaction, delayed, 183
Stretching, on awakening, 87
Stroking, with fingertips, 74, 75
Stuttering, 185
Subconscious, 362. *See also* Unconscious
Subjective reports, 30

Subjective unit of disturbance (SUD), 197, 228, 362
Subjects, 12, 25, 34-37, 42-45, 70, 74, 75, 80, 82, 87, 90, 103, 107, 132
  control, 57
  cultural differences in, 39
  elderly, 37
  expectations of, 207, 354
  female, 37, 45, 176
  foreign-born, 308
  hypnotized, 75, 76, 136
  knowledge of being in an experiment, 320, 321, 323, 327
  male, 176
  negativistic, 52. *See also* Negativism
  screening of, 44
  sex of, 36, 37, 43, 45
  simulating, 90, 102, 103, 109, 115, 125, 127, 128, 132, 134, 141, 152-156, 166, 167, 277, 346
  subjective feelings of, 81, 82, 124, 136, 137, 139, 156
  victimization of, 331, 332
  young children as, 36
Subliminal advertising, 286, 362
Subliminal perception, 386
Successive approximation, method of, 198
SUD. *See* Subjective unit of disturbance
Suffering, 362
Suggested Syllables Test, 29
Suggestibility, 7, 10, 21, 31, 46, 144, 167, 363
Suggestions, 56, 59, 61, 62, 207, 363
  of amnesia, 125, 134
  anti-smoking, 204-211, 256, 338
  authoritarian, 78, 79, 127, 128, 134, 207, 221, 352
  autosuggestion, 352, 362
  cognitive, 85
  confidence building, 338
  of deafness, 104
  direct, 90, 234, 265
  ego building, 224
  emotion generating, 80
  explicit, 82
  ill-advised, 314
  implicit, 82
  indirect, 90, 107, 223, 285, 357
  misinterpretations of, 80
  modification of by subject, 165
  motivational, 144
  pain relief, 242, 243
  permissive, 78, 79, 128, 134, 207, 221, 360
  posthypnotic, 26, 28-31, 75, 76, 124, 126, 131, 163-172, 176, 203, 210, 226, 252, 360
  prehypnotic, 207, 360

Suggestions (*cont.*)
  of relaxation, 204
  of self-confidence, 224
  therapeutic, 206
  uncancelled, 169
  waking, 247, 364
  weight loss, 209, 338
    contraindications for, 209
Suicide, 185, 224, 225, 248, 311
Superego, 186, 200, 310, 354, 360
Supervision
  clinical, 338, 339
  medical, 209, 338
Surgeons, conversations of, 247
Surgery
  brain, 250
  cardiac, 254
  early use of hypnoanesthesia in, 5
  gingival, 257
  gynecological, 251, 269
  lung, 46
  scrotal tumors, 5
  thyroid, 116
Susceptibility, 13, 21-54, 83, 112, 113,
    115, 133, 140, 144-146, 168-170,
    182, 313, 357, 358
  demographic factors in, 33-42
  effect of age on, 36-37
  effect of childhood experiences on, 39-40
  effect of college major on, 38
  effect of drugs on, 46-47
  effect of education on, 38
  effect of IQ on, 37-38
  effect of nationality on, 36, 39
  effect of occupation on, 36, 38
  effect of race on, 36, 39
  effect of religion on, 39
  effect of sex on, 37
  factors affecting, 33-42
Susceptibility scales, 24-31, 58, 182
Symbol, 363
Symbolic material, 229
Symbolic seduction, 316
Sympathetic ear, 303
Symptoms, 194, 195, 201, 363
  direct removal of, 185, 201-211, 269
  dynamic meaning of, 187, 201, 203, 210,
    357, 359
  etiology of, 216
  formation of, 309, 359
  hypnotic generation of, 275
  hysterical, 4, 7. *See also* Reaction, hyster-
    ical
  learning of, 193
  prescription, 221, 222
  substitution, 187, 201-203, 234, 248,
    309, 363

Symptoms (*cont.*)
  ulcer, 202
  withdrawal, 351
Systoles, extra, 92

Tantrums, parent's reaction to, 183, 234
Tape recording
  audio, 70, 71, 119, 123, 127, 144, 146,
    210, 230, 241, 254, 259, 302
  video, 69, 139, 140, 332
Tarnoff case, 225
Task motivation, 10
Task motivational instructions, 32, 55, 101,
    103, 106, 133, 136, 142-146, 149,
    158, 162, 165, 167, 168, 170, 173,
    178, 208, 211, 363
Testimony, hypnotically refreshed, 281-282
Tests
  of creativity, 150-152
  of moral development, 158
  of personality, 42-45
  preinduction, 47-54, 58, 182
    group, 49
    individual, 49
  projective. *See* Projective technique
  screening, 47
  of trance depth. *See* Trance, depth, scales
    of
  word association, 127, 133, 134
Thematic Apperception Test, 42, 43, 125
Theorists
  nonstate, 55, 344
  state, 55, 344
Theory
  Barber's 10, 32, 344, 345
  classical dissociation, 173
  Coe's, 139, 345
  DNA, 342
  Dollard and Miller's, 193, 194, 342
  eclectic, 349
  Einstein's, 349
  Freud's, 186-191
  functions of, 342, 349
  of hypnosis, requirements of, 343
  implicit, 343
  Kohlberg's, of moral development, 158
  neo-dissociation, 130, 172, 175, 359
  Orne's, 10, 344, 346
  Rogerian, 191, 192
  Salter's, 11, 34, 343
  Sarbin's, 10
  social learning, 193, 194
Therapeutic alliance, 223
Therapeutic supervision. *See* Supervision,
    clinical
Therapist
  analytically oriented, 185, 199, 200

Therapist (*cont.*)
  back up, 225
  neurotic needs of, 316
  passive, 192
  prestige of, 14
  sex of, 37
Therapy. *See also* Psychotherapy
  aversive, 199, 231
  behavior, 185, 218. *See also* Behavior,
    modification
  dynamic, 218
  eclectic, 199-201, 212
  ego-stage, 221
  electroshock, 181
  endodontic, 257
  Gestalt, 185, 192-194
  group, 3, 241
  implosive, 230
  insight, 214
  patient's role in, 298
  Rational Emotive. *See* Rational-Emotive
    Therapy
  Rational Stage Directed, 227
  Rogerian, 191, 192
Thought stopping, 231
Threshold. *See* Limen
Thromboangiitis obliterans, 94
Tics, 185, 214
Time
  distortion, hypnotic, 159-163, 212, 297,
    363
    objective effects of, 160-162
  progression, 206
  real, 160, 161
  subjective, 159-163, 362
Tolerance, drug, 351
Torrance Test of Creativity, 151, 152
Tort, 363
Torticollis, 238
Torture, resisting, 283
Training
  analysis, 189
  in hypnosis, 350
Trance, 21-23, 35, 41, 55-57, 61, 68, 79,
    81, 84, 87, 171, 227, 297, 344, 345
  capacity, 13, 21, 23, 34, 42, 363. *See
    also* Susceptibility
  deep, 122, 241
  -deepening techniques, 68, 70, 83-86,
    300
  depth, 22, 23, 56, 69, 85, 90, 117, 125,
    167-169, 213, 268, 297, 363
    scales of, 83-85
  hyperempiric, 57, 344, 357
  induction, 56, 217. *See also* Hypnosis, in-
    duction of
  logic, 81, 108, 109, 363

Trance (*cont.*)
  planary, 84, 360
  productivity, 117, 168, 171, 182
  reinstatement of, involuntary, 163, 164.
    See also Minitrance
  sleeping, 5
  spontaneous, 15, 203, 292, 295, 362
  termination of, 18, 86-88. *See also*
    Awakening
    difficulties in, 18, 87, 88, 309
  utilization, 86
Transcendental meditation, 226, 234. *See
  also* Meditation
Transference, 9, 36, 69, 70, 74, 76, 79,
    148, 178, 189, 193, 194, 207, 212,
    215, 216, 218, 220-222, 225, 227,
    296, 298, 312, 317, 325, 363. *See
    also* Relationship
Transitional object, 158
Tremor, psychogenic, 184
Trichotillomania, 185, 363
True effect, 363

Unconscious, 12, 187, 193, 194, 213, 362,
    363
Urinary retention, psychogenic, 184
Utilization, 222

Vaginismus, 185, 238, 363
Validity, of test, 24, 363
  concurrent, 24
  construct, 24
  predictive, 24
Ventilation, emotional, 212, 217, 218, 261
Verbal compulsion, 28
Verbal inhibition, 25, 26
Vicious cycle, 240, 246, 363. *See also*
    Feedback loop
Violence, on television, 331
Visualizations, 212, 215
Vocal cord nodules, benign, 238
Voice, excessively loud, in children, 269
Voiding, postoperative, 253
Volunteers, 47, 48, 320
Vomiting
  posthypnotic, 310
  postoperative, 253
Voodoo, 181

Waking suggestions. *See* Suggestions, wak-
    ing
Warm-up, 47, 142
Warts, 95, 203, 265, 266
  in immunodeficient children, 265
  juvenile, 208
  multiple, 265

Warts (cont.)
  penile, 265
  spontaneous remissions of, 265
  venereal, 238, 265, 266
weight control, 151, 206-211, 256, 338
Weight reduction, 82, 94, 207-211
Welt, 95
White blood cells, 267
"Will," 17, 19
Within-subjects, repeated measures design,
    275, 364
Witness, 278, 279
  aiding memory of, 279-282

Witness (cont.)
  demeanor of, hypnotically influencing,
    275, 278, 279
  expert, 281
Word picture, 65
Working through, 216

Yoga, 226, 297

Zeigarnik effect, 166, 286, 364
Zeitgeist, 4, 364
Zen, 226, 297
Zoist, 5, 6